KRYGER'S SLEEP MEDICINE REVIEW

THIRD EDITION

KRYGER'S SLEEP MEDICINE REVIEW

A Problem-Oriented Approach

THIRD EDITION

Meir H. Kryger, MD, FRCPC
Professor of Medicine
Yale School of Medicine
New Haven, Connecticut

Russell Rosenberg, PhD, DABSM
CEO
The Atlanta School of Sleep Medicine and Technology
Atlanta, Georgia

Douglas B. Kirsch, MD, FAAN, FAASM
Medical Director, CHS Sleep Medicine
Atrium Health
Charlotte, North Carolina

ELSEVIER

Notice

Practitioners and researchers must always rely on their own experience and knowledge in evaluating and using any information, methods, compounds or experiments described herein. Because of rapid advances in the medical sciences, in particular, independent verification of diagnoses and drug dosages should be made. To the fullest extent of the law, no responsibility is assumed by Elsevier, authors, editors or contributors for any injury and/or damage to persons or property as a matter of products liability, negligence or otherwise, or from any use or operation of any methods, products, instructions, or ideas contained in the material herein.

Previous editions copyrighted 2015 and 2011.

Library of Congress Control Number: 2018966095

Content Strategist: Nancy Duffy
Senior Content Development Specialist: Jennifer Shreiner
Publishing Services Manager: Catherine Jackson
Senior Project Manager: Sharon Corell
Senior Book Designer: Maggie Reid

Last digit is the print number: 9   8   7   6   5   4   3   2   1

1600 John F. Kennedy Blvd.
Ste 1600
Philadelphia, PA 19103-2899

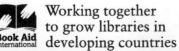

Working together
to grow libraries in
developing countries

www.elsevier.com • www.bookaid.org

Preface

Why another edition of this sleep medicine review book? The short answer is to help identify areas of strength and weakness for all practitioners of the field. The longer answer is that the field has changed. Pediatricians taking care of patients with sleep disorders are handing off care of their now adult patients to other doctors. Home sleep apnea testing is now the norm for first assessment of sleep apnea, there is an update to the classification system (ICSD3), and updates to the scoring manual and new treatments are available. The task of keeping up becomes even more important with the introduction of Maintenance of Certification. Examinations are now offered in many countries. The examinations change with new developments in the field.

At the age of 62, one of the authors, Meir Kryger, decided to take the ABIM sleep medicine board examination. He had previously obtained board certification via the American Board of Sleep Medicine (ABSM) and didn't really need to take the new ABIM exam; nonetheless, he wanted the experience in order to better teach trainees and others preparing for a career in sleep medicine.

The authors have taught at many Board Review sessions and wanted to see the other side—what students and trainees have to go through in preparation for this examination. We were surprised to discover that there really aren't many resources available for examinees that present current standards and scoring techniques and that are in sync with what is expected of a modern sleep medicine practitioner.

Colleagues who have been practicing sleep medicine for many years and are excellent clinicians have confessed hesitancy about taking sleep medicine certification exams. Mainly they were worried that some sections may be too difficult. Pulmonologists worry about neurophysiology and anatomy of the brain, and neurologists are concerned about blood gases, sleep apnea, and CPAP. Yes, the examination is quite diverse, but perceived weakness in one or even a few areas can be overcome.

In preparation for examinations like the sleep boards, you should never rely on a single source of information. You learn from seeing patients, reviewing many polysomnograms, discussing cases with colleagues, working with registered sleep technologists, reading textbooks and journal articles, attending lectures, and challenging yourself with board preparation questions. This book is but one aid in your preparation for the examination. It should not be your only resource, and that is why you will find numerous key references throughout the text. If you have experience in sleep medicine, either through practice or a sleep fellowship, and use the available resources intensely and wisely, you stand an excellent chance of passing the examination.

Recent research in learning suggests that tests offer a very good way to learn and to assess your areas of strength and weakness. Thus an important added benefit of this book is that you will learn more about sleep medicine and therefore take better care of your patients.

Meir H. Kryger, MD, FRCPC
Russell Rosenberg, PhD, DABSM
Douglas Kirsch, MD, FAASM

Acknowledgments

Many people helped in the preparation of this volume, including those listed below.

The staff members at Elsevier who helped this book in its journey were Nancy Duffy, Sharon Corell, Jennifer Shreiner, and many others involved in development, production, and design for both the printed volume and the online content.

Pnina Weiss, Craig Canepari, Stephen Sheldon, and Lynelle Schneeberg contributed some questions and answers.

Acknowledgments

Many people helped in the preparation of this volume, including those listed below.

The staff members at Elsevier who helped this book in its journey were Nancy Duffy, Sharon Corell, Jennifer Shreiner, and many others involved in development, production, and design for both the printed volume and the online content.

Prince Weiss, Craig Canepari, Stephan Sheldon, and Lynelle Schneeberg contributed some questions and answers.

Acknowledgments

Using This Book to Review Sleep Medicine

HOW THE BOOK IS ORGANIZED

The main part of this book is divided into the nine **sections** that correspond to the clinical areas tested by the ABIM sleep medicine certification examination (see Table 2, later in text). This book contains an additional tenth section on pediatrics, a topic that will be covered in several parts of the examination. Most sections contain several subsections with clinical vignettes followed by multiple-choice questions covering diagnosis or management. After the questions section is an **answer section** with detailed explanations. The end of each subsection includes a brief **summary of key learning points**. At the end of the book is a listing of key sources called **Highly Recommended** that form a core of knowledge. In addition, there is a content guide in the **Appendix** for practitioners in Europe (Appendix 3), Japan (Appendix 4), and other countries (Appendix 5), and there is also a content guide for dentists (Appendix 6).

This book is directed to two main groups: those who wish to use the book as a self-assessment and learning tool, and those who are preparing to take initial sleep medicine certification examinations as well as those who are recertifying.

FOR THOSE WISHING TO USE THE BOOK AS A SELF-ASSESSMENT AND LEARNING TOOL

Over the past three decades sleep medicine has evolved into a recognized specialty with board certification. Whereas it used to be a minor academic field with patient assessments carried out in a university hospital, today it is integral to primary care practice. Most patient assessments now take place in the outpatient setting. Even so, sleep specialists are often called on to evaluate inpatients, including patients in the ICU. Although sleep apnea has been the driving force behind the growth in sleep medicine, studying for the boards will make you realize that the field is far more than just OSA and CPAP. You also need to know some neurology, psychiatry, otolaryngology, pharmacology, circadian physiology, pediatrics, and much more.

If you are just getting into the field of sleep medicine—a trainee doing a rotation in sleep medicine or still in your sleep fellowship—*Sleep Medicine Review* will give you a sense of the overall field, where it is heading, what types of patients you will be seeing, and where the research opportunities are. Go through the book from cover to cover and see what interests you most about the field. If you have recently passed the sleep exam, *Sleep Medicine Review* will be a refresher and will help keep you up to speed in your new field. Like all specialties, sleep medicine is constantly evolving; what may have been conventional wisdom just a few years ago may now be wrong. We recommend first reviewing clinical problems you are currently handling. This will help you help your patients and increase your knowledge base.

If you are an experienced sleep medicine practitioner and/or have already passed the sleep medicine exam, this book will help keep you from getting stale. Long-term practitioners run this risk because they tend to see the same types of patients over and over again, often developing expertise in a narrow area (e.g., sleep breathing disorders, movement disorders, or insomnia). *Sleep Medicine Review* presents a wonderful opportunity to study areas that you may not have reviewed for some time. There have been marvelous advances in the field, and we all need to learn about them. We suggest you begin this book by taking the online examination and then focus on areas new to you.

STUDY GUIDE FOR THE ABIM SLEEP MEDICINE CERTIFICATION EXAMINATION

If you are preparing for the sleep medicine examination, you should find this an excellent study guide. The book is divided into major topic areas defined by the certifying boards that make up the certification examination.

The sleep medicine or "board" examination is administered by the American Board of Internal Medicine and so is often called "the ABIM exam." However, it is a joint effort by five board specialties under the umbrella of the American Board of Medical Specialties (ABMS), not to be confused with the old sleep medicine examination, which was administered by the American Board of Sleep Medicine (ABSM). The old ABSM examination is no longer given; in the USA there is currently only one sleep medicine board examination—"the ABIM exam"—and candidates for it may be admitted via prior certification in one of the following ABMS specialties: the American Board of Internal Medicine, the American Board of Psychiatry and Neurology, the American Board of Pediatrics, the American Board of Otolaryngology, the American Board of Family Medicine, or the American Board of Anesthesiology. The examination is the final requirement to become board certified in sleep medicine. The list of requirements for the ABIM version of the exam is as follows*:

- At the time of application, maintain current, valid ABIM certification in internal medicine or a subspecialty
- Satisfactorily complete the requisite formal training requirements
- Demonstrate clinical competence, procedural skills, and moral and ethical behavior in the clinical setting
- Hold a valid, unrestricted, and unchallenged license to practice medicine
- Pass the ABIM Sleep Medicine Certification Examination

Note that the practice pathway for admission to the Sleep Medicine examination, available for the 2007, 2009, and 2011 examinations, is no longer an option. Now, first-time applicants for admission to the examination must fulfill requirements of the *training pathway*, which requires a one-year fellowship. (There are a few exceptions spelled out in the ABIM website under the heading "Candidates for Special Consideration." http://www.abim.org/certification/policies/candidates-for-special-consideration.aspx)

DIFFERENCES BETWEEN THE OLD AND NEW EXAMINATIONS

The now-discontinued American Board of Sleep Medicine examination was much more difficult than the current certification examination. For starters, it was given over 2 days, whereas the ABIM examination is 1 day only. The ABSM exam had two parts; you had to pass Part 1 before taking Part II, and they were given months apart. Part I focused on knowledge of sleep medicine and physiology, and Part II focused on polysomnography and its interpretation. Part II also dealt with technical issues, and the applicant had to know a great deal about instrumentation of the patient, setting up of equipment, and interpretation of what was for many years a paper-based technology. When one of the authors did the ABSM examination in 1997, Part II included going through two 1000-page (yes, on paper) polysomnographic recordings and walking around the room to view a large number of paper or PSG fragments plastered on the walls. There was a high failure rate.

When that examination was initially created, the purpose was to certify that people could *perform* and *interpret* polysomnography. One did not have to be a physician to sit for the examination. For example, many psychologists took the examination and passed. One unintended consequence of the process was that, when people without actual medical training became certified, health systems often employed them not only to interpret polysomnograms, but also to evaluate patients with significant severe medical problems. It was not appreciated that being ABSM certified in sleep medicine was not the same as being certified in a clinical specialty. Now only physicians can take the certification examination, so basic clinical skills are assumed.

---

*List is from http://www.abim.org/~/media/ABIM%20Public/Files/pdf/exam-blueprints/certification/sleep-medicine.pdf

ABIM Exam	2007	2009	2011	2013	2017
Internal Medicine		7226; 88%	7337; 84%	7482; 86%	8265; 90%
Pulmonary Medicine		460; 91%	508; 93%	544; 87%	612; 99%
Sleep Medicine	1882; 73%	2140; 78%	2462; 64%	349; 90%	339; 92%

Table 1 First Time Takers of ABIM Exams (Number; % Passing)

WHO HAS TAKEN AND PASSED THE EXAMINATION?

A total of 1882 people took the first ABIM Sleep Medicine Examination in 2007, and the overall pass rate was 73%. Table 1 shows who took the last five exams and who passed.

Data released in February 2010 about the 2009 examination reported that 2512 people took the sleep examination and 76% of them passed. People taking the examination for the first time had a pass rate of 78%, whereas repeaters had a pass rate of 66%.

RECENT PASS RATES OF THE SLEEP MEDICINE EXAMINATION

The examination has since been given regularly since 2007. Table 1 gives pass rates of first-time takers for these exams compared with pass rates for internal medicine and pulmonary medicine in 2009, 2011, 2013, and 2017 (http://www.abim.org/about/examInfo/data-pass-rates.aspx). Note that the pass rate for sleep medicine was considerably lower (and the number taking the examination considerably higher) when first-time takers included those from the practice pathway. In 2013, when only fellowship-trained physicians could take the sleep examination, the pass rate soared. By February 2014 there were about 5000 doctors holding valid sleep medicine certification by the ABIM.

THE ODDS OF PASSING THE CERTIFICATION EXAMINATION

The following is based on published information from the various certifying bodies and discussions with program directors of accredited programs:

- If applicant has previous ABSM fellowship, about 90%
- If applicant has had accredited training, about 80% to more than 90%

Latest Statistics on Who Is Certified by ABIM

http://www.abim.org/pdf/data-candidates-certified/all-candidates.pdf

Certified by State

http://www.abim.org/pdf/data-candidates-certified/State-Number-of-Certificates-Issued.pdf

CONTENT AREAS OF THE EXAMINATION

The examination covers most topic areas that are likely to be encountered by a sleep medicine practitioner. The ABIM blueprint for the sleep medicine examination is online at https://www.abim.org/~/media/ABIM%20Public/Files/pdf/exam-blueprints/certification/sleep-medicine.pdf.

Reprinted here are parts of the website with some modification of the tables. Also shown are sections in this book that relate to the content areas in the examination. It is important to note that although 60% to 80% of patients in a sleep disorders center likely have a sleep breathing disorder, only 20% of the examination will cover this topic. However, even that number may be misleading, because content related to sleep breathing disorders may be covered in other areas of the examination.

SLEEP MEDICINE CERTIFICATION EXAMINATION BLUEPRINT (FROM THE ABIM WEBSITE)

What Does the Examination Cover?

The exam is designed to evaluate the extent of the candidate's knowledge and clinical judgment in areas in which a sleep medicine specialist should demonstrate a high level of competence. Expertise in the broad domain of sleep disorders, including diagnosis and treatment of both common and rare conditions, will be assessed.

Examination content will be consistent with an established blueprint or table of specifications. The blueprint has been developed by the Sleep Medicine Test Committee, whose members represent the boards sponsoring the exam: the American Board of Internal Medicine, the American Board of Pediatrics, the American Board of Psychiatry and Neurology, the American Board of Otolaryngology, the American Board of Family Medicine, and the American Board of Anesthesiology. The blueprint is used as a guide in developing the examination.

Most questions will be based on patient presentations occurring in settings that reflect current sleep medicine practice. The examination is made up of 240 single-best-answer multiple-choice questions that include patient scenarios that might present in a sleep medicine practice. Clinical information presented may include various images of polysomnograms or results of other tests. The questions are designed to see if you can formulate a differential diagnosis, order appropriate tests, and develop a management plan that might include follow-up.

Questions requiring simple recall of medical facts are in the minority; the majority of questions require integration of basic or clinical information, prioritization of alternatives, and/or clinical judgment in reaching a correct conclusion. Some questions require interpretation of pictorial material, such as polysomnograms and actigrams. In summary, the examination is designed to determine whether you can practice sleep medicine as a specialist.

Content Areas and Their Relative Proportions on the Examination: the Big Picture

Table 2 lists topics covered in a typical Sleep Medicine Certification Examination; actual content on a specific examination may vary. The number of categories was changed from eight to nine for 2019. Questions in pediatrics, pharmacology, sleep evaluation, and organ system physiology, which were previously in their own sections, are now integrated in the above nine categories. Each medical content category from the examination blueprint is listed in boldface in Table 3 along with target blueprint percentage and total number of questions in the category. The percentages in Table 3 describe content of a typical examination and are approximate; actual examination content may vary.

Examination questions in the content areas above may also address clinical topics in pediatric medicine, pharmacology, sleep evaluation, instrumentation and testing and organ system physiology that are important to the practice of sleep medicine specialists. We have added to this volume a section called "Gone, but Not Forgotten," which covers some additional topic areas in pediatrics that may fall between the cracks. A tutorial that has examples of the format of the ABIM examination questions can be found at http://www.abim.org/exam/prepare.aspx.

Table 2 Content Outline of the Certification Examination as of 2018

Medical Content Category	% of Exam	# Questions (Approximate)
Normal Sleep and Its Variants	16%	38
Circadian Rhythm Sleep-Wake Disorders	10%	24
Insomnia	17%	41
Central Disorders of Hypersomnia	12%	29
Parasomnias	7%	17
Sleep-Related Movements	8%	19
Sleep-Related Breathing Disorders	20%	48
Sleep in Other Disorders	5%	12
Instrumentation and Testing	5%	12
Total	100%	240

Adapted from the Sleep Medicine Certification Exam Blueprint, © American Board of Internal Medicine, 2018.

Table 3 Medical Content Category (Relative Percentage and Approximate Number of Questions)

Normal Sleep and Variants	16% of Exam
Sleep-wake mechanisms, neurophysiology Circadian timing Homeostatic sleep regulation Non-rapid eye movement (NREM) sleep mechanism REM sleep regulation Wake neurophysiology	4%
Other physiology Gastrointestinal Pulmonary Endocrine Cardiovascular	<2%
Normal sleep Infancy Childhood Adolescence Adulthood Elder years Pregnancy Menopause	2%
Effects of sleep deprivation Neurocognitive function Mood disturbances Metabolic disturbances	<2%
Scoring and staging Staging and arousals Respiratory events Movement Cardiac Electroencephalogram (EEG) variant	7%

Continued

Table 3 Medical Content Category (Relative Percentage and Approximate Number of Questions)—Cont'd

Normal Sleep and Variants	**16% of Exam**
Circadian Rhythm Sleep-Wake Disorders	**10% of Exam**
Circadian sleep disorders Delayed sleep-wake phase disorder Advanced sleep-wake phase disorder Non-24-hour sleep-wake rhythm disorder (free-running circadian sleep disorder) Irregular sleep-wake disorder	6.5%
Shift work disorder	<2%
Jet lag disorder	<2%
Circadian sleep-wake disorder not otherwise specified, including disruption related to behavior, medical conditions, or drugs or substances	<2%
Insomnia	**17% of Exam**
Short-term insomnia	<2%
Chronic insomnias Chronic insomnia, psychophysiologic subtype Chronic insomnia, paradoxical subtype Chronic insomnia coexisting with mental disorders Chronic insomnia, idiopathic subtype Chronic insomnia due to inadequate sleep hygiene Chronic insomnia of childhood	14% 3.5%
Insomnia related to behavior, medical conditions, or drugs or substances, and isolated symptoms and normal variants associated with reports of insomnia Insomnia related to behavior, medical conditions, or drugs or substances Excessive time in bed Short sleep	2%
Central Disorders of Hypersomnia	**12% of Exam**
Narcolepsy Type 1 (with cataplexy) Type 2 (without cataplexy)	5%
Idiopathic hypersomnia	<2%
Kleine-Levin syndrome (periodic hypersomnia)	<2%
Insufficient sleep syndrome	3%
Hypersomnia due to medical disorders	<2%
Hypersomnia due to medications	<2%
Hypersomnia associated with psychiatric disorders	<2%
Parasomnias	**7% of Exam**
NREM-related parasomnias Confusional arousals Sleep walking Sleep terrors Sleep-related eating disorder	3%
REM-related parasomnias REM sleep behavior disorder Recurrent isolated sleep paralysis Nightmare disorder	3%

Table 3 Medical Content Category (Relative Percentage and Approximate Number of Questions)—Cont'd

Normal Sleep and Variants	16% of Exam
Other parasomnias Exploding head syndrome Sleep-related hallucinations Enuresis Parasomnia due to medical disorders, medications, or substances or unspecified	<2%
Isolated symptoms and normal variants Sleep talking	<2%
Sleep-Related Movements	**8%** of Exam
Restless legs syndrome	3.5%
Periodic limb movement during sleep	2%
Rhythmic movement disorder	<2%
Sleep-related leg cramps	<2%
Bruxism	<2%
Sleep myoclonus Benign sleep myoclonus of infancy Propriospinal myoclonus at sleep onset	<2%
Other-sleep-related movement disorders due to medical disorders, medications, or substances or unspecified and movement related to isolated symptoms and normal variants Other sleep-related movement disorders due to medical disorders, medications, or substances or unspecified Excessive fragmentary myoclonus Hypnagogic foot tremor and alternating leg muscle activation Sleep starts (hypnic jerks)	<2%
Sleep-Related Breathing Disorders	**20%** of Exam
Obstructive sleep apnea Adult obstructive sleep apnea Pediatric obstructive sleep apnea	9%
Central sleep apnea syndromes Central sleep apnea with Cheyne-Stokes breathing Central sleep apnea due to a medical disorder without Cheyne-Stokes breathing Central sleep apnea due to high-altitude periodic breathing Central sleep apnea due to medications or substances Primary central sleep apnea Primary central sleep apnea of infancy Primary central sleep apnea of prematurity Treatment-emergent central sleep apnea	7.5%
Sleep-related hypoventilation disorders Obesity-hypoventilation syndrome Congenital central alveolar hypoventilation syndrome Late-onset central hypoventilation with hypothalamic dysfunction Idiopathic central alveolar hypoventilation Sleep-related hypoventilation due to medications or substances Sleep-related hypoventilation due to medical disorders	2.5%
Sleep-related hypoxemia disorder	<2%
Isolated symptoms and normal variants Snoring Catathrenia	<2%

Continued

Table 3 Medical Content Category (Relative Percentage and Approximate Number of Questions)—Cont'd

Normal Sleep and Variants	16% of Exam
Sleep in Other Disorders	**5% of Exam**
Neurologic disorders Neurodegenerative and neuromuscular disorders Cerebrovascular disorders Sleep-related epilepsy and seizure disorders Congenital disorders Sleep-related headaches Neurodevelopmental disorders	2%
Psychiatric disorders Mood disorders Psychotic disorders Anxiety Substance abuse Other conditions and general topics	2%
Other medical disorders Genetic disorders Endocrine disorders Cardiac disorders Pulmonary disorders Gastrointestinal disorders Hematologic disorders	<2%
Instrumentation and Testing	**5% of Exam**
Electrical components Sensors Filters Analog-to-digital (A-to-D) convertors Display	<2%
Technical aspects of sleep devices Actigraphy Positive airway pressure (PAP) and ventilatory support devices	<2%
Electrical safety	<2%
Artifacts	<2%
Study preparation and testing conditions Polysomnography (PSG) Multiple Sleep Latency Test (MSLT) and Maintenance of Wakefulness Test (MWT) Out-of-center testing	<2%

What's new

UpToDate®

Exam takers are able to use UpToDate®—an online, evidence-based clinical decision support resource—during the Maintenance of Certification (MOC) assessments for certification and recertification. It is recommended that exam takers become familiar with UpToDate® (https://www.uptodate.com/home/uptodate-user-academy-abim-exam).

Longitudinal Knowledge Assessment (LKA®)

This is a new, more convenient, MOC assessment option that doctors can take from their home or workplace over a five-year period. A new exam of 30 questions is available each quarter of the year. Up to 4 minutes is available to answer each question. There is immediate feedback for each question, with references. *The reader is strongly encouraged to visit to learn more about LKA*: https://www.abim.org/maintenance-of-certification/assessment-information/assessment-options/longitudinal-knowledge-assessment/.

There are currently two options for LKA in sleep medicine.

1. The general Sleep Medicine LKA
2. The Sleep Medicine LKA: Obstructive Sleep Apnea (OSA) Emphasis
   o This option has a greater number of questions on OSA. It also includes additional questions on bruxism, snoring, GERD, and home sleep apnea testing. Overall, there is about a 70% overlap with the current general Sleep Medicine blueprint.

Who can take the Sleep Medicine LKA?

- All Sleep board certified physicians, except those in a grace year, can start participating in the LKA in their assessment due year.
- The LKA can be used to regain sleep medicine certification; however, because a decision on performance is not made until the end of the 5th year, a physician will be reported as "Not Certified" until that time. Status will only change at that time if the LKA is passed and all other MOC requirements are met. A physician whose certification has lapsed may use the traditional, 10-year MOC exam to restore certification more quickly.

This is all new so that readers are encouraged to contact ABIM by email (request@abim.org) or telephone (1-(800)-441-ABIM (2246) Monday through Friday, 8:30 a.m. to 6:00 p.m. Eastern Time. Also check the ABIM website: https://www.abim.org/maintenance-of-certification/assessment-information/assessment-options/longitudinal-knowledge-assessment/

How the Traditional Examination Day Will Be Organized

The following information reflects how previous examinations were organized and how future examinations will likely be conducted. You will spend up to 10 hours at the Pearson Vue test site. Up to 8 hours will be spent taking the actual examination, which includes four 2-hour sessions. You don't have to spend the entire 2 hours in the session; you can leave a session early if you have finished it. In the 2018 examination, exam takers who were recertifying had access to UpToDate® in the final three sessions. On the question page there was a button that allowed them to consult UpToDate. Exam takers reported that they used this a lot when it first appeared in the second session but stopped using it because they did not

Table 4 Exam Day Organization	
Activity	**Time***
Registration	Varies
Tutorial	Optional, up to 30 minutes
Instructions and Pledge of Honesty	Up to 10 minutes
First Session	**Up to 2 hours**
Morning Break	Optional, up to 100 minutes (divided among 3 breaks)
Second Session	**Up to 2 hours**
Lunch Break	Optional
Third Session	**Up to 2 hours**
Afternoon Break	Optional
Fourth Session	**Up to 2 hours**
Optional Survey	Up to 10 minutes
Total	**Approximately 10 hours**

*You will have up to 8 hours to answer 240 questions. This averages 2 minutes per question, which is more than enough time to complete the examination.

find it very useful, especially for clinical scenarios. You'll have up to 100 minutes of time that can be divided among three breaks. It's your choice how much time you take at each break. Some people complete each examination session in 60 to 90 minutes and take a short break and a short lunch break, so they are able to leave as early as 4 PM. Others take the maximum amount of time for each activity and may not leave until 6 PM (Table 4).

How your day goes depends on your exam-taking style, your confidence, and your sense of whether additional review of the questions and answers in each session is needed. During the examination you will have the ability to flag questions you want to revisit and to review everything if you have the time available. For some people it may be a race between fatigue and obsession with reviewing. One of the authors found himself very fatigued at the end of the two morning sessions and welcomed the lunch break, during which he had a caffeinated cola beverage (which he usually never drinks after morning).

Distribution of Content Areas and Question Types

There are multiple forms of the exam, and question sequence can vary. The number of questions per section may also vary a bit from the blueprint. The vast majority of questions are structurally simple multiple-choice type. Some questions require opening a second window to examine a PSG fragment. Some questions will seem to come from "left field"; in the 2009 examination there were two questions in which the patient had achondroplasia and one in which the patient had Marfan's syndrome!

TIPS TO HELP YOU PASS THE SLEEP MEDICINE BOARD EXAMINATION
The Testing Facility

The testing facilities have more security than an airport. You will not be able to bring anything with you into the examination room except the clothes you are wearing (not even your watch or your keys). You will likely be supplied with a locker. The exam center may have no food or beverages for sale, so bring a lunch and beverages (juices, water, caffeinated drinks if you use them), plus snacks for the breaks between examination modules. You will be able to store these in your locker or car. Some people also brought earplugs and used them during the examination; there may be 15 people sitting at computer terminals in the exam area, some of whom may have annoying, noisy habits.

Are You a Mac or a PC?

Even if you use an iOS-based Apple computer at home, chances are overwhelming that you use a Windows-based PC at work, so you are familiar with the Windows operating system, the two-button mouse, and the mechanics of opening and closing Windows. If you don't know how to use a PC, take the online exam tutorial (on a PC) that you can download from the Pearson Vue website:

For the PC (http://www.pearsonvue.com/_abimdemo/abim.exe)
For the Mac (http://www.pearsonvue.com/_abimdemo/ABIM_demo_mac.zip)

At this time the examination sites use only PC-based computers!

Taking the Tutorial—You Must Do This!

The tutorial that you downloaded (see immediately above) has two modules: an Overview of Functional Features and a Practice Exam. Go through both modules. The first will show you how to navigate through the examination, pick answers, flag questions, write notes, and open and close windows. The latter is especially important because some content (e.g., PSG fragments or images) may be presented this way.

Certain Rules Will Help You Succeed

In the Months Before the Examination

RULE 1. The Sleep Medicine Board Exam is entirely computer based. It will be held in a high-tech facility designed specifically for examinations. The Pearson Vue facility may be limited in how many individuals can be tested, so you should ***register very early so you can take the exam in the closest testing*** center; otherwise, you might find yourself taking the exam in Wyoming (which is only an advantage if you live in Wyoming). If the testing center is far from your home, you might have to stay near the testing center the night before the examination, or you might have to drive a great distance on the morning of the examination. Don't be sleep deprived when you take the examination. Keep all the paperwork you will n need (e.g., proof of payment, registration, instructions) in one folder.

RULE 2. Make sure you have enough time to study for this examination. Even if you have a great deal of clinical experience, you will have difficulty with parts of the examination if you have not studied. Psychologically it is better to approach this type of examination knowing that you have studied. ***Study for the examination and start early***. Many people start a year before the examination. It is very difficult for people in a busy clinical practice to find the time, but clinical practice alone will not prepare you for this examination. If you are expert in certain areas, focus on the areas in which you are less experienced. Pay attention to the relative percentage of content area being tested on the examination, as presented previously. As you go through the sections in this book, try to pace yourself as you will on the examination.

RULE 3. We were surprised when we learned that the entire examination day could last 10 hours, not counting driving to and from the testing facility. As crazy as it sounds, part of the preparation means developing the stamina to focus on an examination that long. ***Work on your exam-taking stamina*** by doing long practice examinations over long periods of time. After about 3 hours some exam-takers feel fatigued and unfocused and tend to not pay as much attention to the questions. Sometimes one may respond to a question without thinking. Take practice examinations offered by the American Academy of Sleep Medicine on their website because some of the questions were similar to those that were on my examination. Take the practice examinations offered by this book. Do not drive yourself crazy!

RULE 4. Become familiar with the mechanics of the examination and what the computer screens will look like. ***Take the tutorial*** (http://www.abim.org/certification/exam-information/sleep-medicine/exam-tutorial.aspx offered by your board or take the brief tutorial at the beginning of examination day. Sample examinations, like those offered by the American Academy of Sleep Medicine, might be helpful for this. You will have the opportunity to become familiar with the computerized system at the venue where the examination is held. It is always good to know what to expect.

The Night Before the Examination

RULE 5. Look over all the instructions you received from the board and review the instructions from the testing facility. Prepare a folder to include everything you will need. You are now ***getting ready for the big day***. Prepare a lunch, snacks, and beverages that you will need on testing day. This will be your big chance to eat the chocolate you have been craving. Use a mapping or GPS program if you are not familiar with the location of the examination center. It might be helpful to drive to the site a day or two before the examination.

Exam Day: Acing the Examination

RULE 6. If you have not taken practice examinations, ***take the optional tutorial practice examination at the testing site*** so that you become familiar with the screen display, the mouse, etc. You will learn that for some questions you may have to click a tab to bring out additional content related to a question (e.g., a PSG fragment). You will also learn how to flag questions to which you want to return.

RULE 7. It is critical to **allocate your time**. When each session starts, calculate how much time you'll have for each question. About every 20 minutes check to make sure that your pace is not too slow. On the other hand don't race through the exam. Use the time you need to think through the questions. You won't get extra points or a higher level of certification for finishing the exam quickly. Take breaks even if you feel you are not that tired or fatigued. As with sleep deprivation we often underestimate the impact fatigue can have on attention to detail.

RULE 8. It is best to **answer the questions in order**. For each question, if you can eliminate one or more incorrect answers, it is worth guessing. Urban legend has resulted in the following advice: When you have no clue, the longest answer is frequently correct. Also, "All the above" is frequently correct. However, don't spend too much time on questions when you have absolutely no clue about the answer. Flag them and return when you are finished going through the rest of the examination.

RULE 9. Read each question carefully so you **understand what is being asked**. Read the entire question. Every statement in the question is included for a reason—either to help you choose the correct answer or to distract you from answering correctly. Sometimes it helps to ask yourself, "Why are they asking that?"

RULE 10. When you are presented with a PSG or other tracing, make sure you examine the labeling and data for each channel carefully. Also pay attention to the epoch length.

RULE 11. Don't second guess yourself. Once you have picked an answer, don't change it simply because you have time on your hands.

After the Examination

RULE 12. Go home, relax, and apologize to your family for spending so much time preparing for the examination. And don't forget to clean up the mess caused by your study materials strewn all over the house.

RULE 13. Be patient. Your results will be released within 3 months of the last date of the exam. When your results are released, you will receive an e-mail notification with instructions on how to access your Score Report in PDF format in the "My Exams" section of your ABIM Physician Portal.

GET GOING

This book contains sections and subsections that correspond to the content areas of the actual examination. We recommend that you go through the examination questions twice. The number of questions printed in each section is double the number that you will encounter for that topic area on the actual examination. Thus when you finish the entire book you will have finished the equivalent of two examinations. Some of the sections have bonus questions—additional important content.

Important Note About Some Topics

Although the current blueprint for the examination does not mention pediatrics, this is somewhat misleading. We estimate that 5% to 10% of all questions on the examination require some knowledge of pediatric sleep medicine; therefore, ignoring pediatric sleep disorders is not a good idea when preparing for the examination or in keeping up to date in the field. The section "Gone but not forgotten," covers additional pediatric content.

How to Go Through This Book if You Don't Have a Great Deal of Sleep Medicine Experience

1. We suggest that you go through the book cover to cover, starting at the beginning.

2. Answer the questions for each section in one sitting, marking the answers in light pencil (so you can erase the checkmarks). Check the answers to see how you did in that section. Identify the areas of content that need more attention.

3. Review the Summary at the end of each section. Keep track of your score for each section.

4. When you have finished the entire book, you will have completed the equivalent of two complete examinations (480 questions). Calculate your score.

5. Review the topic areas in which you are weak.

6. Do the web-based examinations.

How to Go Through This Book if You Have a Great Deal of Sleep Medicine Experience

1. Do the web-based exams to identify areas of weakness.

2. Go through the book, but first focus on the areas of weakness you have identified.

3. Answer the questions for each section in one sitting, marking the answers in light pencil (so you can erase the checkmarks). Check the answers to see how you did in that section. Identify the areas of content that need more attention.

4. Review the summary at the end of each section. Keep track of your score for each section.

5. When you have finished the entire book, you will have completed the equivalent of two complete examinations (480 questions). Calculate your score.

6. Review the topic areas in which you are weak.

The goal is to obtain at least 75% correct in each of the 10 sections in order to increase the odds of passing.

About the Questions and Content

We understand that your time is valuable and limited, and nobody will ever know everything about sleep medicine. The questions and other content in this book have been chosen to efficiently cover the material that we believe is important and might be on the examination. On the examination itself, the questions generally test one bit of knowledge. Many of the questions in this book are "high value" and may test several different facts. The **Highly Recommended** list is in the Appendix of this volume.

About the Answers

You will note that most of the answers have a brief paragraph that explains why the answer is correct and that contains references if you require them, which will be from one or more of the following:

1. Kryger M, Avidan A, Berry R: *Atlas of Clinical Sleep Medicine*, ed 2, Philadelphia, 2014, Saunders. This will be abbreviated ATLAS2.

2. American Academy of Sleep Medicine (AASM): *International Classification of Sleep Disorders*, ed 3, Darien, Ill., 2014, AASM. This will be abbreviated ICSD3.

3. American Academy of Sleep Medicine: *The AASM Manual for the Scoring of Sleep and Associated Events*, Version 2.5, Darien, Ill., 2018, AASM. This will be abbreviated MANUAL2.

4. Sheldon S, Ferber R, Kryger M, Gozal D: *Principles and Practice of Pediatric Sleep Medicine*, ed 2, Philadelphia, 2014, Elsevier. This will be abbreviated PEDS2.

5. Kryger M, Roth T, Dement W. *Principles and Practice of Sleep Medicine* ed 6, Elsevier, Philadelphia, 2017. This will be abbreviated PPSM6.

6. Published articles or other sources, especially AASM practice guidelines (https://aasm.org/clinical-resources/practice-standards/practice-guidelines/) and provider fact sheets (https://aasm.org/clinical-resources/provider-fact-sheets/).

If you own it, you will be able to access the online version of the *Atlas* directly from the online version of this book.

Highly Recommended Lists

In several places, we refer to resources that we have labeled as **Highly Recommended**, and **the complete list is in Appendix I**. "Highly Recommended" means that we strongly recommend you review and know the material in these sources. Accessing some of the resources mentioned requires membership in the American Academy of Sleep Medicine.

A Note About Illustrations and PSG Fragments in This Volume

The polysomnography fragments and illustrations that were presented in the previous examinations were not of particularly high quality, and it is likely that the display of polysomnographic findings that you are used to (such as those in this book) is much better than what you'll find on the examination. It is likely that the quality of images used in the examination will improve with time.

Disclaimer

Going through this book will not guarantee that you pass the examination. Question types and distribution of questions may change. We have made no attempt to replicate the questions that appear on the exam.

GOOD LUCK!

KRYGER'S SLEEP MEDICINE REVIEW
THIRD EDITION

Normal Sleep and Its Variants

1.1	Sleep-Wake Mechanisms and Neurophysiology

QUESTIONS

A 20-Year-Old Student Pulling an All-Nighter

A 20-year-old student with asthma is cramming for a final exam he will take the next morning. He has studied the entire day and now has decided to study through the night. He becomes extremely sleepy at 4 AM and has two cups of strong coffee.

1. Which neurologic structure is primarily involved in maintaining his alertness?
   A. Ascending reticular activating system
   B. Hypothalamus
   C. Pineal gland
   D. Ventrolateral preoptic (VLPO) nuclei

2. The brain localization for structures that keeps him awake is located in the
   A. Medullary bulb
   B. Midbrain
   C. Pons
   D. Entire brainstem

3. Which of the neurotransmitters below is focused on sleep promotion (as opposed to wakefulness)?
   A. 5-Hydroxytryptamine (5-HT) from serotoninergic neurons in the dorsal raphe nucleus
   B. Acetylcholine from cholinergic neurons in pedunculopontine tegmental and laterodorsal tegmental nuclei
   C. Gamma-aminobutyric acid (GABA) and galanin (GAL) from the VLPO
   D. Norepinephrine from noradrenergic neurons of the ventrolateral medulla and locus coeruleus

4. Pathways of the arousal system reach the cerebral cortex through which neurologic structures?
   A. Cerebellum and pons
   B. Medulla and spinal cord
   C. Pons and medulla
   D. Thalamus, hypothalamus, and basal forebrain

5. Which chemical involved in hunger regulation also has input into the arousal system?
   A. Ghrelin
   B. Insulin
   C. Leptin
   D. Orexin (hypocretin)

6. Which chemical is accumulating in his central nervous system (CNS) to cause sleepiness before he drinks coffee?
   A. Adenosine
   B. Gamma-hydroxybutyric acid (GHB)
   C. Melatonin
   D. Serotonin

7. He drank coffee for its stimulant effect; it works to increase wakefulness by binding to the receptors of which one of the following:
   A. Adenosine
   B. GHB
   C. Melatonin
   D. Serotonin

8. The student becomes jittery about 20 minutes after drinking the coffee and feels his heart beating rapidly. Assuming he is taking all of the following medications, which one is likely producing the tachycardia?
   A. Fluticasone
   B. Montelukast
   C. Prednisone
   D. Theophylline

Daydreamer

A 16-year-old straight-A high school student is referred for evaluation because she no longer focuses well in school. She is seen to "nod off" in class, and her grades have recently plummeted. You learn that she sleeps 8 hours per night but complains of "broken sleep." She sometimes awakens in the middle of the night and then has trouble falling back to sleep. She has also noted a panicky feeling during nocturnal awakenings and states, "I feel someone is in the room, and I can't move." Further history reveals that she has recently started taking afternoon naps and dreams vividly while napping.

9. Her pediatrician believes that she is exhibiting symptoms of a neurologic disease, perhaps multiple sclerosis, and recommends a spinal tap. If a spinal tap were to be performed and the cerebrospinal fluid (CSF) were to be analyzed, what abnormality would likely be found?
   A. Elevated interleukin-6 (IL-6)
   B. Elevated nerve growth factor
   C. Reduced adenosine
   D. Reduced hypocretin

10. The patient's unintended daytime sleep episodes are *most* likely caused by what abnormality?
    A. An underactive ascending reticular activating system
    B. Excessive CNS serotonin levels
    C. Loss of hypocretin neurons
    D. Overactive CNS GABA_A receptors

11. The patient's episodes of awakening during the night, unable to move and sensing that someone is in the room, is characteristic of
    A. Posttraumatic stress disorder (PTSD)
    B. Psychomotor epilepsy
    C. Schizophrenic hallucination
    D. Sleep paralysis

12. What neurologic phenomenon is causing her inability to move when she awakens during the night?
    A. Abnormal discharge from the frontal cortex inhibiting the motor cortex
    B. Excessive adrenergic stimulation causing vasoconstriction of spinal arteries, resulting in ischemia of the spinal motor neurons
    C. Excessive stimulation of the ascending reticular activating system that thus inhibits the motor cortex
    D. Inhibition of motor neurons in the spine by both glycinergic and GABAergic mechanisms

Pandemic of Sleepiness

A 40-year-old patient with acute influenza is noted to have a severe cough and feels extremely sleepy whenever he is awake.

13. Which of the following phenomena is NOT causing sleepiness?
   A. Activation by cytokines of the acute phase response
   B. Viral encephalitis with influenza virus invading hypothalamic cells
   C. Viral ribonucleic acid (RNA) and protein that induces cytokine production within the hypothalamus
   D. Virus replicating in lung cells and inducing production of somnogenic cytokines

14. What is the effect of the infection on sleep architecture?
   A. Enhancement of NREM sleep and inhibition of REM sleep
   B. Increase in wakefulness with inability to consolidate sleep
   C. Marked increase in rapid eye movement (REM) sleep, leading to hallucinations
   D. No systematic effect on the relationship of REM to non-REM (NREM) sleep

15. Which infection-related cytokine/protein is NOT associated with sleepiness?
   A. Brain-derived neurotrophic factor and growth hormone–releasing factor
   B. IL-1β and IL-6
   C. Orexin (hypocretin) and leptin
   D. Tumor necrosis factor and nerve growth factor

16. What is the expected natural history of the sleepiness in this case?
   A. Sleepiness starts within hours of infection and lasts for days to weeks
   B. The sleepiness can become chronic because of damage to the hypothalamus, a condition known as *encephalitis lethargica*
   C. The sleepiness starts after the lung infection begins to resolve and can last months
   D. The sleepiness usually is present only during the prodromal phase

Potpourri

17. A friend likes to drink red wine up to 30 minutes before bedtime about 5 nights a week. He tells you that the wine has an effect on his sleep. Which of the following *best* describes alcohol's effect when taken near bedtime?
   A. Bizarre dreams
   B. Decreased limb movements
   C. Increased REM sleep
   D. Reduced wake after sleep onset (WASO)

18. A waitress drinks three pots of coffee to stay alert and energized on her shift. The reason coffee helps her remain alert is because caffeine is a(n)
   A. Adenosine antagonist
   B. Serotonin antagonist
   C. Norepinephrine agonist
   D. Dopamine reuptake blocker

19. Caffeine has an approximate half-life of
   A. 15 to 30 minutes
   B. 1 to 2 hours
   C. 3 to 5 hours
   D. 6 to 8 hours

20. You are at a social gathering, where someone learns you are a sleep medicine specialist. He brags that he can drink four espresso drinks before bedtime without any effect on his sleep. You reply that caffeine
   A. Has no effect on some people
   B. Reduces REM sleep
   C. Reduces stage N3 sleep
   D. Will eventually cause insomnia

ANSWERS

1. A. Exams (self-assessment or board) often begin with an icebreaker, a question considered to be relatively easy. In this question, *ascending reticular activating system (ARAS)* should appear as the obvious answer. It is important to know the big picture about arousal and initiation of sleep. In 1935, Fredric Bremer, a pioneer in sleep research, showed that if a transection is made between the pons and midbrain of a cat (the preparation is called *cerveau isolé*, literally "isolated brain" in French), there is no arousal, and the animal is comatose. If a transection is made between the lower medulla and the spine, the cat is able to demonstrate wakefulness and sleep. This preparation is known as *l'encéphale isolé. L'encéphale* refers to all the nervous system structures in the cranial vault or skull. In 1949, Moruzzi and Magoun showed that stimulating the structures of the rostral pontine reticular formation (basically in the area between Bremer's two transections) produced a desynchronized (or awake) electroencephalogram (EEG). This area of the brainstem became known as the *ascending reticular activating system.*   (ATLAS2, Ch 3.1)

2. D. This question is a follow-up to the first one. The ARAS begins in the medulla and ascends into the pons and midbrain. This is a type of question in which "all of the above" is often correct.   (ATLAS2, Ch 3.1)

3. C. There are so many chemicals and parts of the brain mentioned that it might make your eyes glaze over. It is desirable to know the sleep-promoting systems and the wakefulness-promoting systems; they are reviewed in the summary that follows. This type of question is relatively easy because you can often get the right answer by a process of elimination. When confronted with such a question, do not panic; look for terms you know and start from there. In this question, you need to know any component of the sleep switch (this includes the VLPO, whose cells contain the inhibitory neurotransmitters GABA and GAL), or you might have to generalize from information you learned from an entirely different topic. For example, you might have remembered that GABA has something to do with sleep from understanding hypnotics. You always know more than you think.   (ATLAS2, Ch 3.1)

4. D. Again, analyze the question, and you will realize that only one of the answers has anything to do with pathways going into the cerebral cortex. There are two pathways of arousal into the cortex from the ARAS: a dorsal route via the thalamus (associated fact: site of spindle formation) and a ventral route via the *basal forebrain* and the *hypothalamus*. The basal forebrain is a ventral structure, and the hypothalamus is ventral and below the thalamus. The hypothalamus is right behind the optic chiasm (associated fact: the *suprachiasmatic nucleus*, the "conductor" of the circadian system "orchestra," is here) and is above the pituitary gland. The hypothalamus secretes many endocrine-releasing factors, and because of its location and function, it links the endocrine and circadian systems.   (ATLAS2, Ch 3.1)

5. D. All these chemical entities are involved in regulation of hunger or energy (or both). *Leptin*, secreted by fat cells, inhibits hunger. *Ghrelin*, produced by cells in the stomach, increases hunger. Insulin is produced in response to high glucose levels. *Orexin* (also called *hypocretin*) is produced by cells in the lateral and posterior hypothalamus and stimulates hunger and wakefulness. Two orexin neuropeptides, orexin A and B, promote arousal and stabilize wakefulness by their effect on the OX-1 and OX-2 receptors. Patients with narcolepsy have reduced orexin-producing cells and are sleepy as a result.

6. A.   It is believed that *adenosine*, an inhibitory neurotransmitter, increases in the nervous system with prolonged wakefulness.

7. A.   Caffeine, a *xanthine*, is a competitive inhibitor of adenosine because it is an antagonist of adenosine receptors in the nervous system. It has structural similarities to adenosine. The net result of blocking the effect of a compound that inhibits CNS function is to stimulate the CNS and promote wakefulness.

8. D.   Theophylline is a xanthine sometimes used to treat asthma. It is one of the metabolites of caffeine. Both caffeine and theophylline can relax bronchial smooth muscle and increase cardiac contractility, heart rate, and blood pressure. Theophylline affects the nervous system through its action as an adenosine receptor antagonist.

9. D.   From the description, this is most likely a case of narcolepsy. Each of the factors mentioned can promote sleepiness or sleep. Although rarely tested for clinical purposes, analysis of CSF in patients with narcolepsy has shown a striking reduction of hypocretin compared with controls.

10. C.   The unintended transition from wakefulness to sleep is related to the fact that hypocretin neurons project widely in the cerebral cortex and stabilize wakefulness. The lack of these neurons results in wakefulness and sleep instability.   (ATLAS2, Ch 3.1)

11. D.   This is a classic description of sleep paralysis. The person awakens, usually from a dream, often with the perception that there is someone else in the room (sometimes a frightening devil-like creature). These events are likely the persistence of REM phenomena (dreaming and motor inhibition) persisting into wakefulness.   (ATLAS2, Ch 7)

12. D.   The motor weakness is related to the neurons of the sublaterodorsal (SLD) nucleus inhibiting motor spinal neurons by glycinergic and GABAergic mechanisms.   (ATLAS2, Ch 3.1) Interestingly, the motor neurons projecting to the diaphragm are spared, and thus the motor atonia does not affect breathing.

13. B.   The sleepiness seen with influenza is seldom caused by infection of cells in the nervous system but rather is brought on by the effect of cytokines that are a response to the infection. Cytokines are proteins and glycoproteins that behave like neurotransmitters and are commonly expressed during infections. The remaining three answers (B, C, and D) are mechanisms that likely do play a role in the sleepiness.   (ATLAS2, Ch 3.5)

14. A.   Infections typically increase NREM sleep (and can increase slow-wave sleep), and they reduce REM sleep.   (ATLAS2, Ch 3.5)

15. C.   This is the type of question in which you might not know much about the topic but can get the right answer from associated bits of knowledge. Orexin is not a cytokine, and leptin, which might be considered a cytokine, is produced by fat cells, and fat cells have nothing to do with infections. Thus, knowing either of these facts could help point to the correct answer. The other answers (B, C, and D) are cytokines that can be increased in infections.   (ATLAS2, Ch 3.5)

16. A.   The sleepiness can start abruptly with infections, sometimes within hours. It is related to cytokine production and will last a few days to a few weeks as the infection resolves. You might have read something about encephalitis lethargica in the distant past, and if so, you wonder whether it could be the correct answer. It is not. Encephalitis lethargica is an encephalitis that affects the junction of the posterior hypothalamus and the midbrain, producing severe hypersomnolence (hence the name *von Economo sleeping sickness*, after the neurologist Constantin von Economo, who described this illness in 1917). Encephalitis lethargica can also cause symptoms such as an inability to move or speak. Between 1915 and 1926, an epidemic of encephalitis lethargica spread around the world; there has been no epidemic of this disease since then, and the cause of the illness was never ascertained (autoimmune and infectious causes have been suggested but never proved). Most victims of encephalitis lethargica died in a coma. Some of the survivors entered into a rigid, Parkinson-like state. This clinical picture was eloquently described by the neurologist Oliver Sacks in his 1973 book *Awakenings* and was also portrayed in the 1990 movie of the same name starring Robin Williams.   (ATLAS2, Ch 3.1, Fig. 3.1–2)

17. A. Many drugs can trigger nightmares and bizarre dreams, including catecholaminergic agents, beta-blockers, antidepressants, barbiturates, and even alcohol. Alcohol is a known sleep disruptor; therefore, it does not reduce WASO or improve sleep consolidation. It is also not known to decrease periodic limb movements.

18. A. Adenosine is thought to be a sleep-inducing neurotransmitter that increases with increasing hours of wakefulness. The mechanism of action of caffeine on wakefulness involves nonspecific adenosine receptor antagonism. Caffeine is a xanthine derivative, which is known to be an A_1 receptor blocker.

19. C. Caffeine is a very rapidly absorbed drug with a half-life of 3.5 to 5 hours.

20. C. Caffeine is known to delay sleep onset and decrease stage N3 sleep. Caffeine has no known effect on REM sleep, and it can be the source of insomnia, but its effects are acute because the drug does not accumulate on a daily basis.

Summary

Highly Recommended

- *Atlas of Clinical Sleep Medicine*, ed 2, Chapter 3.1
- de Lecea L, Huerta R: Hypocretin (orexin) regulation of sleep-to-wake transitions, *Front Pharmacol* 5:16, 2014. eCollection 2014. Free full text is available online at http://www.ncbi.nlm.nih.gov/pubmed/24575043
- *Principles and Practice of Pediatric Sleep Medicine*, ed 2, Chapters 1 to 4 and 6

It is important to understand the structures and mechanisms involved in wakefulness and sleep. Because this topic will make up only about 10 of the 240 questions on the exam, do not spend excessive time reviewing esoteric neural mechanisms. However, the blueprint of the exam includes *circadian timing* in this section even though there is an entire section in the blueprint on circadian rhythm sleep-wake disorders. Thus, later on in this section, we cover the physiologic mechanisms of circadian rhythms with a series of bonus questions.

The topic of drug effects on sleep-wake mechanisms can come up in the therapy of many disorders (e.g., narcolepsy, restless legs, insomnia). Learn the key functions of neurotransmitters so you can predict their impact on sleep-wake functioning. Study the pharmacology of the various drug classes, paying attention to mechanism of action, indications, and impact on sleep parameters (e.g., sleep latency, WASO, REM, N3). It is important to know receptor physiology and the effect of medications on sleep.

Structures and Neurotransmitters Involved in Wakefulness (ATLAS2, Chs 3.1 and 3.2)

- Noradrenergic (NE) neurons of the ventrolateral medulla and locus coeruleus (LC)
- Cholinergic neurons (ACh) in the pedunculopontine and laterodorsal tegmental (PPT/LDT) nuclei
- Serotoninergic neurons (5-HT) in the dorsal raphe nucleus (DR)
- Dopaminergic neurons (DAs) of the ventral periaqueductal gray matter (vPAG)
- Histaminergic neurons (His) of the tuberomammillary nucleus (TMN)
- Orexin neurons in the lateral hypothalamus help stabilize wakefulness and thus prevent unwanted wake-to-sleep transitions

The Two Pathways of Cortical Arousal (ATLAS2, Ch 3.1)

- Dorsal route, through the thalamus
- Ventral route, through the hypothalamus and basal forebrain (BF). The latter pathway receives inputs from the melanin and hypocretin (orexin)–concentrating (MHC) neurons of the lateral hypothalamic area (LH) as well as from GABAergic or cholinergic neurons of the BF

Sleep Switch (ATLAS2, Ch 3.1)

- The VLPO contains cells that contain the inhibitory neurotransmitters GABA and GAL
- The VLPO inhibits input into the components of the ARAS; in turn, the ARAS inhibits the VLPO

REM Switch (ATLAS2, Ch 3.1)

- REM-off neurons in the ventrolateral periaqueductal gray (vlPAG) area and lateral pontine tegmentum (LPT) receive inputs from the VLPO and orexin neurons
- REM-off neurons have a mutually inhibitory interaction with REM-on GABAergic neurons of the ventral sublaterodorsal nucleus (SLD) and the precoeruleus (PC)–parabrachial (PB) nucleus

Structures and Neurotransmitters That Affect REM (ATLAS2, Ch 3.1)

- Cholinergic neurons of the pedunculopontine and laterodorsal tegmental nuclei (PPT-LDT) become REM "on" by inhibiting the LPT. Because these neurons are not in turn directly inhibited by the LPT, they are external to the switch
- Dorsal raphe and noradrenergic locus coeruleus (DR-NLC) neurons activate the REM-off regions but are not inhibited directly by the SLD

Cytokines That Promote Sleep (ATLAS2, Ch 3.5)

- Interleukin (IL)-1β
- IL-6
- Tumor necrosis factor alpha
- Nerve growth factor
- Brain-derived neurotrophic factor
- Growth hormone–releasing factor

Pharmacology of Sleep and Wakefulness (ATLAS2, Ch 6)

- Hypothalamic neurons and adjacent groups of basal forebrain neurons produce the neurotransmitter GABA
- GABA neurons inhibit the firing of cells involved in wakefulness
- GABA inhibits neurons that contain histamine, norepinephrine, serotonin, hypocretin (orexin), and glutamate, and this inhibition promotes sleep
- Hypocretin (orexin) is a neuropeptide that excites the areas in the hypothalamus that produce wakefulness-promoting neurotransmitters

Effects of Drugs on Sleep (ATLAS2, Ch 6)

- Alcohol
  - Decreases sleep latency
  - Disrupts sleep
  - Decreases REM sleep
  - Increases snoring and apnea
- Anticonvulsants
  - Increase sleepiness
  - Can increase N3 sleep
- Antidepressants
  - Suppress REM and prolong REM latency
  - REM rebound may occur after abrupt withdrawal
  - Selective serotonin reuptake inhibitors (SSRIs) can disrupt sleep
  - Low doses of sedating antidepressants are often used (off label) to treat insomnia
  - Antidepressants may cause eye movements outside REM sleep
  - Serotonergic antidepressants can cause restless legs syndrome and REM sleep behavior disorder

- Antihistamines
  - ○ Over-the-counter (OTC) drugs cause sedation
  - ○ Antihistamines do not have a reliable effect on sleep
- Antihypertensive agents
  - ○ Lipophilic beta-blockers can disrupt sleep
  - ○ The most sedative include alpha-adrenergic agonists such as methyldopa and clonidine
  - ○ Some patients taking drugs of this class report nightmares
- Antipsychotics
  - ○ Major effects are increased sedation and improved sleep continuity
  - ○ Newer drugs in this class are being used off label for treating insomnia
  - ○ Mild elevation of N3 may be seen
- Corticosteroids
  - ○ Can cause slight REM suppression
  - ○ Can also disrupt sleep and cause bizarre dreams
- Nicotine
  - ○ Can delay sleep onset
  - ○ Can cause complaints of nonrestorative sleep
  - ○ Nicotine gum has been shown to increase alpha-EEG and reduce N3 sleep
- Opiates
  - ○ Can cause sedation
  - ○ Can disrupt sleep and reduce REM
  - ○ May ameliorate restless legs syndrome
  - ○ May cause sleep hypoventilation
  - ○ May cause central and/or complex sleep apnea
- Hypnotics and sedatives
  - ○ Benzodiazepines decrease sleep-onset latency, improve sleep continuity, and suppress N3 sleep
  - ○ Mild suppression of REM is also possible
  - ○ Newer nonbenzodiazepine hypnotics (e.g., zolpidem, zaleplon, eszopiclone) have little effect on sleep architecture
- Stimulants
  - ○ Increase wakefulness
  - ○ Decrease total sleep time (TST) and stage N3 sleep
  - ○ Amphetamines and cocaine suppress REM sleep
  - ○ Withdrawal causes prolonged periods of sleep and profound REM rebound
- Tetrahydrocannabinol (THC)
  - ○ THC increases TST and stage N3 sleep
  - ○ THC causes mild suppression of REM
  - ○ REM rebound occurs after discontinuation

Clinical Correlations

- REM atonia is produced by SLD neurons via glutamatergic spinal projections to interneurons that inhibit motor neurons in the spine by both glycinergic and GABAergic mechanisms. (ATLAS2, Ch 3.2)
- Hippocampal and cortical activation during REM sleep is generated by glutamatergic inputs from the REM-on region to the medial septum and the BF
- Absence of orexin neurons leads to unintended wake-to-sleep transitions and to the intrusion of REM-sleep phenomena into the awake state
- Agents that antagonize the orexin (both OX-1 and OX-2) receptors have hypnotic properties (Box 1.1-1)

Box 1.1–1 Alphabet Soup

Nothing makes doctors break out in a sweat more quickly than the alphabet soup of neurophysiology and neuroanatomy. Most of us last studied neurophysiology and neuroanatomy in medical school and even then likely found the subjects difficult. There are acronyms galore, from ACh to Gal to OX-1 to RAS to VLPO, along with cells, nuclei, centers, receptors, tracts, and projections found by lesions, electrical stimulation, and other methods. The acronyms tend to be cryptic, mysterious, and nonintuitive. This section will not make you an expert in neuroanatomy and neurophysiology related to sleep, but it is hoped that it will help you gain an understanding of some basic sleep mechanisms. (I like to think that the people writing exam questions may be as baffled as the test takers.)

The first thing to understand is that most of the action controlling sleep and wakefulness occurs in the hypothalamus. Basically, the hypothalamus is the conduit of information that links the nervous and endocrine systems by secreting factors that affect the pituitary gland; the pituitary sits just below the hypothalamus, connected by a stalk of nerve fibers.

Figure 1.1–1 shows the main areas involved in NREM sleep and wakefulness. It is not complete (see the summary for additional detail) but is provided to help you learn the locations of the main anatomic structures involved in sleep and wakefulness. The blue boxes are structures involved mainly in promoting sleep. The red boxes are structures involved primarily in maintaining wakefulness.

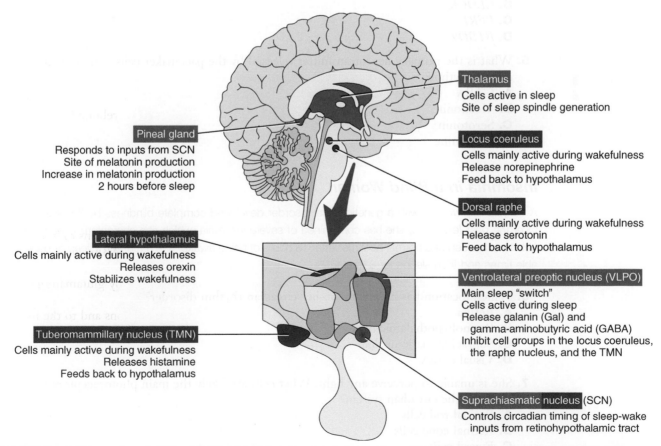

Thalamus
Cells active in sleep
Site of sleep spindle generation

Pineal gland
Responds to inputs from SCN
Site of melatonin production
Increase in melatonin production
2 hours before sleep

Locus coeruleus
Cells mainly active during wakefulness
Release norepinephrine
Feed back to hypothalamus

Dorsal raphe
Cells mainly active during wakefulness
Release serotonin
Feed back to hypothalamus

Lateral hypothalamus
Cells mainly active during wakefulness
Releases orexin
Stabilizes wakefulness

Ventrolateral preoptic nucleus (VLPO)
Main sleep "switch"
Cells active during sleep
Release galanin (Gal) and
   gamma-aminobutyric acid (GABA)
Inhibit cell groups in the locus coeruleus,
   the raphe nucleus, and the TMN

Tuberomammillary nucleus (TMN)
Cells mainly active during wakefulness
Releases histamine
Feeds back to hypothalamus

Suprachiasmatic nucleus (SCN)
Controls circadian timing of sleep-wake
   inputs from retinohypothalamic tract

FIGURE 1.1–1 Sleep-wake regulation—the big picture (see Box 1.1–1). From: Kryger MH, Avidan A, Berry R. *Atlas of clinical sleep medicine.* 2nd ed. Page 22 Philadelphia: Saunders; 2014.

BONUS QUESTIONS ON CIRCADIAN MECHANISMS AND NEUROPHYSIOLOGY

Not Sleepy at Bedtime

An 18-year-old high school senior is referred because of difficulty awakening in the morning, falling grades, and concerns that she will not get into college. She just is not sleepy at normal bedtime and cannot fall asleep until 3 AM. On weekends, she sleeps until early afternoon and then feels great the rest of the day.

1. What is the *most* likely diagnosis?
   A. Delayed sleep phase disorder
   B. Advanced sleep phase disorder
   C. Sleep-onset insomnia
   D. Free-running circadian rhythm

2. Where are the cells located that synchronize the circadian timing of her sleep-wake pattern?
   A. Optic chiasm
   B. Visual cortex in the occipital lobe
   C. Hypocretin nucleus
   D. Suprachiasmatic nucleus

3. Which of the following structures helps synchronize her circadian system?
   A. Rod cells
   B. Cone cells
   C. Retinohypothalamic tract
   D. Anterior pituitary gland

4. Which of the following is *not* involved in generating this patient's circadian rhythm?
   A. *ARNTL (formerly BMAL1)*
   B. *CLOCK*
   C. *PER1*
   D. *BTBD9*

5. What is the primary neurotransmitter released by the pacemaker cells that control the circadian rhythm?
   A. GABA
   B. Melatonin
   C. Serotonin
   D. Dopamine

Insomnia in a Blind Woman

A 39-year-old woman with a genetic visual disorder developed complete blindness by 35 years of age. Over the past few years, she has complained of severe insomnia, which she characterizes as not being able to fall asleep at a normal bedtime. After 18 hours of being awake, she often falls asleep at unpredictable times and then sleeps for 8 hours.

6. Which location has no impact on her circadian rhythm disorder?
   A. Retina
   B. Retinohypothalamic tract
   C. Suprachiasmatic nucleus
   D. Visual cortex

7. She is unable to perceive any light. What cells are likely the main photoreceptors that synchronize the circadian system?
   A. Retinal rod cells
   B. Retinal cone cells
   C. Foveal cells
   D. Ganglion cells

8. This patient's suprachiasmatic nucleus (SCN) is unsynchronized to external light, yet the SCN still has outputs to the
   A. Cerebral cortex
   B. Thalamus
   C. Hypothalamus
   D. Pineal gland

9. If you measured her body temperature continuously over several weeks, you would find
   A. No pattern but random variations in temperature
   B. Temperature oscillation at a period of 22 to 23 hours
   C. Temperature oscillation at a period of 24 to 25 hours
   D. Stable temperature without oscillation

10. The *correct* circadian diagnosis in this patient is
    A. Advanced sleep-wake phase disorder
    B. Delayed sleep-wake phase disorder
    C. Non–24-hour sleep-wake rhythm disorder
    D. Irregular sleep-wake rhythm disorder

ANSWERS

1. **A.** This brief history is classic for a circadian rhythm sleep disorder, which has been previously classified as a delayed sleep phase type (and before that, a syndrome). Note that it is no longer officially called a *syndrome*; the term *disorder* is used to describe it in the third edition of the *International Classification of Sleep Disorders* (ICSD3). Knowledge of circadian rhythm sleep disorders is important; questions about them will be on the exam. (ATLAS2, Ch 9.1)

2. **D.** The best answer is the SCN. This nucleus is in the hypothalamus just above the optic chiasm (hence the designation *suprachiasmatic*). The nucleus is the "conductor" that directs and synchronizes the "orchestra" that creates the circadian rhythm of the various endocrine and physiologic systems of the body. (ATLAS2, p 22)

3. **C.** The retinohypothalamic tract carries information from the eye (melanopsin-containing ganglion cells in the retina) to the hypothalamus (hence the designation *retinohypothalamic* tract), where the SCN is located. In medical school, you learned about rods and cones, which are necessary for vision. However, they are not involved in circadian physiology. (ATLAS2, p 35)

4. **D.** The language of genetics is complex; our knowledge of how genes affect circadian rhythmicity is evolving, and the names of some genes change. A human gene is generally indicated by all capital letters, but the same gene in mammals is not (e.g., *PER1* vs *Per1*). Mammalian clock genes include three Per (for period) genes: *Per1*, *Per2*, and *Per3*; two cryptochrome genes: *Cry1* and *Cry2*; and *Tim*, *Clock*, *Bmal1*, and *Csnk1e*. These are all expressed in suprachiasmatic neurons. These genes and the proteins they produce interact to form negative and positive autoregulatory transcription–translation feedback loops that define the molecular machinery of the circadian oscillator. The incorrect answer is *BTBD9*, which has been linked to periodic limb movements of sleep. (ATLAS2, p 34)

5. **A.** Although GABA is the right answer, you might be tempted to pick melatonin because it has something to do with the circadian system and is used to treat circadian disorders. Approach questions like this, for which you might not have a clue as to the correct answer, by ruling out what you know. Here, for example, you should be able to rule out serotonin and dopamine, thus increasing your odds of answering correctly.

6. **D.** The first three structures listed play a role in transmitting visual information to the SCN, the latter being the location of the circadian pacemaker. After the pathways that carry visual information bifurcate in the optic chiasm, the pathways (from the rods and cones) that continue to the visual cortex play no role in synchronizing the circadian system. Thus, people with cortical blindness or those with blindness related to abnormalities in the visual cortex can have normally synchronized circadian systems.

7. D.   Besides the rods and cones, the retina also has ganglion cells that contain the protein melanopsin, which functions as a photoreceptor. Axons of rods and cones become the retinohypothalamic tract (RHT), which ends in the SCN. The RHT in the SCN releases glutamate, which leads to increased expression of *PER1* and *PER2*. The SCN contains cellular oscillators that are normally coupled but that can oscillate independently. It is also emerging that almost all cells in all tissues of the body contain the machinery to produce circadian rhythms.

8. C.   There are projections from the SCN to the adjacent subparaventricular zone (SPZ). There is a secondary projection to the dorsomedial hypothalamic nucleus (DMH), which projects to other brain regions that regulate sleep and wakefulness. There are also projections from the SCN to the paraventricular hypothalamic nucleus (PVH) to regulate corticosteroid secretion and synthesis of melatonin (see Summary). Normally, the SCN would send out alerting signals when it is daytime and a sleep signal at night, but in this blind patient, the signals would not be synchronized to light and darkness cues, and the patient's circadian rhythm would be free running.

9. C.   Without synchronization with light-dark cycles, the patient will demonstrate the normal period of the human free-running circadian rhythm. The consensus at this time is that the free-running period in humans (called *tau*) is between 24 and 25 hours and is closer to 24 than 25 hours. If presented with a choice on the exam, select the value that is larger than and closest to 24 hours. The nonentrained period of most plants and animals maintained under constant darkness and temperature is almost always close to 24 hours (hence the term *circadian*, or about 1 day) and is rarely less than 23 hours or greater than 25 hours.

10. C.   It is important to know the differences between the major circadian disorders. The names of the circadian rhythm sleep-wake disorders seem to change about every 5 years. This patient has a pattern, but it is unsynchronized to light-dark cycles. This is in contrast to people who have no pattern (truly random times of sleep and wakefulness), such as those with dementia, brain injury, or neurocognitive impairment. The difference between answers C and D is that in the latter, there is no pattern.   (ATLAS2, Ch 9; ICSD3, pp 189–224)

Summary

Highly Recommended

- *Atlas of Clinical Sleep Medicine*, ed 2, Chapters 3.3 and 9

It is important to understand the structures and mechanisms involved in circadian physiology. Although the exam blueprint combines circadian physiology with other mechanisms controlling sleep, it is important to understand these mechanisms, and the questions on circadian physiology have been added as a bonus.

Types of Rhythms That Affect Sleep

- Circadian: About 1 day or 24 hours
- Ultradian: The 80- to 110-minute REM-NREM cycle
- Infradian: Greater than 24-hour cycles

The Two-Process Model

- Is an interaction of   (ATLAS2, p 36)
  - Process S: Sleep homeostasis (the less time asleep, the greater the drive to sleep)
  - Process C: Regulation by the circadian system
  - Zeitgebers (time synchronizers), which are:
    - Photic (light)
    - Nonphotic (timing of eating and drinking, social interactions, environmental temperature)

Control of the Circadian System

- The master pacemaker is the SCN in the hypothalamus just above the optic chiasm; it has two main functions   (ATLAS2, p 36):
  - Alerting of the CNS and controlling of circadian rhythms
  - Synchronizing the circadian system
    - Light → melanopsin-containing ganglion cells → retinohypothalamic tract → SCN of hypothalamus
- Receptors in the SCN include   (ATLAS2, p 36):
  - Melatonin 1 (MT1) (whose stimulation decreases the alerting signal from the SCN)
  - Melatonin 2 (MT2) (whose stimulation synchronizes the circadian system)
- The genes and proteins that interact to regulate circadian timing include   (ATLAS2, p 34):
  - Genes
    - Three *PER* (period) genes: *PER1, PER2, PER3*
    - *ARHGEF5* (formerly *Tim*)
    - CLOCK
    - ARNTL (formerly Bmal1)
    - Csnk1e (formerly CK1e)
    - Two cryptochrome genes (CRY1 and CRY2), which are expressed in suprachiasmatic neurons
  - These genes and the proteins they produce interact to form negative and positive autoregulatory transcription-translation feedback loops that define the molecular machinery of the circadian oscillator.

Relationship Between Time and Core Body Temperature

- The declining portion of the core body temperature (CBT) starts near the beginning of the sleepy phase of the circadian rhythm.   (ATLAS2, p 135)
  - It is difficult to fall asleep unless body temperature is falling
- The increasing portion of the CBT starts near the beginning of the awake phase of the circadian rhythm
  - It is difficult to wake up unless body temperature is increasing

Dim-Light Melatonin Onset

- In normal subjects, dim-light melatonin onset (DLMO) is between 8 PM and 10 PM.   (ATLAS2, p 135)
  - DLMO is several hours earlier in patients with advanced sleep phase disorder
  - DLMO is several hours later in patients with delayed sleep phase disorder

Circadian Rhythm and Aging

- In neonates, sleep is polyphasic
- In adolescents, a delayed sleep phase can develop
- In older people, an advanced sleep phase with reduced amplitude can develop

Circadian, Endocrine, and Physiologic Interactions

- Reviewed in Chapter 3.9 of ATLAS2

Circadian Rhythm Sleep Disorders

- Reviewed in Section 2 of this volume

1.2   Other Physiology

A Medical Student Volunteers for an Experiment

A 23-year-old first-year med student volunteers for an experiment designed to evaluate metabolism during sleep. The researcher explains that the test will involve measurement of various metabolic functions while awake and asleep.

1. The medical student accepts (reluctantly) a rectal probe and an intravenous (IV) catheter. The IV line is connected to a machine that automatically draws aliquots of blood for testing every 15 minutes. Even with the IV and rectal probe, he manages to sleep several consecutive nights while data are collected. The first set of data analyzed is core body temperature. What statement best describes his thermoregulation during sleep?
   A. Absent in REM
   B. Inhibited in slow-wave sleep
   C. Inhibited in all stages of sleep
   D. Unchanged from his awake state

2. As the student falls asleep, there are changes in his core body temperature. Which statement best describes one of those changes?
   A. There is heat conservation, and body temperature increases
   B. There is heat loss via the skin
   C. Vasoconstriction occurs, leading to an increase in body temperature
   D. Vasodilation occurs, leading to an increase in body temperature

3. What will *most* likely be found when cortisol levels are measured?
   A. Lowest cortisol level around midnight
   B. Lowest level last third of the night
   C. Lowest level around noon
   D. Cortisol level does not vary significantly over 24-hour day

4. What will *most* likely be found when growth hormone (GH) levels are measured?
   A. Lowest level around midnight
   B. Highest level last third of the night
   C. Highest level in first third of the night
   D. GH does not vary significantly over 24-hour day

5. GH release is *most* strongly related to
   A. Slow-wave sleep
   B. REM sleep
   C. Output of the suprachiasmatic nucleus
   D. Duration of prior wakefulness

BONUS QUESTIONS

6. What will *most* likely be found when the researcher studies the effects of repetitive noise during sleep?
   A. Increase in nocturnal growth hormone (GH) levels
   B. Increase in nocturnal prolactin (PRL) levels
   C. Decrease in nocturnal levels of both GH and PRL
   D. Decrease in thyroid-stimulating hormone (TSH) levels

7. Which of the following hormones is *most* strongly modulated by both circadian and homeostatic sleep processes?
   A. Thyroid-stimulating hormone (TSH)
   B. Growth hormone (GH)
   C. Prolactin (PRL)
   D. Blood glucose concentration

8. On EKG, the student is found to have sinus arrest during sleep. During what sleep stage is this *most* likely to occur?
   A. N1
   B. N2
   C. N3
   D. REM

Overcaffeinated and Overweight

A 42-year-old male software engineer is referred to the Sleep Disorders Center for history of daytime sleepiness. His body mass index is 42, and his neck collar size 17.5 inches. His Epworth Sleepiness Scale score is 20 of 24 (normal <10 of 24). Because of daytime sleepiness, he drinks up to 8 cups of coffee each day. History includes symptoms suggesting a duodenal ulcer. He has an overnight sleep study that shows the following data:

Sleep onset latency	4 minutes
Total sleep time	490 minutes
Percent of total sleep time in	
N1	1%
N2	40%
N3	40%
REM	19%
Percent sleep time with snoring	40%
Indices (per hour of sleep)	
AHI	6 events/hr
PLMS	6/hr
Arousals	6/hr

9. Based on these data, what would you advise the referring physician?

A. The findings are typical for obstructive sleep apnea, and a continuous positive airway pressure (CPAP) titration is recommended

B. His sleepiness is explained by the periodic leg movements of sleep (PLMS); a history of restless legs syndrome should be explored

C. The findings are typical of sleep deprivation, and that issue should be explored

D. The sleep architecture findings are typical of upper airway resistance syndrome (UARS), and CPAP titration is recommended

10. Given the above findings, what change in hormone level would you *most* likely find?

A. Reduced thyroxin

B. Increased melatonin

C. Increased ghrelin

D. Increased leptin

11. What change in his glucose metabolism would you expect to find?

A. Reduced insulin secretion in response to glucose load

B. Increased insulin secretion in response to glucose load

C. Hypoglycemia

D. No changes in glucose metabolism are expected

12. Which of the following statements is *most* correct concerning the effect of sleep and circadian rhythm on gastric acid production or gastroesophageal reflux (GER)?

A. Neither sleep nor circadian rhythm has an effect on gastric acid production

B. Gastric acid production peaks just before awakening in the morning

C. Gastric acid production has circadian variability, with peaks occurring between 10 PM and 2 AM

D. GER is maximal during REM sleep

ANSWERS

1. A. Most automatically controlled homeostatic mechanisms are maintained during non-REM (NREM) sleep, but homeostasis seems absent for many systems during REM sleep, including the system controlling temperature. For example, shivering occurs during NREM sleep but does not occur in REM sleep.   (ATLAS2, pp 37–38) Interestingly, hot flashes in menopausal women do not occur during REM sleep. Body temperature is controlled primarily by cells in the preoptic anterior hypothalamic nuclei, which are located very near the VLPO and the suprachiasmatic nucleus, emphasizing the interrelationship between regulation of sleep, temperature, and circadian rhythms.

2. B. Body temperature decreases with sleep onset, so answers A, C, and D are incorrect. The onset of sleepiness in the evening is associated with vasodilatation resulting in heat loss. (PPSM6, p 220, Chapter Highlights) It has been shown that people with cold hands and feet are prone to have insomnia; thus, dysfunctional thermoregulation may play a role in interfering with the sleep onset.   (PPSM6, p 228, Clinical Pearl)

3. A. The lowest cortisol level is around midnight and the highest level in the last third of the night. Assessing cortisol production by measuring levels at midnight and in the morning has been done for decades in the clinical setting. This timing of cortisol production has also been determined in sleep deprivation. Changes in cortisol level are more closely related to time than to the awake or sleep state.   (ATLAS2)

4. C. GH production peaks in the first third of the night in the sleeping subject. During a night of sleep deprivation, there is no peak growth hormone level.   (ATLAS2, p 59, Figs. 3.90–3.92, and PPSM6, p 204)

5. A. GH is released during the first slow-wave sleep cycle, usually within minutes of SWS onset. The elevation in GH concentration is more robust in males than females. (Females exhibit more frequent daytime pulses.)   (PPSM6, p 204)

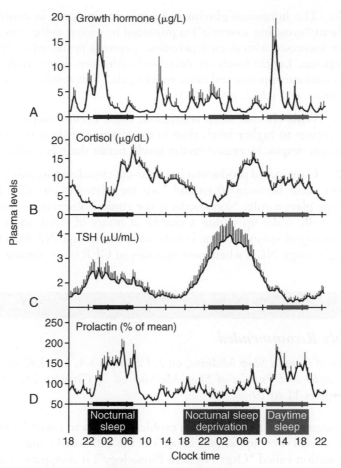

FIGURE 1.2–1 Question 4.

6. C. GH and PRL concentrations are strongly sleep dependent, with only weak circadian modulation. Fragmenting sleep with artificial awakenings, particularly when they interfere with slow-wave sleep, will inhibit nocturnal release of GH and PRL and therefore lower nocturnal levels.

7. A. TSH exhibits a clear circadian pattern, with peaks occurring nocturnally in the absence of sleep. Sleep deprivation is accompanied by supranormal peak levels, indicating an interaction in which sleep processes normally exert a damping effect on circadian-induced release.   (PPSM6, p 204)

8. D. When a question is based on something going wrong during sleep and you are asked what stage of sleep, it seems the answer is usually REM. During REM sleep, healthy people sometimes demonstrate abnormal breathing patterns, or apneas, and (as in this example) sinus arrest. Sinus arrest is likely caused by a surge of parasympathetic activity. (Guilleminault C, Pool P, Motta J, Gillis AM. Sinus arrest during REM sleep in young adults. *N Engl J Med* 311(16):1006-1010, 1984)

9. C. The clue to the correct diagnosis in this case is the marked increase in stage N3 sleep (40%, but normal N3 is about 20% of adult sleep time). Such a large amount of slow-wave sleep is usually found in recovery sleep after sleep deprivation but can also be caused by certain medications. In the presence of a significant sleep breathing abnormality or a movement disorder causing many arousals, one would expect a reduction in SWS and REM sleep.

10. C.   The hormones ghrelin and leptin are involved in control of appetite. Ghrelin (think about "growling stomach") is produced by gastric cells; it increases appetite. Ghrelin levels are increased with sleep deprivation. Leptin is produced by fat cells and normally suppresses appetite. Leptin levels are decreased with sleep deprivation. Thus, sleep deprivation tends to increase appetite and cause weight gain. This result has been shown in both children and adults   (ATLAS2, pp 56–58)

11. B.   With chronic sleep restriction, there occurs insulin resistance. After meals, glucose increases to higher levels than in the absence of sleep restriction. This increase in glucose occurs despite increased insulin levels, hence there is insulin resistance.   (PPSM6, Ch 20)

12. C.   Gastric acid production has clear-cut circadian variability. It is unclear whether the peaks that occur between 10 PM and 2 AM are related to circadian factors alone or whether sleep stage plays a role. Noteworthy is the clinical observation that patients with duodenal ulcer typically wake up within a couple of hours of sleep onset with ulcer symptoms. Lower esophageal sphincter tone is reduced more in stage N2 sleep than in REM, and not surprisingly, stage N2 is when most episodes of GER occur during sleep.

Summary

Highly Recommended

- *Atlas of Clinical Sleep Medicine*, ed 2, Chapters 3.4, 3.5, 3.8, and 3.9
- *Principles and Practice of Sleep Medicine* ed 6, Chapter 20; Abstracts and Clinical Pearls of Chapters 11 to 19

Nonrespiratory physiology is a problematic area to cover for the sleep boards because it is so broad yet will show up on only about 3 of the 240 board exam questions. The very first blueprint had a section called "Organ System Physiology"; it disappeared in the next blueprint. It is back in the current blueprint as "Other Physiology." (The exam committee seems to have difficulty in deciding what to do with this. We have added some bonus questions to help cover this large area of knowledge. Your review should focus on the physiology that has most direct clinical application (i.e., respiratory and endocrine). In this section, even though we present twice as many questions as on the examination, all topic areas could not be covered. Some of the high-value topic areas will be mentioned here. At the end of the day, keep in mind that the exam is geared toward clinical sleep medicine and that most of the questions, even those dealing with physiology, will likely have some clinical implications.

Physiologic Regulation

- Pituitary hormones (ATLAS2, Ch 3.10; PPSM5, Ch 26)
  - All hormones show diurnal variation
  - Primarily linked to circadian rhythm
    - Adrenocorticotropic hormone (ACTH)
  - Primarily linked to sleep
    - GH (to SWS) and PRL
  - Somewhat inhibited by sleep
    - TSH
- Endocrine function (ATLAS2, Ch 3.9)
  - Sleep deprivation increases appetite because of
    - Increase in ghrelin
    - Decrease in leptin
  - Sleep deprivation leads to obesity
    - Sleep deprivation causes insulin resistance
- Metabolic rate
  - Related to arousal state
    - Decreases with depth of NREM sleep
    - Increases in REM

- Thermoregulation
  - ○ Thermostat located in preoptic anterior hypothalamic area
  - ○ Mechanisms of control of body temperature
    - To conserve energy (to raise temperature)
      - ◆ Vasoconstriction
      - ◆ Piloerection
      - ◆ Shivering
    - To lose energy (to lower temperature)
      - ◆ Sweating
      - ◆ Panting
    - Related to sleep state
      - ◆ Homeostasis present in NREM sleep
      - ◆ Homeostasis inhibited in REM sleep
  - ○ Clinical implications
    - Night sweats common in hypermetabolic states (hyperthyroidism, infections)
    - Hot flashes in menopausal women do not occur during REM
- Cardiovascular (ATLAS2, Ch 3.7; PPSM6, Chs 13 and 14)
  - ○ Circulatory homeostasis
    - Related to sleep stage
      - ◆ NREM sleep: relative autonomic *stability* in heart rate, rhythm, and blood pressure
      - ◆ REM sleep: relative autonomic *instability* in heart rate, rhythm, and blood pressure
    - Phasic REM–related changes
      - ◆ Surges in sympathetic tone and heart rate
      - ◆ Decreases in coronary flow in patients with coronary artery disease
    - Tonic REM–related changes
      - ◆ Parasympathetic tone increases may result in rate decrease or sinus arrest
      - ◆ In patients with long QT3 syndrome, may lead to torsades de pointes
  - ○ Cerebral blood flow
    - Decreases in NREM
    - Increases in REM (to match increased metabolic rate of brain in this stage)
- Gastrointestinal   (ATLAS2, Ch 15.3)
  - ○ Gastric acid secretion has circadian variability with peak between 10 PM and 2 AM
  - ○ Related to sleep stage
    - Lower esophageal sphincter (LES) tone lower in NREM than REM sleep
    - GER more frequent in NREM sleep
- Respiratory physiology: see p 220 of this volume
- Cytokines: see p 7 of this volume

1.3   Normal Sleep

QUESTIONS

A Pregnant Internist

An internist is pregnant with her first child. Before pregnancy, her body mass index (BMI) was 24. At 36 weeks' gestation, her weight gain is normal, but she has begun to snore and manifest restless leg syndrome symptoms.

1. Which of the following conditions is she *most* likely to have during sleep?
   A. Hypoxemia
   B. Hypoventilation
   C. Hypocapnia
   D. Apnea

2. Snoring in pregnancy increases the pregnancy-related risk of
   A. Increased fetal size
   B. Hypertension
   C. Elevated infant Apgar scores
   D. Gestational diabetes

3. Fetal sleep near term (at 38–40 weeks of gestation) is typically
   A. Mostly REM sleep
   B. Time linked to maternal sleep
   C. Associated with absence of effort to breathe
   D. Absent

4. The term *polyphasic sleep* identifies sleep that
   A. Occurs multiple times day or night
   B. Occurs only during the daytime
   C. Occurs with early-onset REM
   D. Occurs any time it is dark

5. Which feature of sleep architecture in infants is *incorrect*?
   A. Appearance of sleep spindles by 9 weeks of age
   B. Disappearance of the trace-alternant pattern by 6 weeks of age
   C. K complexes that appear by 12 weeks of age
   D. Poor differentiation of NREM stages until 12 months of age

6. The typical 1-year-old child is *most* likely to
   A. Sleep up to 10 hours out of every 24-hour period
   B. Take two naps during the day
   C. Enter REM sleep (stage R) at sleep onset
   D. Have central apneas one to five times per hour of sleep

7. Up until what age is napping common in children?
   A. 1 to 2 years
   B. 2 to 4 years
   C. 4 to 5 years
   D. 7 to 9 years

8. In school-age children, slow-wave sleep (stage N3) is likely to occur
   A. During the first third of the night
   B. During the middle third of the night
   C. During the last third of the night
   D. 90 minutes after sleep onset

Older and Wiser but With Trouble Sleeping

A 77-year-old man complains of restless sleep and awakening early in the morning with an inability to fall asleep again.

9. As people age, which of the following increases?
   A. REM sleep as a percentage of TST
   B. Slow-wave sleep as a percentage of TST
   C. Sleep efficiency
   D. Resistance to sleep deprivation

10. REM sleep in older adults
   A. Occurs at sleep onset
   B. Is minimal or absent
   C. Diminishes less than slow-wave sleep in older adults
   D. Is less fragmented with aging

ANSWERS

1. C. Snoring occurs in about 30% of pregnant women and is due in part to edema in the nasal passage and to pharyngeal hypotonia. However, obstructive sleep apnea is relatively uncommon, as are hypoventilation (hypercapnia) and hypoxemia. In contrast, practically all pregnant women hyperventilate by the third trimester because of high progesterone levels. (ATLAS2, p 356)

2. B. Snoring in pregnancy increases the risk for pregnancy-induced hypertension (pre-eclampsia). Babies born to snoring mothers are small and have lower Apgar scores than babies born to nonsnoring mothers. (ATLAS2, p 356; Table 16.2–1 reviews sleep throughout pregnancy and is a must.)

3. A. Indeed, fetuses do sleep, and most of the sleep appears to be REM sleep. A fetus at 30 weeks' gestation spends 80% of her or his sleep time in "active" or REM sleep. (ATLAS2, p 89)

4. A. *Polyphasic sleep* refers to several sleep bouts that occur both during the day and at night. This pattern is found in newborns and in some animals. In newborns, circadian entrainment eventually occurs, and then most sleep occurs at night. This pattern is also seen in older adults in institutions who might lack circadian entrainment and can therefore develop an irregular sleep-wake disorder. (ATLAS2, p 94)

5. D. In the newborn period, roughly half the time is spent in REM sleep; the remainder is spent in NREM sleep. At this age, the NREM stages are not well characterized electrophysiologically, and the term *nondeterminant sleep* is often used to describe the pattern. One transient pattern that is seen is a trace-alternant pattern. (ATLAS2, p 89; PEDS2, Ch 1)

6. B. It is important to know the relationship between sleep and age. A 1-year-old child no longer enters sleep via REM, sleeps 10 to 16 hours out of 24, and has about two naps a day. An apnea index greater than 1 (one hypopnea or apnea per hour) is considered abnormal in this age group. (ATLAS2, p 89, Table 4–2; PEDS2, Ch 1)

7. C. By the time a child is about 6 years old, napping should no longer occur. Imagine if there were naps in first grade! The persistence or return of napping in a child older than 6 years usually indicates sleep deprivation or that the child has developed a sleep disorder. (ATLAS2, p 89)

8. A. Slow-wave sleep usually occurs in the first third of the night in all age groups. The percentage of sleep spent in slow-wave sleep is highest in children and decreases with age. (ATLAS2, p 86)

9. D. Resistance to sleep deprivation surprisingly increases with age. Slow-wave sleep as a percentage of total sleep time decreases more in men than women. (ATLAS2, p 86)

10. C. REM sleep diminishes much less than slow-wave sleep in older people, but the REM episodes may be more fragmented. (ATLAS2, p 90)

Summary

Highly Recommended

■ *Atlas of Clinical Sleep Medicine*, ed 2, Chapter 4.2

The topic of sleep and aging is important, because it overlaps other areas that include pediatrics and polysomnography (PSG) findings. Below are sleep characteristics of each age you should know.

Sleep by Age Range (ATLAS2, pp 85-97, and Table 4.2–1)

- Newborns
  - ○ Sleep 16 to 18 hours of each 24 hours; 5 to 10 hours of this is napping
  - ○ Sleep is polyphasic
  - ○ 50% of sleep occurs in REM
- At 2 to 3 months
  - ○ Sleep spindles start to appear
- At 3 to 4 months
  - ○ Major sleep period is at night
- At 4 to 4.5 months
  - ○ Stages N1, N2, and N3 can be ascertained
- At 5 months
  - ○ K complexes start to appear
- At 1 year
  - ○ Sleeps 13 to 15 hours of every 24 hours; 2 to 3 hours of this is napping
  - ○ 30% of sleep is in REM
- At 2 years
  - ○ Sleeps 12 to 14 hours of every 24 hours; 1.5 to 2.5 hours of this is napping
  - ○ 25% of sleep is in REM (percentage remains constant with further aging)
- At 3 to 5 years
  - ○ Sleeps 11 to 13 hours of every 24 hours; 0 to 2.5 hours of this is napping
- At 5 to 12 years
  - ○ Sleeps 9 to 12 hours of every 24 hours; no napping
- At 13 to 20 years
  - ○ Sleeps 8 to 9 hours of each 24 hours; no napping
  - ○ Delay in sleep phase can occur
- At 20 to 65 years
  - ○ Large decline in amplitude of slow-wave sleep (SWS)
  - ○ Slow but progressive decline in SWS as percentage of total sleep time
  - ○ Deterioration of sleep with menopause (about age 50 years)
- Older than 65 years
  - ○ Napping returns
  - ○ Advance in sleep phase is common
  - ○ Difficulty initiating and maintaining sleep occurs
  - ○ Sleep is fragmented with increased awakenings
  - ○ Melatonin production is decreased
  - ○ Sleep deteriorates with deterioration of overall health

Sleep in Women

- Pregnancy
  - ○ Table 1.3–1
- Postpartum
  - ○ See last row of Table 1.3–1
- Menopause
  - ○ Prevalence of obstructive sleep apnea (OSA) increases compared with men of similar age
  - ○ Hot flashes interfere with sleep; they are not present in REM sleep
  - ○ Sleep abnormalities due to depression increase

REFERENCES

Grigg-Damberger M, Gozal D, Marcus CL, et al. The visual scoring of sleep and arousal in infants and children. *J Clin Sleep Med*. 2007;3(2):201–240.

Kryger MH, Avidan A, Berry R. *Atlas of clinical sleep medicine*. 2nd ed. Chapter 4. Philadelphia: Saunders; 2014.

Sheldon SH, Ferber R, Gozal D, Kryger MH, eds. *Principles and practice of pediatric sleep medicine*. 2nd ed. Philadelphia: Elsevier; 2005.

Shepertycky MR, Banno K, Kryger MH. Differences between men and women in the clinical presentation of patients diagnosed with obstructive sleep apnea syndrome. *Sleep*. 2005;28(3):309–314.

Table 1.3–1 Features of Sleep Disturbances in Pregnancy and Postpartum

Trimester	Complaints	PSG Findings	Hormonal Correlates	Sleep Disorders[a]
First (mo 1–3)	Excessive daytime sleepiness, insomnia, urinary frequency	↑ Naps ↑ TST ↑ Wake time ↓ SWS	↑ Progesterone: hyperventilation, sedation, smooth muscle relaxation ↑ Prolactin ↑ REM ↑ Estrogen Melatonin not affected[b]	Snoring, OSA Less bruxism than baseline More sleep starts
Second (mo 4–6)	↑ Awakenings	↓ SWS ↓ REM	↑ Progesterone ↑ Estrogen	Snoring, OSA More sleep paralysis Less somnambulism Less somniloquy
Third (mo 7–9)	Three to five awakenings per night, ↓ daytime alertness, leg cramps, dyspnea, backache, heartburn, abdominal discomfort, fetal movement, frequent nocturia	↓ TST ↓ SWS ↓ REM ↑ WASO ↑ Stage 1 sleep	↑ Estrogen ↓ Progesterone at parturition Oxytocin at parturition Lower cortisol	Snoring, OSA Preeclampsia Restless legs Leg cramps Recurrence of somnambulism More sleep paralysis
Preeclampsia	Poor sleep, nausea, edema, headaches, dizziness, changes in vision, sleepiness	↑ Sleep fragmentation ↑ Time out of bed ↑ Body movements	↑ Cytokines ↑ CRP ↑ TNF	Snoring, OSA
Postpartum[c]	Poor sleep	↓ TST[d] ↓ REM ↓ REM latency ↓ Stage 2 sleep ↑ SWS ↑ Awake time ↓ Sleep efficiency	↓ Estrogen ↓ Progesterone	Blues: 50%–80% Depression:10%–20% Psychosis (rare): 0.1%

[a]Narcoleptic symptoms can continue during pregnancy.
[b]Beta human chorionic growth hormone, renin, nitric oxide, interleukin-1, tumor necrosis factor (TNF), and interferon may also facilitate sleepiness.
[c]Multiparous mothers have fewer symptoms compared with primiparous mothers.
[d]Mothers caring for premature infants with more wake after sleep onset (WASO) and even less total sleep time (TST).
CRP, C-reactive protein; *OSA*, obstructive sleep apnea; *PSG*, polysomnography; *REM*, rapid eye movement; *SWS*, slow-wave sleep.
From Kryger MH, Avidan A, Berry R: *Atlas of clinical sleep medicine*, ed 2, Philadelphia, 2014, Saunders; Table 16.2–1.

1.4 Sleep Deprivation

QUESTIONS

An Acutely Sleep-Deprived Surgeon

A 64-year-old surgeon, Dr. K, flies to Indonesia immediately after he learns of an earthquake there. After arriving, not having recovered from jet lag, he operates continuously on one patient after another for about 48 hours, amputating gangrenous extremities. He has been gulping down food and water between cases.

1. After being awake for 48 hours, Dr. K is likely to have all of the following *except*
   A. Irritability
   B. Difficulty in concentrating
   C. Visual hallucinations
   D. Auditory hallucinations

2. Although his manual dexterity seemed unimpaired, Dr. K started to make errors such as illogical triaging of cases and performing operative procedures in the wrong sequence. Abnormal activity in what part of his brain is likely causing these mistakes?
   A. Broca's area
   B. Prefrontal cortex
   C. Parietal lobe
   D. Temporal lobe

3. Examination of Dr. K's blood would show
   A. Normal growth hormone level
   B. Hypoglycemia
   C. Reduced cortisol levels
   D. Increased thyroid activity

4. Others on the surgical team insisted Dr. K have a full night's sleep before continuing to operate because he was endangering patients. Dr. K, on the other hand, thought he just needed a nap. Of the following statements, which is *most* correct?
   A. Dr. K needs 1 night of recovery sleep before he is alert again
   B. Dr. K needs 3 nights of recovery sleep before he is alert again
   C. If Dr. K were 24 years old, 1 night of recovery sleep would suffice
   D. If Dr. K took a 4-hour nap, it would restore alertness

5. If this surgeon's recovery night sleep was monitored by polysomnography, what sleep stage impact would be observed?
   A. Increase in percentage of time spent in REM sleep
   B. Increase in percentage of time spent in slow-wave sleep
   C. Increase in percentage of time spent in slow-wave sleep and REM sleep
   D. Increased REM sleep and reduced slow-wave sleep

6. During recovery sleep, Dr. K would have which of the following medical findings?
   A. A decrease in plasma glucose
   B. A reduction in adrenocorticotropic hormone (ACTH)
   C. Increased production of growth hormone (GH)
   D. Increased thyroid (thyroxine T_4) activity

The Chronically Sleep-Deprived Surgeon

After 48 hours of being awake, Dr. K sleeps 12 hours, takes a day off from operating, and then sleeps 8 hours the next night. On awakening, he feels great and starts to operate again. He promises the surgical team he will get some sleep every night and settles on a routine of sleeping 4 hours, then staying awake for 20 hours, operating on the continual stream of cases.

7. After 4 nights of sleeping 4 hours per night, what would you expect to find in his *awake* EEG?
   A. Increase of power in the delta range
   B. Increase of power in the alpha range
   C. Decrease of power in the theta range
   D. No change in his awake EEG

8. What changes in sleep architecture would you find during his fourth night of 4-hour sleep?
   A. Increased REM sleep percent
   B. Increased SWS percent
   C. Similar increases in REM and SWS percent
   D. No change in the percentage of the sleep stages

9. Dr. K insisted that with this sleep schedule, he did not feel sleepy during the daytime and he could safely operate. What mean sleep latency would you likely find if Dr. K had a multiple sleep latency test (MSLT) after the fourth night of sleeping only 4 hours a night?
   A. 20 minutes
   B. 15 minutes
   C. 10 minutes
   D. 5 minutes

10. On the fourth day of Dr. K's sleeping 4 hours each night, what would you expect if you measured his performance using the psychomotor vigilance task (PVT)?
    A. PVT lapses would be similar in degree to the findings after 3 days of no sleep
    B. PVT lapses would be greater than after 3 days of no sleep
    C. PVT lapses would be in the range seen in normal subjects sleeping 8 hours a night
    D. PVT lapses would be about the same as if he had slept for 6 hours each night but much greater than if he had slept 8 hours each night

ANSWERS

1. **D.**   Auditory hallucinations are an uncommon manifestation of chronic sleep deprivation. Personality changes and symptoms of psychopathology become apparent with prolonged sleep loss. Hallucinations occur in up to 80% of subjects; they are generally visual and different from the more common auditory hallucinations found in schizophrenia.

2. **B.**   Acute sleep deprivation leads to abnormal executive function, which results from loss of function of regions in the prefrontal cortex. This area of the brain plays a role in temporal memory (planning, organization, prioritization). There is also impairment of newly acquired skills and decrement in the ability to perform complex tasks.

3. **D.**   Thyroid activity is increased, suggesting a hypermetabolic state. (Continuous sleep deprivation in rodents ultimately led to their death. However, the rodents behaved as though they were hypermetabolic, increasing their food intake but losing weight.) Secretion of GH appears linked to SWS; thus absence of sleep would result in decreased GH levels. Cortisol may be increased after a night of total sleep deprivation.

4. **A.**   Because Dr. K is in his 60s, a full night of recovery sleep is sufficient to restore his alertness to baseline. One night is not sufficient in young adults, who usually need 2 or more nights to recover after chronic sleep deprivation.

5. **B.**   By far, the most impressive change during recovery sleep in older people is a substantial increase in the percentage of SWS. There occurs a reduction in both REM latency and percentage of REM sleep.

6. **C.**   With recovery from acute sleep loss, there is an increase in both ACTH and GH, the latter from the rise in SWS during recovery (GH increases in SWS). The increase in thyroid function that occurred during the prolonged wakefulness would not be expected to continue with recovery.

7. **A.**   With chronic sleep restriction, an overall slowing of the awake EEG occurs that reflects increased homeostatic drive. Thus, delta power (3.75–4.5 Hz) is increased. There is also an increase in theta power, thought to reflect "spectral leakage" from the changes in delta power. These might reflect a tendency toward microsleeps. Alpha power decreases.

8. **B.**   The body tries to maintain SWS. Thus, with chronic sleep deprivation, conservation of the amount of SWS occurs at the expense of the other NREM stages and REM sleep.

9. **D.**   There is progressive decrease in mean sleep latency after successive nights of restricted sleep, and after 4 nights, the mean latency would be expected to be abnormally low. Interestingly, subjective assessments of sleepiness might not parallel objective impairment as measured by the MSLT or performance tests. Generally, sleep-deprived patients tend to overestimate their level of alertness.

10. D.   After the first 4 nights of sleeping 4 hours per night, PVT results indicate more lapses than in the 8-hour sleep condition but the same as in subjects sleeping 6 hours per night. By the seventh night of 4-hour sleep, the lapses are greater than with 6-hour sleep. By 2 weeks of 4-hour sleep, the results would be similar to 3 consecutive nights of no sleep. Thus, with chronic sleep loss comes a progressive worsening of function.

Summary

Highly Recommended

Atlas of Clinical Sleep Medicine, ed 2, Chapter 5.
   Sleep deprivation is important in clinical practice, and some of this content overlaps with other sections. Expect about 10 questions covering this topic on the exam.

Acute Total Sleep Deprivation

- Effects
  - ○ Memory impairment (short-term memory is affected more)
  - ○ Impairment of executive function (prefrontal lobe: planning, prioritization, organization)
  - ○ Daytime sleepiness
  - ○ Changes in waking EEG
    - • Decreased alpha activity
    - • Increased delta and theta activity
  - ○ Increased thyroid activity but few other metabolic changes noted
  - ○ Increases in IL-1 and IL-6
- Recovery sleep
  - ○ Performance generally normalizes within 1 to 3 nights of normal sleep
  - ○ MSLT shows recovery occurs more quickly in older than in younger people
  - ○ An increase in SWS shows, but REM sleep may be unchanged or reduced

Chronic Sleep Deprivation

- Effects
  - ○ Abnormal awake EEG
    - • Increased delta and theta power
    - • Decreased alpha power
  - ○ Changes in sleep architecture: conservation of SWS
  - ○ Progressive sleepiness as measured by the MSLT
  - ○ Progressive decrements in performance as measured by PVTs
  - ○ Impaired driving performance
  - ○ Subjective assessment of sleepiness can underestimate sleepiness and impairment
  - ○ Metabolic changes
    - • Elevation of evening cortisol and sympathetic activity and impaired glucose tolerance
    - • Obesity
    - • Increased cardiovascular events, morbidity, and likely mortality; effects are likely mediated by increased C-reactive protein (a marker of increased cardiovascular risk)

QUESTIONS

You, the Technologist

In preparation for the sleep board exam, you decide to spend part of the night in the sleep lab. Your goal is to assist the technologist in setting up a sleep study on one of your patients.

1. For the EEG lead placements, you will use the 10-20 system. This means you place the electrodes
   A. So that there are 20 derivations (two from each electrode)
   B. Either 10% or 20% of the distance between a given pair of skull landmarks
   C. Either 10 or 20 mm from specific skull landmarks
   D. Somewhere between 10 and 20 nm into the scalp

2. After explaining the test to your patient, your first task is to place electrodes for the recommended EEG derivations. These are
   A. F4-M1, C4-M1, O2-M1
   B. F4-M2, C4-M2, O2-M2
   C. F3-M1, C3-M1, O1-M1
   D. Fz-Cz, Cz-Oz

3. Next, to detect eye movements, you place electrodes 1 cm below the left eye outer canthus (E1) and 1 cm above the right eye outer canthus (E2). This placement will give the recommended electrooculogram (EOG) derivations, which are
   A. E1-M2 and E2-M2
   B. E1-M2 and E2-M1
   C. E1-M2 and E2-E1
   D. E1-E2 and E2-E1

4. Recording of eye movements during polysomnography is possible because
   A. The cornea is electrically positive with respect to the retina
   B. The retina is electrically positive with respect to the cornea
   C. Gross eye movements generate electrical signals that differ slightly owing to the distance of each eye to the recording electrode
   D. Eye movements generate static electricity by rubbing on nearby tissue

5. You next attach leads for the electromyogram (EMG) that will be used for sleep staging purposes; they are attached to the
   A. Lower legs
   B. Thighs
   C. Chin
   D. Forehead

6. After the patient falls asleep, you help monitor the channels. You enjoy figuring out the EEG patterns, knowing that they can be distinguished by all of the following *except*
   A. Frequency: the number of cycles per second (Hz)
   B. Amplitude: measured by voltage
   C. Shape of the waveform
   D. Sinusoidal or waxing and waning pattern over 5 or more seconds
   E. Distribution: the location where the waveform is normally most prominent

7. The three distinct states of consciousness for a normal subject are
   A. Wakefulness, REM sleep, and deep sleep (N3)
   B. Wakefulness, REM sleep, and NREM sleep
   C. REM sleep, light sleep (N1 and N2), and deep sleep (N3)
   D. Wakefulness, transition to sleep, and sleep

8. The three distinct states of consciousness are identified by
   A. Clinical observation plus EEG
   B. EEG, EOG, and EMG
   C. EEG alone
   D. EEG plus video of the subject sleeping

9. Which EEG waveform is NOT commonly used to differentiate and classify sleep stages?
   A. Alpha
   B. Beta
   C. Delta
   D. Theta

10. The term *relatively low-voltage, mixed frequency pattern* for the EEG *most* closely describes which sleep stage?
   A. N1
   B. N2
   C. N3
   D. R

11. Delta activity includes brainwaves with a frequency less than 4 Hz. Within this group, *slow waves* are defined as
   A. Synonymous with delta activity
   B. Peak-to-peak amplitude greater than 75 μV and frequency 0.5 to 2.0 Hz
   C. Frequency 0.5 to 2.0 Hz, any amplitude
   D. Peak-to-peak amplitude greater than 75 μV, frequency less than 4 Hz

12. The sleep-staging nomenclature in the American Academy of Sleep Medicine (AASM) manual, version 2.5 (referenced in this text as MANUAL2), includes all of the following stages *except*
   A. N1
   B. N2
   C. N3
   D. N4
   E. REM

13. All of the following are true about scoring an EEG arousal *except*
   A. It requires either an associated body movement or a respiratory event
   B. It requires an abrupt shift of EEG frequency that lasts at least 3 seconds
   C. It must be preceded by at least 10 seconds of stable sleep
   D. In REM, it requires a concurrent increase in submental EMG lasting at least 1 second

14. The requirement of increase in submental EMG to score arousal in REM sleep is necessary because:
   A. Alpha activity (8–13 Hz) is not seen in REM
   B. The background EEG in REM is predominantly alpha activity
   C. Alpha bursts routinely appear during REM sleep and do not necessarily represent pathology
   D. The chin EMG has a higher digital sampling rate than the EEG

15. The epoch in Figure 1.5–1 shows transition from
   A. Wakefulness to stage N1
   B. N1 to N2
   C. N1 to REM
   D. N2 to REM

16. Which of the following is *true* about the artifact shown in the PSG fragment (Fig. 1.5–2)?
   A. Can result from high electrode impedance, a poor electrical connection, or excessive current leakage from nearby electrical equipment (e.g., computers, televisions)
   B. Has the same frequency as electrocardiogram (ECG) artifact
   C. Is usually indistinguishable from perspiration artifact
   D. Is best avoided by use of a 60-Hz filter

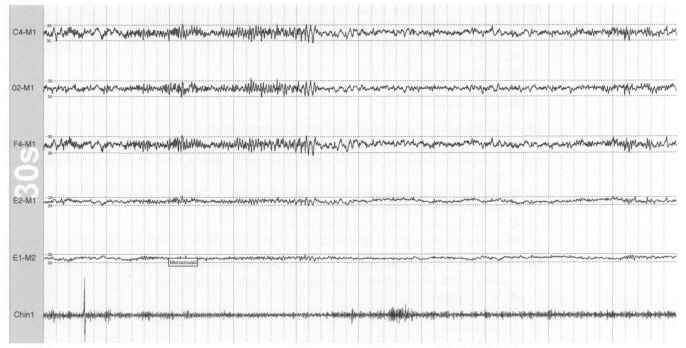

FIGURE 1.5–1 Question 15.

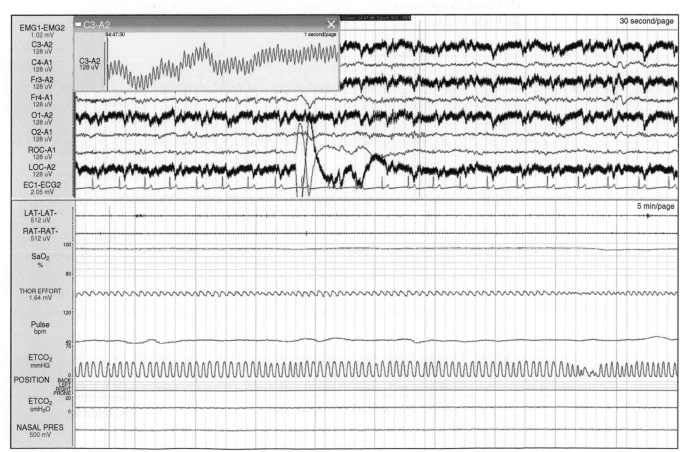

FIGURE 1.5–2 Question 16. (From ATLAS2, Fig. 19–111)

17. In PSG, most of the recorded signals are amplified by alternating current (AC) amplifiers. A few signals are amplified by direct current (DC) amplifiers. Which of the following is recorded by a DC amplifier in the PSG?

 A. EEG

 B. EOG

 C. ECG

 D. Pulse oximetry

18. All of the following are true about the K complex *except*

 A. It is defined as a well-delineated negative sharp wave immediately followed by a positive component standing out from the background, with a total duration of 0.5 second or longer

 B. For an arousal to be associated with a K complex, it must commence no more than 1 second after termination of the K complex

 C. It can be used to score an epoch as stage N2

 D. In the absence of a sleep spindle, a K complex must be present to score an epoch as N2

19. Figure 1.5–3 is a 30-second epoch. The large waves seen in channel F4-M1 in the first 3 seconds of this epoch (from beginning to first solid vertical line) are

 A. K complexes

 B. Vertex sharp waves

 C. Slow waves

 D. Delta waves

20. Figure 1.5–4 shows a 30-second epoch. The large waves seen in all three EEG channels (F4-M1, C4-M1, and O2-M1) in the first 3 seconds of this epoch (from beginning to first solid vertical line) are

 A. K complexes

 B. Slow waves

 C. Vertex sharp waves

 D. REM artifact

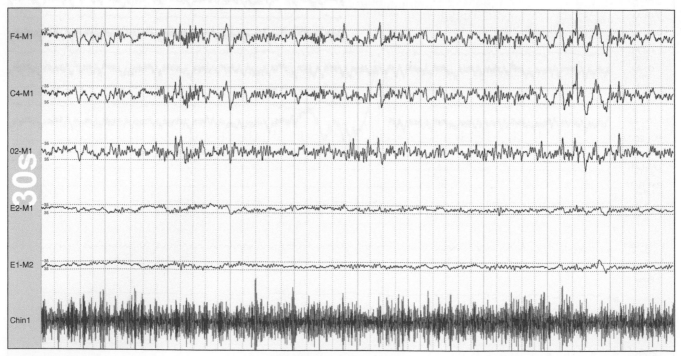

FIGURE 1.5–3 Question 19.

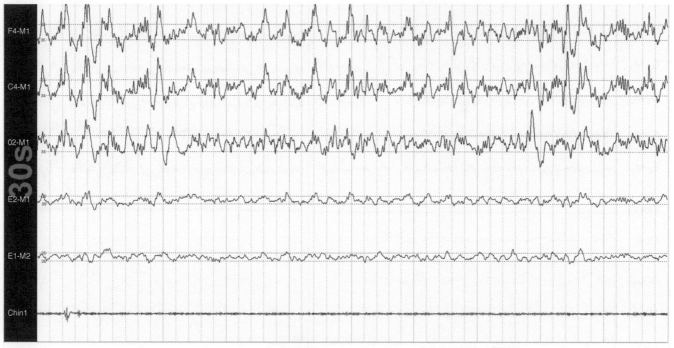

FIGURE 1.5–4 Question 20.

21. To score respiratory events in adults, all of the following are true *except*
   A. Oronasal thermal sensor is recommended to detect absence of airflow and score an apnea
   B. Nasal air pressure transducer is recommended to detect airflow reduction and score a hypopnea
   C. Inductance plethysmography is recommended to detect respiratory effort
   D. To score an apnea, a drop in the peak thermal sensor excursion by at least 70% of baseline must be evident

22. According to the AASM manual, which of the following is NOT a criterion for scoring an apnea?
   A. There is a drop in the peak signal excursion by 90% or greater of pre-event baseline using an oronasal thermal sensor
   B. There is a drop in the peak signal excursion by 90% or greater of pre-event baseline using a positive air pressure (PAP) device flow during a titration study
   C. The duration of the 90% or greater drop in sensor signal is 10 seconds or longer
   D. There is a drop of at least 3% in SaO_2 attributable to the apnea event

23. Figure 1.5–5, *A*, demonstrates
   A. Obstructive apnea
   B. Hypopnea
   C. Respiratory effort–related arousal (RERA)
   D. Normal breathing

24. Figure 1.5–5, *B*, demonstrates
   A. Obstructive apnea
   B. Hypopnea
   C. RERA
   D. Normal breathing

25. All of the following may be seen in the waking stage *except*
   A. Alpha rhythm
   B. Eye blinks
   C. Reading eye movements
   D. REM
   E. K complexes

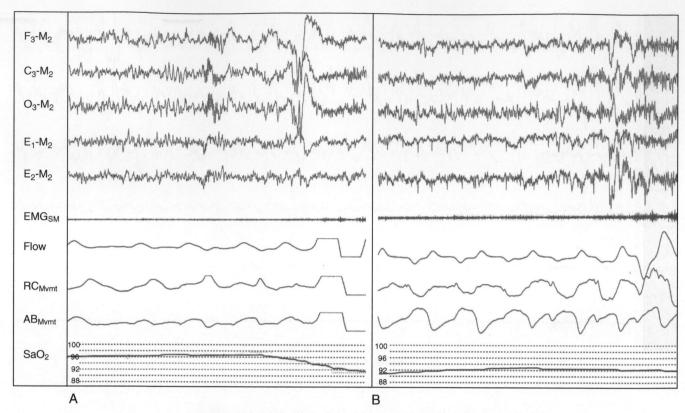

FIGURE 1.5–5 Questions 23 and 24. (From ATLAS2, Fig. 18–14)

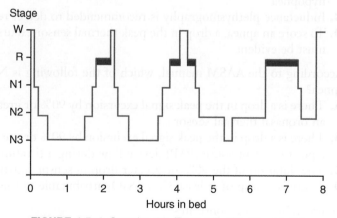

FIGURE 1.5–6 Question 26. (From ATLAS2, Fig. 4.2–25)

26. A normal sleep hypnogram for a child is shown in Figure 1.5–6. A principal difference compared with adults is that adults have
 A. More REM sleep
 B. Less REM sleep
 C. More slow-wave sleep
 D. Less slow-wave sleep

27. Considering normal sleep, which statement is *most* accurate?
 A. REM occurs in several discrete periods, lengthening as the sleep progresses
 B. Deep sleep tends to concentrate in the latter part of the sleep cycle
 C. Wake after sleep onset (WASO) occupies about 15% of the sleep cycle
 D. REM latency is about 30 to 60 minutes

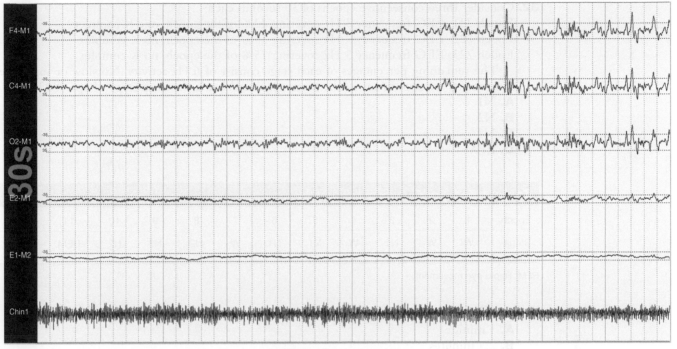

FIGURE 1.5–7 Question 29.

28. Alpha rhythm is BEST seen in the EEG during
  A. Stage N1
  B. Stage N3
  C. Wakefulness with eyes open
  D. Wakefulness with eyes closed

29. The 30-second epoch in Figure 1.5–7 shows what stage of sleep?
  A. N1
  B. N2
  C. N3
  D. REM

30. The transition from wakefulness to stage N1 sleep may be associated with all of the following *except*
  A. Slow-rolling eye movements
  B. Low-amplitude, mixed-frequency EEG in the range of 4 to 7 Hz
  C. Appearance of vertex sharp waves
  D. Alpha activity in the frontal lobe EEG

31. During a 30-second epoch, the first 23 seconds have a baseline EEG frequency of 7 Hz. The EEG frequency then shifts to 11 Hz on the 28th second. Slow eye movements are seen throughout the epoch. This epoch should be scored as
  A. Awake
  B. N1
  C. N2
  D. N3
  E. REM

32. Consider three consecutive epochs of 30 seconds each:
Epoch 221: EEG frequency 3 Hz covering 22% of the epoch, one K complex
Epoch 222: EEG frequency 3 Hz covering 55% of the epoch, no K complex
Epoch 223: EEG frequency 3 Hz covering 75% of the epoch, no K complex
   The remaining percentages of each stage consist of 6 Hz activity. No slow or rapid eye movements are seen in any of the three epochs. What is the sleep stage of epoch 223?
   A. N1
   B. N2
   C. N3
   D. REM

Table 1.5–1 For Questions 33 and 34

Epoch	1	2	3	4	5	6	7	8	9	10	11	12
Stage	W	W	N1	W	N1	N1	W	N2	N2	N2	REM	REM

REM, Rapid eye movement.

33. In Table 1.5–1, each epoch is 30 seconds. When is sleep onset?
   A. 1 minute
   B. 2.5 minutes
   C. 4 minutes
   D. 6 minutes

34. In Table 1.5–1, what is the REM onset?
   A. 3.5 minutes
   B. 4.0 minutes
   C. 5.0 minutes
   D. 5.5 minutes

BONUS QUESTIONS

35. Regarding alpha-delta sleep shown in Figure 1.5–8, choose the *most* correct combination of statements lettered A through D.
   1. Consists of 15% to 20% delta activity superimposed on prominent alpha activity
   2. Alpha portion usually 1 to 2 Hz slower than waking alpha
   3. Often believed to be a marker for nonrestorative sleep
   4. Often seen in patients with musculoskeletal pain
   A. 1, 3, and 4 only
   B. 3 and 4 only
   C. 2, 3, and 4 only
   D. 1, 2, 3, and 4

36. The transition from a low-voltage awake stage to N1 is characterized by
   A. Slow eye movements of greater than 500 ms
   B. Sleep spindles
   C. Delta waves
   D. Rapid eye movements of less than 500 ms

37. Which of the following is NOT specifically recommended by the AASM for detecting hypoventilation during a PSG?
   A. PcO_2 measured in arterial blood gas
   B. PcO_2 measured via an end-tidal CO_2 sensor
   C. PcO_2 measured via transcutaneous CO_2 sensor
   D. Combination of apnea for longer than 30 seconds with a concomitant drop of SaO_2 greater than 3%

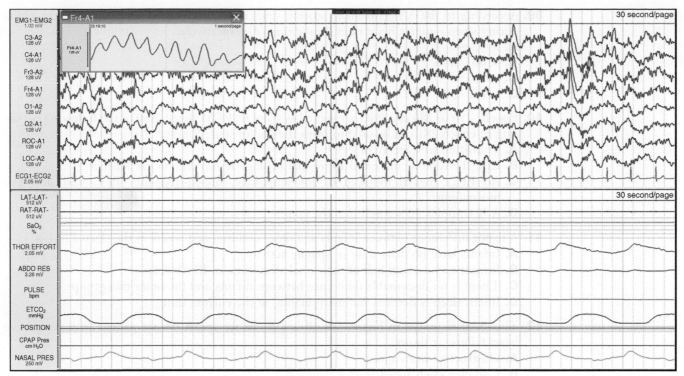

FIGURE 1.5–8 Question 35.

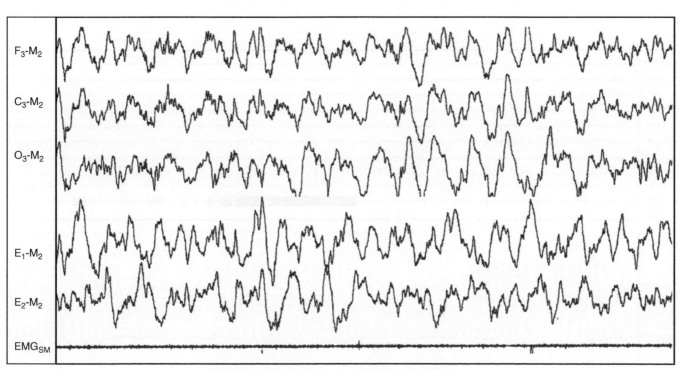

FIGURE 1.5–9 Question 38. (From ATLAS2, Fig. 18–7)

38. What is the sleep stage in Figure 1.5–9?
    A. W
    B. N1
    C. N2
    D. N3
    E. REM

39. According to the AASM manual, scoring sinus tachycardia and sinus bradycardia in adults during sleep requires heart rates (beats/min) of, respectively,
   A. >90, <40
   B. >100, <40
   C. >90, <50
   D. >100, <50

40. Epochs 250 to 280 of a PSG are scored as stage R (REM sleep). Any of the following occurring in epoch 281 can be used to mark the end of stage R *except*
   A. Transition to stage W or N3
   B. Chin EMG tone increased above that of stage R and criteria for N1 met
   C. An EEG arousal followed by low-amplitude, mixed-frequency EEG and slow eye movements
   D. A K complex 20 seconds into the epoch

41. A major difference between infants and older children and adults in the sleep EEG is
   A. Infants have no delta wave or spindle activity
   B. Infants spend about half of their total sleep time in REM sleep
   C. There is no discernable difference between infants and the other two groups
   D. Infant sleep is deemed "uninterpretable" at the current time

42. The sleep fragment in Figure 1.5–10 is a 5-minute epoch from a patient with congestive heart failure; it shows
   A. Obstructive sleep apnea
   B. Complex sleep apnea
   C. Cheyne-Stokes breathing
   D. None of the above

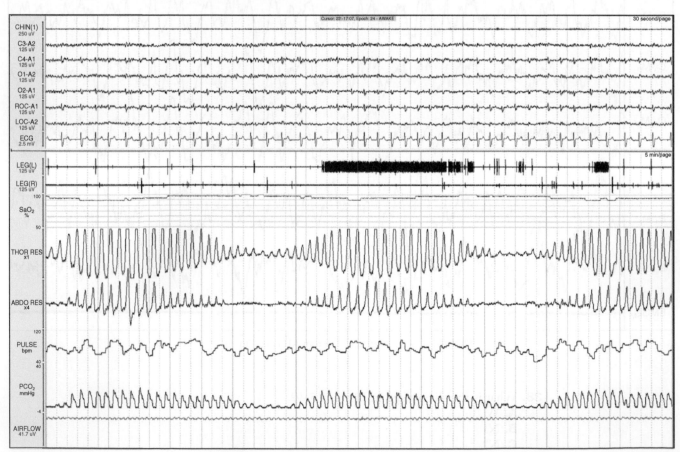

FIGURE 1.5–10 Question 42. (From ATLAS2, Fig. 19–44)

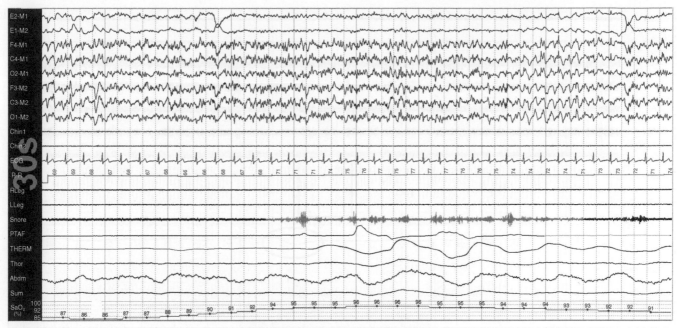

FIGURE 1.5–11 Questions 43 and 44.

43. A new sleep technologist is concerned about PSG abnormalities in the epoch in Figure 1.5–11. What do the EEG channels show?
   A. The patient is having a seizure
   B. The patient is in stage 2 NREM sleep (stage N2)
   C. The patient is in NREM slow-wave sleep (stage N3)
   D. The patient is in REM sleep (stage R)

44. What breathing pattern abnormalities are present in Figure 1.5–11?
   A. The abnormalities are too short to be scored
   B. The start of the epoch shows a central apnea, and the end shows an obstructive apnea
   C. The start of the epoch shows an obstructive apnea, and the end shows a hypopnea
   D. Two hypopneas are shown

45. Figure 1.5–12 is a 10-minute epoch from a PSG. What is shown by the information in the box and oval?
   A. RERA
   B. Hypopnea
   C. Obstructive apnea
   D. Central apnea

46. Figure 1.5–13 is a 10-minute epoch from a PSG. What is the *most* likely abnormality shown?
   A. Mixed apnea
   B. Hypopnea
   C. Obstructive apnea
   D. Central apnea

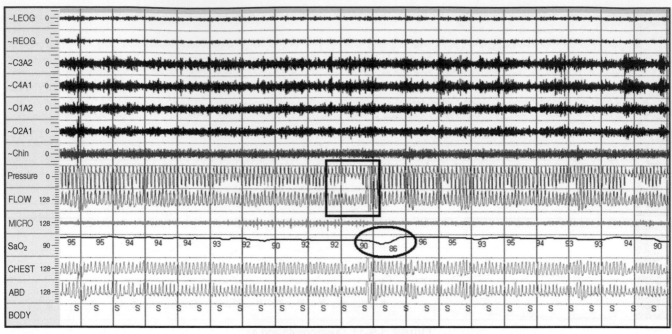

FIGURE 1.5–12 Question 45.

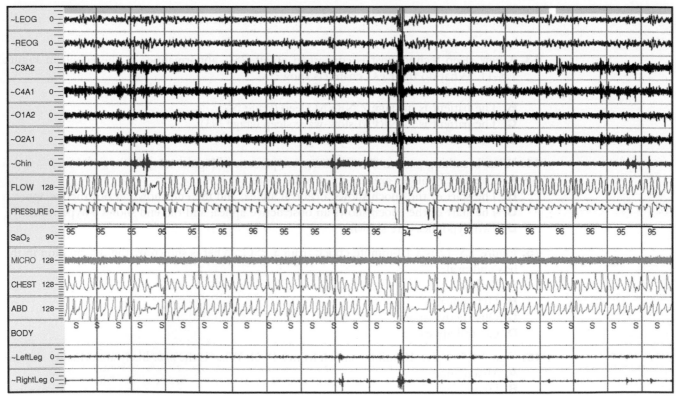

FIGURE 1.5–13 Question 46.

Questions 47 and 48 refer to the following five epochs numbered 345 through 349.

345: Contains a spindle and a K complex

346: Major body movements for 20 seconds; the other 10 seconds contain alpha rhythm

347: Contains a spindle

348: Major body movements for 18 seconds; no alpha rhythm seen

349: Contains a K complex

47. How should you score epoch 346?
  A. W
  B. N1
  C. N2
  D. N3

48. How should you score epoch 348?
  A. W
  B. N1
  C. N2
  D. N3

ANSWERS

1. B. The 10-20 method of EEG electrode placement was developed in 1958. Percentages are used, rather than absolute distances, to allow for normal variations in head shape and size. Figure 1.5–14 shows the 10-20 placement of electrodes. For example, T3 is placed 10% of the distance from M1 to M2, C3 is placed 20% of the distance from T3, CZ is 50% of the distance from M1 or M2, and C4 is 20% of the distance from CZ. Other electrodes are similarly placed 10% to 20% of the distance from the inion or nasion or points in between. Older nomenclature labeled M1 and M2 (mastoid) as A1 and A2 (auricular), respectively. The new nomenclature is promulgated in MANUAL2.

2. A. The recommended derivations are frontal right (F4)–mastoid left (M1), central right (C4)–mastoid left (M1), and occipital right (O2)–mastoid left (M1; see Fig. 1.5–14). Answers B and C have frontal, central, and occipital electrodes connected to the same-side mastoid electrode, which is *not* recommended. Answer D has only two derivations; at least three are recommended. When the electrode set in Answer A is used, back-up electrodes (in case of malfunction) are recommended at F3, C3, O1, and M2 to allow display of F3-M2, C3-M2, and O1-M2.   (MANUAL2)

3. A. Both eyes are referenced to the right mastoid electrode, M2.   (MANUAL2)

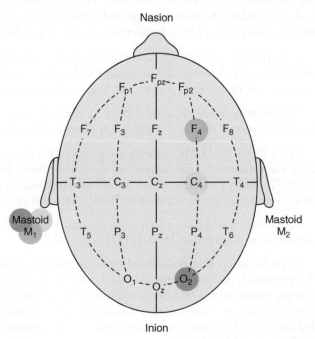

FIGURE 1.5–14 Answers 1 and 2. (From ATLAS2, Fig. 18–2)

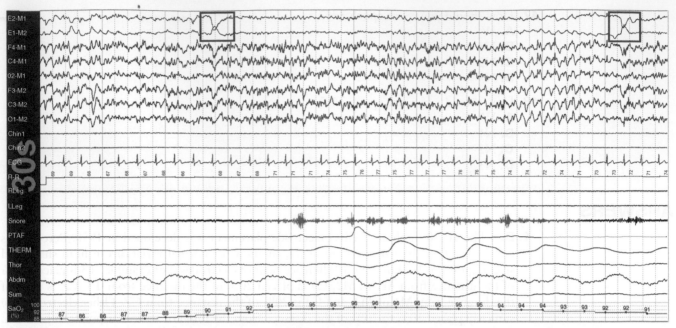

FIGURE 1.5–15 Answer 4.

4. A. The cornea is electrically positive with respect to the retina. When eye movements occur, the EOG channel tracing shows the movements because of this electrical difference. Thus, a rightward movement of the right eye causes the cornea of the right eye to move closer to the recording electrode, which is the right outer canthus (ROC); this movement generates a positive voltage (the pen moves downward by convention, as shown in E2-M1 of the PSG epoch in Fig. 1.5–15). At the same time, the cornea of the left eye moves away from the left outer canthus (LOC), and this generates a negative voltage (the digital tracing moves upward by convention; E1-M2 in the epoch). The EOG tracings show two separate instances of rapid eye movement (*red boxes*). In both instances, the eyes move conjugately toward the ROC electrode.

5. C. The standard EMG derivation for sleep staging requires a chin electrode placed 1 cm above the inferior edge of the mandible. That electrode is referenced to a second electrode placed 2 cm below the inferior edge and either 2 cm to the right or left of midline. (If referenced to the right, a left-side electrode is placed as a backup and vice versa.)

6. D. EEG patterns are distinguishable by frequency, amplitude, shape, and distribution (e.g., occipital, frontal). A sinusoidal or waxing and waning pattern over 5 seconds or more may be artifact, and in any case, it does not help in interpreting the EEG.

7. B. Wakefulness, REM sleep, and NREM sleep are considered three distinct states of the CNS, and a normal subject goes through all three in a given 24-hour period.

8. B. EEG, EOG, and EMG activity are essential for sleep staging. In a standard PSG, they require (as minimum) three derivations for EEG activity (six electrodes), one derivation for chin EMG activity (two electrodes), and two derivations for eye movements (four electrodes). Back-up electrodes are in addition to these minimum requirements.

9. B. Beta waves, which have a frequency greater than 13 Hz, are not used in the classification or diagnosis of sleep stages W, N1, N2, N3, or REM.

10. A. Stage N2 sleep is characterized by sleep spindles or K complexes, not by the baseline EEG. Previously defined as stages 3 and 4 NREM sleep, they are now combined into a single N3 stage, characterized by large-amplitude slow waves (<2 Hz) that occupy at least 20% of the epoch. The term "low voltage, mixed frequency" is also characteristic of REM sleep (now called *stage R*), which must also have rapid eye movements and/or low-voltage EMG on the chin channel.   (MANUAL2)

11. B.   For scoring stage N3, slow waves must occupy 20% or more of the epoch, meeting the definition as stated.   (MANUAL2)

12. D.   Since the AASM's 2007 revision of the classic 1968 sleep-stage scoring manual by Allan Rechtschaffen and Anthony Kales, NREM stages 3 and 4 have been combined into a single stage, N3. A PSG epoch is scored as stage N3 if it includes 20% or more of slow-wave activity (≥6 seconds for a 30-second epoch). *Slow waves* are defined as waves of 0.5 to 2.0 Hz and peak-to-peak amplitude greater than 75 μV, measured over the frontal region. (Note that for purposes of staging N3, slow waves represent a subset of delta activity, defined as EEG waves with a frequency of less than 4 Hz.)

13. A.   The AASM manual states, "Score arousal during sleep stages N1, N2, N3, or R if there is an abrupt shift of EEG frequency including alpha, theta, and/or frequencies greater than 16 Hz (but not spindles) that lasts at least 3 seconds, with at least 10 seconds of stable sleep preceding the change. Scoring of arousal during REM requires a concurrent increase in submental EMG lasting at least 1 second." Both occipital and central derivations are to be incorporated when scoring arousals. The AASM manual also notes that scoring an arousal does not require (and cannot be based on) other information such as body movements or respiratory events.   (MANUAL2)

14. C.   The background EEG activity for REM is a relatively low-voltage, mixed-frequency pattern, but alpha bursts routinely appear and do not necessarily indicate arousals or any pathology. The digital sampling rate for both EEG and EMG is the same: 500 Hz is desirable, and 200 Hz is minimal.   (MANUAL2)

15. A.   In this 30-second epoch (see Fig. 1.5–1), the distance between the solid vertical lines is 3 seconds. In the first 13 seconds, alpha rhythm (8–13 Hz) is seen, so this part is an awake stage. Then there is an abrupt change to low amplitude and mixed frequency with predominance of theta waves (4–7 Hz) plus slow, rolling eye movements (leads E2-M1 and E1-M2), characteristic of stage N1. There are no spindles or K complexes, so you cannot score N2. Finally, the lack of rapid eye movements and the relatively large-amplitude chin EMG rule against REM sleep. Because more than half the epoch is stage N1, the epoch should be scored as N1.

16. A.   This fragment (see Fig. 1.5–2) shows 60-Hz interference. The inset shows 1 second of a single EEG channel. The cause in this example is lead A2 because the artifact was found in all channels that included this lead. ECG artifact usually manifests as the ECG in some other channel. Because heart rate is normally 60 to 100 beats/min, it should not be mistaken for an artifact that is 60 cycles per second. Perspiration artifact is a slow, rhythmic waveform that often coincides with breathing. The best way to avoid 60-Hz artifact is to make sure all electrodes are properly applied and that there are no nearby electrical devices that might leak current. Ideally, a 60-Hz filter should not be necessary.

17. D.   EEG, EOG, ECG, and EMG appear as rapidly fluctuating voltages within a specific frequency bandwidth, and they require the use of both high- and low-frequency filters that are part of AC amplifiers. On the other hand, some signals are slowly fluctuating and can be picked up by DC amplifiers that do not require a low-frequency filter; examples are pulse oximetry and respiratory rate. Respiratory rate can also be amplified by an AC amplifier whose low-frequency filter is set to 0.1 Hz (the high-frequency filter is set to 15 Hz).   (Butkov and Lee-Chiong, 2007; MANUAL2)

18. D.   If a K complex appears in any epoch without an accompanying arousal, that epoch is scored as N2. All subsequent epochs with low amplitude and mixed frequency are scored as N2 even if they do not manifest a K complex or spindle unless they contain an arousal or meet criteria for stage N3 or REM.   (MANUAL2)

19. A. The K complex is a well-delineated negative sharp wave (upward deflection) immediately followed by a positive component (downward deflection) standing out from the background, with total duration of at least 0.5 second. Amplitude is not a criterion. Note that none of the waves in Figure 1.5–3 reaches 75 µV in peak-to-peak amplitude, the criterion for slow waves. The four large waves in the first 3 seconds are all K complexes. A vertex sharp wave is a sharply contoured, negative deflection (upward on EEG) that stands out from the background; vertex waves appear most often in central leads placed near the midline and are characteristically seen in stage N1. Slow waves have high amplitude (at least 75 µV) and low frequency (no more than 2 Hz), are a subset of delta (1 to 4 Hz) activity, and are the defining characteristics of stage N3 sleep.

20. B. Slow waves. Note the high peak-to-peak amplitude (≥75 µV) and low frequency (≤2 Hz). Slow waves are a subset of delta (1–4 Hz) activity and are the defining characteristics of stage N3 sleep. See the answer to Question 19 for discussion of the K complex. K complexes are at least 0.5 second, and amplitude is not a criterion.

21. D. Different sensors are recommended for scoring apneas versus hypopneas. For apnea detection, a thermal sensor (thermistor or thermocouple) is recommended. Thermal sensors detect changes in air temperature, which reflect airflow. Cooler air (room temperature) is inhaled, and warmer air (body temperature) is exhaled, and this change is transduced to a deflection in the thermal airflow channel. An *apnea* is defined as a drop in the peak thermal sensor excursion by at least 90% of baseline. A nasal pressure transducer is more sensitive than a thermistor or thermocouple, and it can better detect hypopneas.   (MANUAL2)

22. D. The AASM manual states: "Score a respiratory event as an apnea when BOTH of the following criteria are met:
a. There is a drop in the peak signal excursion by ≥90% of preevent baseline using an oronasal thermal sensor (diagnostic study), PAP device flow (titration study), or an *alternative* apnea sensor (diagnostic study).
b. The duration of the ≥90% drop in sensor signal is ≥10 seconds."
Drop in SaO$_2$ is not a criterion for scoring apneas (Fig. 1.5–16).

23. B. The AASM manual has two criteria for scoring a hypopnea, Rules 1A and 1B. *Both* require a 30% or more drop of peak signal excursions compared with baseline *and* a duration of 10 or more seconds. 1A also requires a 3% or more drop in SaO$_2$ from pre-event baseline *or* the event is associated with an arousal. 1B requires a 4% or more drop in SaO$_2$ from pre-event baseline and no arousal. The two rules are mutually exclusive when scoring a single study; that is, you can use one or the other, but not both, in the same study.   (MANUAL2)

24. B. Panel B also shows a hypopnea by Rule 1B: a 30% drop in peak signal excursion for at least 10 seconds plus an arousal (seen in EEG leads). Note that SaO$_2$ did not drop.

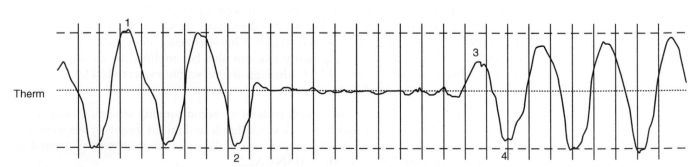

FIGURE 1.5–16 Answer 22. (From AASM Technologist's Handbook, Fig. 41)

25. E. Not part of the awake stage, a K complex is instead a criterion for stage N2. The AASM manual lists five criteria for scoring the awake stage:
- ○ **Alpha rhythm:** Trains of sinusoidal 8- to 13-Hz activity recorded over the occipital region with eye closure, attenuating with eye opening
- ○ **Eye blinks:** Conjugate vertical eye movements at a frequency of 0.5 to 2 Hz present in wakefulness with the eyes open or closed
- ○ **Reading eye movements:** Trains of conjugate eye movements consisting of a slow phase followed by a rapid phase in the opposite direction as the individual reads
- ○ **REMs:** Conjugate, irregular, sharply peaked eye movements with an initial deflection usually lasting less than 500 ms. Although REMs are characteristic of stage R sleep, they may also be seen in wakefulness with eyes open when individuals scan the environment.
- ○ **Slow eye movements (SEMs):** Conjugate, reasonably regular, sinusoidal eye movements with an initial deflection usually lasting longer than 500 ms.

26. D. Adults have less SWS compared with children. Figure 1.5–17 shows a typical hypnogram from a young adult. SWS continues to decrease with age. For people aged 20 to 29 years, SWS occupies about 15.5% of sleep time; for those older than 60 years, about 5% of sleep time is SWS. SWS represents the most dramatic change in sleep stage from childhood to old age. Other changes include a decline in REM and an increase in WASO. These changes are shown graphically in Figure 1.5–18.   (Pressman, 2002, Ch 1)

27. A. "Deep sleep" refers to stage N3 because the arousal threshold is highest in this stage of sleep. Stage N3 concentrates in the first part of the sleep cycle. WASO increases with age, ranging from about 3% in young adults to about 11% in older adults. *REM latency* is defined as the time from sleep onset to the first epoch of REM; it is normally about 90 to 120 minutes. See Figure 1.5–18.   (Pressman, 2002, Ch 1)

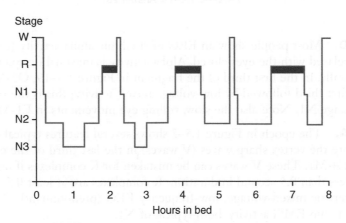

FIGURE 1.5–17 Answer 26. (From ATLAS2, Fig 4.2-25)

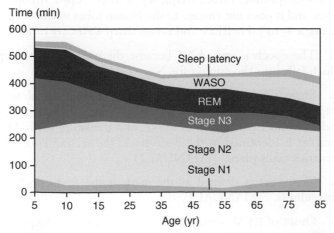

FIGURE 1.5–18 Answers 26 and 27. (From ATLAS2, Fig. 4.2–28)

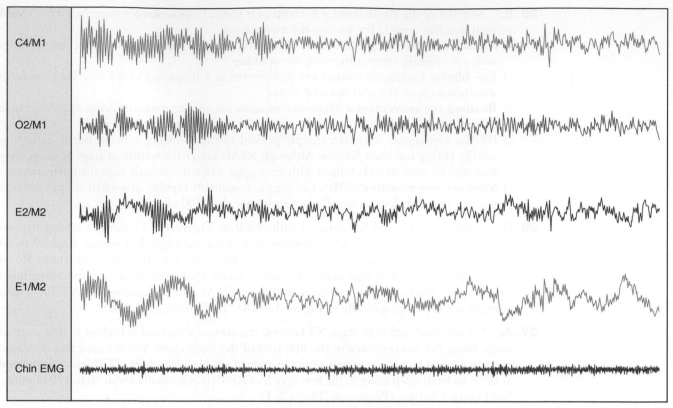

FIGURE 1.5–19 Answer 28.

28. D. Most people show an EEG of rhythmic alpha activity (in the range of 8–13 Hz) when relaxed with the eyes closed. Alpha activity is maximal occipitally but also often occurs centrally. In the first third of the fragment in Figure 1.5–19, O2-M1 shows alpha activity in the first third followed by low-voltage mixed activity; this is the transition from wakefulness to stage N1. Note also the slow, rolling eye movements in E1-M2.

29. A. The epoch in Figure 1.5–7 shows several features typical of stage N1. Most prominent are the vertex sharp waves (V waves) in the last third of the epoch of channels F4-M1 and C4-M1. These V waves can be mistaken for K complexes if not measured; whereas they are less than 0.5 second in duration, K complexes are at least 0.5 second. Also note the characteristic mixed-voltage, low-frequency EEG (predominantly 4–7 Hz) and the large amount of chin EMG activity, both typical of N1.

30. D. The transition to sleep is associated with attenuation of alpha rhythm that is replaced by low-amplitude, mixed-frequency activity. Alpha rhythm is strongest over the occipital lobes, and it does not change to the frontal lobes when sleep occurs. Slow, rolling eye movements; a 4- to 7-Hz EEG; and vertex sharp waves are often seen in stage N1.   (MANUAL2)

31. B. The epoch is scored N1 because the majority of the epoch has a frequency of 7 Hz, which falls into the criteria for N1.   (MANUAL2)

32. B. Stage N2 can be scored when one or more K complexes are unassociated with arousals. Stage N2 is concluded when an arousal takes place or a transition to wakefulness, a major body movement, a transition to N3, or a transition to REM occurs. Therefore, when the K complex is identified in the first epoch, the second epoch is scored N2 until one of these scenarios takes place.   (MANUAL2)

33. A. *Sleep onset* is defined as the start of the first epoch scored as any stage other than wakefulness.   (MANUAL2)

34. B. Onset of REM is measured from the onset of sleep to the beginning of the first REM epoch.

35. D. An EEG pattern of alpha intrusion into NREM sleep was first noted in patients with psychiatric disorders. The pattern was described as a mixture of 5% to 20% delta waves (>75 μV, 0.5–2 Hz) combined with relatively large amplitude, alphalike rhythms (7 to 10 Hz). The alpha rhythms are usually 1 to 2 Hz slower than waking alpha. A similar pattern has been related to the complaint of nonrestorative sleep in patients with musculoskeletal pain or fibromyalgia. Although epochs with alpha-delta sleep are not scored as such (this epoch is N3), the EEG pattern should be noted in the PSG report.

36. A. SEMs are conjugate, reasonably regular, and sinusoidal with an initial deflection that usually lasts longer than 500 ms. They are characteristic of stage N1. Sleep spindles are characteristic of stage N2. Delta waves are seen in stage N3, and REMs of less than 500 ms are seen in the REM stage.   (MANUAL2)

37. D. For detection of hypoventilation during a diagnostic study, you can use arterial, transcutaneous, or end-tidal PcO_2. You cannot use duration of apnea, no matter how long. (MANUAL2)

38. D. Figure 1.5–9 depicts 30 seconds of PSG activity characterizing stage N3 sleep; to score stage N3, at least 20% of the epoch must show slow-wave activity.   (MANUAL2)

39. A. Note that these are arbitrary definitions and differ from the awake state, in which *tachycardia* (in adults) is usually defined as more than 100 beats/min and *bradycardia* as less than 60 beats/min.   (MANUAL2)

40. D. To score epoch 281 as the end of stage R, the K complex would have to occur in the first half of the epoch. In this example, epoch 281 would be scored R, and the next epoch would be N2 unless it met criteria scoring for another stage.   (MANUAL2)

41. B. One of the major differences in the sleep EEG of infants compared with older children and adults is that infants spend about twice as much time in REM sleep.   (PEDS2, p 20)

42. C. The 5-minute epoch shows the typical waxing and waning (crescendo-decrescendo) of tidal volume seen in Cheyne-Stokes breathing. Note that the green airflow line is flat; this is because the airflow channel is measuring nasal flow, and the patient is mouth breathing. Note also that the PcO_2 channel is measuring end-tidal PcO_2 both orally and nasally, and thus it nicely displays the waxing and waning breathing pattern.

43. D. The most striking feature in Figure 1.5–11 is the synchronized activity (all the EEG channels change together) toward the end of the epoch (see the red box in Fig. 1.5–20). Close inspection of the waveforms (the green ovals in the figure) shows that some of the waves have notches; these are sawtooth waves (so called because they resemble teeth on a saw). The usual frequency of sawtooth waves is 2 to 6 Hz, so they can appear as theta waves (4–7 Hz). Sawtooth waves are characteristic of stage R, but they are not required to identify this stage.

44. C. The thermal sensor is used to define apnea (see the *therm* channel shown by the purple line in Fig. 1.5–20), and the pressure sensor (*PTAF*, above *therm*) is used to define a hypopnea. Hypopneas and apneas in adults are scored if the duration is 10 seconds or longer. Inductance plethysmography is used for the effort channels (or esophageal manometry, which is not used in clinical labs). *Airflow* and *effort* define the two types of apneas. In an *obstructive apnea*, there is respiratory effort. In a *central apnea*, respiratory effort is absent. A *mixed event* begins with central apnea features (no airflow, no respiratory effort) and ends with obstructive features (no airflow, respiratory effort present). Two sets of rules define hypopnea (see the answer to Question 23).   (MANUAL2)

45. B. This 10-minute epoch shows the standard features of a hypopnea: reduction in airflow to at least 30% of baseline in the pressure transducer signal and a 4% or greater drop in SaO_2 (low SaO_2 = 86% in this epoch). Note the difference in the pressure transducer and thermal sensor channels. The former changes significantly (and makes the diagnosis possible); the latter changes very little. Whereas thermal sensors are used to monitor for apneas, pressure transducers are used to monitor for hypopneas.   (MANUAL2)

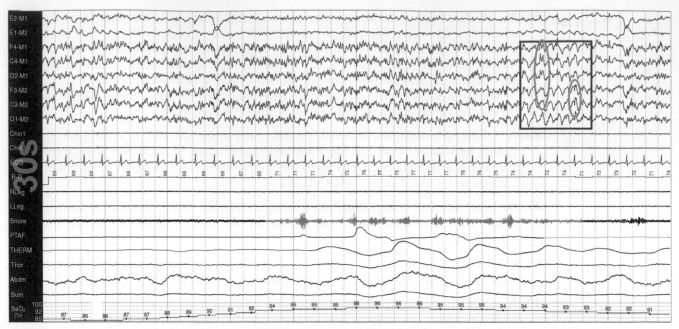

FIGURE 1.5–20 Answers 43 and 44.

46. B.   Note the difference between the pressure channel and the flow (thermal) channel. The pressure channel shows almost complete flow cessation, but the thermal channel shows only a small decrease in flow. So is it an apnea or a hypopnea? It is not an apnea because the thermal flow channel does not show cessation of airflow. Can this be scored as a hypopnea because the decrease in SaO_2 is only 1%? (It requires at least a 3% drop.) Note that immediately after the decreased waveform in the pressure channel, a spike appears in the EEG channels; this is an arousal. (Also note the leg jerk in the leg channels.) You can score this event as a hypopnea because an arousal associated with a 30% or more drop in signal excursion meets the MANUAL2 criteria for hypopnea. Under *D. Scoring of Hypopneas* of the AASM manual, 1A.c states hypopnea can be scored if there is "a ≥3% oxygen desaturation from preevent baseline *or* the event is associated with an arousal."

47. A.   The rule states that if alpha rhythm is present for any part of the epoch with a "major body movement," the epoch is scored as stage W.   (MANUAL2)

48. C.   The rule states that if alpha rhythm is not discernable in an epoch with major body movements, the epoch is scored the same stage as the epoch that follows it. In this case, epoch 349 contains a spindle and a K complex, which indicate stage N2; hence, N2 is also the score for epoch 348 (Boxes 1.5–1 and 1.5–2).

Box 1.5–1 How to Examine a Polysomnogram on a Board Exam

Step 1. Look at the entire image. The most striking finding may be a distractor. In Figure 1.5–21, the most obvious finding is in the snoring channel, with loud snores. These may have nothing to do with the question (e.g., What is the sleep stage?). Always circle back to the question being asked. If at any point you can answer the question confidently without using the most obvious finding, you can ignore that finding.

Step 2. Make sure you have determined (or know from the question) what the epoch length is. A polysomnogram (PSG) can have a split screen with the top and bottom showing different lengths, as shown in Figure 1.5–22. In this fragment, the top is 30 seconds, and the bottom is 2 minutes.

Step 3. Examine the channels recorded in the montage. This will be the first clue about what type of study is being shown. It is clear from examining the montage that this study is being done on continuous positive airway pressure (CPAP) and is therefore not solely a diagnostic study (Fig. 1.5–23).

Step 4. Examine the scales of the quantitative channels. In Figure 1.5–24, we see the patient is on CPAP (pressure is 19 cm H_2O) and oxygenation is adequate (SaO_2 = 99%).

Step 5. Look for artifacts and distractors. In Figure 1.5–25, the PTAF and THERM are flat because they are not being recorded (this is a CPAP study, and the pressure level from the CPAP machine is being recorded). At this point, you actually know enough to answer the question being asked. There are, of course, artifacts (electrocardiograph [ECG] in the chin and electroencephalograph [EEG] channels) and other interesting findings, but do not waste your time on them because you have already answered the question.

Step 6. As a final step, you might have to look for a specific finding to answer the question. In this example (Fig. 1.5–26), you see a flattening of the C-flow (flow measured by the CPAP machine) and snoring noise, both indicating flow limitation, which answers the question.

Step 7. In the real world, when you interpret a PSG, you will go through the history, the tech notes, and steps 1 through 6 and then look at other channels (legs, EEG, ECG) for abnormalities.

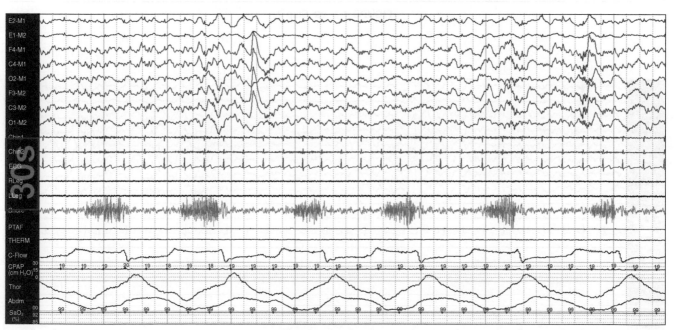

FIGURE 1.5–21 Step 1.

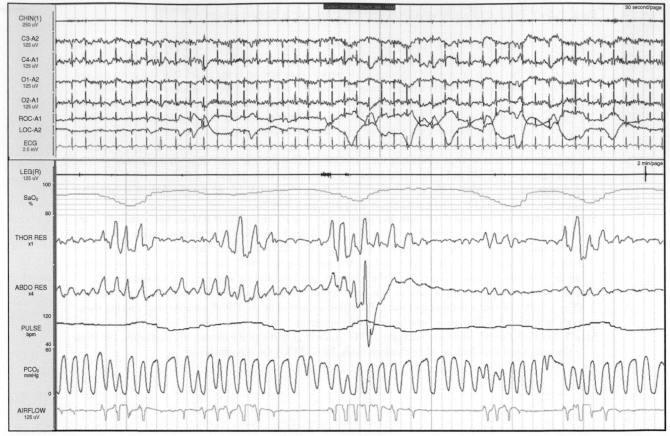

FIGURE 1.5–22 Step 2.

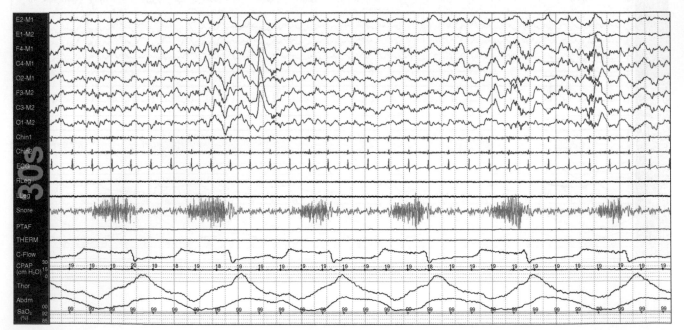

FIGURE 1.5–23 Step 3.

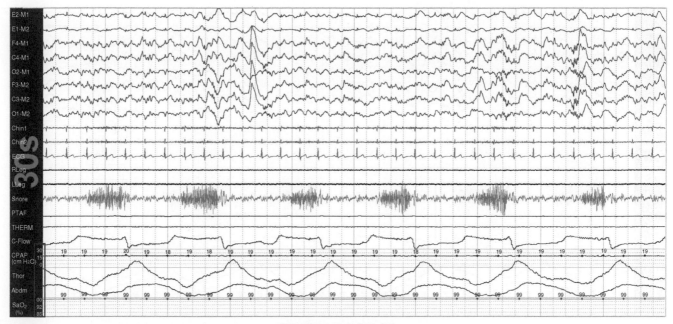

FIGURE 1.5–24 Step 4.

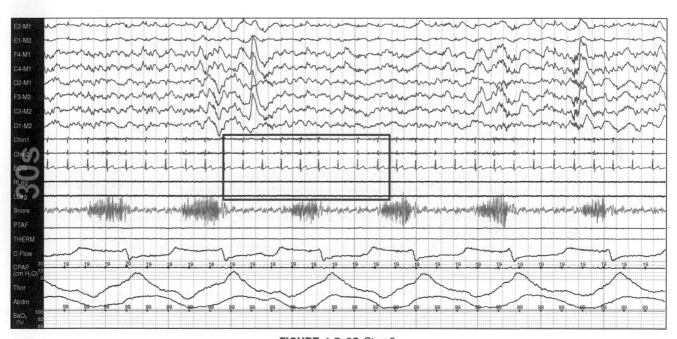

FIGURE 1.5–25 Step 5.

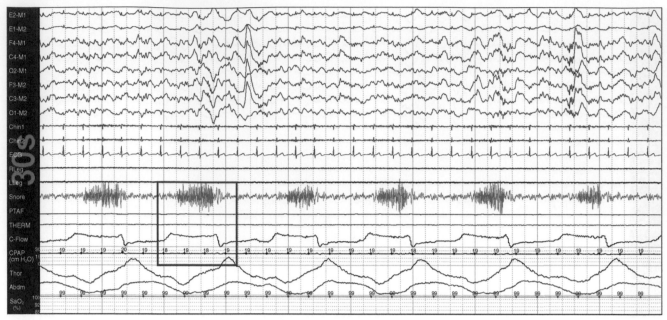

FIGURE 1.5–26 Step 6.

Box 1.5–2 Six Steps in Determining the Rapid Eye Movement Stage (Stage R)

Step 1. Three features define rapid eye movement (REM) sleep, or stage R. The first is the presence of a low-amplitude, mixed-frequency pattern in the electroencephalography (EEG) channels (*red rectangle*, Fig. 1.5–27). This is nonspecific and can also be found in stage N1.

Step 2. Second is low or absent chin electromyography (EMG) tone (*red rectangle*, Fig. 1.5–28).

Step 3. Third is REMs. REMs are often sharply peaked, with the initial deflection being less than 0.5 second (*red boxes*, Fig. 1.5–29).

Step 4. Look for other features of REM that *are not* required for staging. Sawtooth waves are found exclusively in REM; these are notched waves and can be seen in the EEG channels.

- There may also be short (<0.25 second) twitches or transient muscle activity noted in the chin and leg EMGs
- Breathing may become irregular in normal subjects and in patients with Cheyne-Stokes breathing. Cardiac rhythm may become erratic

Step 5. Look for continuation of REM. After REM is scored in an epoch, it continues to be scored in subsequent epochs, even when eye movements are not seen *if* chin tone remains low, EEG continues to show mixed frequency, *and* there are no K complexes or sleep spindles.

Step 6. Look for the end of REM. REM is no longer scored if another stage is scored. K complexes or sleep spindles mean stage N2 is present. An arousal followed by slow eye movements means stage N1 is present. (Specific rules for continuing and ending REM scoring are provided in MANUAL2, pp 26–30.)

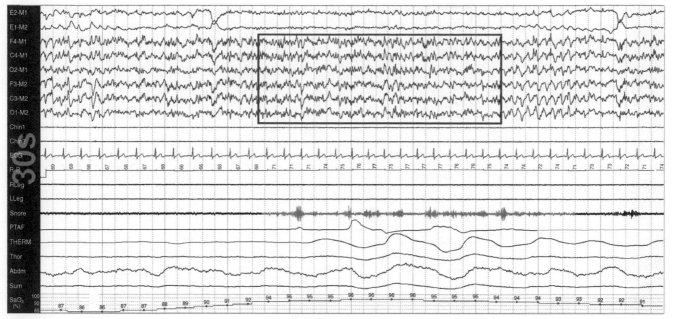

FIGURE 1.5–27 Step 1.

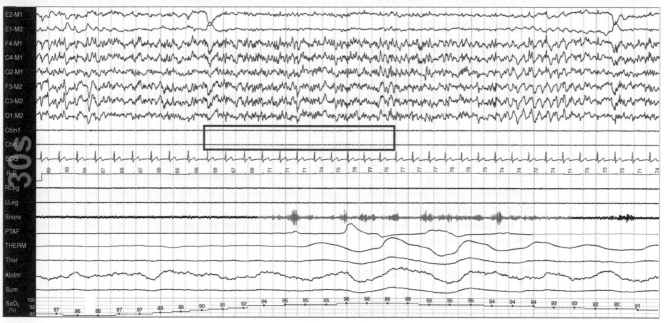

FIGURE 1.5–28 Step 2.

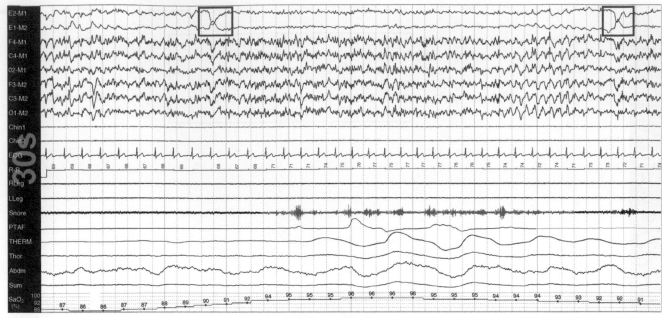

FIGURE 1.5–29 Step 3.

Highly Recommended

■ *AASM Manual for the Scoring of Sleep and Associated Events: Rules, Terminology and Technical Specifications*, Version 2.5
■ *Atlas of Clinical Sleep Medicine*, ed 2, Ch 18
■ *Technologist's Handbook for Understanding and Implementing the AASM Manual for the Scoring of Sleep and Associated Events: Rules, Terminology, and Technical Specifications*, 2009

Your knowledge of methods, rules, and event scoring will be addressed throughout the exam in a variety of questions. Sleep staging dovetails with event rules, so some overlap occurs; you cannot stage the PSG unless you can identify common waveforms, such as alpha rhythm, K complexes, and slow-wave sleep. Expect many questions on the examination that require knowledge of sleep staging.

You must know in detail the AASM rules for scoring and staging published in version 2.5 and now updated online.

Polysomnography Methods

■ 10-20 EEG electrode placement
   ○ Recommended derivations: F4-M1, C4-M1, and O2-M1
   ○ Alternative derivations: Fz-Cz, Cz-Oz, and C4-M1
■ EOG placement
   ○ Where the electrodes are placed (outer canthi)
      • Both eyes are referenced to M2.
   ○ Source of voltage for recording EOG
      • Cornea is electrically positive with respect to the retina
   ○ When right and left eyes move toward the right electrode
      • Positive voltage in right EOG (E2-M2), pen moves downward by convention
      • Negative voltage in left EOG (E1-M2), pen moves upward by convention
■ EMG placement
   ○ Chin EMG for stage scoring
      • Chin electrode 1 cm above the inferior edge of the mandible
      • Reference electrode 2 cm below the inferior edge and either 2 cm to the right or left of midline

- ○ Leg EMG for leg movements
  - • Anterior tibialis muscle, electrodes 2 to 3 cm apart
- ■ Inductance plethysmography for chest and abdominal movement (not piezoelectric belts)
- ■ Nasal and oral thermistor and nasal pressure sensor
  - ○ Thermistor for apneas
  - ○ Nasal pressure sensor for hypopneas

Rules and Event Scoring

- ■ Epoch length
  - ○ Standard is 30 seconds, but longer epochs are often used to display breathing events
- ■ PSG display
  - ○ To display the raw data for scoring on a screen, the AASM recommends a 15-inch screen size, 1600 pixels horizontal, and 1050 pixels vertical
  - ○ Be aware of channel labeling; always check labeling of derivations when looking at the EEG
  - ○ Alpha rhythm is more prominent in occipital derivations
  - ○ Slow waves and K complexes are more prominent in frontal derivations
  - ○ Spindles are more prominent with central derivations
- ■ EEG and EOG waveforms
  - ○ K complex (Fig. 1.5–30)
    - • Well-delineated negative sharp wave (upward deflection by convention) immediately followed by a positive component that stands out from the background EEG
    - • Total duration, 0.5 seconds or longer
    - • Usually maximal over the frontal regions
  - ○ Slow waves (Fig. 1.5–31)
    - • High amplitude (≥75 μV) and low frequency (≤2 Hz)
    - • Subset of delta (1 to 4 Hz) activity
    - • Defining characteristics of stage N3
  - ○ Alpha activity (Fig. 1.5–32)
    - • 8- to 13-Hz rhythm
    - • Most prominent in occipital leads
    - • Thought to be generated by the cortex
    - • Used as marker for relaxed wakefulness and CNS arousals

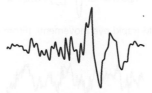

FIGURE 1.5–30 K complex. (From ATLAS2, Table 18–2)

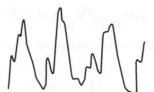

FIGURE 1.5–31 Slow waves. (From ATLAS2, Table 18–2)

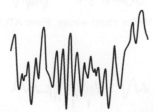

FIGURE 1.5–32 Alpha activity. (From ATLAS2, Table 18–2)

- Theta activity (Fig. 1.5–33)
  - 4 to 7 Hz
  - Typically prominent in central and temporal leads
  - Seen in both stage N1 and REM sleep
  - Sawtooth waves in this range
- Rapid eye movement (Fig. 1.5–34)
  - Conjugate saccades that occur during stage R (REM sleep)
  - Sharply peaked with initial deflection usually less than 0.5 seconds in duration
- Slow eye movements (Fig. 1.5–35)
  - Conjugate, usually rhythmic, rolling eye movements with initial deflection more than 0.5 seconds in duration
  - Typically in stage N1
- Vertex sharp waves (Fig. 1.5–36)
  - Sharply contoured, negative deflection (upward on EEG) that stands out from the background
  - Most often in central leads placed near the midline
  - Characteristically seen in stage N1
- Sleep spindle (Fig. 1.5–37)
  - Phasic burst of 11- to 16-Hz activity
  - Prominent in central scalp leads
  - Typically lasts for 0.5 to 1.0 seconds
  - Scalp representation of thalamocortical discharges

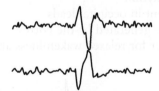

FIGURE 1.5–33 Theta activity. (From ATLAS2, Table 18–2)

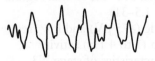

FIGURE 1.5–34 REM (rapid eye movement). (From ATLAS2, Table 18–2)

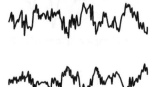

FIGURE 1.5–35 SEM (slow eye movements). (From ATLAS2, Table 18–2)

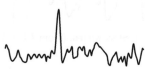

FIGURE 1.5–36 Vertex sharp waves. (From ATLAS2, Table 18–2)

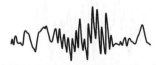

FIGURE 1.5–37 Sleep spindle. (From ATLAS2, Table 18–2)

Rules for Scoring Sleep

- Sleep staging rules for adults (MANUAL2, section IV, part 1)
  - Stages of sleep
    - Stage W
      - Alpha rhythm (8–13 Hz) with eyes closed
      - Eye blinks
      - Reading eye movements
      - Rapid eye movements on occasion (when scanning environment)
    - Stage N1
      - Slow eye movements
      - Alpha rhythm is attenuated, replaced by low-amplitude, mixed-frequency rhythm
      - Vertex waves
    - Stage N2
      - K complex: negative sharp wave followed by a positive component; total duration, 0.5 seconds or longer
      - Sleep spindles: train of distinct waves 11 to 16 Hz; duration, 0.5 seconds or longer
    - Stage N3
      - Slow waves (0.5–2.0 Hz; peak to peak >75 Hz measured over frontal regions) occupy 20% or more of epoch
    - Stage R
      - REMs
      - Low chin EMG
      - Sawtooth waves
  - Artifacts
    - 60-Hz interference (60-Hz filter last resort)
    - Sweat artifact
    - ECG artifacts (can appear in any channel)
  - Arousals
    - Abrupt shift in EEG frequency that lasts at least 3 seconds, with at least 10 seconds of stable sleep preceding

Rules for Scoring Abnormal Events

- Cardiac rules (MANUAL2)
  - Sinus tachycardia (in adults): more than 90 beats/min
  - Sinus bradycardia (age 6 years through adult): less than 40 beats/min
  - Asystole (age 6 years to adult): longer than 3 seconds between heartbeats
  - Wide-complex tachycardia
  - Narrow-complex tachycardia
- Periodic limb movements
  - Minimum number of consecutive movements is four
  - Minimum period length between movements is 5 seconds
  - Maximum period length between movements is 90 seconds
  - Movements on two different legs separated by less than 5 seconds are counted as a single leg movement
- Movement rules (MANUAL2, section VII)
  - Movement time no longer scored
  - Major body movement (MBM)
- Movement and muscle artifact obscuring EEG more than half of the epoch to the extent that stage cannot be determined
  - Score epoch with MBM as W, N1, N2, N3, or REM
    - If alpha rhythm is seen in any part of the epoch with MBM, score as W
    - Otherwise, if the epoch before or after is W, score the epoch with MBM as W
    - Otherwise, score the epoch the same stage as the epoch *after* the MBM

- Respiratory rules in adults (MANUAL2, section VIII)
  - Apnea criteria
    - Use the thermistor channel to document
    - Score when there is at least a 90% decrease in thermistor flow for at least 9 seconds of a 10-second apnea (see the answer to Question 22)
  - Hypopnea criteria; two different rules: 1A and 1B
    - 1A. Score a respiratory event as a hypopnea if *all* of the following criteria are met:
      - The peak signal excursions drop by 30% or greater of pre-event baseline using nasal pressure (diagnostic study), PAP device flow (titration study), or an alternative hypopnea sensor (diagnostic study)
      - The duration of the 30% or greater drop in signal excursion is 10 seconds or more
      - A 3% or greater oxygen desaturation from pre-event baseline occurs or the event is associated with an arousal
    - 1B. Score a respiratory event as a hypopnea if *all* of the following criteria are met:
      - The peak signal excursions drop by 30% or greater of pre-event baseline using nasal pressure (diagnostic study), PAP device flow (titration study), or an alternative hypopnea sensor (diagnostic study)
      - The duration of the 30% or greater drop in signal excursion is 10 seconds or more
      - A 4% or greater oxygen desaturation from pre-event baseline occurs
  - RERA criteria (MANUAL2)
    - If electing to score RERAs, score a respiratory event as a RERA if a sequence of breaths lasts 10 or more seconds and is characterized by increasing respiratory effort or by flattening of the inspiratory portion of the nasal pressure (diagnostic study) or PAP device flow (titration study) waveform, leading to arousal from sleep; the event is a RERA when the sequence of breaths does not meet criteria for an apnea or hypopnea
    - RERAs are an "option" for scoring (i.e., not recommended)
    - RERAs are added to the apnea/hypopnea index (AHI) to determine respiratory disturbance index (RDI)
  - Hypoventilation (MANUAL2)
    - Score hypoventilation during sleep if *either* of the following occurs:
      - Arterial PcO_2 (or surrogate) increases to a value greater than 55 mm Hg for 10 or more minutes
      - An increase of greater than or equal to 10 mm Hg in arterial PcO_2 (or surrogate) occurs during sleep (compared with an awake supine value) to a value that exceeds 50 mm Hg for 10 or more minutes
- Respiratory rules in children (MANUAL2)
  - Apnea criteria
    - Event lasts for at least two missed breaths
    - A 90% fall in signal amplitude occurs for 90% of the respiratory cycle compared with baseline
    - Continued respiratory effort occurs throughout the period of decreased airflow
  - Hypopnea criteria
    - At least 50% fall in nasal pressure signal *and*
    - Lasts for at least two missed breaths *and*
    - Fall in nasal pressure must last for at least 90% of the hypopnea duration *and*
    - The event is associated with arousal, awakening, or at least 3% O_2 desaturation
  - Hypoventilation criteria
    - Properly calibrated and validated end-tidal PcO_2 or transcutaneous PcO_2 monitoring are acceptable surrogates for following $PacO_2$
    - If end-tidal CO_2 is used, it is crucial to obtain the plateau in waveform
    - Score hypoventilation if PcO_2 is less than 50 mm Hg for more than 25% of the sleep time (Box 1.5–3)

Box 1.5–3 Don't Forget

- The cornea is electrically positive with respect to the retina. When eye movements occur, the electrooculogram (EOG) channel tracing shows the movements because of this electrical difference
- The standard electromyogram (EMG) derivation for sleep staging requires a chin EMG. This is used for scoring REM sleep (low amplitude during REM). In contrast, leg EMGs are used to score leg movements
- Electroencephalogram (EEG) patterns are distinguishable by frequency, amplitude, shape, and distribution (e.g., occipital, central, frontal)
- Wakefulness, non-REM (NREM) sleep, and REM sleep are considered three distinct states of the central nervous system, and the normal subject goes through all three during a sleep study. These states are distinguishable on the PSG by just three sets of derivations: EEG, EOG, and chin EMG
- In a typical sleep study, EEG uses three derivations (F4-M1, C4-M1, and O2-M1), EOG uses two derivations (E1-M2 and E2-M2), and chin EMG uses one derivation. Each derivation involves two electrodes: the *recording electrode* and the *reference electrode*
- Staging of sleep is based on a set of well-defined rules outlined in this section and detailed in the AASM manual (MANUAL2; see References). Full knowledge of this manual is a must for the exam
- Apnea is scored when there is a ≥90% decrease in thermistor flow for ≥9 seconds of a 10-second apnea (see answer to Question 22 for clarification of this often confusing point)

- Hypopnea: There are two sets of definitions (see earlier under *Respiratory rules in adults*)
- Apnea-hypopnea index (AHI) includes all apneas plus hypopneas, with the latter scored by *either* the recommended or alternative methods; you cannot use both to determine any patient's AHI. The level of AHI is then used to determine the severity of a sleep apnea (could be obstructive and/or central sleep apnea). Medicare criteria for reimbursement of CPAP is based on the AHI and clinical features
- Scoring of respiratory effort–related arousals (RERAs) is optional. Some labs include RERAs in the respiratory disturbance index (RDI), which is therefore more inclusive than the AHI. However, sometimes labs use RDI interchangeably with AHI. AHI and RDI should not be reported without defining how they are derived
- Medicare (CMS) uses the term *RDI* in its CPAP Decision Memo but does not define it. Many sleep specialists think that CMS meant RDI to be synonymous with AHI
- Flattening on a nasal pressure channel or a CPAP flow channel indicates flow limitation. If there is also amplitude reduction with a requisite drop in SaO_2, hypopnea can be scored. Otherwise, it might represent a RERA. If flattening occurs in a CPAP flow channel, it usually indicates a need for an increase in pressure
- End-tidal or transcutaneous CO_2 monitoring is recommended to diagnose hypoventilation in children but not in adults
- Two sets of rules are used to define *hypopnea*: recommended and alternative. Criteria in either set must be met to score hypopneas in a PSG; they cannot be mixed in a given study. (MANUAL2, p 59)

Sleep Staging

- EEG, EOG, and EMG activity is essential for sleep staging.
  - Standard PSG
    - Three derivations for EEG (six electrodes)
    - One derivation for chin EMG activity (two electrodes)
    - Two derivations for eye movements (four electrodes)
    - Back-up electrodes are in addition to these minimum requirements.
- The natural progression from wakefulness to REM
  - Wakefulness
    - About 5% of the sleep period (WASO) in adults; increases with age
    - Alpha rhythm, eye blinks
  - Stage N1
    - Occupies about 4% to 5% of sleep time in adults
    - Attenuation of alpha rhythm
    - Replaced by low-amplitude, mixed-frequency activity in more than 50% of the epoch
    - Vertex waves
  - Stage N2
    - Occupies about 50% of sleep time in adults
    - Either of the following in the first half of the epoch or in the last half of the previous epoch:
      - K complexes
      - Sleep spindles
  - Stage N3
    - Percentage of N3 declines with age: about 15.5% in young adults, down to about 5% in persons older than 60 years
    - Slow waves (0.5–2.0 Hz peak-to-peak amplitude >75 μV) occupy 20% or more of the epoch

○ Stage R
  • Occupies about 25% of sleep time in adults
  • Rapid eye movements
  • Low chin EMG
  • Low voltage, mixed frequency (often with sawtooth waves, although not needed for scoring REM)
■ Changes in sleep stages with aging, childhood to old age (ATLAS2, Fig. 4.2–23)
  ○ Increase in WASO
  ○ Not much change in N1
  ○ Some decrease in REM sleep
  ○ Not much change in N2
  ○ Marked decrease in N3
    • This is the most striking change among all sleep stages
    • In addition to having more N3 sleep, children have slow waves with a very high amplitude compared with adults
    • In children, the other stages more closely resemble those of adults
■ Continuation rules
  ○ N2 continues if subsequent epochs show low amplitude, mixed frequency without K complexes or sleep spindles
  ○ N2 ends with an arousal or with transition to stage W, N3, or R or with a major body movement followed by SEMs. (MANUAL2)
  ○ R continues if EEG continues to show low-amplitude, mixed-frequency activity without K complexes or sleep spindles, and chin EMG tone remains low
  ○ R ends. (MANUAL2)
  ○ Epochs are at transition between N2 and R. (MANUAL2)
■ Major body movement (MBM)
  ○ Epochs are scored with MBM based on:
    • Alpha-rhythm part of epoch: score as W
    • No alpha rhythm: W before or after, score epoch with MBM as W
    • Otherwise, score same stage as epoch that follows
  ○ Pediatric scoring has some differences compared with adults (MANUAL2)
■ Alpha-delta sleep
  ○ Alpha portion usually 1 to 2 Hz slower than waking alpha
    • Often seen in patients with fibromyalgia or musculoskeletal pain
    • May be associated with nonrestorative sleep (Box 1.5–4)

Box 1.5–4 Don't Forget

- Attenuation of alpha sleep into a low-amplitude, mixed-frequency sleep is a hallmark of transition from W to N1. However, alpha sleep is not always present in humans, and the AASM has specific rules for scoring the transition to sleep in such situations (see MANUAL2)
- Alpha rhythm is present most prominently over the occipital lobe, delta waves and K complexes are present most prominently over the frontal lobes, and sleep spindles are most prominent over the center of the brain
- Normally, there is progression of rapid eye movements (REMs) throughout the sleep cycle, manifesting as three or four discrete REM periods, each progressively longer
- REMs help define stage R, where they are accompanied by a low-amplitude chin electroencephalography (EEG). However, they may also be seen in stage W, as patients scan the room or read a book; in this case, chin electromyography is very active
- Slow, rolling eye movements are seen in stage N1, and they help to define the transition from W to N1
- One of the major differences in the sleep EEG of infants compared with older children and adults is that newborn infants spend about 50% of total sleep time in REM sleep
- Sawtooth waves are characteristic of stage R, but they are not required to identify it
- The thermal sensor is used to define apnea. The nasal pressure sensor is used to define hypopneas
- If alpha rhythm is present for any part of the epoch with a major body movement, score the epoch as stage W

REFERENCES

American Academy of Sleep Medicine. *A technologist's handbook for understanding and implementing the AASM manual for the scoring of sleep and associated events: rules, terminology and technical specifications.* Darien, Ill.: American Academy of Sleep Medicine; 2009.

American Academy of Sleep Medicine. *International classification of sleep disorders.* 3th ed. Darien, Ill.: American Academy of Sleep Medicine; 2014.

American Academy of Sleep Medicine. *The AASM manual for the scoring of sleep and associated events: rules terminology and technical specifications,* Version 2.5 or higher. Darien, Ill.: American Academy of Sleep Medicine; 2014.

Butkov N, Lee-Chiong T. *Fundamentals of sleep technology.* Philadelphia: Lippincott Williams & Wilkins; 2007.

Kryger MH, Avidan A, Berry R. *Atlas of clinical sleep medicine.* 2nd ed. Philadelphia: Saunders; 2014.

Pressman MR. *Primer of polysomnogram interpretation.* Boston: Butterworth Heinemann; 2002.

Rechtschaffen A, Kales A. *A manual of standardized terminology, techniques and scoring system for sleep stages of human subjects.* Washington, D.C.: US Dept of Health, Education, and Welfare; National Institutes of Health; 1968.

Sleep-Wake Timing

QUESTIONS

A 22-Year-Old Man With Excessive Daytime Sleepiness

A 22-year-old man who recently graduated from Georgia Tech in Atlanta with an engineering degree comes to the sleep clinic with severe excessive daytime sleepiness. He is very concerned about poor work performance and has a history of sleepiness dating back to his early teens that has worsened since he began his engineering job. To combat the sleepiness, he drinks 8 to 10 high-caffeine energy drinks a day, mostly before noon. On weekends, he feels "pretty alert" most of the time. When he lived at home, his parents used to think he was lazy because on weekends, he slept until 3 PM. However, he always made good grades in school. Apart from depression, his medical history is unremarkable. He is currently taking fluoxetine 20 mg at bedtime. History does not suggest cataplexy or sleep paralysis.

1. What should the next step be?
   A. All-night polysomnography (PSG)
   B. All-night PSG followed by a maintenance of wakefulness test (MWT)
   C. All-night PSG followed by a multiple sleep latency test (MSLT)
   D. Two-week sleep diary

2. The patient reports that he only sleeps 4 hours per night except on weekends, when he might sleep 10 to 12 hours. Based on the information in the case description, which of the following is the *least* likely diagnosis?
   A. Narcolepsy
   B. Delayed sleep-wake phase disorder (DSWPD)
   C. Paradoxic insomnia
   D. Psychophysiologic insomnia

3. Concerning dim-light melatonin onset (DLMO), which of the following would be consistent with DSWPD?
   A. DLMO occurs at about noon
   B. DLMO occurs after 10 PM
   C. DLMO occurs randomly
   D. DLMO occurs at about 8 AM

4. DSWPD can be caused by all of the following *except*
   A. Traumatic brain injury
   B. Behavioral factors alone
   C. Hypersensitivity to nighttime suppression of melatonin by light
   D. Endogenous circadian system dysfunction

5. The *most* effective treatment for DSWPD is
   A. Bright light exposure in the evening
   B. Bright light exposure in the morning
   C. 1 mg of melatonin upon awakening
   D. Chronotherapy

6. Patients with DSWPD have
   A. Increased ability to compensate for sleep loss compared with normal control participants
   B. Decreased ability to compensate for sleep loss compared with normal control participants
   C. Identical ability to compensate for sleep loss compared with normal control participants
   D. Sleep loss recovery that is only possible during daytime hours

7. Which of the following disorders is *most* often familial?
   A. DSWPD
   B. Non–24-hour sleep-wake rhythm
   C. Irregular sleep-wake rhythm disorder
   D. Advanced sleep-wake phase disorder (ASWPD)

A 68-Year-Old Woman With Early Morning Awakening

A 68-year-old woman comes to the sleep clinic with a history of sleep maintenance insomnia and early morning awakenings. This problem began 5 years earlier with the unexpected death of her husband. Her final awakening is usually around 3:30 AM; then she often lies in bed, frustrated because she cannot return to sleep. She is 5 feet, 3 inches tall and weighs 185 lb. She is unaware of snoring but does complain of daytime fatigue. Current medications include metoprolol 50 mg/day and three drugs at bedtime: esomeprazole 20 mg, atorvastatin 10 mg, and trazodone 100 mg. She denies depression but has occasional bouts of intense anxiety, especially in crowds and on airplanes.

8. The *most* important clinical issue to explore at this point is
   A. Snoring and possible apnea
   B. Anxiety disorder
   C. Habitual sleep-wake schedule
   D. Depression history

9. If you suspect ASWPD, you would conduct a PSG
   A. At the usual in-and-out-of-bed times for the laboratory
   B. At the patient's desired sleep and wake times
   C. At the patient's habitual in-and-out-of-bed times
   D. No criteria have been established for using PSG in ASWPD

A PSG is conducted from 10 PM to 6:30 AM with the following results:

Sleep latency = 4 minutes; total sleep time (TST) = 5 hours; sleep efficiency = 72%; apnea-hypopnea index (AHI) = 8 events/hr; periodic limb movement (PLM) arousal index = 3/hr. No electrocardiograph (ECG) or electroencephalograph (EEG) abnormalities are seen.

10. Based on these findings, you should
    A. Initiate a continuous positive airway pressure (CPAP) titration
    B. Increase trazodone to 150 mg
    C. Reduce trazodone to 50 mg and add 2 mg of eszopiclone at bedtime
    D. Consider other clinical factors

11. Treating ASWPD should include
    A. Morning bright light therapy
    B. Chronotherapy, delaying sleep by 3 hours per day
    C. Evening melatonin
    D. Morning melatonin

12. In patients with ASWPD,
    A. The DLMO is much later than normal
    B. Core body temperature (CBT) variation is decreased
    C. The DLMO is significantly earlier than normal
    D. Core body temperature nadir is 5 hours before sleep offset

13. The best way to diagnose ASWPD objectively is with
    A. Actigraphy
    B. PSG
    C. Core temperature
    D. Sleep diary

A 42-Year-Old Man Who Cannot Keep a Job

A 42-year-old man comes to the sleep clinic with complaint of an irregular sleep schedule. He was recently fired from work for tardiness. To assess his sleep-wake schedule, you ask him to wear an actigraph for 2 weeks. The results are shown in Figure 2–1.

14. This patient demonstrates a sleep-wake schedule consistent with
   A. DSWPD
   B. ASWPD
   C. Non–24-hour sleep-wake disorder
   D. Irregular sleep-wake rhythm disorder

15. Patients with the sleep-wake pattern shown in Figure 2–1 are rarely
   A. Older than 45 years
   B. Blind persons with no retinas
   C. Supersensitive to light
   D. Normal sighted

16. Factors that can influence a patient's circadian rhythm include all of the following *except*
   A. Light-dark cycle
   B. Watching a favorite TV show at the same time daily
   C. Using sedating antidepressants
   D. Morning exercise

17. Bright light therapy for non–24-hour sleep-wake disorder is
   A. Effective only in sighted persons
   B. Not as good as vitamin B_{12}
   C. Not as effective as a consistent dose of melatonin in the morning
   D. Worth considering in persons with no light perception

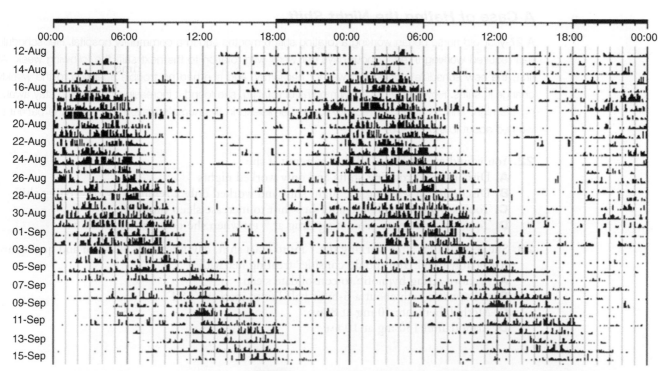

FIGURE 2–1 Questions 14 to 17.

A 12-Year-Old Girl With Insomnia and Daytime Sleepiness

A 12-year-old girl comes to the clinic with difficulty initiating and maintaining sleep. She also has involuntary sleep episodes in school. The problem began about a year ago, after she was involved in a car accident; she sustained head trauma and was hospitalized for 2 weeks. Before the accident, she was a good student with no sleep complaints. She has fully recovered from the accident and has only a small forehead scar from the injury. Her mother thinks the sleep problem is related to hormonal changes associated with puberty. Actigraphy shows a highly variable sleep-wake schedule that is divided into four short blocks throughout the day.

18. The *most* likely diagnosis is
  A. DSWPD
  B. Shift-work sleep disorder
  C. Non–24-hour sleep-wake disorder
  D. Irregular sleep-wake rhythm disorder

19. The pathogenesis of this condition includes all of the following *except*
  A. Reduced exposure to light-dark signals
  B. Suprachiasmatic nucleus (SCN) dysfunction
  C. Morning melatonin release
  D. Low levels of physical activity during the 24-hour cycle

20. One of the *most* successful treatments for irregular sleep-wake rhythm disorder has been
  A. Chronotherapy, bright light therapy, vitamin B_{12}, and hypnotics
  B. Melatonin and bright light therapy
  C. Melatonin alone
  D. Stimulus control, bright light therapy, and zolpidem

21. Circadian rhythm disorders are common in the following medical disorders *except*
  A. Hepatic encephalopathy
  B. Parkinson disease
  C. Type 2 diabetes
  D. Dementia

A Case of Hating the Night Shift

A 27-year-old nurse began working a rotating shift 6 months ago in a community hospital. Her schedule has required working three 12-hour days per week with rotation to the next shift the following week. At first, the new schedule worked out well for her family, and she had no trouble adapting to the weekly change in shifts. However, after a few months of rotating, she found it increasingly difficult to stay awake on the night shift. A coworker recently found her asleep in the nurse's station, and now the patient is worried about losing her job.

22. You would expect her condition to remit if she
  A. Discontinued rotating shifts and only worked nights
  B. Discontinued working the night shift and worked only a regular day or evening shift
  C. Took a hypnotic at home after her shift to increase sleep time
  D. Took a wakefulness-promoting drug at 7 PM when she does the night shifts

23. She reports that after working the 7 PM to 7 AM shift, daytime sleep duration and quality are reasonably good. You should consider treating her with
  A. A short-acting hypnotic to consolidate sleep
  B. A hypnotic with about a 6-hour half-life to increase TST
  C. Methylphenidate 10 mg at 8 PM
  D. Armodafinil 150 mg at 10 PM

24. Which one of the following actions would be *most* advisable for a patient with a shift-work–type disorder?
    A. Get to sleep soon after the night shift is over
    B. Go to bed 5 hours after getting off the night shift
    C. Allow a modest amount of sunlight in the sleeping room
    D. Increase the room temperature during the sleep period by 3° to 5°F

Grandma and Grandpa Will Not Meet for Dinner

Robert invites his 68-year-old grandfather, Bill, and 67-year-old grandmother, Susan, for dinner to his favorite restaurant. He suggests they meet at 7:30 PM Friday night, but they ask him to make it at 5 PM because they typically get ready for bed by 7:30 to 8 PM. Bill usually wakes up at 4 AM, and Susan is awake by 5 AM. Bill is distressed about the early awakenings and recently asked his primary care physician for a sleeping pill to try to extend his sleep time. This pattern of early to bed and early to rise began for both grandparents in their early 60s. They were expecting to be able to sleep in later after they retired from work at 65 years of age.

25. Given this information, what is the grandparents' *most* likely diagnosis?
    A. DSWPD
    B. Irregular sleep-wake rhythm disorder
    C. Non–24-hour sleep-wake disorder
    D. ASWPD

26. About what time would you expect Bill's DLMO to occur?
    A. 4:00 AM
    B. 2:00 AM
    C. 6:00 PM
    D. 7:30 PM

27. About what time would you expect Bill's core body temperature minimum (CBTmin) to occur?
    A. 1:00 AM
    B. 4:00 AM
    C. 12:00 AM
    D. 11:00 PM

28. Although you know there is inadequate data to support using melatonin for ASWSD, your patient wants to try it anyway. You decide to prescribe 3 mg of melatonin for Bill. At what time do you suggest he take it?
    A. At bedtime
    B. Midnight
    C. 3:00 PM
    D. 6:00 AM

29. What is a possible cause of this disorder?
    A. Early morning walks
    B. Lack of exposure to morning light
    C. No light perception
    D. Intact, overpowering *CLOCK* genes that promote early awakenings

Charlie Cannot Hold Down a Job

Charlie, age 37 years, was in a serious motor vehicle accident 4 years ago that caused loss of the ability to see and perceive light. He was trained as an engineer and has a degree from Georgia Tech. After extensive rehabilitation, he qualified to return to work. However, he found it difficult to get to sleep. His primary care physician thought the problem was caused by the psychological trauma of losing sight, so his physician prescribed an antidepressant. Even so, Charlie found it more and more difficult to stick to a regular sleep-wake schedule. Some nights he found it "nearly impossible" to sleep. The sleep problem became so intense that his work began to suffer, and his poor work performance was attributed to depression. His physician increased the antidepressant without improvement in mood or sleep. Charlie decided to take disability because he could not produce quality work owing to poor sleep.

30. What is the *most* likely diagnosis?
   A. Shift-work disorder
   B. Irregular sleep-wake rhythm disorder
   C. Non–24-hour sleep-wake disorder
   D. ASWPD

31. This disorder is characterized by
   A. Sleep-wake rhythms that are progressively longer than 24 hours
   B. Progressive delays in sleep-wake schedules by 1 to 2 hours per day
   C. A steady drift of the sleep period by 4 to 7 hours each day
   D. Mostly in-phase rhythms with acute out-of-phase periods

32. The pathophysiology is
   A. Almost always head trauma
   B. Tumor in the SCN
   C. Absence of light information to the brain
   D. Melatonin depletion

33. The best initial treatment strategy is
   A. Tasimelteon 20 mg administration upon awakening
   B. Melatonin 0.5 mg upon awakening
   C. Melatonin 3 mg 1 hour before desired bedtime
   D. Melatonin 0.5 mg every 4 hours while awake

Dad Threw a Bucket of Water on His Son

A 17-year-old high school junior is an A student but has been late to school 37 times this year. The student and his parents have had to meet with school officials on several occasions, and there is a risk of expulsion. His parents believe the problem is that their son is oppositional. They sent him to a psychologist, who reported that their son is extremely bright but is not being challenged academically. His parents decided that he would not be able to drive the family car unless he consistently awakened in time for school. This plan failed, leaving his parents at their wits' end. They cajoled and threatened and removed his driving privilege; still, the problem persisted. One morning, the father became so frustrated that he went into his son's room at 7 AM and threw a bucket of water on him. The son jumped out of bed and began hitting his father with his fists. This combative behavior upon awakening was uncharacteristic and had never happened before. As a result of the continued tardiness and aggressive behavior, a psychiatric consultation was scheduled.

34. What is the *most* likely diagnosis?
   A. DSWPD
   B. Irregular sleep-wake rhythm disorder
   C. Non–24-hour sleep-wake disorder
   D. Rapid eye movement (REM) behavior disorder

35. Which symptom is *most* common in this disorder?
   A. Difficulty staying alert in the afternoon
   B. Difficulty staying alert in the evening
   C. Difficulty getting to sleep before midnight
   D. Sleeping beyond 10 hours most nights

36. Treatment should be
   A. Bright light for 30 minutes upon awakening
   B. Evening bright light for 30 minutes
   C. Bright light for 30 minutes shortly after CBTmin
   D. Zolpidem 10 mg at 11 PM

37. Which of the following would likely make symptoms worse?
   A. 3 mg of melatonin at 6 AM
   B. 3 mg of melatonin at 8 PM
   C. Bright light exposure at 7 AM
   D. Temazepam 30 mg qhs

38. How long does it take for the human biological oscillator to complete one cycle, also known as *Tau*?
   A. 26.3 hours
   B. 24.2 hours
   C. 21.3 hours
   D. 23.9 hours

39. Which assessment is *not* useful to make the diagnosis?
   A. Actigraphy
   B. Sleep diary
   C. Core body temperature monitoring
   D. PSG

Assistant Secretary of State Falls Asleep at an Important Dinner

The Ambassador to Japan complains of excessive daytime sleepiness. He recently fell asleep at a fundraising dinner for the president in Washington, DC. He was terribly embarrassed by the incident and decided to seek medical help; this was not the first time he had an involuntary sleep episode. He travels overseas a great deal for his job, and recent trips to China and Japan were particularly demanding. He often feels sleepy in meetings and has trouble sleeping at night. He can rarely sleep on a plane and has a history of snoring. He is 5 feet, 9 inches tall and weighs 210 lb.

40. Given this information, what is the *most* likely diagnosis?
   A. DSWPD
   B. Jet lag disorder
   C. Non–24-hour sleep-wake disorder
   D. Shift-work disorder

41. Symptoms of this disorder usually include
   A. Difficulty sleeping on a plane
   B. Impairment of daytime functioning
   C. Excessive sleeping on planes
   D. A sleep-wake rhythm of greater than 25.5 hours

42. This disorder only occurs when
   A. Crossing four or more time zones
   B. Crossing at least two time zones
   C. Traveling from west to east
   D. Traveling from east to west

43. It is usually easier to tolerate travel that is
   A. Westward travel of four time zones
   B. Westward travel of eight time zones
   C. Eastward travel of four time zones
   D. Eastward travel of six time zones

44. To adapt to a flight from New York to London, the *best* strategy is to
- **A.** Stay up later by 1 hour for four nights before the trip
- **B.** Take 10 mg of melatonin at 8 PM for four mornings before the trip
- **C.** Go to bed earlier by 1 hour four nights before the trip
- **D.** Get bright light exposure in the late afternoon and evening walking around London

CNN Reporter Falls Asleep at the Wheel

A CNN reporter in Atlanta regularly appears on the 5 AM (Eastern Standard Time) international news. She needs to be at the studio by 3:45 AM for makeup and to review stories. She lives about 45 minutes away and has to leave the house by 3:00 AM, so she wakes up most mornings at 2 AM having gone to bed at 7 PM. She does the show 5 days a week, on Monday, Tuesday, Thursday, Friday, and Saturday. On her days off, she sleeps in to about 7:30 AM. During a recent trip to the studio one morning, she fell asleep at the wheel, went off the road, and hit a telephone pole. The airbag deployed, and she did not sustain any serious injuries.

45. What is the *most* likely diagnosis?
- **A.** Jet lag disorder
- **B.** Irregular sleep-wake rhythm disorder
- **C.** Shift-work disorder
- **D.** Advance sleep-wake phase disorder

46. Assuming she has circadian alignment with her work schedule, at what time is her dim light melatonin onset (DLMO).
- **A.** 4:00 AM
- **B.** 2:00 AM
- **C.** 5:00 PM
- **D.** 12:00 AM

47. For an individual working the night shift, which treatment strategy is appropriate?
- **A.** Bright light at the end of the shift
- **B.** Bright light exposure at the beginning of the shift
- **C.** Modafinil or armodafinil at 10:00 AM
- **D.** Bright light exposure on the way home from work

48. Individuals working night or rotating shifts have been shown to be at increased risk of all of the following *except*
- **A.** Obesity
- **B.** Family disturbances
- **C.** Breast cancer
- **D.** Dementia

ANSWERS

1. D.   This case of a young man presenting with excessive daytime sleepiness poses an interesting diagnostic challenge. The onset of symptoms suggests narcolepsy or a circadian rhythm disorder. He has poor sleep hygiene, and his sleepiness could be caused by chronic insufficient sleep. No sleep-wake schedule data are included, so before ordering a PSG, a 2-week sleep diary is the logical next step. The diary or even 2 weeks of actigraphy could provide very useful information regarding his habitual sleep schedule.

2. A.   The least likely diagnosis is narcolepsy because he has evidence of a circadian rhythm disorder, including an irregular sleep schedule and history such that with 12 hours of sleep on weekends, he feels fully alert the rest of the day. The patient also denies cataplexy and sleep paralysis, which are symptoms of narcolepsy, and there is no history of sleep attacks. Paradoxic insomnia, also known as *sleep state misperception insomnia*, and psychophysiologic insomnia are unlikely, but given the history, they are more plausible than narcolepsy. Finally, idiopathic hypersomnolence is a possibility, but that is not an option here. (ICSD3, pp 143–188)

3. B. The phase response curve (PRC) for melatonin is shifted about 180 degrees from that of light. DLMO usually occurs in the late afternoon or early evening for conventional sleepers without a phase delay or an advance. In patients with DSWPD, melatonin onset is usually 10 PM or later.

4. B. Although behavioral factors can play a substantial role in initiating and maintaining a delayed sleep pattern, they are not considered to be the primary cause of the disorder. In most cases, the patient cannot initiate sleep at more conventional hours, even when sleep hygiene is vastly improved. Social interaction and use of caffeine in the evening can perpetuate the delayed sleep phase pattern, making it particularly hard to resolve.

5. B. The PRC indicates that whereas light given after the temperature nadir produces a phase advance, light given before the temperature nadir produces a phase delay. The closer to the switch point on the PRC for bright light exposure, the stronger the effect. Patients with delayed sleep phase have a delayed temperature rhythm, so advancing it requires morning light. There are no well-established protocols for light duration and timing. However, light presented at an intensity of 2500 to 10,000 lux for 30 to 60 minutes per day at the appropriate time usually produces the desired effect. (Morgenthaler et al, 2007)

6. B. Evidence shows that alterations in the homeostatic regulation of sleep might play a role in DSWPD, and compared with control participants, these patients show a decreased ability to compensate for sleep loss during the subjective day and the first hours of subjective night. Alterations in circadian timing and impaired sleep recovery contribute to symptoms of insomnia and excessive sleepiness in DSWPD. Sleep architecture seems to be nearly normal when patients with DSWPD sleep during their habitual sleep times. (Uchiyama et al, 1999)

7. D. Some evidence supports a genetic basis to DSWPD. In a few cases, the syndrome is familial and has an autosomal-dominant mode of inheritance. Additional support for a genetic basis for DSWPD comes from reports of polymorphisms in circadian genes such as *PER3*, the arylalkylamine *N*-acetyltransferase gene *AANAT*, human leukocyte antigen (HLA) genes, and *CLOCK*. However, the strongest support for a familial disorder is for ASWPD, and several cases of familial ASWPD can be found in the literature; these families show a clear autosomal-dominant mode of inheritance of ASWPD, and genetic analysis of these familial cases shows heterogeneity of this disorder between and even within large families. Gene polymorphisms have been identified in the circadian clock gene *PER2* in a large family with ASWPD. (Ancoli-Israel et al, 2001; Satoh et al, 2003; Toh et al, 2001)

8. C. We are told of the onset of insomnia related to her husband's death 5 years earlier. We know she does not have acute insomnia because the duration is longer than 90 days. We need to know her habitual sleep-wake times to discern the pattern before proceeding with additional studies or treatment. (ICSD3, pp 19-48)

9. D. PSG is not required for diagnosing or characterizing insomnia, and no criteria have been established for using the PSG in ASWPD. However, if obstructive sleep apnea is also suspected in either condition, a PSG is indicated.

10. D. Not enough clinical information is provided in this scenario. Habitual time in bed is important. Snoring and apnea are potentially important clinical issues, yet without knowing whether chronic sleep deprivation is due to an early morning insomnia, it is not possible to know whether the other PSG results (AHI = 8) are relevant.

11. D. A good way to understand the effects of light and melatonin on sleep phase is to remember that melatonin "pulls" the rhythm toward the time of administration, and light "pushes" it away from time of exposure. In a case of ASWPD, morning melatonin is appropriate if it is taken several hours after the core body temperature nadir in the morning. Auger et al., Clin Sleep Med 2015; 11(10): 1199-1236. (Lewy et al, 1998)

12. C. DLMO is significantly earlier in patients with ASWPD compared with normal participants.

13. A. Actigraphy is the correct answer because PSG is neither indicated nor required to make the diagnosis. Core body temperature recording could establish an advanced circadian rhythm, but it is impractical for the majority of sleep clinics or laboratories. Sleep diaries are self-report measures, and although they correlate with objective measures, they are not as reliable. (ICSD3, pp 198-203)

14. C. This image (see Fig. 2–1) is of a double raster plot of a patient's activity level obtained from an actigraph. The double raster plot replicates the past 24 hours on the next line down on the left side of the image. The areas with dark bars represent activity or wakefulness, and the areas without bars represent periods of quiescence or sleep. The pattern of activity is shifting to the right, or phase delaying, on a daily basis. A free-running disorder known as non–24-hour sleep-wake disorder is characterized by successive delays of the sleep-wake schedule, which is chronic.

15. D. The non–24-hour sleep-wake pattern, characterized by the actigraph plots in Figure 2–1, are similar to those seen in participants placed in a constant-routine experimental environment where light-dark, social, and other cues—known as *zeitgebers*, or "time givers"—are controlled or made unavailable. Sighted persons in normal environmental conditions are highly unlikely to have this sleep-wake pattern. (ICSD3, pp 209-214)

16. C. Antidepressants—including selective serotonin reuptake inhibitors, monoamine oxidase inhibitors, and tricyclic antidepressants—are not known to influence circadian rhythms. Other factors that include exposure to light-dark cues, behavioral routines, and exercise have been shown to affect circadian rhythms.

17. D. Light therapy for non–24-hour sleep-wake disorder has been shown to be effective in some persons with no light perception. It remains possible for the melanopsin-containing ganglion cells in the retina to accept and transmit the light signals to the SCN. Light is known to have a more powerful effect on circadian rhythms than exogenous melatonin. (Czeisler et al, 1995)

18. D. The symptoms described in this case are consistent with irregular sleep-wake rhythm disorder. Sleep is usually broken into several shifts without a regular pattern. It is possible that the head trauma caused a dysfunction in the processes that help establish a regular sleep-wake pattern. In DSWPD, the pattern is consistent and fixed, but with the free-running type of circadian sleep disorder, the sleep-wake pattern is continually drifting later each day. (ICSD-3, pp 204-208)

19. C. Irregular sleep-wake rhythm disorder is thought to be due to a dysfunction of the central nervous system area that regulates circadian rhythms, most likely the SCN. Because the disorder is rare, melatonin release patterns in this population are not well established, so we have to assume the release pattern is abnormal. Reduced exposure to zeitgebers could also be involved in the etiology.

20. A. Irregular sleep-wake rhythm disorder is very difficult to treat. The most effective strategy described in the literature is a combination approach with chronotherapy, bright light treatments, vitamin B_{12} supplementation, and hypnotics. (Okawa et al, 1990; Yamadera et al, 1996)

21. C. Circadian rhythm disorders are often comorbid with medical and psychiatric disorders. However, there is no evidence that diabetes affects circadian rhythms.

22. B. Shift-work sleep disorder resolves when the worker discontinues the night shift and establishes a regular day or evening shift. This commonsense approach is rarely accepted by patients because they have often selected the night shift for social or economic reasons. Patients who are required to work the night shift might seek a medical exemption to work only day or evening shifts.

23. D. She does not complain of poor sleep, so a hypnotic is not a good choice. Also, when patients have severe sleepiness on their shift, improved sleep duration does not usually resolve the sleepiness. The first-line approach is modafinil or armodafinil. Armodafinil has been approved by the Food and Drug Administration for treating shift-work sleep disorder.

Studies in the sleep laboratory, as well as in simulated work environments, have shown armodafinil to be effective for treating excessive sleepiness associated with working on the night shift or rotating shifts.

24. A. It is advisable to tell patients with shift-work sleep disorder to avoid morning light and to get into a dark, quiet, cool room as soon as possible after their shift ends. Sunlight after the night shift can cause a phase advance, and the light itself can have an alerting effect, making it difficult to fall asleep. Additionally, areas on the PRC known as *wake maintenance zones* show when the probability of sleeping is considerably reduced owing to circadian wake drive.

25. D. ASWPD is characterized by an inability to stay awake past 8:00 PM, and early morning awakening is often a complaint. ASWPD is more often seen in individuals in the sixth decade of life and older, rarely before that. The prevalence is not known but is thought to be about 1% of this age group. PSG is required for diagnosis and should be normal, as is the TST. (ICSD3, pp 198-203)

26. C. DMLO is a useful circadian marker that occurs about 2 to 3 hours before habitual bedtime.

27. A. CBTmin usually occurs 2 to 3 hours before sleep offset. For individuals without a circadian rhythm disorder, this is usually 4 to 5 AM. The reduced core body temperature correlates with melatonin production or suppression. One way to compute CBTmin is to identify DLMO and add 7 hours.

28. D. This patient's sleep cycle is advanced, so to delay the morning melatonin is appropriate even though the AASM position paper on Advance Sleep Wake Phase Disorder concluded there was inadequate evidentce for using melatonin as well as prescribed sleep-wake scheduling, timed physical activity/exercise, strategic avoidance of light, sleep-promoting medications, wakefulness promoting medications, other somatic interventions, or combination treatments. Some caution for sedation should be taken in giving anyone melatonin during waking hours.

29. A. Light exposure during very early morning hours is likely to cause a phase advance. Phase shifting can occur when light exposure is before or after the CBTmin. To move the sleep-wake schedule later, bright light exposure should be in the evening.

30. C. Non–24-hour sleep-wake disorder occurs in 50% of blind individuals. It is characterized by successive delays of the sleep-wake schedule. Entrainment does not occur, and patients often complain of sleep-onset problems as well as daytime sleepiness. Because the circadian rhythm is free running, most complaints occur when the rhythm is out of phase with desired sleep-wake times. (ICSD3, pp 209-214)

31. B. Light exposure causes melatonin suppression. In blind individuals without light perception, this suppression does not occur, which allows an intrinsic phase delay to take place. The internal circadian rhythm is slightly longer than 24 hours, and light is the most powerful zeitgeber. (ICSD3, pp 209-214)

32. C. Without light exposure to the retina, a phase delay can occur.

33. C. To establish entrainment, a dose of melatonin 1 hour or so before bedtime is appropriate. The ideal dose has not been established and studies have evaluated doses from 0.5 to 10 mg. Melatonin administered at other times may "pull" the circadian rhythm in an undesired direction. Tasimelteon 20 mg taken about 1 hour before bedtime is also an MT receptor agonist that may be used. (Neubauer et, al, Drugs Today, 2015.)

34. A. Patients with DSWPD complain of an inability to get to sleep at a socially desirable time. Their sleep-wake rhythm is out of sync, and they have trouble waking up in time for school or work. Despite their best efforts, sleep before midnight is rare except with significant sleep deprivation. People with DSWPD are often viewed as lazy or oppositional. Drugs or alcohol can be a part of the clinical picture, and family discord is common. (ICSD3, pp 191-198)

35. C. The late sleep-wake schedule may begin as voluntary, but the delayed sleep phase patient cannot reset earlier without treatment. Sleep is perfectly normal at undesired hours. Sleep-onset difficulties are present, but the most troublesome aspect is difficulty with waking early. A family history is present in about 40% of cases.   (ICSD3, pp 191-198)

36. C. Bright light "pushes" the rhythm earlier in cases of DSWPD. The ideal timing is shortly after CBTmin, but this strategy is often impractical unless a family member can assist the patient by waking her or him at the appropriate time. The light exposure duration is not well established, but 30 minutes has consistently been shown to impact rhythms.

37. A. Melatonin "pulls" the rhythm, so morning administration would be inappropriate. Evening administration of melatonin at a few hours before expected bedtime is the best strategy.

38. B. *Tau* refers to the normal circadian length, which is 24.2 hours.

39. D. According to the ICSD3, the diagnosis of advanced or delayed sleep phase is appropriately diagnosed using a sleep diary or actigraphy. Core body temperature can also be used but is for the most part impractical in a clinical setting. One night of PSG does not offer enough data to support a circadian rhythm disorder.   (ICSD3, pp 101-203)

40. B. Jet lag occurs when eastward or westward travel spans several time zones. The core issue is desynchrony between body time and environmental clock time. The disorder causes problems with excessive sleepiness, alertness, and daytime functioning.   (ICSD3, pp 220-224)

41. B. Jet lag does not occur in all individuals who travel across times zones. It is a temporary condition that resolves because of adaptation to the new time zone or a rapid return to the original zone. The severity of symptoms is often influenced by behaviors of the traveler. Daytime function can be significantly impaired.

42. B. Jet lag does not occur if there is no transmeridian travel, and ICSD3 criteria require transmeridian travel across two or more time zones. The symptoms and pathophysiology have nothing to do with being on a plane.   (ICSD3, pp 220-224)

43. A. Circadian rhythm for normal healthy adults is slightly greater than 24 hours (about 24.2 hours). This rhythm predisposes toward a phase delay of the sleep-wake cycle. When traveling in a westward direction across time zones, adaptation requires a phase delay, but traveling in an eastward direction requires a phase advance; it is therefore easier to tolerate westward travel. If travel requires crossing more than eight time zones, the direction of travel has less impact on the ease of adaptation.

44. C. Traveling New York to London involves an eastward flight. Adaptation to the new environmental time for eastward flights requires a phase advance of the sleep-wake rhythm of 5 hours. Although it may be impractical to go to bed early and wake earlier for several nights before the trip, it is a phase-advance strategy that could be useful.

45. C. Shift-work disorder can involve rotating shifts, night shifts, or early shifts that result in partial night and day schedules combined.

46. D. DLMO is a useful circadian marker. It occurs about 2 to 3 hours before habitual bedtime. In this reporter's case, habitual bedtime is 7:00 PM.

47. B. Bright light at the workplace is a valuable strategy if timed properly. It should be provided at the beginning of the shift. Wakefulness-promoting drugs can be prescribed for increasing alertness at desired times, but taken too late in the day, they may result in sleep difficulties. Bright light exposure at the end of a night shift could also inhibit sleep onset if the sleep attempt is made shortly after arriving home.

48. D. Substantial data indicate that several organ systems may be negatively affected by rotating or night shift work. No data suggest that working night or rotating shifts increases the risk of dementia.

Summary

Highly Recommended

- Auger RR, Burgess HJ, Emens JS, et al: Clinical practice guideline for the treatment of intrinsic circadian rhythm sleep-wake disorders: Advanced sleep-wake phase disorder (ASWPD), delayed sleep-wake phase disorder (DSWPD), non-24-hour sleep-wake rhythm disorder (N24SWD), and irregular sleep-wake rhythm disorder (ISWRD). An update for 2015. *J Clin Sleep Med*. 11(10):1199–1236, 2015. (Download "Intrinsic CRSWD Decision Tree" from AASM website)
- *International Classification of Sleep* Disorders, ed 3, pp 199–224
- Morgenthaler TI, Lee-Chiong T, Alessi C, et al: Practice parameters for the clinical evaluation and treatment of circadian rhythm sleep disorders: an American Academy of Sleep Medicine report, *Sleep* 30:1445–1459, 2007
- Quera Salva MA, Hartley S, Léger D, et al: Non-24-Hour Sleep-Wake Rhythm Disorder in the Totally Blind: Diagnosis and Management. *Front Neurol*. 2017 Dec 18;8:686

Circadian rhythm sleep disorders are commonly seen in clinical practice, and you can expect at least 24 questions on this topic. However, content related to this topic may be found in other sections of the examination, for example, in the basic science sections that cover sleep mechanisms and circadian physiology (e.g., the physiology of the SCN) and pharmacology (e.g., ramelteon, melatonin, and modafinil). Thus, knowledge of this topic is essential.

Epidemiology

- DSWPD
  - Reported more often as appearing in adolescence
  - Few studies exist with regard to prevalence; may be 7% in adults and adolescents
- ASWPD
  - Considered to be less prevalent than DSWPD
  - Seen more in older adults
  - Estimated prevalence of 1% in middle-aged adults
- Non–24-hour sleep-wake disorder
  - This type is considered to be rare in sighted persons
  - 50% to 70% of blind persons are not well entrained to a 24-hour sleep-wake rhythm
  - Non–24-hour sleep-wake disorder can be diagnosed in 13% to 18% of blind persons
- Irregular sleep-wake rhythm disorder
  - Unknown prevalence
  - More often seen in patients with comorbid neurologic disorders
- Shift-work disorder
  - Seen in 2% to 5% of shift workers

Pathophysiology

Behavioral preference may play a role but is not a primary factor.
- DSWPD
  - Inability to phase-advance sleep schedule despite consequences
  - Hypersensitivity to nighttime suppression of melatonin by bright light
  - Genetic basis: polymorphisms in circadian genes
  - Factors of the sleep homeostatic process might play a role
- ASWPD
  - Inability to phase-delay sleep schedule despite consequences
  - Abnormal phase response curve
  - Rhythm shorter than 24 hours
  - Gene polymorphisms have been identified in some families with the disorder

- Non–24-hour sleep-wake disorder
  - Seen in some forms of blindness
  - Absence of light exposure
  - Dampened melatonin rhythm
  - Reduced exposure to social cues
- Irregular sleep-wake rhythm disorder
  - Reduced exposure to light
  - Reduced exposure to social cues
- Shift-work disorder
  - Maladaptation to rotating or night shift
  - No entrainment to night-wake and day-sleep schedule

Diagnostic Methods and Requirements

- DSWPD
  - Clinical history
    - Difficulty getting to sleep before 2 or 3 AM
    - Difficulty waking up in the morning
  - Actigraphy or sleep diary
- ASWPD
  - Clinical history
    - Difficulty staying up past 7 or 8 PM
    - Distressed by early morning awakening
  - Actigraphy or sleep diary
- Non–24-hour sleep-wake disorder
  - Clinical history
    - No sleep-wake cycle entrainment
    - Sleep period delays by 2 to 3 hours each cycle
    - Misalignment 3 out of 4 weeks per month
  - Actigraphy or sleep diary
- Irregular sleep-wake rhythm disorder
  - Clinical history
    - Unpredictable sleep-wake schedule
    - Sleep is usually broken into three to four blocks around the 24-hour cycle
  - Actigraphy or sleep diary
- Shift-work disorder
  - Clinical history
    - Occurs in rotating or night shift workers
    - Insomnia during daytime and/or excessive sleepiness on night shift

Treatment

- DSWPD
  - Sleep hygiene
  - Bright light in the morning
  - Melatonin 5 to 7 hours before desired sleep-onset time
  - Chronotherapy is difficult but can be effective
- ASWPD
  - Sleep hygiene
  - Bright light in the evening
  - Melatonin in the morning at or near the desired waking time
  - Chronotherapy is difficult but can be effective
- Non–24-hour sleep-wake disorder
  - Should include multimodal treatment (Quera, 2017)
    - Bright light
    - Vitamin B_{12}

- Rapid-released melatonin or tasimelteon taken about 1 hour before desired bedtime. Treatment should start about when the patient's time of falling asleep roughly aligns with the desired bedtime. The optimal dose for melatonin has not been established, and there are data for doses ranging from 0.5 to 10 mg. Tasimelteon (the trade name is Hetlioz) is a melatonin agonist approved in the United States and Europe for non–24-hour sleep-wake disorder. Dosing is 20-mg capsule once a day, before bedtime, at the same time every night.
  - Sleep hygiene
- Irregular sleep-wake rhythm disorder
  - Should include multimodal treatment
    - Bright light
    - Vitamin B$_{12}$
    - Melatonin
    - Sleep hygiene
- Shift-work disorder
  - Sleep hygiene
  - Nonbenzodiazepines to promote daytime sleep
  - Wakefulness-promoting drugs (modafinil and armodafinil) for staying alert on night shifts
    - Be alert for potential adverse effects such as increased insomnia during daytime sleep attempts
    - Be alert for rash or other allergic reactions

REFERENCES

American Academy of Sleep Medicine. *International classification of sleep disorders*. ed 3. Darien, Ill.: American Academy of Sleep Medicine; 2014.

Ancoli-Israel S, Schnierow B, Kelsoe J, Fink R. A pedigree of one family with delayed sleep phase syndrome. *Chronobiol Int*. 2001;18:831–840.

Czeisler CA, Shanahan TL, Klerman EB, et al. Suppression of melatonin secretion in some blind patients by exposure to bright light. *N Engl J Med*. 1995;332:6–11.

Lewy AJ, Bauer VK, Ahmed S, et al. The human phase response curve (PRC) to melatonin is about 12 hours out of phase with the PRC to light. *Chronobiol Int*. 1998;15:71–83.

Morgenthaler TI, Lee-Chiong T, Alessi C, et al. Practice parameters for the clinical evaluation and treatment of circadian rhythm sleep disorders: an American Academy of Sleep Medicine report. *Sleep*. 2007;30:1445–1459.

Neubauer DN. Tasimelteon for the treatment of non-24 hour sleep wake disorder. *Drugs Today (Barc)*. 2015;51(1):29–35.

Okawa M, Mishima K, Nanami T, et al. Vitamin B$_{12}$ treatment for sleep–wake rhythm disorders. *Sleep*. 1990;13:15–23.

Quera Salva MA, Hartley S, Léger D, et al. Non-24-hour sleep-wake rhythm disorder in the totally blind: diagnosis and management. *Front Neurol*. 2017;8:686.

Sack RL, Auckley D, Auger RR, et al. Circadian rhythm sleep disorders: part II, advanced sleep phase disorder, delayed sleep phase disorder, non 24 hour sleep wake disorder, and irregular sleep–wake rhythm. An American Academy of Sleep Medicine review. *Sleep*. 2007;30:1484–1501.

Satoh K, Mishima K, Inoue Y, et al. Two pedigrees of familial advanced sleep phase syndrome in Japan. *Sleep*. 2003;26:416–417.

Toh KL, Jones CR, He Y, et al. An *hPer2* phosphorylation site mutation in familial advanced sleep phase syndrome. *Science*. 2001;291:1040–1043.

Uchiyama M, Okawa M, Shibui K, et al. Poor recovery sleep after sleep deprivation in delayed sleep phase syndrome. *Psychiatry Clin Neurosci*. 1999;53:195–197.

Yamadera H, Takahashi K, Okawa M. A multicenter study of sleep–wake rhythm disorders: clinical features of sleep–wake rhythm disorders. *Psychiatry Clin Neurosci*. 1996;50:195–201.

Insomnia

QUESTIONS
Where Does One Begin?

A 50-year-old woman presents with the complaint of "insomnia." She was always a good sleeper until she had her first child at 33 years of age, and then she developed difficulty initiating and maintaining sleep. At age 35 years, she started the selective serotonin reuptake inhibitor (SSRI) antidepressant fluoxetine, which she still takes. Her sleep greatly improved when she started the SSRI, but 6 months ago, she again developed trouble staying asleep. She has no trouble falling asleep; in fact, she falls asleep the minute her head hits the pillow. However, she typically, wakes up after 3 to 4 hours and is then "wide awake," sometimes for hours. She feels very tired during the day but does not nap. Her periods have become irregular, but she denies hot flashes or night sweats. She lives with her husband and two teenage daughters, and her home life seems calm and stable. She works in real estate part time but denies stress or anxiety over the bad real estate market, stating "My husband is a good provider. I've never been happier, never had less stress. Then bang, out of the blue, I start having sleep problems." She denies racing thoughts but admits that in the middle of the night, she can perseverate on not being able to return to sleep. She is concerned she is "wrecking" her health and worries about this as she lies in bed trying to get back to sleep. Overall, she estimates obtaining only 5 hours of sleep a night. Her only surgery has been a tonsillectomy at age 6 years. Her only medication is the SSRI, and she has gained 20 lb in the past 2 years. She does admit that about 1 year ago, her husband started complaining about her snoring. She saw her physician recently and states, "All my blood work came back normal." On physical examination, you note she is overweight with a body mass index (BMI) of 30 and a neck circumference of 16 inches. Oropharyngeal exam shows a Mallampati 4 throat opening, and she has no tonsils. The rest of the examination is unremarkable.

1. The *most* likely type of insomnia is
   A. Adjustment insomnia
   B. Idiopathic insomnia
   C. Paradoxical insomnia
   D. Psychophysiologic insomnia

2. Which aspect of her presentation is the *least* common feature of chronic insomnia?
   A. In the past, her insomnia improved with the SSRI
   B. She first had sleep problems when she had children
   C. She is having sleep difficulty as she enters menopause
   D. She does not nap

3. As you review her sleep hygiene, you learn more about her evening habits. Which habit is *most* likely contributing to her maintenance insomnia?
   A. She eats cheese and crackers 2 hours before bedtime
   B. She often sips wine in bed to help her relax
   C. She watches the evening news in the living room before going to bed and admits that the stories often upset her
   D. She and her husband listen to classical music as they go to sleep

4. What other disorder is likely contributing to her sleep-maintenance insomnia?
   A. Depression
   B. Narcolepsy
   C. Obstructive sleep apnea (OSA)
   D. Obesity hypoventilation syndrome

5. You order a polysomnogram (PSG). Which of the following findings would be *least* surprising?
   A. Her total sleep time (TST) was 7 hours, 45 minutes
   B. She has central sleep apnea with Cheyne-Stokes respirations
   C. She has an increase in her amount of rapid eye movement (REM) sleep
   D. She has increased electromyography (EMG) tone during REM

6. According to the *International Classification of Sleep Disorders* (ed. 3 [ICSD3]), which one of the following subtypes of insomnia would *not* be classified as a chronic insomnia?
   A. Insomnia due to a mental disorder
   B. Insomnia due to a medical condition
   C. Insomnia due to a drug or substance
   D. Insomnia due to sleep-disruptive environmental circumstances

7. The ICSD3 diagnostic criteria for chronic insomnia disorder requires that the symptoms be present for at least
   A. 1 month
   B. 3 months
   C. 6 months
   D. 12 months

8. Which test has a very high specificity and sensitivity in diagnosing chronic insomnia?
   A. Polysomnography (PSG)
   B. Multiple sleep latency test (MSLT)
   C. Maintenance of wakefulness test (MWT)
   D. Sleep laboratory tests are not indicated for insomnia

9. What is the single *most* useful tool in assessing an insomnia complaint?
   A. Actigraphy
   B. Sleep diary
   C. Beck Depression Inventory
   D. 8 AM serum cortisol

Worried About Having an Awful Disease

A 30-year-old woman is referred to the sleep center by her psychiatrist for an evaluation of "refractory insomnia." She has a history of generalized anxiety and attention-deficit/hyperactivity disorder (ADHD). She has taken paroxetine and methylphenidate for years. The patient appears a bit anxious and somewhat tired but not chronically ill or in any distress. Early in the interview, she shares a fear about a disease she read about on the Internet, fatal familial insomnia.

10. Which of the following statements about fatal familial insomnia is *false*?
   A. It is an exceedingly rare disease
   B. Intravenous immunoglobulin (IVIG) can be useful in prolonging life
   C. It is a neurodegenerative prion disease
   D. Loss of sleep spindles is a common electroencephalograph (EEG) finding on PSG

You learn that she is an aspiring actress and works until 3 AM as a waitress. In the daytime, she often has auditions or rehearsals. During the daytime, she says, "I feel great and am too busy to worry about being tired as long as I don't have some awful disease." She then adds, "If I am having a bad day, I just take a little extra Ritalin."

11. Which feature of her story makes you suspect that she might *not* have insomnia?
    A. She is not giving herself adequate opportunity to sleep
    B. She does not report daytime impairment
    C. She has an anxiety disorder for which she sees a psychiatrist
    D. She may be abusing stimulant medication
    E. A and B

12. The prevalence rate of chronic insomnia disorder varies widely depending on the study; for the general population, the rate *most* commonly quoted in the sleep literature is
    A. 10%
    B. 20%
    C. 30%
    D. 40%

13. Which nonpharmacologic therapy is often successful in treating insomnia?
    A. Freudian psychoanalysis
    B. Jungian dream interpretation
    C. Cognitive behavioral therapy (CBTi)
    D. Eye movement desensitization and reprocessing (EMDR)

14. Which of the following is associated with an increased risk for chronic insomnia?
    A. Increasing age
    B. Female gender
    C. Psychiatric disorders
    D. Chronic medical disorders
    E. All of the above

The Teenager Who Could Not Fall Asleep

A 17-year-old high school senior is brought to the sleep center by his mother because of "insomnia" and excessive daytime sleepiness (EDS). He goes to bed at midnight but cannot fall asleep until approximately 2 AM. He must then wake up at 6:30 AM to make his first advanced-placement class at 7:45 AM. He is very tired during the day and often falls asleep in class. On weekends or during vacation, he stays up just as late, but because he can sleep as long as he wants (often 9 or 10 hours), he then does not feel tired while he is awake.

15. What is the *most* likely diagnosis?
    A. Narcolepsy
    B. Adjustment insomnia
    C. Short-term insomnia
    D. Delayed sleep-wake phase disorder (DSWPD)

Always a Lousy Sleeper

A 33-year-old man presents to the sleep center with a long history of "insomnia." He reports difficulty falling asleep since childhood. He has seen many doctors, including more than one sleep physician, and thinks that he has "tried every medication," including prescription, over-the-counter (OTC), and "herbal" remedies. Some of these drugs helped for a while but then ceased working. You mention Cognitive Behavioral Therapy for Insomnia (CBTi) as a possible treatment, and he claims to "know all about it." He proceeds to tell you about his changes in "sleep hygiene" and how it has not helped his sleep at all. His primary care physician (PCP) has recently diagnosed depression.

16. You explain to him that besides sleep hygiene, CBTi involves all of the following components *except*
  A. Stimulus-control therapy
  B. Sleep-restriction therapy
  C. Hypnosis
  D. Cognitive restructuring
  E. Relaxation training

17. He is interested in CBTi but asks if it is better to combine it with medication, especially in cases of severe insomnia. You explain
  A. Some studies show that medication is better for long-term treatment of insomnia, but CBTi is better for short-term treatment
  B. Most studies show that medication is a far superior treatment in the short term, but CBTi is only slightly superior in long-term treatment of insomnia
  C. Most studies show that CBTi and hypnotic medications are equally efficacious in short-term treatment, but CBTi produces far superior results over the long term
  D. Studies have been inconsistent. Some show that CBTi produces better treatment, but others show medications are better at improving sleep, but unlike CBTi, they come with the risk of tolerance and addiction

18. What is the purpose of stimulus-control therapy?
  A. To consolidate sleep and increase sleep efficiency by curtailing time in bed (TIB)
  B. To reassociate the bed and bedroom with sleep
  C. To reduce somatic tension
  D. To change faulty beliefs and attitudes that perpetuate among patients with insomnia

19. What is the purpose of sleep-restriction therapy?
  A. To consolidate sleep and increase sleep efficiency by curtailing TIB
  B. To reassociate the bed and bedroom with sleep
  C. To reduce somatic tension
  D. To change faulty beliefs and attitudes that perpetuate among patients with insomnia

20. What is the purpose of cognitive restructuring?
  A. To consolidate sleep and increase sleep efficiency by curtailing TIB
  B. To reassociate the bed and bedroom with sleep
  C. To reduce somatic tension
  D. To change faulty beliefs and attitudes that perpetuate among patients with insomnia

21. Recently, his primary care physician (PCP) prescribed a medication that would do "double duty"; the patient was told it should help him sleep and treat his depression. Which medication did his physician likely prescribe?
  A. Trazodone
  B. Zaleplon
  C. Clonazepam
  D. Suvorexant

Because it was having no effect on either his insomnia or depression, his primary care physician stopped the first drug, started him on a new medication for depression, and referred him to your sleep clinic. You see him after he has taken the new drug for 5 nights straight. He quotes the primary care physician (who was quoting a seminar expert), saying that the second antidepressant "should have no effect on sleep." However, the patient reports the new antidepressant has made his initiation insomnia even worse.

22. Which medication is he *most* likely taking?
  A. Mirtazapine
  B. Paroxetine
  C. Amitriptyline
  D. Bupropion

23. Which subtype of insomnia does he have?
   A. Psychophysiologic insomnia
   B. Physiologic (organic) insomnia
   C. Insomnia due to a mental disorder
   D. Idiopathic insomnia

24. He states that he had a "bad reaction" to zolpidem that did not involve rash or anaphylaxis. Which adverse reaction are you *most* concerned about?
   A. Compulsive behaviors
   B. Seizure
   C. Anterograde amnesia
   D. Urinary retention

25. Which herb is *not* touted as a sleep aid?
   A. Basil flower
   B. Valerian root
   C. Chamomile
   D. Kava kava

26. Which OTC medication has proven effective in treating insomnia?
   A. Melatonin
   B. L-Tryptophan
   C. Doxylamine
   D. Diphenhydramine

27. Which of the following hypnotics has demonstrated the *lowest* risk for tolerance and addiction?
   A. Zaleplon
   B. Ramelteon
   C. Zolpidem
   D. Suvorexant

28. In which disorder is there supportive evidence that melatonin improves sleep?
   A. Maintenance insomnia
   B. Shift-work disorder
   C. Circadian rhythm disorder, non–24-hour sleep-wake disorder
   D. All of the above
   E. B and C

Waking Too Early

A 76-year-old woman who is a retired psychiatrist reports to the sleep center with the complaint of "early morning awakening." She wakes each day at 4 AM. This upsets her because she says, "I don't want to start the day in the cold dark." She seeks your help in figuring out whether she has a "primary sleep disorder or depression."

29. What is the *most* important question to ask to understand the nature of her "early morning awakening"?
   A. Does she feel sad?
   B. Does she have suicidal ideations?
   C. What time is she going to bed?
   D. Has she lost interest in activities she normally enjoys?

On further questioning, she admits to multiple awakenings during the night with difficulty returning to sleep. She is tired in the daytime and sometimes naps. She is also being treated for hypertension, chronic obstructive pulmonary disorder, and osteoarthritis.

30. Of the following medications she takes, which one(s) could be causing or exacerbating her sleep problem?
- **A.** Metoprolol
- **B.** Prednisone
- **C.** Ibuprofen
- **D.** All of the above

31. Which medication(s) can cause daytime drowsiness and fatigue, with or without an insomnia complaint?
- **A.** Beta-blockers
- **B.** Alpha$_1$-agonists
- **C.** Alpha$_2$-blockers
- **D.** Adenosine blockers

She admits using alprazolam for many months, until her primary care physician became alarmed because of escalating doses and asked her to stop the drug. He told her that because alprazolam is a short-acting benzodiazepine, there should be no risk of withdrawal symptoms.

32. What *most* likely happened when she stopped alprazolam abruptly?
- **A.** Her original insomnia symptoms returned at their original severity level
- **B.** For the first 2 nights, her insomnia symptoms were much worse, and then they returned to their original level
- **C.** She developed new symptoms, such as heart palpitations, anxiety, and gastrointestinal (GI) distress that lasted for several weeks
- **D.** None of the above

33. Which of the following neurotransmitters promotes wakefulness?
- **A.** Orexin (hypocretin)
- **B.** Gamma-aminobutyric acid (GABA)
- **C.** Dopamine
- **D.** Acetylcholine
- **E.** A, C, and D

34. Caffeine is a wakefulness-promoting agent because
- **A.** It is a histamine agonist
- **B.** It increases serum levels of substance P
- **C.** It is an adenosine-receptor antagonist
- **D.** It increases the release of glutamate from the reticular formation

35. Which statement is the *most* correct explanation for the difference between benzodiazepine-receptor agonists (BzRAs) and nonbenzodiazepine BzRAs?
- **A.** Whereas benzodiazepines act on GABA$_A$, the nonbenzodiazepine BzRAs act on GABA$_B$
- **B.** Compared with benzodiazepines that act nonselectively on the GABA$_A$ receptor, the nonbenzodiazepine BzRAs have a selective affinity for the alpha$_1$ subunit on GABA$_A$ receptors
- **C.** Whereas benzodiazepines act on GABA$_A$ receptors found in the thalamus, the nonbenzodiazepine BzRAs act on the GABA$_A$ receptors located in the reticular formation
- **D.** Whereas benzodiazepines act on benzodiazepine receptors found on the GABA-receptor complex, nonbenzodiazepine BzRAs bind to benzodiazepine receptors found on the serotonin-receptor complex

36. Which pharmacologic effect is lost with the nonbenzodiazepine BzRAs compared with the BzRAs?
- **A.** Anxiolysis
- **B.** Amnesia
- **C.** Anticonvulsant properties
- **D.** A, B, and C

The Insomnia That Will Not Go Away

A 60-year-old woman presents to the sleep clinic with a 5-year history of difficulty falling asleep. She has always been a light sleeper, just like her mother, but her sleep problems really began when her husband died suddenly 5 years ago. During the acute grief phase, she had trouble going to sleep and found that she was afraid to be alone in the house. She started leaving most of the lights on at night, including several table lamps in the bedroom. She moved the TV into the bedroom "to take my mind off things" and started allowing her 80-lb Labrador retriever to sleep with her "to keep me company." She often has a highball late at night to help her relax. She claims that she has been "getting by" but that the past 6 months have seen further deterioration in her sleep, and she is only sleeping 4 to 5 hours a night.

37. Which neurocognitive or neurophysiologic model *best* describes this scenario?
  A. Two-process model (process C and process S) for the sleep-wake cycle
  B. Spielman's three-P model
  C. The physiologic model of hyperarousal
  D. None of the above

She has been using zolpidem 20 mg for the past 2 years in addition to her nighttime beverage of whiskey and ginger ale. Recently, because the 20 mg was not working anymore, she has increased the dose to 30 mg (without the whiskey) and now is worried about drug effects.

38. Which treatment is *most* effective in discontinuing hypnotics in patients with hypnotic dependence?
  A. CBTi combined with hypnotic taper
  B. Psychoanalysis with accelerated hypnotic taper
  C. Slow taper over 10 weeks followed by 6 months of disulfiram along with frequent follow-up
  D. Closely supervised medication taper that allows ad libitum use of low-dose hypnotic

39. Which statement *best* describes paradoxical intention?
  A. As part of relaxation training, patients at first attempt to become as stressed as possible before letting go of all worries
  B. As the final step in sleep-restriction therapy, patients tell themselves that they are only allowed to sleep 4 hours when really they can sleep 7 to 8 hours
  C. As part of stimulus-control therapy, patients are told to find the least comfortable place in the house, such as the bathroom floor, and try to sleep there at night
  D. As part of cognitive restructuring, patients are instructed to attempt to stay awake for 30 minutes when they get into bed, even if they are very sleepy

40. Which of the following is an essential recommendation given as part of CBTi?
  A. Go to bed when sleepy every night and have a fixed wake time
  B. Have a flexible wake time that allows approximately 7 hours of sleep
  C. Keep naps to 30 minutes
  D. Keep the bedroom dark and warm

41. What percentage of patients complaining of insomnia also have a psychiatric disorder?
  A. 10% to 20%
  B. 20% to 30%
  C. 40% to 50%
  D. 70% to 80%

42. In which patient population has hypnotic medication *not* been shown to be a superior treatment when compared with CBTi?
  A. Depressed patients with comorbid insomnia
  B. Patients older than 55 years
  C. Chronic pain patients with comorbid insomnia
  D. 12-year-old patients with comorbid insomnia

43. Chronic insomnia can increase the risk of all of the following *except*
  A. Cervical cancer in women
  B. Depression
  C. Work-related fatalities
  D. Cognitive errors

44. Which condition is the *greatest* predictor for developing insomnia?
  A. Fibromyalgia
  B. Major depressive disorder
  C. Generalized anxiety disorder
  D. Bipolar disorder

45. Which condition will people with insomnia *most* likely develop?
  A. Fibromyalgia
  B. Major depressive disorder
  C. Generalized anxiety disorder
  D. Bipolar disorder

46. What would you likely find on polysomnography (PSG) if a patient has both insomnia and depression?
  A. Decreased REM, long REM latency, early morning awakening
  B. Increased REM, long REM latency, early morning awakening
  C. Increased slow-wave sleep (SWS), short REM latency, early morning awakening
  D. Short REM latency, more REM later in the night, and early morning awakening

47. Which statement is *true* regarding morbidity and mortality data?
  A. Patients with insomnia report a similar reduction in quality of life as that of patients with congestive heart failure (CHF)
  B. All studies to date show an association between insomnia and increased mortality rates
  C. Newer data from longitudinal studies show that mild insomnia might extend people's lives
  D. People with chronic insomnia have fewer work-related accidents, which is thought to be secondary to their hyperarousal and hypervigilance

48. Which of the following statements is *not* true?
  A. Insomnia can be caused by a central nervous system (CNS) stimulant or depressant
  B. About 15% of insomnia cases have no identifiable precipitant or cause
  C. Because of irregular sleep patterns in infants, the earliest age to consider for the diagnosis of chronic insomnia disorder in a child is 6 months
  D. Insomnia patients typically show abnormal daytime alertness when tested with the MSLT

A Case of Waking Up Four Times a Night

A 48-year-old woman presents to your clinic with a 10-year history of insomnia. Many years ago, she was treated with barbiturates but was concerned about addiction. She has no difficulty going to sleep but awakens frequently at night and has trouble reinitiating sleep. Her overall health is good, although she has been told she snores if she has a glass of wine about 1 hour before bedtime. Answer the following series of questions.

49. You think about prescribing a hypnotic. Which of the following medications is *least* likely to be useful in her case?
  A. Eszopiclone
  B. Zolpidem
  C. Ramelteon
  D. Zaleplon

50. Barbiturates affect sleep architecture by
  A. Increasing REM sleep
  B. Decreasing N3 sleep
  C. Increasing N3 sleep
  D. Decreasing REM

51. She undergoes a PSG and is found to have only 3% stage N3 sleep, which you attribute to one of her medications. Which one is the *most* likely cause?
A. The barbiturate
B. The benzodiazepine
C. The monoamine oxidase inhibitor (MAOI)
D. The SSRI

52. She is also found to have no REM sleep on the PSG, possibly because of one of her medications. Which of the following drug classes is the *most* powerful REM suppressor?
A. Tricyclic antidepressants (TCAs)
B. MAOIs
C. SSRIs
D. Serotonin antagonists

53. Which of the following is *true* about zolpidem in the treatment of insomnia?
A. The half-life is about 6 hours
B. The drug has a relative affinity for type 2 GABA$_A$ receptors
C. There is no food effect
D. Peak plasma is at about 1.5 hours

Call From a Psychiatrist

You receive a call from a psychiatrist colleague who is planning to treat a 22-year-old man with schizophrenia. The psychiatrist wants to start an antipsychotic to help him obtain deeper sleep.

54. All of the following antipsychotic drugs increase N3 sleep *except*
A. Olanzapine
B. Haloperidol
C. Ziprasidone
D. Quetiapine

55. The psychiatrist also plans to prescribe an anxiolytic but has concerns about its effect on daytime alertness. Which of the following drugs is *not* known to induce sleepiness?
A. Diazepam
B. Alprazolam
C. Buspirone
D. Mirtazapine

The Overcaffeinated Waitress

56. A waitress drinks three pots of coffee to stay alert and energized on her shift. The reason caffeine helps her remain alert is
A. Caffeine is an adenosine agonist
B. Caffeine is an adenosine antagonist
C. Caffeine is a norepinephrine agonist
D. Caffeine blocks reuptake of dopamine

57. Caffeine has an approximate half-life of
A. 3 to 5 hours
B. 15 to 30 minutes
C. 6 to 8 hours
D. 1 to 2 hours

58. You are at a social gathering. One of the partygoers hears you are a sleep medicine specialist. He brags to you that he can drink four espresso drinks before bed without an effect on subsequent sleep. What should you tell him?
A. Caffeine has no effect on some people
B. Caffeine consumption will eventually cause insomnia
C. Caffeine reduces REM sleep
D. Caffeine reduces N3 sleep

59. An 82-year-old patient with a 5-year history of insomnia involving onset and maintenance problems tells you he is taking Tylenol PM (acetaminophen and diphenhydramine) at bedtime, which has not improved his condition. The *most* likely reason for this is

    A. Diphenhydramine has little effect on reducing sleep-onset latency

    B. Diphenhydramine can reduce objective TST

    C. Diphenhydramine makes most people feel groggy for up to 30 minutes after sleep offset

    D. Diphenhydramine does not reduce objective nighttime awakenings

60. A pediatrician is caring for an 8-year-old boy with a long history of sleep-onset insomnia. Behavioral intervention has been unsuccessful, and the parents are upset because their child is having problems with performance at school. The pediatrician decides to try a low dose of chloral hydrate to treat the insomnia. Chloral hydrate can affect sleep architecture by

    A. Increasing REM latency

    B. Reducing N3 sleep

    C. Increasing N3 sleep

    D. Chloral hydrate has no impact on N3 or REM sleep.

Insomnia, the Old and the New

One of your patients has successfully been treated for insomnia with zolpidem 10 mg at bedtime. He takes the drug about 30 minutes before bedtime, 5 nights per week. Two months into treatment, he reports that his sleep is good on nights he takes the drug. He usually reads for about 1 hour before bed and finds the book on his chest the next morning. While pleased with treatment, he complains of having no recall of what he read the night before.

61. Decrements in memory function are *most* likely from benzodiazepine receptor agonists that have a strong affinity to

    A. $GABA_A$ $alpha_1$

    B. $GABA_A$ $alpha_2$

    C. $GABA_A$ $alpha_3$

    D. $GABA_A$ $alpha_4$

62. Because of the memory problems, you decide to switch him to low-dose doxepin, also approved by the US Food and Drug Administration (FDA) for insomnia. The peak plasma level of low-dose doxepin is at 1.5 to 4 hours after ingestion. Most improvement with this drug is

    A. In reducing sleep-onset latency

    B. In the last third of the sleep period

    C. In the second third of the sleep period

    D. In the first part of the sleep period

63. Before switching him to doxepin, you considered trazodone because it is less expensive. Compared with zolpidem, trazodone has

    A. Identical 4- to 6-month efficacy on sleep parameters on PSG

    B. No durable efficacy on sleep parameters on PSG measures

    C. Significantly reduced efficacy beyond 1 week

    D. Improved sleep-maintenance effect seen only after a week of nightly administration

Other Medications That Affect Sleep

64. A patient with a blood pressure of 160/110 mm Hg is started on a beta-blocker. His cardiac symptoms are vastly improved, but he complains of insomnia. Beta-blockers can affect sleep by

    A. Increasing melatonin release

    B. Decreasing melatonin release

    C. Inhibiting GABA release at the ventrolateral preoptic nucleus (VLPO)

    D. Having high affinity for 5-HT receptors

65. A patient's internist prescribed an H_2 antagonist for gastroesophageal reflux disease (GERD) and a benzodiazepine receptor agonist for insomnia. The H_2 antagonist drug significantly reduced the reflux episodes. However, the patient complains of an unwanted adverse effect (daytime sleepiness) during his follow-up visit. Of the following H_2 histamine receptor antagonists, which one is *most* likely to cause the significant adverse effects in patients taking a hypnotic?
   A. Cimetidine
   B. Ranitidine
   C. Famotidine
   D. Nizatidine

66. A 55-year-old patient reports that since starting ibuprofen for minor joint pains, her sleep has become fragmented, with awakenings at night and difficulty returning to sleep. Nonsteroidal antiinflammatory drugs (NSAIDs) can cause sleep disruption by
   A. Increasing the synthesis of prostaglandin D_2
   B. Suppressing melatonin release
   C. Enhancing normal decrease in core body temperature
   D. Directly acting as a GABA antagonist

A Case of Sunday Night Insomnia

A 28-year-old woman presents to the clinic with a complaint of poor sleep. She typically gets in bed with lights out at 10 PM, but about twice a week, it takes her hours to fall asleep. It seems to always occur on Sunday nights. Once asleep, she may wake once to go to the bathroom but then is able to reinitiate sleep within minutes. As a result of the insomnia, her mood has been poor, and she has had difficulty getting along with coworkers.

67. What is the *most* likely diagnosis, according to the ICSD3?
   A. Short-term insomnia disorder
   B. Chronic insomnia disorder
   C. Paradoxical insomnia
   D. Other insomnia disorder

68. Which hypnotic and dosage is *most* appropriate for this pattern of insomnia?
   A. Zolpidem 10 mg as needed (prn)
   B. Zolpidem 5 mg prn
   C. Eszopiclone 3 mg nightly
   D. Temazepam 15 mg prn

69. You decide to suggest behavioral treatment. Which of the following is unlikely to be of much help compared with drug monotherapy?
   A. Stimulus control
   B. Sleep restriction
   C. Sleep hygiene
   D. Relaxation therapy

70. You give the patient samples of a medication, but she calls the next day stating she woke with a "funny metallic-like taste in her mouth." Which medication was it?
   A. Zolpidem
   B. Quetiapine
   C. Diazepam
   D. Eszopiclone

71. After a few weeks, the patient also develops a problem staying asleep, waking at 2:00 AM and again at 4:00 AM, and taking about 1 hour to get back to sleep after each awakening. Which FDA-approved hypnotic would be *least* likely to help this type of insomnia?
   A. Doxepin
   B. Eszopiclone
   C. Temazepam
   D. Ramelteon

Retirement Ruined His Sleep

John is a 67-year-old man with a 5-year history of sleep-onset insomnia and sleep-maintenance problems. About the same time the sleep disturbance began, he decided to retire from his job at the Centers for Disease Control and Prevention in Atlanta. He worked for 20 years in the security department. The difficulty with sleep occurs 6 or 7 nights per week. He likes to read the news on his laptop until bedtime and checks emails at night if he wakes up, hoping his 29-year-old daughter has sent him a message from her home in Europe.

72. What is the *most* likely subtype insomnia diagnosis according to the ICSD3?
   A. Short-term insomnia disorder
   B. Chronic insomnia disorder
   C. Paradoxical insomnia
   D. Other insomnia disorder

73. What initial behavioral advice are you going to give to John?
   A. Wear blue-colored glasses at night to negate the light from the laptop
   B. Wear amber-colored glasses at night to negate the light from the laptop
   C. Try stimulus-control therapy only after sleep onset
   D. Wear amber-colored glasses for 1 hour upon awakening

74. During a subsequent office visit, you find out that John tries to make up for lost sleep by staying in bed until 10 AM, giving him an 11-hour opportunity for sleep. What advice should you give him about this schedule?
   A. Take afternoon naps rather than staying in bed longer
   B. Restrict bedtime to no more than 7 to 8 hours
   C. Increase temazepam to 30 mg at bedtime
   D. As long as weather permits, take an evening walk in an attempt to enhance sunlight exposure

75. Which of the following assessments would be best for making the diagnosis of insomnia?
   A. PSG
   B. Sleep diary
   C. Sleep app on smartphone
   D. Insomnia Severity Index

Fear of Standing Before a Crowd

A 49-year-old woman with a 1.5-month history of insomnia 5 nights per week has been taking 10 mg of zolpidem at bedtime for 3 weeks. The insomnia began shortly after she found out that her job at Coca-Cola was going to involve public speaking. Anxiety over this task became progressively worse, and she began to engage in compulsive eating at night about 1 hour after falling asleep. She was seen by a psychiatrist, who prescribed escitalopram 10 mg at bedtime. She continued taking zolpidem for insomnia.

76. What is the *most* likely subtype insomnia diagnosis according to the ICSD3?
   A. Short-term insomnia disorder
   B. Chronic insomnia disorder
   C. Paradoxical insomnia
   D. Other insomnia disorder

77. What would you do next?
   A. Reduce the dose or eliminate the zolpidem
   B. Eliminate the escitalopram
   C. Increase the dose of escitalopram
   D. Increase the bedtime dose of zolpidem

78. Which of the following is *not* usually a side effect of BzRAs?
    A. Sleep eating
    B. Anterograde amnesia
    C. Ataxia
    D. Increased anxiety

79. The medication treatment is becoming less effective, so you ask for a CBTi consultation. The patient undergoes therapy and continues taking the hypnotic. Which of the following is *most* correct?
    A. The combination of treatments is always better than monotherapy
    B. CBTi will lose its effectiveness within 1 week of discontinuation
    C. The hypnotic withdrawal will cause significant rebound insomnia
    D. CBTi alone continues to show benefits weeks after treatment has been terminated

80. The patient complains of fatigue and lack of energy. There was a hint of OSA in her history, so she undergoes a PSG and an MSLT. What mean sleep latency would you expect from an insomniac on an MSLT, assuming the PSG was not indicative of sleep-disordered breathing?
    A. Less than 5 minutes
    B. 6 to 8 minutes
    C. 10 to 12 minutes
    D. 6 to 8 minutes with one sleep-onset REM period (SOREMP)

Potpourri

81. You decide to develop a new drug for treating insomnia. To ensure success, which of the following pharmacologic mechanisms should your drug have?
    A. $GABA_A$ receptor antagonism
    B. $5\text{-}HT_{2A}$ receptor agonism
    C. $5\text{-}HT_{2A}$ receptor antagonism
    D. Orexin receptor agonism

82. A friend likes to drink red wine up to 30 minutes before bed about 5 nights a week. He tells you that the wine does indeed have an effect on his sleep. Which of the following is an expected impact on sleep when adults drink alcoholic beverages close to bedtime?
    A. Bizarre dreams
    B. Increased REM sleep
    C. Reduced wakefulness after sleep onset (WASO)
    D. Decreased limb movements

ANSWERS

1. D. This patient has chronic insomnia. General criteria for this diagnosis include difficulty initiating or maintaining sleep for 3 months or longer; some daytime problem associated with the insomnia, such as fatigue, sleepiness, impaired school or work performance, and behavioral problems; and the sleep difficulty occurs despite adequate opportunity for sleep. The ICSD3 discusses many subtypes of chronic insomnia, of which psychophysiologic insomnia is the most common. The essential feature is a state of hyperarousal or hypervigilance and a negative conditioned response whereby the patient's sleep environment is stimulating rather than soothing. Most patients admit to racing thoughts or perseverations; these are often about life stressors, but most commonly the obsessive thoughts center on the sleep difficulty itself, thus further exacerbating the patient's anxiety surrounding sleep. People with psychophysiologic insomnia often characterize themselves as lifelong poor sleepers. It is also common that life stressors or life transitions cause an adjustment insomnia that then develops into a chronic insomnia. This patient clearly does not fit adjustment insomnia because of its 6-month course and lack of an obvious precipitating event. This is not idiopathic insomnia because that diagnosis requires a history of insomnia starting in infancy or childhood. This is not paradoxical insomnia, also known as *sleep-state misperception*; these patients misperceive how much sleep they actually obtain. She reports averaging 5 hours of sleep per night, but patients with paradoxical insomnia report "no sleep for 2 weeks" or sleeping only "1 to 2 hours a night," which is inaccurate and also incompatible with their level of functioning. Actigraphy data can help reorient a patient's sleep perception. (ATLAS2, pp 151-155; ICSD3, pp 19-47)

2. A.   It is unusual for a patient to show improvement with antidepressant use even if the insomnia began at the time of the depression. It used to be commonly assumed that insomnia was simply a symptom of the depression and that if we treated the "underlying cause"—the depression—the insomnia would naturally resolve. Studies have now shown that insomnia is the symptom least likely to remit with treatment of depression, even when all other symptoms have resolved. The standard of care now is to treat the insomnia along with the depression. It should also be noted that SSRIs and most antidepressants can disturb sleep and sleep architecture; for example, they can decrease REM sleep. The other answers are common features of psychophysiologic insomnia. (ATLAS2, pp 155-158)

3. B.   Alcohol is a soporific, but as it metabolizes, this effect begins to wane. Often after 3 to 4 hours of sleep, a person who fell asleep from alcohol wakes up and then has difficulty returning to sleep. If she ate a snack with a high glycemic index 1 to 2 hours before bed, then that might contribute to sleep-maintenance problems, but it is unlikely that cheese and crackers play a big role. If either the news stories or the music in the bedroom were to disturb her sleep, they would both likely cause trouble initiating sleep, but they would not cause sleep-maintenance insomnia.

4. C.   There should be a strong suspicion for OSA in this patient. She snores, falls asleep immediately, reports weight gain, and is perimenopausal, which greatly increases her risk for OSA. (The prevalence of OSA in menopausal women is equal to that of men of similar age.) On physical examination, she has a large neck and a crowded oropharynx. Women with OSA are much more likely than men to present with a chief complaint of insomnia. OSA can, of course, be comorbid with insomnia. However, given this history, it is possible that treating sleep apnea and refraining from alcohol near bedtime will solve her sleep-maintenance difficulties. There are no symptoms of depression. Waking up after 3 to 4 hours does not constitute early morning awakening. There is no evidence of narcolepsy, whose sine qua non is excessive daytime sleepiness, often with sleep attacks, and whose pathognomonic symptom is cataplexy. A BMI of 30 is unlikely to lead to obesity hypoventilation syndrome, and if that diagnosis were present, she would likely manifest inadvertent sleep attacks during the day. (ATLAS2, pp 152-154)

5. A.   A hallmark of psychophysiologic insomnia is that patients sleep better when not in their own bed; they even sleep better in the sleep lab and often remark on this. This makes sense because it is a conditioned insomnia; the patient's own sleep environment elicits an arousal response. Do not misinterpret this phenomenon as paradoxical insomnia, in which patients report levels of sleep too low for their level of functioning. The most appropriate reason to order a PSG in this patient is the suspicion of OSA, not central sleep apnea (CSA). It would be surprising to find CSA with Cheyne-Stokes breathing without a history of CHF or stroke, and it is also much more common in men. You would expect her REM sleep to be decreased, not increased, in the setting of likely OSA and because she is taking an SSRI. Increased EMG during REM sleep is usually associated with REM sleep behavior disorder (RBD), although it can be an isolated finding; still, it is not a diagnosis you would expect in this case. She reports no dream-enacting behavior, and RBD is most commonly seen in men older than 60 years. (ATLAS2, p 155, Table 10-1)

6. D.   According to the ICSD3, "Chronic insomnia should be discriminated from situational sleep difficulties arising from sleep-disruptive environmental circumstances." The other conditions are considered subtypes of chronic insomnia. (ICSD3, pp 19-47)

7. B.   Although a diagnosis of chronic insomnia requires symptoms lasting at least 3 months, be aware that short-term insomnia can last more than 1 month but less than 3 months. Therefore, do not use duration as your primary diagnostic criterion. (ICSD3, pp 19-47)

8. D.   Insomnia is primarily a clinical diagnosis. PSG is not recommended by the American Academy of Sleep Medicine (AASM), and you should only order it when you suspect another disorder such as sleep-disordered breathing, a parasomnia, periodic limb movement disorder (PLMD), and so on. Two helpful diagnostic tools for insomnia are the sleep diary and actigraphy.   (ATLAS2, p 392)

9. B.   Actigraphy can be helpful if you suspect paradoxical insomnia, and it can be useful in distinguishing insomnia from delayed sleep-wake phase disorder. However, it is not used routinely, but all patients who complain of insomnia should be encouraged to fill out a sleep log or diary for 2 to 4 weeks. Given the high prevalence of comorbid psychiatric disorders, especially depression and anxiety, depression screening with a questionnaire such as the Beck Depression Inventory is often part of a thorough workup but is not recommended for all patients. Cortisol levels are not a routine part of an insomnia workup.   (ATLAS2, pp 392-393)

10. B.   There is no treatment for fatal familial insomnia (FFI). FFI is usually fatal within 6 to 12 months of presentation. It is a progressive neurodegenerative prion disease that has both familial and sporadic forms. PSG shows loss of sleep spindles. FFI is a rare disorder, but do not be surprised if at least one question about it appears on the board exam.   (ATLAS2, p 234)

11. E.   General criteria for insomnia require "adequate opportunity and circumstances for sleep" as well as "daytime impairment." The fact that a patient might have a comorbid psychiatric diagnosis should not dissuade you from diagnosing insomnia. The former notion of insomnia as being secondary to a psychiatric or medical disorder has been replaced by the concept that insomnia is often comorbid with psychiatric and medical disorders. This new way of conceptualizing the relationship between insomnia and other disorders encourages physicians to treat the comorbid insomnia rather than assume that it will resolve with treatment of the psychiatric or medical disorder. The nosology of the ICSD3 includes "insomnia due to drug or substance." Stimulant abuse is common in teens and young adults even when it is prescribed for an indicated disorder.   (ICSD3, pp 19-47)

12. A.   Prevalence estimates of insomnia vary widely depending on the definition used. The ICSD3 states that the prevalence of chronic insomnia is about 10%. The prevalence of transient insomnia symptoms is much higher, at 30% to 35%.   (ICSD3, p 30)

13. C.   CBTi is a well-established treatment modality that consists of many elements, including stimulus control, sleep restriction, relaxation training, cognitive therapy, and sleep hygiene education. Neither Freudian nor Jungian psychoanalysis nor any dream interpretation has been shown to improve insomnia. Eye movement desensitization and reprocessing (EMDR) is psychotherapy that attempts to integrate past trauma. It is not used by behavioral sleep specialists as treatment for insomnia.   (ATLAS2, p 157, Table 10-3)

14. E.   Prevalence for chronic insomnia in the general population is about 10%, but it is higher in women, older people, and in those with psychiatric and medical disorders. According to the ICSD3, "[chronic insomnia] may occur at any age but is more commonly diagnosed in older adults, most likely due to age-related deterioration in sleep continuity and increase in medical comorbidities and medication use that increase insomnia risk."   (ATLAS2, p 364; ICSD3, p 30; Ohayon and Roth, 2003)

15. D.   Delayed sleep-wake phase disorder (DSWPD), one of the circadian rhythm disorders, should be in the differential diagnosis when patients complain of trouble getting to sleep. There are several clues in this scenario that DSWPD is more likely than either adjustment insomnia or short-term insomnia: First, there is no evidence of a conditioned arousal response to his sleep environment. Second is the patient's age; DSWPD is most prevalent in teens and young adults. The third clue is that he sleeps well on weekends and vacations, awakens refreshed, and feels alert throughout the day. While in school, he is sleep deprived during the week, and this, rather than narcolepsy, likely explains his daytime somnolence.   (ICSD3, pp 191-198)

16. C.   CBTi is a multicomponent treatment approach for insomnia that studies have shown is often more effective than medication. Although some psychologists use hypnosis, hypnosis is not a component of CBTi and has not been proven to help insomnia. Sleep restriction and stimulus-control therapy, along with relaxation therapy and sleep hygiene education, are components of CBTi.   (Morin et al, 2006)

17. C.   Most head-to-head trials show that hypnotics and CBTi are equally effective in the short term but that CBTi produces better long-term control of insomnia symptoms. One study showed that CBTi was associated with a greater benefit than zopiclone. The National Institutes of Health (NIH) State of the Science Conference statement concluded that CBTi is as effective as medication for short-term treatment of chronic insomnia and that benefits of CBTi, in contrast to medication, may last well beyond the termination of treatment.   (Sivertsen et al, 2006; NIH, 2005)

18. B.   Stimulus-control therapy involves a set of instructions designed to reassociate the bed and bedroom with drowsiness and sleep rather than hyperarousal and wakefulness. Patients are instructed to only go to bed when they are sleepy, to get out of bed if they lie awake for more than 15 minutes, to use the bedroom only for sleeping (i.e., no TV, computer, or reading), to arise at the same time every morning, and to avoid napping. Answer A describes sleep-restriction therapy. Answer C describes relaxation therapy. Answer D describes cognitive restructuring.   (Morin et al, 2006)

19. A.   Sleep-restriction therapy is designed to create more consolidated and more efficient sleep by curtailing TIB. Usually several weeks of a patient's sleep diary are reviewed to ascertain the average amount of sleep per night. If the patient is spending 8 hours in bed but reports sleeping only 6 hours on average, the sleep window (from lights out to final rising) would be restricted to 6 hours until the patient raises the sleep efficiency to 85%. The sleep window is extended by 15 to 30 minutes each time the patient achieves good sleep efficiency until the optimal sleep duration is achieved. Caution should be used with restricting the sleep window to 5 hours or less with any patient, and such severe restriction should not be recommended to anyone with a history of mania.   (Morin et al, 2006)

20. D.   Cognitive restructuring aims to challenge and change misconceptions about sleep and faulty beliefs about insomnia.   (ATLAS2, p 157, Table 10-3)

21. A.   Trazodone, although not a sedative or a hypnotic, is the most widely prescribed sleeping pill in the United States. It is FDA approved as an antidepressant but is rarely used for that purpose because at therapeutic doses (300 to 400 mg/day), it tends to be sedating and may cause orthostatic hypotension. The typical dose for sleep is 50 to 150 mg a night. Zaleplon, along with zolpidem and eszopiclone, is a nonbenzodiazepine BzRA. The BzRAs have no antidepressant effect. Suvorexant is a relatively new hypnotic. The mechanism of action is as an orexin antagonist. Suvorexant is approved for sleep onset and maintenance insomnia. It does not have an indication for depression.   (ATLAS2, pp 105-112; Herring et al, 2016)

22. D.   Bupropion is an atypical antidepressant that primarily inhibits the reuptake of norepinephrine and dopamine. Compared with other antidepressants, it is least likely to disturb sleep architecture. However, bupropion can have a mild stimulatory effect and therefore should be taken in the morning, not before bed, as in this case. Paroxetine can disturb sleep, and insomnia is a reported side effect, so it would not be the drug with "no effect on sleep." Both amitriptyline and mirtazapine are antidepressants that, like trazodone, are widely prescribed for sleep because of their side effect of sedation, so it is unlikely either one would worsen sleep-initiation insomnia.

23. D.   The essential feature of idiopathic insomnia is onset of the sleep disturbance in childhood or infancy. This case is not insomnia caused by a mental disorder because the insomnia well precedes the depression diagnosis.   (ICSD3, pp 19-46)

24. C.   Anterograde amnesia, amnesia for events that occur after administration of the drug, is a well-described side effect of zolpidem. Parasomnias and amnesia are known to occur with all the BzRAs. They are worrisome side effects because people can engage in potentially dangerous behavior such as sleepwalking, sleep driving, and sleep eating. Higher doses are associated with a higher prevalence of amnestic events. Most sleep specialists would immediately stop the medication if it caused an amnestic event. Compulsive behaviors are a side effect of dopamine agonists used in the treatment of restless legs syndrome (RLS). Seizures are a concern with bupropion because the drug lowers the seizure threshold. Urinary retention is an anticholinergic side effect seen in patients taking TCAs and antihistamines.

25. A. All of these except basil flower have been promoted as sleep aids. Only valerian has been well studied and found to improve sleep, but the effect is small. Kava kava and chamomile are sold as sleep aids, but there is no evidence they are better than placebo. Kava kava can cause serious liver damage and should be used with caution, as should all herbal remedies. (Morgenthaler et al, 2006)

26. A. Melatonin is a naturally occurring hormone synthesized from tryptophan and released from the pineal gland. Its levels are highest at night, and secretion can be suppressed by ordinary room light (100 lux). Melatonin has been shown to improve insomnia when compared with placebo. L-Tryptophan is an essential amino acid and a precursor of serotonin, which in turn is converted to melatonin. No studies have shown L-tryptophan to be effective for insomnia. OTC tryptophan was banned for many years in the United States after a 1989 outbreak of eosinophilia myalgia syndrome was thought to have been caused by contaminated tryptophan. OTC tryptophan is again available (it has always been available by prescription). Diphenhydramine and doxylamine are both sedating antihistamines that are not well studied but are known to cause significant drowsiness. In fact, they tend to be so sedating that many people have residual sedation the next day. Owing to daytime grogginess, along with the anticholinergic side effects (dry mouth and eyes, urinary retention, constipation, and ataxia), these drugs are not usually recommended as sleep aids. There is also concern for a paradoxical effect sometimes reported in very sick and very old patients. (ATLAS2, pp 105-112)

27. B. Ramelteon is a melatonin receptor agonist that seems to have no potential for tolerance or addiction. Zaleplon and zolpidem are nonbenzodiazepine BzRAs, which have been labeled to have addiction potential. Suvorexant, an orexin antagonist, has a warning on its label about the potential for addiction. (Herring et al, 2016; ATLAS2, p 109)

28. E. There are few good randomized, controlled trials comparing melatonin with placebo. Studies to date that evaluate its efficacy as a hypnotic show that the most consistent results occur when endogenous melatonin levels are low. A few studies show that it can be effective in treating the circadian misalignment often experienced by totally blind persons. (Kostoglou-Athanassiou, 2013)

29. C. Before exploring whether the patient's "early morning awakening" is secondary to depression or a primary sleep disorder, be sure the symptom is accurate. "Early morning awakening" is meant to describe an awakening after an insufficient amount of sleep *and* the inability to return to sleep. If she states that she goes to sleep at 11 PM and consistently wakes at 5 AM feeling unrefreshed but unable to return to sleep, she has a type of insomnia. You should then explore whether it is comorbid with a psychiatric disorder such as depression or anxiety. If, on the other hand, you find out that she is going to bed at 8 PM with the same wake time, then she has advanced sleep-wake phase disorder (ASWPD) rather than insomnia. ASWPD may also be comorbid with a depressive disorder, but there is not as strong an association between circadian rhythm problems and psychiatric disorders as there is with circadian rhythm disorders and insomnia. (ATLAS2, pp 365-367; Sutton, 2014)

30. D. Beta-antagonists, corticosteroids, and NSAIDs can all have the side effect of insomnia.

31. A. Side effects of beta-blockers include both insomnia and daytime sleepiness and fatigue. Answers B and C are a bit of a trick. Alpha$_1$ (not alpha$_2$) blockers (e.g. Prazosin and other …osins) and alpha$_2$ (not alpha$_1$) agonists (e.g., clonidine) are associated with somnolence and fatigue. Other classes of medications that are associated with complaints of somnolence and fatigue include antidepressants, especially TCAs; anxiolytics; antiarrhythmics; antiepileptics; first-generation antihistamines; and antiparkinson medications.

32. B.   This question tests your understanding of the possible discontinuation effects of hypnotics. Answer B describes rebound insomnia, which is a worsening of symptoms relative to the baseline complaint that only lasts for 1 or 2 nights. Answer A describes recrudescence, which is a return of the original symptom at the original severity level. Answer C describes withdrawal syndrome, which by definition involves new symptoms and lasts from several days to several weeks. Rebound insomnia is more likely to occur after high doses of short- and intermediate-acting BzRAs, as in this case with short-acting alprazolam. On the other hand, withdrawal syndrome is more common with long-acting BzRAs.

33. E.   All of these neurotransmitters except GABA can promote wakefulness. Additional wakefulness-promoting neurotransmitters are norepinephrine, glutamate, and serotonin. This is not to say that these neurotransmitters are simply "off" or downregulated during sleep. In fact, many of them—such as norepinephrine, acetylcholine, and serotonin—are involved in modulating the REM-on, REM-off neurons. The major neurotransmitters that promote sleep are GABA, galanin, melatonin, and adenosine.   (ATLAS2, pp 113-166)

34. C.   Caffeine is a stimulant because it blocks the adenosine receptor, and adenosine promotes sleep. The other answers are different mechanisms by which a substance could promote wakefulness.   (ATLAS2, p 116)

35. B.   All the BzRAs bind to the GABA$_A$ receptor, but the nonbenzodiazepines have a higher affinity for the alpha$_1$ subunit. There is a GABA$_B$, but neither benzodiazepines nor nonbenzodiazepine BzRAs bind to it. There are GABA receptors on cells in both the thalamus and the reticular formation, but this does not explain the pharmacologic differences of these drugs. Answer D is complete nonsense.   (ATLAS2, p 106)

36. A.   The anxiolytic and myorelaxant properties are lost because they are not mediated by the alpha$_1$ subunit. Treatment effects such as amnesia and antiepileptic properties are still present.   (ATLAS2, p 108, Fig. 6-3)

37. B.   The three-P model attempts to account for how acute insomnia becomes chronic by positing *predisposing*, *precipitating*, and *perpetuating* factors. This model has been criticized for failing to address the concept of conditioned arousal, which helps explain why insomnia can persist even when maladaptive perpetuating strategies have been eliminated.   (ATLAS2, p 150)

38. A.   CBTi has been shown to be a very effective treatment in benzodiazepine-dependent patients.   (Morin et al, 2004)

39. D.   Paradoxical intention aims to defuse performance anxiety and address the conditioned failure to sleep when appropriate by having the patient attempt to stay awake, rather than try to fall asleep, even though it is bedtime and the patient is sleepy.   (Morin et al, 2006)

40. A.   Stimulus-control therapy (a component of CBTi) recommends that patients only go to bed when they are sleepy, not at a set bedtime, and that they keep a firm waking time. It also includes no napping so as to allow the homeostatic drive to sleep to build throughout the day. Sleep hygiene education informs patients that most people sleep better in a dark, cool place.   (Morin et al, 2006)

41. C.   Anxiety disorders are the most common psychiatric disorder, followed closely by depression. Much of the sleep literature quotes prevalence rates for psychiatric disorders among people with insomnia at around 50%.   (ATLAS2, pp 154 and 364)

42. D.   CBTi has been shown to be effective in all these patient groups, and it is standard treatment for insomnia in older adults. Hypnotics are not FDA approved for pediatric populations.   (Taylor and Pruiksma, 2014)

43. A.   All are associated with insomnia except cervical cancer. There is an association between shift work and breast cancer, but no data link cervical cancer to insomnia.

44. B.   Longitudinal data collected at Stanford University show that persons with major depressive disorder have a relative risk of 3.8 of developing insomnia within a 3-year time frame.

The relative risk of developing insomnia was 2.6 among those with anxiety disorders and 1.8 among those who had chronic pain. (Ohayon, 2009)

45. B.   Data from the Stanford study show that the relationship between insomnia and depression is bidirectional. Participants who had insomnia but who did not have a major depressive disorder at baseline had a relative risk of 2.1 of developing a major depressive disorder and a relative risk of 1.9 of developing an anxiety disorder. (Ohayon, 2009)

46. D.   These PSG findings are common in depression, which is often comorbid with insomnia. Keep in mind that PSG is not indicated for the routine evaluation of insomnia. PSG is only indicated if you suspect a sleep disorder other than, or in addition to, insomnia or if the patient fails to respond to insomnia treatment. (ATLAS2, pp 154 and 365)

47. A.   Morbidity data for insomnia consistently show increased medical and psychiatric illness, an increase in work-related and traffic accidents, higher absenteeism, higher health care utilization, and reduced quality of life. Insomnia data have not consistently shown an increase in mortality, and no data show insomnia to confer longevity benefits. (Morin, 2004)

48. D.   According to the ICSD3, "results of the Multiple Sleep Latency Test (MSLT) usually show normal daytime alertness. In several studies, patients with insomnia have longer mean MSLT values than control subjects, suggesting hyperalertness or arousal. A minority of insomnia patients, particularly older adults with insomnia, have reduced mean MSLT values indicating increased sleepiness. Such a finding should prompt consideration of other concurrent sleep disorder such as obstructive sleep apnea." (ICSD3, p 35)

49. C.   All of the drugs listed in this question are FDA-approved hypnotic agents. The patient has difficulty with sleep maintenance. Eszopiclone has been shown to improve sleep maintenance and to reduce sleep latency. Zolpidem reduces sleep latency but does not have a substantial effect on maintenance. Zaleplon has an ultrashort half-life and does not improve sleep maintenance. However, these last two drugs are occasionally given off label in the middle of the night, as long as there are at least 4 hours remaining in the sleep period. Ramelteon is only labeled for sleep-onset insomnia and would not be useful or appropriate for use in the middle of the night. (ATLAS2, p 105)

50. D.   Barbiturates and ethanol, to some degree, increase sleep-spindle activity. With regard to sleep architecture, barbiturates are very potent REM suppressors.

51. B.   In contrast to the barbiturates, the benzodiazepines are potent suppressors of N3 sleep. Barbiturates are powerful REM suppressors. Ethanol, benzodiazepines, and barbiturates may increase spindle activity. Benzodiazepines and nonbenzodiazepines mildly suppress REM sleep.

52. B.   TCAs and SSRIs do suppress REM sleep but not to the degree that MAOIs do. Some PSG studies show almost complete elimination of REM in patients taking MAOIs, and MAOIs increase concentrations of serotonin, norepinephrine, and dopamine.

53. D.   Zolpidem is a rapidly absorbed insomnia drug with a half-life of 1.5 to 2.4 hours. The drug has selectivity for the type 1 $GABA_A$–benzodiazepine receptor. There is a significant decrease in absorption if taken with food in the gut. (ATLAS2, p 106)

54. D.   Only a few PSG studies have been done of antipsychotics in healthy control participants, and none have been done in schizophrenic patients. Olanzapine, quetiapine, and ziprasidone decrease sleep latency and improve sleep continuity. REM suppression is variable with these drugs and has not been well documented. Increases in N3 sleep are usually seen in patients taking antipsychotics, with the exception of quetiapine. (ATLAS2, p 367)

55. C.   Diazepam and alprazolam are benzodiazepines and therefore bind to $GABA_A$ receptors. Mirtazapine is an antidepressant with sleep-enhancing qualities because of antagonism of adrenergic (alpha$_1$ and alpha$_2$), serotoninergic (5-HT$_2$ and 5-HT$_3$), and histaminergic (H$_1$) receptors. Buspirone is an anxiolytic drug that is a 5-HT$_{1A}$ receptor partial agonist. It does not have sedating properties. (ATLAS2, p 112)

56. B.   Adenosine is thought to be a sleep-inducing neurotransmitter that builds with hours of wakefulness. The mechanism of action of caffeine on wakefulness involves nonspecific adenosine receptor antagonism. Caffeine is a xanthine derivative, which is known to be an A_1 receptor blocker.   (ATLAS2, p 115)

57. A.   Caffeine is a rapidly absorbed drug with a half-life of 3.5 to 5 hours.   (ATLAS2, p 115)

58. D.   Caffeine is known to delay sleep onset and decrease N3 sleep. Caffeine has no known effect on REM sleep, and it can be the source of insomnia, but its effects are acute because the drug does not accumulate on a daily basis.

59. D.   Diphenhydramine is an antihistamine; therefore, it can cause drowsiness. This OTC drug is not known to reduce TST. Patients report reduced sleep-onset latency; however, diphenhydramine does not reduce objective awakenings as measured by PSG.   (ATLAS2, p 111)

60. D.   Chloral hydrate is commonly used as a hypnotic in children. It is rapidly converted by alcohol dehydrogenase in the liver to the active compound trichloroethanol, which acts at the barbiturate-recognition site on $GABA_A$ receptors. The drug has a half-life of approximately 5 to 10 hours. Effects on sleep include reduction in sleep latency and improvement in sleep continuity. There is no significant effect on REM or N3 sleep. Surprisingly little published data support its use.

61. A.   In an animal model, studies using knock-in technology in mice indicate that the $alpha_1$ subunit can mediate both sedation and memory effects of benzodiazepine agonists.   (ATLAS2, p 108)

62. B.   Low-dose doxepin is FDA approved for treatment of insomnia. The studies carried out with doxepin have demonstrated evidence of self-reported and PSG efficacy in reducing sleep-onset latency and improving sleep maintenance, with most of the effects on maintenance of sleep. The therapeutic effects appear to be largest in the last third of the night.   (ATLAS2, p 109)

63. C.   In subjects with primary insomnia, trazodone was studied using a parallel group, 2-week study design. Trazodone 50 mg, zolpidem 10 mg, and placebo were compared. Several self-report sleep parameters were significantly improved compared with placebo for both trazodone and zolpidem in the first week of treatment; however, by the second week, these differences were not significant. No published study has examined PSG outcomes with trazodone in patients with primary insomnia.   (ATLAS2, p 111)

64. B.   Beta-blockers can cause CNS adverse effects that include tiredness, fatigue, insomnia, nightmares, depression, mental confusion, and psychomotor impairment. Sleep disturbance appears to be more common with the more lipophilic drugs. Beta-antagonists are known to decrease melatonin release, and this could account for the increase in sleep disruption.

65. A.   Cimetidine, ranitidine, famotidine, and nizatidine—all H_2 antagonists—are not known to impair CNS function because these compounds do not cross the blood-brain barrier easily. Cimetidine can slow the clearance of some benzodiazepine-receptor agonists, which can make carryover effects of hypnotics more of a problem. Ranitidine can produce some of the same adverse effects, although not to the same degree seen with cimetidine.

66. B.   NSAIDs can negatively affect sleep because they suppress the normal surge in melatonin release, decrease the synthesis of prostaglandin D_2, and attenuate the normal nocturnal decrease in body temperature.

67. D.   The ICSD3 criteria for chronic insomnia disorder include the occurrence of the sleep disturbance at least three times per week. Whereas chronic insomnia disorder must have a duration of 3 months or more, short-term insomnia has a duration criterion of less than 3 months with no frequency criterion. This patient's history is consistent with chronic insomnia disorder.   (ICSD3, pp 19-47)

68. B. For women, the recommended zolpidem dose is 5 mg. There is no need for nightly dosing because the patient is aware of her high-risk nights for insomnia.

69. C. Sleep hygiene refers to a group of behaviors that should be reviewed with the patient and possibly altered as part of a behavioral treatment for insomnia. It is a necessary therapy, yet it is inadequate when used alone.

70. D. Eszopiclone can cause patients to experience a sour or metallic taste upon awakening. However, most patients do not discontinue the treatment because of this adverse effect.

71. D. Doxepin, temazepam, and eszopiclone can increase sleep maintenance or decrease WASO. Ramelteon is a melatonin agonist that has only demonstrated an ability to reduce sleep-onset latency.   (ATLAS2, p 109)

72. B. The ICSD3 criteria for chronic insomnia include the occurrence of the sleep disturbance at least three times per week. Whereas chronic insomnia disorder must have a duration of 3 months or more, short-term insomnia has a duration criterion of less than 3 months with no frequency criterion. This patient's history is consistent with chronic insomnia disorder.   (ICSD3, pp 19-47)

73. B. Exposure to a light-emitting screen before bedtime is poor sleep hygiene and causes circadian rhythm issues. Computer screens, TVs, and cell phone screens all emit blue light, which is known to suppress melatonin and therefore could delay sleep onset. Amber-colored glasses can be used to block blue light yet still allow the viewer to see the screen.

74. B. Many patients make the mistake of increased TIB in the hope that they will get more sleep. Reducing TIB to 7 hours from 11 is consistent with sleep-restriction therapy, which has a goal of increasing sleep efficiency.   (ATLAS2, p 157)

75. B. When used properly, a sleep diary can be very useful for assessment and follow-up. Patients should be encouraged to complete the diary on a daily basis and not a week at a time. PSGs are not recommended for routine evaluation of insomnia. The Insomnia Severity Index (ISI) is a validated self-report measure, but it is not usually used for making a diagnosis in clinical practice. As of this writing, wearable devices that contain accelerometers that can function as actigraphs have not been validated to use in the clinic setting.

76. B. Despite the parasomnia, this is a case of chronic insomnia disorder. The ICSD3 criteria for chronic insomnia include the occurrence of the sleep disturbance at least three times per week. Whereas chronic insomnia disorder must have a duration of 3 months or more, short-term insomnia has a duration criterion of less than 3 months with no frequency criterion.   (ICSD3, pp 19-47)

77. A. Zolpidem is known to have sleepwalking, sleep eating, or sleep driving as adverse effects. Although also a risk, another hypnotic from another drug class should be considered.

78. D. BzRAs are not known to increase anxiety. However, they can cause parasomnias, ataxia, and memory difficulties.

79. D. Withdrawal can cause insomnia intensity to return to baseline. Long periods of rebound are not seen with the most recent hypnotics. CBTi is a durable therapy that can be effective long after therapy has concluded.

80. C. People with insomnia typically do not score in the abnormal range on the MSLT. In fact, people with insomnia are hyperaroused and often fail to initiate sleep during MSLT naps. Having a mean sleep latency of 10 to 12 minutes is within normal limits and is not indicative of pathologic sleepiness.

81. C. $GABA_A$ receptor antagonists, $5\text{-}HT_{2A}$ receptor agonists, and orexin (hypocretin) receptor agonists can all promote wakefulness. $5\text{-}HT_{2A}$ receptor antagonists promote sleepiness and therefore could be developed to treat insomnia. Orexin receptor antagonists have been developed to treat insomnia, and one such agent was approved by the FDA in 2014.   (ATLAS2, p 112)

82. A. Many drugs can trigger nightmares and bizarre dreams, including catecholaminergic agents, beta-blockers, antidepressants, barbiturates, and even alcohol. Alcohol is a known sleep disruptor; therefore, it does not reduce WASO, nor does it improve sleep consolidation. It is also not known to decrease periodic limb movements.

Summary

Highly Recommended

- *Atlas of Clinical Sleep Medicine*, ed 2, Chapters 6, 10, and 17
- *International Classification of Sleep Disorders*, ed 3, Insomnia section, pp 19-46
- Atkin T, Comai S, Gobbi G. Drugs for insomnia beyond benzodiazepines: pharmacology, clinical applications, and discovery. *Pharmacol Rev.* 2018. Apr;70(2):197-245

Topics You Should Know

Insomnia

Insomnia is an important topic, and you can expect about 40 questions (17% of the exam) on this topic on the examination. However, remember that insomnia questions can overlap with questions related to other topics, such as pharmacology, movement disorders, and psychiatric disorders. Expect questions on the topics mentioned in the blueprint: adjustment insomnia, psychophysiologic insomnia, paradoxical insomnia, insomnia due to psychiatric disorders, insomnia due to medical disorders and/or medications and drugs, and insomnia due to poor sleep hygiene. You might encounter the term *comorbid insomnia*, a designation becoming more commonly used.

Epidemiology

- Age range
  - ○ Overall prevalence of chronic insomnia for the general population: 10% to 15%
  - ○ Prevalence in children and adolescents: 10%
  - ○ Prevalence in persons older than 65 years: 35% to 50%
- Risk factors
  - ○ We need better longitudinal studies, but cross-sectional data show that insomnia is more common in women, older adults, unmarried people, unemployed people, and people with medical or psychiatric conditions

Classification

The ICSD3 lists three subtypes of insomnia: chronic insomnia disorder, short-term insomnia disorder, and other insomnia disorder.

Chronic Insomnia Disorder (ICSD3, p 21)

Criteria 1 through 6 must be met.

1. The patient reports, or the patient's parent or caregiver observes, one or more of the following:
   A. Difficulty initiating sleep
   B. Difficulty maintaining sleep
   C. Waking up earlier than desired
   D. Resistance to going to bed on an appropriate schedule
   E. Difficulty sleeping without parent or caregiver intervention

2. The patient reports, or the patient's parent or caregiver observes, one or more of the following related to the nighttime sleep difficulty:
   A. Fatigue or malaise
   B. Attention, concentration, or memory impairment
   C. Impaired social, family, occupational, or academic performance
   D. Mood disturbance or irritability
   E. Daytime sleepiness
   F. Behavioral problems (e.g., hyperactivity, impulsivity, aggression)
   G. Reduced motivation, energy, or initiative
   H. Proneness for errors or accidents
   I. Concerns about or dissatisfaction with sleep

3. The reported sleep-wake complaints cannot be explained purely by inadequate sleep opportunity (i.e., enough time is allotted for sleep) or inadequate circumstances for sleep (i.e., the environment is safe, dark, quiet, and comfortable)

4. The sleep disturbance and associated daytime symptoms occur at least three times per week

5. The sleep disturbance and associated daytime symptoms have been present for at least three months

6. The sleep-wake difficulty is not better explained by another sleep disorder

Short-Term Insomnia Disorder (ICSD3, p 41)

■ The primary difference between chronic insomnia disorder and short-term insomnia disorder is that the sleep disturbance and associated daytime symptoms have been present for less than 3 months

Other Insomnia Disorder (ICSD3, p 46)

■ Other insomnia disorder is for individuals who complain of difficulty initiating and maintaining sleep and yet do not meet the full criteria for either chronic insomnia disorder or short-term insomnia disorder

Insomnia Subtypes (ICSD3, p 26)

■ The ICSD3 now lists the following as subtypes, but the validity and reliability of using this nosology last described in the ICSD2 have been questioned. Note that there are differences between ICD 10-CM and ICSD3. Billing for services requires ICD 10-CM. ICD 10 includes codes for primary insomnia (F51.01), adjustment insomnia (F51.02), paradoxical insomnia (F51.03), psychophysiologic insomnia (F51.04), and insomnia due to other mental disorder (F51.05). These ICD-DM are billable or specific codes that can be used to indicate a diagnosis of insomnia subtype for reimbursement purposes
   ○ Childhood-onset insomnia
     • Essential feature is lifelong sleeplessness with onset in infancy or childhood
     • Attributed to an abnormality in the neurologic control of the sleep-wake cycle for many areas of the wakefulness-promoting reticular activating system as well as in sleep-promoting areas such as suprachiasmatic nuclei, raphe nuclei, and medial forebrain areas
   ○ Psychophysiologic insomnia
     • Caused by a maladaptive conditioned response in which the patient learns to associate the bed environment with heightened arousal rather than sleep
     • Onset is often associated with an event that causes acute insomnia, with the sleep disturbance persisting despite resolution of the precipitating factor

○ Paradoxical insomnia (sleep-state misperception)
  ● Paradoxical insomnia with reports of severe insomnia without supporting objective evidence such as daytime sleepiness or correlating PSG findings
○ Adjustment insomnia (acute)
  ● Associated with an identifiable stressor lasting only a few days to several weeks but no longer than 3 months
○ Secondary insomnia
  ● Secondary insomnia refers to what we now call *comorbid insomnia*, which accounts for the majority of insomnia cases
    ◆ These are insomnias that are comorbid with medical and/or psychiatric disease
      ● Insomnia due to a mental disorder
        ◆ Mood disorders, most notably depression and anxiety (Sutton, 2014)
      ● Insomnia due to a medical disorder
        ◆ Pain disorders
        ◆ Heart disease
        ◆ Lung disease
      ● Insomnia due to drug or substance
      ● Inadequate sleep hygiene
      ● Behavioral insomnia of childhood (sleep-onset association type or limit-setting type)

Pathophysiology (ATLAS2, p 150)

■ The etiology and pathophysiology are not well understood
■ Insomnia is considered a disorder of hyperarousal, or, alternatively, it is conceptualized as a failure of wakefulness inhibition
■ Four models attempt to explain how hyperarousal is responsible for insomnia: (1) physiologic, (2) cognitive, (3) neurocognitive, and (4) behavioral
■ Homeostatic dysregulation and circadian dysrhythmia may also be important contributing factors

Clinical Presentation

■ Sleep complaints
  ○ "Insomnia" or "trouble falling asleep"
  ○ Frequent awakenings or early morning awakenings
  ○ Nonrestorative or light sleep
  ○ Difficulty functioning in occupational, educational, or social settings
  ○ Reduced overall quality of life
  ○ Patients usually express considerable anxiety and distress about their sleep problems
■ Nonsleep complaints
  ○ Either in addition to the sleep complaint or in the absence of a sleep complaint
  ○ Symptoms can include:
    ● Headache
    ● GI distress
    ● Chronic pain
    ● Accidents
    ● Fatigue
    ● Depressed mood
    ● Irritability
    ● Cognitive impairment
    ● Anxiety
    ● Obsessive thinking
    ● Muscle tension
    ● Fibromyalgia symptoms

Differential Diagnosis

- Primary sleep disorder other than insomnia, for example, sleep-disordered breathing, RLS, PLMD, shift-work disorder, circadian rhythm disorder, and parasomnias
- Psychiatric disorder (e.g., depression, anxiety)
- Medical disorder (e.g., chronic pain, lung disease, heart failure, endocrine disease)

Diagnostic Workup

- Thorough sleep history and detailed medical, substance, and psychiatric history along with a thorough physical exam
- Psychological testing as indicated
- Sleep diary for 1 to 4 weeks
- Actigraphy for 1 to 2 weeks
  - Can offer some measure of objective data
  - Very useful when paradoxical insomnia is suspected
- PSG if a sleep disorder other than insomnia is suspected
- Consider blood tests if signs and symptoms raise suspicion for a medical disorder

Treatment (ATLAS2, pp 155-158)

- Nonpharmacologic
  - Cranial electrical stimulation: approved by FDA but controversial
  - CBTi is a multimodal treatment approach that has proven to be just as effective as medication in short-term follow-up and to be superior to medication in long-term follow-up. (Sutton, 2014)
  - Stimulus control
  - Sleep restriction
  - Relaxation techniques (e.g., progressive muscle relaxation, guided imagery, biofeedback)
  - Sleep hygiene education
  - Cognitive therapy (of which paradoxical intention is a subset)
- Pharmacologic   (ATLAS2, pp 105-111; Ioachimescu and El-Sohl, 2012; Atkin, 2018)
  - Benzodiazepines: Know whether a given benzodiazepine is short, intermediate, or long acting
  - Nonbenzodiazepine hypnotics
    - Zolpidem
    - Eszopiclone
    - Zaleplon (much shorter acting than the other two above)
    - Suvorexant (dual orexin receptor antagonist)
  - Antidepressants
    - Doxepin
    - Trazodone
    - Amitriptyline
  - Antipsychotics
    - Quetiapine
    - Olanzapine
  - Antihistamines: diphenhydramine
- Herbs and supplements
  - Melatonin
  - Valerian root
  - Passion flower
  - Chamomile

Prognosis

- Chronic insomnia tends to have a remitting-relapsing course
- Long-term prognosis is best with CBTi

Morbidity and Mortality

- Morbidity
  - Increased risk for depression, anxiety, substance use and abuse, work-related and traffic accidents, and cognitive decline
- Mortality
  - Data are more equivocal
  - Unclear whether we can extrapolate from the short-sleep literature in which numerous studies show increased mortality with sleep durations less than 6 to 6.5 hours

REFERENCES

American Academy of Sleep Medicine. *International classification of sleep disorders.* 3rd ed. Darien, Ill.: American Academy of Sleep Medicine; 2014.

Atkin T, Comai S, Gobbi G. Drugs for insomnia beyond benzodiazepines: pharmacology, clinical applications, and discovery. *Pharmacol Rev.* 2018;70(2):197–245.

Buysse DJ. Insomnia. *JAMA.* 2013;309(7):706–716.

Herring WJ, Connor KM, Ivgy-May N, et al. Suvorexant in patients with insomnia: results from two 3-month randomized controlled clinical trials. *Biol Psychiatry.* 2016;79(2):136–148.

Ioachimescu OC, El-Solh AA. Pharmacotherapy of insomnia. *Expert Opin Pharmacother.* 2012;13(9):1243–1260.

Koffel EA, Koffel JB, Gehrman PR. A meta-analysis of group cognitive behavioral therapy for insomnia. *Sleep Med Rev.* 2014;pii: S1087-0792(14)00048-3.

Kostoglou-Athanassiou I. Therapeutic applications of melatonin. *Ther Adv Endocrinol Metab.* 2013;4(1):13–24.

Kryger MH, Avidan A, Berry R. *Atlas of clinical sleep medicine.* 2nd ed. Philadelphia: Saunders; 2014.

Morgenthaler T, Kramer M, Alessi C, et al. American Academy of Sleep Medicine. Practice parameters for the psychological and behavioral treatment of insomnia: an update. An American Academy of Sleep Medicine report. *Sleep.* 2006;29(11):1415–1419.

Morin CM. Cognitive-behavioral approaches to the treatment of insomnia. *J Clin Psychiatry.* 2004;65(suppl 16):33–40.

Morin CM, Bastien C, Guay B, et al. Randomized clinical trial of supervised tapering and cognitive behavior therapy to facilitate benzodiazepine discontinuation in older adults with chronic insomnia. *Am J Psychiatry.* 2004;161(2):332–342.

Morin CM, Bootzin RR, Buysse DJ, et al. Psychological and behavioral treatment of insomnia: update of the recent evidence (1998-2004). *Sleep.* 2006;29(11):1398–1414.

National Institutes of Health. National Institutes of Health state of the science conference statement on manifestations and management of chronic insomnia in adults, June 13-15, 2005. *Sleep.* 2005;28(9):1049–1057.

Ohayon MM. Observation of the natural evolution of insomnia in the American general population cohort. *Sleep Med Clin.* 2009;4(1):87–92.

Ohayon MM, Roth T. Place of chronic insomnia in the course of depressive and anxiety disorders. *J Psychiatr Res.* 2003;37:9–15.

Shekelle P, Cook I, Miake-Lye IM, et al. *The effectiveness and risks of cranial electrical stimulation for the treatment of pain, depression, anxiety, PTSD, and insomnia: a systematic review [Internet].* Washington (DC): Department of Veterans Affairs (US); 2018. Available from: http://www.ncbi.nlm.nih.gov/books/NBK493132/.

Sivertsen B, Omvik S, Pallesen S, et al. Cognitive behavioral therapy vs zopiclone for treatment of chronic primary insomnia in older adults: a randomized controlled trial. *JAMA.* 2006;295(24):2851–2858.

Sutton EL. Psychiatric disorders and sleep issues. *Med Clin North Am.* 2014;98(5):1123–1143.

Taylor DJ, Pruiksma KE. Cognitive and behavioural therapy for insomnia (CBT-I) in psychiatric populations: a systematic review. *Int Rev Psychiatry.* 2014;26(2):205–213.

Central Disorders of Hypersomnolence

4.1   Narcolepsy

QUESTIONS

Call to 911

A 22-year-old nursing student is referred to the neurology clinic with an unusual history. She had been lying lengthwise on her couch with her head propped up, watching a TV comedy program, when her husband found her apneic and cyanotic, yet she appeared to be awake with her eyes wide open. She did not respond when he called out to her. He immediately called 911 and then rolled her onto the floor to do cardiopulmonary resuscitation (CPR), when she suddenly started to breathe. She was able to speak and was alert and oriented. She stated that she had never lost consciousness. Emergency medical technicians arrived within 5 minutes, quickly examined her, and found normal vital signs. Assuming she had a seizure, they suggested she see a neurologist. The patient's medical history includes severe daytime sleepiness, which started around age 15 years, and recurrent episodes of knee buckling, especially when arguing. She has otherwise been healthy.

1. What is the *most* likely diagnosis?
   A. Epilepsy
   B. Cardiac arrhythmia
   C. Transient ischemic attack
   D. Narcolepsy with cataplexy

2. The woman has a 30-minute nap every day right after lunch. Which statement about these naps is likely to be *true*?
   A. She feels refreshed for 1 to 3 hours after the naps
   B. She dreams infrequently or not at all during naps
   C. She is likely to stop breathing during these naps
   D. She has been noted to twitch during naps

3. Which symptom is the patient *least* likely to have?
   A. Vivid dream imagery at sleep onset
   B. Cataplexy
   C. Sleep paralysis
   D. Enuresis

4. What statement is *most* correct concerning the sleep of narcolepsy patients?
   A. Sleep apnea is common
   B. Sleep paralysis occurs in more than 90%
   C. Stage R comes late in the sleep period
   D. Sleep disruption is common

5. Which statement about the patient's disease is *true*?
   A. After symptoms manifest, narcolepsy is a lifelong condition
   B. Narcolepsy symptoms do not improve with age
   C. It is strongly linked to autoimmune disorders
   D. Cataplexy is found in fewer than 5% of cases

6. Which set of findings would *most* strongly support the diagnosis of narcolepsy in this patient?
   A. Polysomnography (PSG) showing sleep efficiency greater than 90%; multiple sleep latency test (MSLT) showing a mean latency of 4 minutes; 1 sleep-onset rapid eye movement period (SOREMP)
   B. PSG showing rapid eye movement (REM) latency of 180 minutes with more than 6 hours of sleep; MSLT showing a mean latency of 5 minutes; 1 SOREMP
   C. PSG showing a REM latency of 45 minutes with more than 6 hours of sleep; MSLT showing a mean latency of 5 minutes; 2 SOREMPs
   D. PSG showing a REM latency of 90 minutes with more than 6 hours of sleep; MSLT showing a mean latency of 3 minutes; 0 SOREMPs

Collapsing at Baseball Games

A 29-year-old man has a 15-year history of severe daytime sleepiness and episodes of "falling spells." At baseball games, he sometimes falls to the ground when cheering. His family doctor recently diagnosed narcolepsy and started him on fluoxetine 20 mg in the morning to control what he believed to be cataplexy. No response was seen after 4 days, so he was referred to the sleep clinic.

7. Why was the fluoxetine not effective in reducing cataplexy?
   A. The dose was too small
   B. Inhibition of adrenergic uptake is an effective treatment, but fluoxetine is a selective serotonin reuptake inhibitor (SSRI) with little effect on adrenergic reuptake
   C. The fluoxetine should have been taken at bedtime
   D. It takes 2 weeks for fluoxetine to be effective

8. Which of the following medications is *most* likely to be effective in treating the cataplexy?
   A. Atomoxetine
   B. Modafinil
   C. Prazosin
   D. Propranolol

9. The patient is started on modafinil, 200 mg in the morning. After 1 week, he reports little improvement in the sleepiness and no effect on the cataplexy. What is the next step?
   A. Increase the dose of modafinil to 400 mg, either as one dose in the morning or 200 mg in the morning and 200 mg at noon
   B. Switch to methylphenidate sustained release, 20 mg in the morning
   C. Switch to dextroamphetamine sustained release, 15 mg in the morning
   D. Switch to armodafinil, 100 mg in the morning

10. With the adjustment of stimulant medication, the patient has some improvement in sleepiness, but the cataplexy is still severe. What is the next step in therapy?
    A. Reassure the patient. Adding any additional medication will offer little benefit
    B. No additional medication is warranted because no medication is approved by the Food and Drug Administration (FDA) for cataplexy
    C. Add clomipramine at bedtime
    D. Add sodium oxybate at bedtime and another dose 4 hours later

11. What cerebrospinal fluid (CSF) abnormality is likely to be found in this patient?
    A. CSF hypocretin-1 level less than 110 pg/mL
    B. CSF orexin level greater than 110 pg/mL
    C. High histamine levels
    D. Low serotonin levels

The Devil Is in the Details

A 19-year-old woman is referred because of four frightening episodes occurring over the preceding year. In each episode, she awakens unable to move and is aware of a gnomelike creature hovering over her bed. She cannot visualize the creature's face but senses it is about to attack her. Despite the fear, she is unable to verbalize or move for about 5 minutes. These episodes occur about 90 minutes after she falls asleep. When she is finally able to move, there is relief but also concern about going back to sleep. However, the episode has not repeated on the same night. She denies any other symptoms and has no daytime sleepiness. Her aunt has narcolepsy.

12. What is the likely diagnosis?
    A. Psychogenic state
    B. Psychomotor seizure
    C. Narcolepsy
    D. Isolated sleep paralysis

13. The patient's doctor prescribes sodium oxybate, assuming that she has a form of narcolepsy. She takes it for three nights and then stops, deciding it is not prudent to take medication for a symptom that occurs so infrequently. Instead, she takes three herbal products from the health food store to help her sleep: valerian, kava, and chamomile. About 2 months later, her 18-year-old brother, a weightlifter, is brought to the emergency department (ED) with low blood pressure and hypercapnic respiratory failure. The ED physician believes that he might have overdosed on some medication, and a toxic panel is ordered. Which of the medications is a possible cause of her brother's respiratory failure?
    A. Valerian
    B. Sodium oxybate
    C. Chamomile
    D. Kava

14. What is the *most* likely reason her brother would want to take one of these medications?
    A. To get "high"
    B. To sleep
    C. To enhance physical performance
    D. To improve memory

Blame It on the Ex-Boyfriend

A 5'4", 122-lb (body mass index [BMI], 20.9), 20-year-old college student presents to her family physician with a complaint of "low energy," poor sleep, and daytime sleepiness. The problems began about 1 year ago when she broke up with her boyfriend. A few months earlier, before the breakup, she had presented to the same internist at the university with symptoms (fever, headache, sore throat, and lethargy that were likely caused by a bout of the flu. Her friends tell her she looks sleepy and depressed. She has great difficulty completing school work and routinely falls asleep in class. In recent months, she has been dropping items from both her right and left hands when surprised. These dropping episodes do not seem to be associated with an awareness of muscle weakness or fatigue.

15. Which of the following are *least* likely to explain her symptoms?
    A. Depression
    B. Narcolepsy
    C. Strep throat
    D. Chronic insomnia

16. Which of the following best explains the onset of narcolepsy in those who have contracted the flu?
    A. Autoimmune destruction of hypocretin cells
    B. Autoimmune destruction of dopamine cells
    C. Destruction of gamma-aminobutyric acid (GABA) cells in the ventrolateral preoptic nucleus (VLPO)
    D. Evidence that the flu may result in a small number of cases of narcolepsy has not been established

17. Which of the following narcolepsy symptoms can closely be linked to autoimmune response from H1N1 infections?
   A. Sleep paralysis
   B. Sleep attacks
   C. Cataplexy
   D. Automatic behavior

18. The patient's physician believes the symptoms are caused by the breakup with the patient's boyfriend and her subsequent depression. She is prescribed a selective norepinephrine reuptake inhibitor (SNRI) and returns to the clinic 4 weeks later. What would you predict about the patient's status at this point?
   A. Her mood is much better, and her sleepiness has resolved
   B. She reports having been in a recent "fender bender" because she fell asleep at the wheel
   C. Her mood has improved, and there have been continued episodes of dropping things since she began treatment
   D. She has reconciled with her boyfriend, and she does not want to continue with the antidepressant

The Case of a Sleepy Attorney

A 5'3", 185-lb (BMI, 33.5), 32-year-old women who works full time as a real estate attorney presents to a physician with sleep attacks, which she reports to be getting more frequent. As a result, she no longer drives. Her law practice has suffered, and she only works 1 day a week. She struggled with sleepiness in law school but was able to get by taking caffeine pills. In high school, she was diagnosed with attention-deficit/hyperactivity disorder (ADHD) and was prescribed a long-acting form of methylphenidate, which significantly diminished her sleepiness and sleep attacks. The methylphenidate caused her to be anxious and have palpitations, so she discontinued and never followed up for additional treatment. A sleep medicine specialist has her undergo a PSG, which results in an apnea/hypopnea index (AHI) of 35/hr. Her rapid eye movement (REM) latency is 14 minutes. MSLT results are a mean sleep latency of 8.8 minutes across 5 naps. REM was evident only in nap 2.

19. What is her diagnosis?
   A. Narcolepsy
   B. Narcolepsy and obstructive sleep apnea (OSA)
   C. ADHD and OSA
   D. OSA

20. What should you do first?
   A. Prescribe sodium oxybate
   B. Have her retested for ADHD
   C. Repeat PSG and MSLT
   D. Prescribe continuous positive airway pressure (CPAP) and follow

A Sleepy Narcoleptic on Treatment

A 31-year-old narcoleptic patient has been taking 250 mg of armodafinil, resulting in moderate success in reducing daytime sleepiness. The sleepiness is so severe on awakening that she has to delay her drive to work until the armodafinil kicks in. You prescribe 10 mg of dextroamphetamine to be taken immediately upon awakening.

21. The mechanism of action of amphetamines is to directly
   A. Increase activity in histamine neurons
   B. Increase activity in the dopamine system
   C. Increase activity in the orexin system
   D. Increase activity in VLPO neurons

22. The patient's previous sleep specialist prescribed clomipramine for treatment of cataplexy. Tricyclic antidepressants (TCAs) interact with all of the following *except*
    A. Dopamine receptors
    B. Serotonin receptors
    C. Acetylcholine receptors
    D. Histamine receptors

23. Regarding laboratory tests for diagnosing narcolepsy, all of the following are true *except*
    A. About 12% to 38% of the general population is positive for HLA-DQB1*06:02, so human leukocyte antigen (HLA) typing alone is not diagnostic for narcolepsy
    B. About 99% of patients with cataplexy are HLA-DQB1*06:02 positive, so a negative test result essentially eliminates the possibility of hypocretin deficiency
    C. About 95% of patients with CSF hypocretin deficiency have a positive MSLT result and cataplexy
    D. In a majority of patients with narcolepsy with cataplexy (type 1 narcolepsy), CSF hypocretin will be less than 210 pg/mL

24. All of the following are true of cataplexy *except*
    A. It usually is not the first symptom of type 1 narcolepsy and typically occurs weeks to months after the onset of excessive sleepiness
    B. In the vast majority of attacks, the cataplexy is bilateral
    C. The incidence of narcolepsy with cataplexy is 0.02% to 0.18% in the United States
    D. Respiratory muscles are often involved in children with cataplexy

---

ANSWERS

1. D. She has narcolepsy with cataplexy. An important clue that makes the first three answers unlikely is that she never lost consciousness. Features also suggestive of narcolepsy are the history of severe sleepiness starting in her teens and recurrent episodes of buckling of the knees, a classic description for cataplexy. (It is always important to read the entire question and each possible answer carefully.) In this scenario, she developed cataplexy while watching a comedy program, losing tone of her neck's strap muscles. The ensuing anatomic position of her head and neck led to an obstructed upper airway. Note that *narcolepsy with cataplexy* (narcolepsy type 1) is distinct from *narcolepsy without cataplexy* (narcolepsy type 2). Type 1 (with cataplexy) is a hypocretin deficiency believed to be pathogenetic. (ICSD3, pp 146-155)

2. A. Naps are generally very refreshing in patients with narcolepsy, and prescription of strategically timed naps is an important part of treatment. After a nap, patients with narcolepsy often become more alert and energetic for up to several hours. This is in contrast to patients with sleep apnea or idiopathic hypersomnia (IH), in whom the feeling of sleepiness generally does not improve much after napping.

3. D. Enuresis is not a feature of narcolepsy. The classic tetrad of narcolepsy includes sleepiness, cataplexy, sleep paralysis, and hypnagogic hallucinations. Other common symptoms include disrupted nocturnal sleep and automatic behavior.

4. D. Sleep disruption and the complaint of insomnia are common and are often not elicited when taking the history. Sleep paralysis has been reported to occur in 40% to 80% of patients with narcolepsy. REM sleep can occur much earlier than the typical 90 minutes after sleep onset, including within 15 minutes of sleep onset. REM sleep that occurs within 15 minutes of sleep onset is called a *sleep-onset REM period* (SOREMP). It used to be that two SOREMPS in the MSLT were needed to make a diagnosis of narcolepsy. Revised diagnostic criteria now allow a SOREMP in the PSG preceding the MSLT to substitute for one SOREMP in the MSLT. Thus, one SOREMP in the preceding PSG and one SOREMP in the MSLT will satisfy the two-SOREMP criteria for diagnosing narcolepsy. (ICSD3, p 159)

5. A.   After symptoms of narcolepsy manifest, which often begins during the teenage years, the condition is lifelong. There is some evidence that sleepiness and cataplexy may attenuate in older patents.   (Dauvilliers Y, Gosselin A, Paquet J, Touchon J, Billiard M, Montplaisir J. Neurology Jan 2004, 62(1):46-50.) Cataplexy is found in at least 60% of cases and is a necessary component to diagnose type 1 narcolepsy. Type 2 narcolepsy is caused by a deficiency of hypothalamic hypocretin (orexin) signaling. Cataplexy is defined as "more than one episode of generally brief (<2 min), usually bilaterally symmetric sudden loss of muscle tone with retained consciousness. The episodes are precipitated by strong emotions, usually positive, with almost all patients reporting some episodes precipitated by emotions associated with laughter."   (ICSD3, p 147) Although it is hypothesized that an autoimmune process may be responsible for the loss of hypocretin neurons, there has been no rigorous association with any specific autoimmune disorder. Knowledge of narcolepsy and its symptoms, pathophysiology, and treatment will be tested in several sections of the exam.   (ATLAS2, Ch 11.1)

6. C.   In the context of a supporting clinical history, the finding during the MSLT of a mean sleep latency of 8 minutes or less and two or more SOREMPs is considered diagnostic of narcolepsy. Alternatively, the two-SOREMP requirement can be satisfied with one SOREMP in the PSG preceding the MSLT and just one SOREMP in the MSLT. Low hypocretin (≤110 pg/mL) in the CSF is diagnostic of narcolepsy with cataplexy and may be used instead of the MSLT to confirm the diagnosis.   (ICSD3, p 146)

7. B.   In both animal models of narcolepsy and in humans with the disease, inhibition of adrenergic uptake improves cataplexy. Dopamine and serotonin reuptake inhibition is not very effective. Fluoxetine is a serotonin reuptake inhibitor.

8. A.   Drugs that inhibit adrenergic uptake (protriptyline, desipramine, viloxazine, atomoxetine) are often effective in improving cataplexy. Atomoxetine is an SNRI approved for use in ADHD. Modafinil has no effect on cataplexy. Prazosin, an alpha$_1$-antagonist, dramatically aggravates canine narcolepsy-cataplexy. This question is an example in which you deduce an answer by knowing which answers are incorrect.

9. A.   The dose of modafinil could be increased to 400 mg before treating the patient with either methylphenidate or dextroamphetamine. Armodafinil is the R-isomer of modafinil; a dose of 100 mg would be no more effective than 200 mg of modafinil.   (ATLAS2, p 173, Table 11.1–1; PPSM 6, pp 469-470 and 879-880)

10. D.   Sodium oxybate (gamma-hydroxybutyric acid [GHB]) is highly effective in treating cataplexy in narcolepsy, and it also improves daytime sleepiness. Before the availability of sodium oxybate, antidepressants such as clomipramine were widely used for this indication.

11. A.   Hypocretin, also called *orexin*, is produced by a small number of cells in the lateral hypothalamus. The hypocretin-producing cells are markedly decreased or absent in patients with narcolepsy with cataplexy, and cells may be damaged as part of an autoimmune process. Hypocretin levels in the CSF are reduced (<110 pg/mL), and low histamine levels have been reported in patients with hypersomnia.

12. D.   This is a classic description of isolated sleep paralysis. The episodes are generally uncommon, and treatment is usually reassurance. The episodes do not portend a later diagnosis of narcolepsy.

13. B.   Sodium oxybate in high doses can lead to respiratory failure. GHB, the "street" version of the medication, has been linked to deaths from overdose. Abuse of sodium oxybate is actually uncommon because a large amount of salt (sodium) added to the liquid product gives it a very unpleasant taste.

14. C.   Sodium oxybate increases slow-wave sleep, which is associated with increased growth hormone secretion. Some athletes will use illicit GHB as a performance-enhancing product. The kava plant (*Piper methysticum*) is used to produce a drink with sedative properties, which is consumed to relax without disrupting mental clarity. However, kava can cause liver failure, and its use is regulated in some countries.   (Sarris et al, 2011; Van Cauter et al, 2004)

15. D. She does not have a complaint of difficulty initiating and maintaining sleep, so insomnia is not likely the cause of symptoms. People with insomnia, in addition to nighttime sleep difficulties, often are "hyperaroused" and rarely have involuntary sleep episodes.

16. A. Narcolepsy is strongly associated with the HLA-DQB1*06:02 genotype. Other risk genes, such as T-cell receptor α chain and purinergic receptor subtype 2Y11, are also implicated. Interest in narcolepsy has increased since the epidemiologic observations that H1N1 infection and vaccination are potential triggering factors for hypocretin cell destruction, and an increase in the incidence of narcolepsy after the pandemic AS03 adjuvanted H1N1 vaccination in 2010 from Sweden and Finland supports the immune-mediated pathogenesis. (Partinen et al, 2014)

17. C. The pathophysiology of narcolepsy type 1 (with cataplexy) is best explained by loss of hypocretin. The hypocretin cell loss is caused by an autoimmune response.

18. B. Although some antidepressants are used to treat cataplexy, they have not been shown to reduce excessive sleepiness or sleep attacks.

19. D. This could be a case that eventually unveils itself as OSA with narcolepsy, but the data are not supportive. An early REM latency can occur in untreated OSA patients, and this patient's MSLT results were not precisely consistent with a narcolepsy ICSD3 diagnosis. When there is severe OSA, the sleep laboratory data are often not definitive.

20. D. The most rational approach is to treat the sleep-disordered breathing and reevaluate in 1 to 2 months.

21 B. Amphetamines target release of catecholamines (both dopamine and norepinephrine) and inhibit reuptake from presynaptic terminals. Increasing activity in the VLPO would cause sleepiness.   (ATLAS2, Table 11.1–1)

22. A. TCAs affect several neurotransmitter receptors, including serotonin, norepinephrine, acetylcholine, and histamine. There is no known interaction with dopamine receptors.

23. D. In a majority of patients with type 1 narcolepsy, the CSF hypocretin will be 110 pg/mL or less, or less than one third of the mean values obtained in normal subjects. The other statements are all true.   (ATLAS2, Fig. 11.1–5; ICSD3, p 146)

24. D. Characteristic of cataplexy is that respiratory muscles are not involved in children or adults.

Summary

Highly Recommended

- *Atlas of clinical sleep medicine*, 2nd ed, Chapter 11.1
- Dauvilliers Y, Barateau L: Narcolepsy and other central hypersomnias. *Continuum (Minneap Minn)*. Aug;23(4, Sleep Neurology):989-1004, 2017
- De la Herrán-Arita AK, García-García F: Current and emerging options for the drug treatment of narcolepsy, *Drugs*. 73(16):1771–1781, 2013
- *International classification of sleep disorders*, 3rd ed, pp 146-161

Narcolepsy—Key Points

Although you can expect only about 12 specific narcolepsy questions on the exam, you will likely encounter many more questions for which an understanding of this condition is helpful (e.g., about REM sleep, the MSLT, drugs used in treatment, "sleep attacks"). Thus, it is important that you have a solid understanding of narcolepsy and cataplexy.

Forms of Narcolepsy

- The three main forms of narcolepsy are
  - Narcolepsy with cataplexy (associated with hypocretin deficiency), type 1 narcolepsy
  - Narcolepsy without cataplexy, type 2 narcolepsy
  - Secondary narcolepsy, found in a variety of conditions
    - After central nervous system (CNS) trauma
    - With genetic disorders
      - ◆ That cause mainly CNS abnormalities: Niemann-Pick type C, autosomal-dominant cerebellar ataxia, Norrie disease (blindness and hearing loss), Coffin-Lowry syndrome (mental retardation and cardiovascular defects)
      - ◆ That also cause sleep breathing disorders: myotonic dystrophy, Prader-Willi syndrome
    - With lesions in the brain: neoplastic, inflammatory, neurodegenerative

Epidemiology

- Narcolepsy with cataplexy prevalence varies geographically, affecting, for example,
  - 1 of 4000 people in Western Europe and the United States
  - 1 of 600 people in Japan
  - 1 of 500,000 people in Israel
- The prevalence of narcolepsy without cataplexy is not well known
  - Makes up 10% to 50% of narcolepsy cases

Core Features

- Sleepiness
- Cataplexy (in the type associated with hypocretin deficiency)
  - Induced by laughter (87%)
  - Induced by joking (73%)
  - Induced by anger (68%)
- Hallucinations
  - Hypnagogic (at sleep onset)
  - Hypnopompic (on awakening)
- Sleep paralysis
- Disrupted nocturnal sleep
- Onset most often in teenage years

Pathophysiology and Genetics

- Narcolepsy with cataplexy
  - Associated with human leukocyte antigen (HLA)-DQB1*0602
  - Found in 25% of people without narcolepsy
  - Autoimmune loss of hypocretin (orexin) cells in hypothalamus
  - Deficiency of hypocretin-1 in CNS is causal
- Narcolepsy without cataplexy
  - Pathophysiology is unclear
- Secondary narcolepsy
  - Low or intermediate hypocretin-1 levels may be seen in many disorders associated with narcolepsy
    - Myotonic dystrophy
    - Multiple sclerosis
    - Prader-Willi syndrome
    - Autosomal-dominant cerebellar ataxia
    - Traumatic brain injury
    - Mass lesions involving hypothalamus

Diagnosis (ICSD3)

- Type 1 (narcolepsy with cataplexy)
  - ○ For at least 3 months, daily periods of irrepressible need to sleep
  - ○ Cataplexy (see answer to Question 5) *and* a mean sleep latency ≤8 minutes with two or more SOREMPs on MSLT or one SOREMP on the preceding nocturnal PSG plus one SOREMP on the MSLT; *or*
  - ○ CSF hypocretin ≤110 pg/mL
- Type 2 (narcolepsy without cataplexy); must meet all of the following:
  - ○ For at least 3 months, daily periods of irrepressible need to sleep
  - ○ A mean sleep latency ≤8 minutes with two or more SOREMPs on MSLT or one SOREMP on the preceding nocturnal PSG plus one SOREMP on the MSLT
  - ○ If measured, CSF hypocretin is >110 pg/mL *or* the hypersomnolence and/or MSLT findings are not better explained by other causes
  - ○ REM latency may be short
- MSLT
  - ○ Four or five naps in test; performed after preceding PSG
  - ○ For proper interpretation, ICSD3 (p 152) lists specific conditions that precede the MSLT (e.g., free of confounding drugs for 2 weeks, etc.)
  - ○ Confirm pathologic sleepiness with mean sleep latency of 8 minutes or less
  - ○ Two or more SOREMPs *or* one SOREMP in the PSG preceding the MSLT and one SOREMP in the MSLT
- Measurement of hypocretin-1 level in CSF
  - ○ May substitute for MSLT in type 1 narcolepsy
  - ○ Low level (≤110 pg/mL) is diagnostic
- HLA-DQB1*0602 determination
  - ○ Of limited diagnostic usefulness
  - ○ Found in 25% of people without narcolepsy

Treatment

- General measures
  - ○ Take short scheduled naps
  - ○ Follow a regular sleep schedule
  - ○ Get an appropriate amount of nighttime sleep
  - ○ If patient is a student, notify teachers
  - ○ If patient is a driver, caution patient (or parent) and comply with local department of motor vehicle (DMV) regulations
- Children's drug dosages vary with age and weight
  - ○ For sleepiness, prescribed in order based on response:
    - Modafinil 100 to 400 mg or armodafinil 150 to 250 mg in the morning
    - Sodium oxybate 4.5 to 9 g at night in divided doses
    - Methylphenidate 10 to 30 mg/day, depending on whether the sustained-release preparation is used, in the morning and during the day as needed
    - Atomoxetine 10 to 25 mg in the morning
  - ○ For cataplexy
    - Sodium oxybate 4.5 to 9 g at night in divided doses
    - Venlafaxine 75 to 150 mg in the morning
- Adults
  - ○ For sleepiness, prescribed in order based on response
  - ○ Many experts start patients on both modafinil and sodium oxybate initially
    - Modafinil 100 to 400 mg or armodafinil 150 to 250 mg in the morning
      - ◆ May reduce levels of steroidal contraceptives, cyclosporine, and triazolam
    - Sodium oxybate 4.5 to 9 g at night in divided doses
    - Methylphenidate 10 to 30 mg/day, depending on whether a sustained-release preparation is used, in the morning and during the day as needed
    - Atomoxetine in teenagers: start at 0.5 mg/kg and increase to 1 to 1.2 mg/kg within 1 week

○ For sleepiness not responsive to the medications above
  • Dextroamphetamine
  • Dexedrine
○ For cataplexy
  • Sodium oxybate 4.5 to 9 g at night in divided doses
  • Venlafaxine 75 to 150 mg in the morning

Although not FDA approved at this writing, additional pharmacologic treatments are in development for narcolepsy, including pitolisant, solriamfetol, and alternative forms of sodium oxybate (longer acting, reduced sodium content).

REFERENCES

American Academy of Sleep Medicine. *International classification of sleep disorders.* 3rd ed. Darien, Ill.: American Academy of Sleep Medicine; 2014.

Kryger MH, Avidan A, Berry R, eds. *Atlas of clinical sleep medicine.* 2nd ed. Philadelphia: Saunders; 2014.

Kallweit U, Bassetti CL. Pharmacological management of narcolepsy with and without cataplexy. *Expert Opin Pharmacother.* 2017;18(8):809–817.

Lopez R, Dauvilliers Y. Pharmacotherapy options for cataplexy. *Expert Opin Pharmacother.* 2013;14(7):895–903.

Partinen M, Kornum BR, Plazzi G, et al. Narcolepsy as an autoimmune disease: the role of H1N1 infection and vaccination. *Lancet Neurol.* 2014;13(6):600–613.

Sarris J, Laporte E, Schweitzer I. Kava: a comprehensive review of efficacy, safety, and psychopharmacology. *Aust N Z J Psychiatry.* 2011;45.

Van Cauter E, Latta F, Nedeltcheva A, et al. Reciprocal interactions between the GH axis and sleep. *Growth Horm IGF Res.* 2004;14(supplA):S10–S17.

4.2   Idiopathic Hypersomnia

Comparisons

In comparing narcolepsy with IH, link the features in questions 1 through 5 with the following:

  A. Narcolepsy
  B. Idiopathic hypersomnia
  C. Both conditions
  D. Neither condition

1. Excessive daytime sleepiness

2. Presence of cataplexy

3. REM-related phenomena common (e.g., sleep paralysis, hallucinations)

4. Reports of remission

5. Naps are frequently restorative.

ANSWERS

1. C.   (ATLAS2, p 160)

2. A.   (ATLAS2, p 160)

3. A.   (ATLAS2, p 160)

4. B.   (ATLAS2, p 160)

5. A.   (ATLAS2, p 160)

Summary

Idiopathic Hypersomnia—Key Points

Expect two or three questions about this topic on the examination.
- Conclusive epidemiologic studies have not been conducted
- Disease onset occurs most often during adolescence or young adulthood
- A familial background is often present, but rigorous studies are still lacking
- The key manifestation is hypersomnolence
- It is often accompanied by sleep of long duration and debilitating sleep inertia
- PSG followed by an MSLT is mandatory, as well as a 24-hour PSG or a 2-week actigraphy in association with a sleep log to ensure a total 24-hour sleep time longer than or equal to 660 minutes, when the mean sleep latency on the MSLT is longer than 8 minutes
- MSLT is neither sensitive nor specific, the PSG diagnostic criteria require continuous readjustment, and biological markers are still lacking

Diagnosis and Course

- Idiopathic hypersomnia is most often a chronic condition, although spontaneous remission may occur
- Based on neurochemical, genetic, and immunologic analyses as well as on exploration of the homeostatic and circadian processes of sleep, various pathophysiologic hypotheses have been proposed
- Differential diagnosis involves a number of diseases, and it is not yet clear whether IH and narcolepsy type 2 are not the same condition

Idiopathic Hypersomnia (ICSD3, pp 161-166)

- Epidemiology
  - Rare
  - 50 per million people
- Clinical features
  - Onset ages: most often 10 to 30 years
  - Sleepiness
    - Constant
    - Naps prolonged
    - Naps not refreshing
    - 2 to 3 hours of sleep inertia in the morning
    - May be aggressive after awakening
- Diagnosis   (ICSD3, pp 161-166)
  - Sleepiness is present for at least 3 months
  - Cataplexy is absent
  - MSLT shows fewer than two SOREMPs
  - MSLT mean sleep latency ≤8 minutes, or total 24-hour sleep time is ≥660 minutes
  - Insufficient sleep time is ruled out
  - Findings are not better explained by another disorder or use of drugs
- Treatment
  - No consistently effective treatment is available
  - Modafinil response is less robust than in narcolepsy
  - Works best in patients with long sleep times

Treatment

The treatment of IH has mirrored that of the sleepiness of narcolepsy type 1 or 2. Recent studies using drugs that antagonize GABA have been used and are under development.

REFERENCES

Billiard M. Idiopathic hypersomnia. *Neurol Clin.* 1996;14:573.
Trotti LM, Saini P, Bliwise DL, et al. Clarithromycin in γ-aminobutyric acid-related hypersomnolence: a randomized, crossover trial. *Ann Neurol.* 2015;78:454.
Trotti LM, Saini P, Koola C, et al. Flumazenil for the treatment of refractory hypersomnolence: clinical experience with 153 patients. *J Clin Sleep Med.* 2016;12:1389.
American Academy of Sleep Medicine: International classification of sleep disorders, ed 3, Darien, Ill., 2014, American Academy of Sleep Medicine. pp 161-166.

4.3	**Sleepiness With Hypersexuality**

QUESTIONS

A 12-year-old boy, previously well, had a brief illness for which headache was a prominent symptom. A few days later he developed severe daytime sleepiness, which lasted about 5 days; during this period, he slept for about 14 hours each day. About 2 months later, the daytime sleepiness suddenly returned, and he began sleeping about 15 hours a day. He also developed a voracious appetite and gained 10 lb in 2 weeks and started to snore. The sleepiness and increased appetite symptoms resolved after 2 weeks. While awake, he would also sometimes hallucinate, and at other times, he would masturbate in front of family members.

1. What is the suspected diagnosis and why?
   A. Kleine-Levin syndrome (periodic hypersomnia)
   B. Recurrent hypersomnia; the episodes of sleepiness are separated by periods of normal sleep and behavior
   C. OSA; the boy snores and is obese and sleepy
   D. Schizophreniform reaction; he has hallucinations
   E. Narcolepsy; this is suggested by his age, the sleepiness, and the hallucinations

2. How would you manage the patient during the phases when his sleep is normal?
   A. Use an antipsychotic agent such as risperidone or haloperidol to prevent further episodes
   B. Use low-dose (100 mg/day) modafinil
   C. Reassure the patient and the family
   D. Use low-dose (7.5 mg/day) prednisone because this is an autoimmune disorder

3. How would you manage the patient during the phases when he sleeps excessively and has abnormal behavior?
   A. Use an antipsychotic agent such as risperidone or haloperidol
   B. Use high-dose (400 mg) modafinil
   C. Reassure the patient and the family
   D. Use high-dose (60 mg) prednisone because this is an autoimmune disorder

ANSWERS

1. A. The description is classic for recurrent hypersomnia or Kleine-Levin syndrome (*not* Kleine-Levin; the syndrome is named after early 20th-century reports by German neurologist Will Kleine and American psychiatrist Max Levin). (ICSD3, pp 166-170)

2. C. No intervention is known to change the course of the illness.

3. C. No intervention is known to change the course of the illness. In most cases, the episodes of sleepiness resolve within 1 to 4 years. Readers should note that lesions in the hypothalamus (e.g., tumors) can cause severe sleepiness, but the sleepiness is generally continuous and without spontaneous resolution.

Summary

Recurrent Hypersomnia (ICSD3, pp 166-170)

Expect one or two questions about this topic on the examination.
- Kleine-Levin syndrome
  - Epidemiology
    - Rare
    - Starts in teenage years
    - Much more common in male patients
  - Clinical features
    - Recurrent episodes of hypersomnia
      - Sleeping up to 18 hours a day
      - Lasting a few days to weeks
      - Occurs between 1 and 10 times a year
    - Hyperphagia during episodes
    - Hypersexuality during episodes
    - Abnormal behavior
      - Confusion, irritability, aggression, hallucinations
    - Normal sleep and behavior between episodes of hypersomnia
  - Course
    - Duration of episodes is from 1 to several years (average, ~4 years).
  - Treatment
    - There is no effective FDA-approved treatment.   (Huang et al, 2010)
      - Stimulants can have unwanted psychiatric effects
      - Case reports have described positive outcomes.   (Arnulf et al, 2018)
        - With gabapentin
        - With carbamazepine
        - With lithium (to reduce frequency of episodes)
        - With intravenous steroids (to reduce duration of episodes)

REFERENCES

Arnulf I, Groos E, Dodet P. Kleine-Levin syndrome: a neuropsychiatric disorder. *Rev Neurol (Paris)*. 2018;174(4):216–227.
Huang YS, Lakkis C, Guilleminault C. Kleine-Levin syndrome: current status. *Med Clin North Am*. 2010;94(3):557–562.

4.4 Insufficient Sleep Syndrome

QUESTIONS

Always Sleeping

A 24-year-old man was recently referred for evaluation because of a drowsy-driving automobile crash on his morning commute to work. He often goes to sleep after coming home from work at 4 PM and does not awaken until 5:30 AM. He goes to bed at 10 PM, awakens at 4:30 AM, and has a 1-hour commute before his work as a municipal bus driver. He is on a split shift: his first shift is from 6 AM to noon, and the second shift goes from 3 to 7 PM; in between, he is at the bus terminal, killing time. He denies hypnagogic hallucinations, cataplexy, and sleep paralysis, and his family history is entirely negative. He takes no medications. An overnight sleep study showed he spent 8.9 hours in bed and slept 8.2 hours and during 37.7% of sleep time showed findings similar to those in Figure 4.4–1.

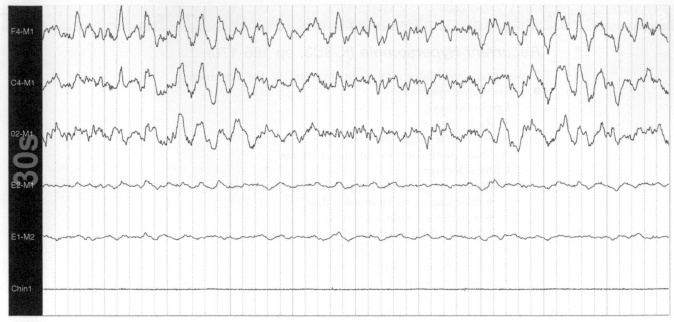

FIGURE 4.4–1 Questions 1 and 2.

1. What does Figure 4.4–1 show?
- **A.** Seizure activity
- **B.** Stage R sleep
- **C.** Stage N3 sleep
- **D.** Spindling

2. About this finding, which statement is *most* correct?
- **A.** Any time spent with this finding is considered abnormal
- **B.** The percentage is within normal limits
- **C.** The percentage is much greater than one would expect in a 24-year-old adult
- **D.** The percentage is much less than one would expect in a 24-year-old adult

3. The patient spent 22% of the night with findings similar to those shown in Figure 4.4–2. What does this figure show?
- **A.** Seizure activity
- **B.** Stage R sleep
- **C.** Stage N3 sleep
- **D.** Prozac eyes

4. Which statement is *most* correct about this finding?
- **A.** Any time spent with this finding is considered abnormal
- **B.** This finding is within normal limits
- **C.** This finding is much greater than one would expect in a 24-year-old adult
- **D.** This finding is much less than one would expect in a 24-year-old adult

5. The patient spent 65.6% of the night with findings similar to those in Figure 4.4–3. What does this figure show?
- **A.** Vertex sharp wave
- **B.** Seizure activity
- **C.** K complex
- **D.** Alpha waves

6. About this finding, which statement is *most* correct?
- **A.** Any time spent with this finding is considered abnormal
- **B.** The percentage is within normal limits
- **C.** The percentage is much greater than one would expect in a 24-year-old adult
- **D.** The percentage is much less than one would expect in a 24-year-old adult

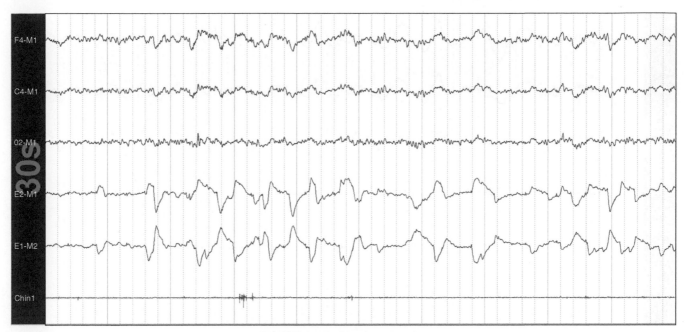

FIGURE 4.4–2 Questions 3 and 4.

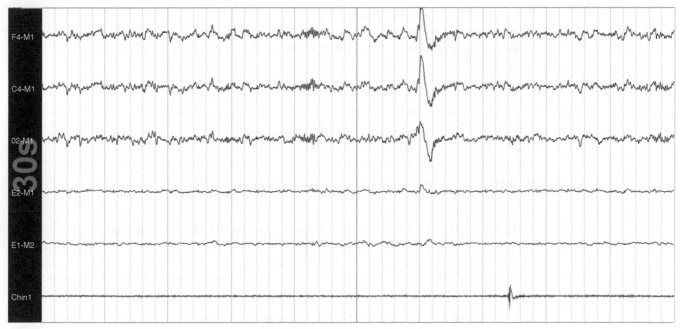

FIGURE 4.4–3 Questions 5 and 6.

Blacking Out at Red Lights

A 48-year-old Manhattan taxi driver has been "blacking out" at red lights, and after crashing into a parked car, he is referred for a sleep evaluation. He has a BMI of 38 and a neck collar size of 19 inches. His history includes snoring but no witnessed apneas. To stay awake, he drinks 10 cups of coffee a day. He starts his daily shift at 4 AM and ends at 7 PM and lives about 40 minutes away from Manhattan. His Epworth Sleepiness Scale (ESS) score is 4 of 24, pulse 90/min and regular, and blood pressure 150/95 mm Hg.

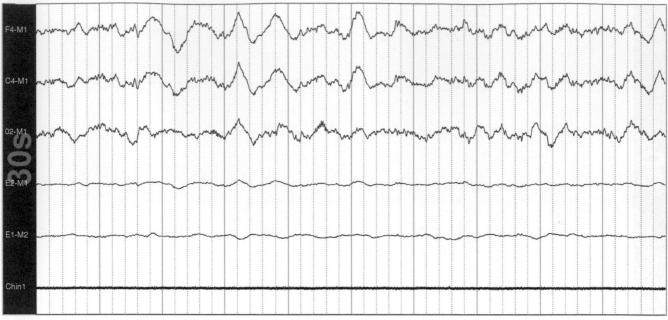

FIGURE 4.4–4 Question 7.

7. What would you recommend?
   A. Advise the patient to sleep at least 7 hours per day and to return if his sleepiness remains
   B. Perform an MSLT to document sleepiness because he is a hazard on the road
   C. Start him on modafinil
   D. Perform an overnight comprehensive PSG

The patient has an overnight PSG, and 40% of the recording is similar to Figure 4.4–4. The sleep study showed:

Sleep: Latency = 2 min; efficiency = 94%; stage R latency = 70 min; non-REM (NREM) sleep = 80% of sleep time; stage R = 20%; arousal index = 7/hr; periodic limb movement (PLM) index = 4/hr

Breathing: AHI = 4 events/hr; RDI = 6 events/hr; low SaO_2 = 93%

8. What would you do next?
   A. Order MSLT to rule out narcolepsy because the REM latency was short
   B. Arrange for a CPAP titration study
   C. Refer to a neurologist to evaluate for epilepsy
   D. Reassure the patient that his problem is sleep deprivation, and strongly suggest that he sleep more—or else

9. The patient returns 1 month later, requesting a prescription for modafinil. He now sleeps 8 hours a night and has done so for more than 2 weeks yet is still "blacking out" at red lights. He tried a few modafinil pills provided by another taxi driver and thought they helped him. What would you do next?
   A. Prescribe modafinil
   B. Order an MSLT alone
   C. Order a maintenance of wakefulness test (MWT)
   D. Repeat the PSG followed by an MSLT

10. What metabolic factors may explain the patient's obesity?
   A. Low levels of ghrelin
   B. Low levels of leptin
   C. High levels of thyroid hormone
   D. Low levels of growth hormone

Sleepy Computer Programmer

A 35-year-old computer programmer has been cited for poor work performance, including falling asleep at his desk. He comes in with his wife, who says the problem has been noticeable the past few months; his first citation was 1 month ago, and she is concerned he is about to be fired. In your office, he manifests flat affect but answers questions appropriately. His wife says he snores, and she has not witnessed any apneas. She reports that he sleeps "at least 8 hours every night." She helps him fill out the ESS form; the score is 16 of 24. His BMI is 31, and his neck circumference is 16.5 inches. There is a history of depression in college, for which he was briefly prescribed an antidepressant, but he is not currently taking any medications. You send him for an overnight PSG followed the next morning by an MSLT. The results showed that he slept 7 hours out of 7.5 hours during the study time. The AHI revealed 5.9 events per hour and low SaO_2 at 89%. His average sleep latency on the MSLT was 13.5 minutes, and no SOREMPs were recorded.

11. The *most* likely diagnosis is
   A. Narcolepsy
   B. Idiopathic hypersomnolence
   C. Hypersomnia associated with a psychiatric disorder
   D. OSA

12. The definitive test for diagnosing hypersomnolence associated with a psychiatric disorder is
   A. MSLT
   B. Beck Depression Inventory
   C. Diagnosis of bipolar disorder or major depression in patient with hypersomnolence, normal PSG, and normal MSLT
   D. No test is definitive

Sleepy Graduate Student

A 23-year-old graduate student is evaluated for excessive daytime sleepiness (EDS). She has no significant health problems, but her ESS score is 17 of 24, and she complains of frequently falling asleep in seminars. She reports that her sleep is erratic because she goes to bed late and sometimes has to get up early for school. On weekends, she will often "sleep in until 10 or 11 AM." There is no history of cataplexy. Her father uses CPAP, and the patient thinks she may have OSA. Her BMI is 24. She has a live-in boyfriend and no history of heavy snoring or witnessed apneas. Because of her concern, you order a PSG followed by an MSLT.

  She arrived at the sleep lab late and was not ready to start the study until after midnight. She slept a total of 5 hours and 20 minutes. Her AHI showed 2.4 events per hour and low SaO_2 at 92%. Her PLM index was increased at 27 movements per hour, and her arousal index was 15 arousals per hour. In the MSLT, latency to onset of sleep, averaged over five naps, was 5.4 minutes. She had two SOREMPs in these five naps.

13. The *most* likely cause for her excessive daytime sleepiness (EDS) is
   A. Narcolepsy without cataplexy
   B. Periodic limb movement disorder
   C. Idiopathic hypersomnolence
   D. Insufficient sleep syndrome

14. Which of the following statements is *most* correct about insufficient sleep syndrome?
   A. A familial pattern is discernible in most patients
   B. It is a subset of delayed sleep phase disorder that is common among adolescents
   C. When present in middle-aged or older people, it is a circadian rhythm disorder
   D. The diagnosis is made when a trial with longer sleep periods eliminates the patient's symptoms

ANSWERS

1. C.   This is stage N3, or slow-wave sleep (SWS).

2. C.   It would be expected that a 24-year-old adult would spend 20% to 25% of sleep time in stage N3, or SWS. A value of about 37.7% would be considered normally high.

3. B.   This is classic REM sleep (stage R) with a mixed frequency electroencephalogram (EEG), eye movements, and absent chin muscle tone. *Prozac eyes* are pendulous movements that can be seen in patients taking SSRIs in all stages of sleep. These were first described with fluoxetine.   (Armitage et al, 1995)

4. B.   The time is in the normal range for REM sleep.

5. C.   To the right of the center of the epoch is a K complex. To the left is a sleep spindle. These are visible in the three EEG channels.

6. C.   This is stage N2, and one would expect a 24-year-old adult to spend only about 50% of the total sleep time (TST) in this stage.

7. D.   A comprehensive PSG is the correct answer because not only is the patient sleep deprived, but he is also at high risk of having sleep apnea. MSLT alone is not indicated in patients with sleep deprivation (except at times for medicolegal reasons). Modafinil is not indicated for sleep deprivation. Although answer A appears reasonable, because of the risk of sleep apnea, it is not. Note that the ESS is low, which reflects the fact that a patient whose job depends on alertness might lie to "pass the test" or drink large amounts of caffeine.

8. D.   This is stage N3, or SWS. A substantial portion of the fragment reveals slow waves (Fig. 4.4–5). Sleep deprivation is the cause of the findings (SWS rebound), and no additional evaluation is required at this time. The official term for this is *behaviorally induced insufficient sleep syndrome*. The "or else" refers to the fact that to protect the public's and the patient's safety, he could be reported to the authorities.

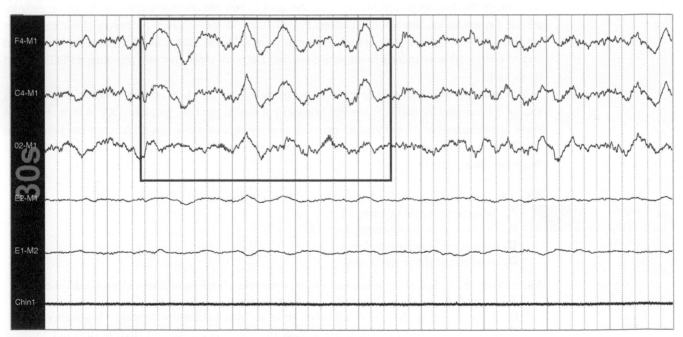

FIGURE 4.4–5 Answer 8.

9. D. This scenario occurs commonly. There is no indication to perform a PSG if only insufficient sleep is suspected. However, if the patient states that he is sleeping an appropriate amount of time and still has severe sleepiness, an evaluation is in order. In this case, the next step would be a PSG followed by an MSLT. There is night-to-night variation, and perhaps a repeat study will show apnea (in which case the MSLT would be canceled). Or the MSLT might confirm pathologic sleepiness and will perhaps even show SOREMPs. The next step for this patient would be to schedule a PSG followed by an MSLT. (ISCD3, pp 182-186)

10. B. Leptin, a hormone secreted by adipocytes, acts on centers in the hypothalamus, suppressing food intake and stimulating energy expenditure. Ghrelin is a hormone produced by cells of the gastrointestinal tract, and it results in hunger (think of a growling stomach). Insufficient sleep has been shown to cause high levels of ghrelin, resulting in increased hunger. Sleep deprivation leads to reduced leptin and increased ghrelin.

11. C. Hypersomnia with a psychiatric disorder can only be diagnosed if the patient has a psychiatric disorder. In this case, there is history of depression, and the initial encounter suggests depression is significant. The other two criteria needed to make this diagnosis are symptoms for at least 3 months and symptoms not better explained by another sleep disorder. He meets all three criteria. The PSG is near normal; an AHI of 5.9 would not explain his daytime sleepiness. His MSLT results do not meet criteria for narcolepsy or IH. (ICSD3, pp 179-181)

12. D. No definitive test exists for this diagnosis. Most important is to rule out other common causes of sleepiness, particularly insufficient sleep and medication side effects. The diagnosis is based on history, ruling out other conditions, and a confirmed psychiatric disorder. The patient was referred to a psychiatrist for treatment of major depression.

13. D. Technically speaking, an MSLT is not valid if the patient begins the test with insufficient sleep. SOREMPs can appear in the setting of insufficient sleep, and in that situation, they cannot be used to diagnose narcolepsy. A minimum of 6 hours of sleep the night before is the threshold for doing an MSLT. Periodic limb movement disorder (PLMD) may cause EDS if the movements are associated with excessive arousals; in this patient's case, the arousal index was in the normal range (<20/hr). Idiopathic hypersomnolence can only be diagnosed when the sleep latency is 8 minutes or less on MSLT *and* the patient has had sufficient sleep before the test. In this case, there is abundant evidence for insufficient sleep syndrome: her own history, plus the PSG data. This patient really did not need the PSG and MSLT; a detailed sleep diary (kept by the patient or, if available, via actigraphy) would have confirmed insufficient total sleep over 24 hours.

14. D. No familial pattern is present to diagnose insufficient sleep syndrome. Delayed sleep phase disorder (DSPD) may lead to insufficient sleep, but the two are considered separate diagnoses; the latter is not considered a circadian disorder in any age group. The diagnosis is secure if longer sleep time corrects the problem. Note that "the diagnosis of insufficient sleep syndrome may be especially difficult to make in subjects who have a physiologic need for unusually large amounts of sleep." (ICSD3, pp 182-185)

Summary

Insufficient Sleep Syndrome, or Behaviorally Induced Insufficient Sleep Syndrome (ICSD3, pp 182-186)

Expect about seven questions on this topic on the exam.
- Diagnosis
  - Present at least 3 months
  - Sleep duration below population norms

○ PSG (not required for diagnosis)
  • High sleep efficiency
  • Might have SOREMPs
  • Can have increased stage 3 sleep
○ MSLT (not required for diagnosis)
  • Mean sleep latency ≤8 minutes
  • One or more SOREMPs can occur.

REFERENCE

Armitage R, Trivedi M, Rush AJ. Fluoxetine and oculomotor activity during sleep in depressed patients. *Neuropsychopharmacology*. 1995;12:159–165.

4.5   Hypersomnia Due to Medical Disorders

Sleepy After a Football Game

A military veteran is seen in the sleep disorders center because he has severe daytime sleepiness and does not believe he can safely drive a car. The symptoms started several weeks after sustaining a concussion in a football game; he thought he had recovered from the concussion. Computed tomography and magnetic resonance imaging MRI of his brain are normal. He has a BMI of 29 and a snoring history but no witnessed apneas. His ESS score is 22 of 24.

1. What is your next step?
   A. PSG followed by MSLT if the PSG results are normal
   B. MSLT alone because OSA is unlikely here
   C. MWT alone
   D. Clinical trial of modafinil

The following results were obtained on testing:

Sleep: Latency = 1 min; stage R latency = 70 min; stage N1 = 1% of sleep time; stage N2 = 49%; stage N3 = 25%; stage R = 25%; arousal index = 5/hr; PLM index = 1.2/hr

Breathing: AHI = 4 events/hr; RDI = 6 events/hr; low SaO_2 = 93%

MSLT: Mean sleep latency = 2 min; SOREMPs = 0

2. Given these results, what would you do next?
   A. Tell the patient that no therapy works for his problem
   B. Arrange a psychiatric evaluation
   C. Repeat high-resolution imaging of the hypothalamic area
   D. Begin a clinical trial of modafinil

BONUS QUESTIONS

Sleepiness Despite CPAP

Moderate OSA has been diagnosed in a 54-year-old man after a PSG. He has a BMI of 37 and a neck circumference of 18.5 inches. A second night in the lab reveals an optimal CPAP of 14 cm H_2O, which is prescribed. He returns 60 days later, and the download of data from his CPAP machine indicates he is using it an average of 6 hours per night, 6 nights per week. He tells you that his sleepiness has improved since he began CPAP but that on some days he is still severely sleepy, even when he has used CPAP the night before. To objectively measure his sleepiness, you order an MSLT, which shows a mean sleep latency of 6.5 minutes. His ESS score is 15 of 24. You then prescribe 200 mg of modafinil.

3. Modafinil for treating residual sleepiness associated with OSA has been found to
   A. Increase sleep latency on the MSLT by 1 to 2 minutes compared with baseline
   B. Increase sleep latency on the MSLT by 5 to 10 minutes compared with baseline
   C. Decrease the ESS score on average by 2 points
   D. Decrease the ESS score on average by 5 points

4. The patient returns to see you 2 weeks later, and his sleepiness has resolved; however, he complains of side effects from taking the drug. Which one of the following adverse events associated with modafinil is *least* likely?
   A. Headache
   B. Chest pain
   C. Rash
   D. Severe depression

5. All of the following are true about the R-enantiomer of modafinil, armodafinil, *except*
   A. It has a longer half-life
   B. It has the same potency
   C. It has been approved by the FDA for treating EDS associated with narcolepsy, OSA, and shift-work disorder
   D. It has a similar side effect profile

ANSWERS

1. A.   A patient who has had a traumatic brain injury (TBI) and who has sleep complaints requires an evaluation. Of 57 patients studied 3 months after TBI, 39% had abnormal sleep study results. Of patients with abnormal sleep, 23% had sleep apnea, 3% had posttraumatic hypersomnia, 5% had narcolepsy, and 7% had periodic limb movement syndrome (PLMS). Objective excessive daytime sleepiness with sleep latency less than 10 minutes on the MSLT was found in 21% of the patients.   (Castriotta et al, 2009)

2. D.   Technically, the correct answer is A because no drug has been shown to work consistently for TBI hypersomnia. However, the only randomized trial published to date shows sporadic but inconsistent improvement with modafinil. Thus, a clinical trial is indicated, although it is unlikely to be successful. Interestingly, when apneas, hypopneas, and snoring were eliminated by CPAP in TBI patients found to have OSA, there was no significant change in MSLT scores.   (Jha et al, 2008; Castriotta et al, 2009; Castriotta et al, 2011; Borghol et al, 2018)

3. A.   In a double-blind, placebo-controlled study of patients who have OSA and residual excessive sleepiness while compliant with CPAP therapy, modafinil at doses of 400 mg improved objective measures of alertness on the MSLT by 1.2 minutes (sleep latency was 8.6 minutes compared with 7.4 minutes at baseline). Although this improvement on the MSLT is small, it does represent a statistically significant signal that modafinil improves alertness.   (Black and Hirshkowitz, 2005)

4. D.   The most common adverse event with modafinil is headache, which is not usually a problem if the dose is increased gradually. No significant cardiovascular adverse effects have been reported from treatment in the clinical trials, except with a previous history of cardiovascular sensitivity to activating or stimulant medications. In these cases, palpitations and chest pain have been reported. A few cases of severe allergic reactions resulting in rashes have been documented.

5. B.   Compared with modafinil, armodafinil has a longer half-life and is approximately two times more potent when steady state is achieved. It has the same FDA indications as modafinil and a similar side effect profile.   (ATLAS2, Table 11.1–1)

Summary

Posttraumatic Hypersomnia

- Pathophysiology
  - Trauma results in loss of hypocretin (orexin) neurons. (Baumann et al, 2009)
- Clinical features
  - Sleepiness occurs after head trauma
  - Sleepiness may be persistent
- Treatment
  - No established treatment (Jha et al, 2008; Borghol et al, 2018)

REFERENCES

Baumann CR, Bassetti CL, Valko PO, et al. Loss of hypocretin (orexin) neurons with traumatic brain injury. *Ann Neurol.* 2009;66:555–559.

Black JD, Hirshkowitz M. Modafinil for treatment of residual excessive sleepiness in nasal continuous positive airway pressure–treated obstructive sleep apnea/hypopnea syndrome. *Sleep.* 2005;28:464–471.

Borghol A, Aucoin M, Onor I, et al. Modafinil for the improvement of patient outcomes following traumatic brain injury. *Innov Clin Neurosci.* 2018;15(3–4):17–23.

Castriotta RJ, Atanasov S, Wilde MC, et al. Treatment of sleep disorders after traumatic brain injury. *J Clin Sleep Med.* 2009;5:137–144.

Castriotta RJ, Murthy JN. Sleep disorders in patients with traumatic brain injury: a review. *CNS Drugs.* 2011;25: 175–185.

Jha A, Weintraub A, Allshouse A, et al. A randomized trial of modafinil for the treatment of fatigue and excessive daytime sleepiness in individuals with chronic traumatic brain injury. *J Head Trauma Rehabil.* 2008;23(1):52–63.

4.6   Hypersomnia Due to Medications

A Patient on Many Drugs

A 58-year-old woman is referred to you by her primary care physician for EDS, to "rule out sleep apnea." Her ESS score is 15 of 24. She is obese with a BMI of 33, but there is no history of witnessed apneas. She thinks her sleep is sufficient, "probably 7 to 8 hours a night." You learn she has a psychiatric disorder and is taking Xanax, Seroquel, trazodone, and an opiate for chronic pain syndrome. You mention the possibility of medication side effects, but she states she has been on these drugs "for years."

1. The *best* next step is to
  A. Order a PSG
  B. Stop at least two of the drugs
  C. Prescribe modafinil
  D. Have her keep a detailed sleep diary and return in 2 weeks

Female, Forty, and ...

A 40-year-old woman with a BMI of 36 kg/m² is referred to the sleep disorders center. She has a 5-year history of severe daytime sleepiness and snoring. Her ESS score is elevated, at 19 of 24. For several months, she has been taking clonazepam, taken as needed during the daytime, and amitriptyline at night. She also takes medications for major depressive disorder (MDD) and anxiety and denies that the medications worsened her daytime sleepiness. Her overnight sleep study showed these data:

Sleep: Latency = 9 min; stage R latency = 240 min; stage N1 = 4% of sleep time; stage N2 = 75%; stage N3 = 1%: stage R = 20%; arousal index = 5/hr; periodic limb movement (PLM) index = 12/hr

Breathing: AHI = 4 events/hr; respiratory disturbance index (RDI) = 6 events/hr; low SaO₂ = 93%

2. What is the *most* likely cause of her daytime sleepiness?
  A. Upper airway resistance syndrome
  B. Periodic limb movements
  C. MDD
  D. Her medications

3. The referring clinician was concerned that her nocturnal leg movements might be clinically significant and wanted to treat them. What should you recommend?
  A. Clonazepam at bedtime
  B. Consider switching from amitriptyline to bupropion
  C. Stopping antidepressant therapy
  D. Adding pramipexole

4. Another 40-year-old-woman, also with a BMI of 36, is referred to the sleep disorders center with a several-year history of severe daytime sleepiness and snoring. For several months, she has taken clonazepam for insomnia and amitriptyline for depression before bedtime. The referral letter indicates that she is being treated for MDD and anxiety, but these medications have had no effect on her sleepiness. The referring physician requests a nocturnal PSG. What do you recommend?
  A. An MSLT to document sleepiness objectively
  B. A clinical trial of autotitrating CPAP in a range from 5 to 12 cm H$_2$O
  C. An overnight PSG
  D. A clinical trial of modafinil, and if that is not helpful, a PSG

5. A sleep study is done with the following results:

Sleep: Latency = 9 min; stage R latency = 240 min; stage N1 = 14% of sleep time; stage N2 = 75%; stage N3 = 1%; stage R = 10%; arousal index = 36/hr; PLM index = 12/hr

Breathing: AHI = 34 events/hr; RDI = 44 events/hr; low SaO$_2$ = 83%

After a CPAP titration study, the patient is started on CPAP. In addition to CPAP, what would you recommend?

  A. Stop the clonazepam at night, and reassess the patient's need for antidepressants after 2 weeks
  B. Stop the antidepressant therapy
  C. Continue the clonazepam
  D. Add modafinil to treat the sleepiness

ANSWERS

1. A. The best way to answer the referral question is conduct a PSG. Given you have the expertise, taking the time to unwind her even from two of the psychotropic drugs could be a lengthy process.

2. C. The likeliest cause is MDD, which is diagnosed when the patient has had two or more major depressive episodes. It is beyond the scope of this volume to review the diagnosis of depression, but symptoms of MDD include depressed mood every day for at least 2 months and loss of interest in almost all activities. Another symptom is hypersomnia or insomnia every day. In this patient, the sleepiness preceded the use of the medication, although both MDD and the medication could cause sleepiness. The AHI, periodic limb movement index (PLMI), and arousal index are not sufficiently abnormal to explain the daytime sleepiness.   (ICSD3, pp 179-181)

3. B. The presence of leg movements per se is not an indication that they should be treated. There is certainly no indication that restless legs syndrome (RLS) is present and therefore no indication to prescribe pramipexole. Because the arousal index is normal, there is no reason to prescribe clonazepam at bedtime. Because virtually all antidepressants except bupropion have been associated with a movement disorder (RLS symptoms, motor restlessness, or PLMs) and because the antidepressant does not appear to be working, a trial of bupropion might be considered.

4. C. Female patients with sleep apnea are very likely to be treated for depression. Some are depressed, but for some, it is a misdiagnosis that may deter you from doing a PSG and finding OSA. Insomnia is also a common presenting symptom of women with OSA. A clinical trial of CPAP would not be indicated because a diagnosis of apnea has not been made, and insurance companies would not pay for the equipment without an objective diagnosis. It would be inappropriate to use modafinil at this point of management.

5. A. Stopping the antidepressant is not indicated because the patient could be depressed. Clonazepam can worsen apnea and could be stopped. Modafinil should not be used at this point in management.

| 4.7 | **Hypersomnia Associated With Psychiatric Disorders** |

A 68-year-old, 5′10″, 222-lb (BMI, 32) male patient is referred to you for hypersomnolence likely caused by OSA. According to his wife, he has a long history of snoring but no witnessed apneas. He is not hypertensive, but there is a history of depression for which he was taking doxepin 75 mg at bedtime. He has been taking the doxepin for more than 20 years, and his internist has maintained him on it because it reportedly relieved the depression. The patient reports feeling very sad and depressed because of the recent loss of his son in a motor vehicle accident.

QUESTIONS

1. After taking a careful history, what should you do first?
   A. Order an HSAT or in-lab PSG
   B. Withdraw him from the doxepin and start an SNRI
   C. Refer him for grief therapy to a psychologist
   D. Order a PSG and MSLT

The PSG demonstrates that patient has an AHI of 18 with a low SaO_2 of 87%. At the follow-up visit, he admits to drinking three or four glasses of bourbon most evenings. The night of the PSG, he did not ingest alcohol.

2. What is the proper first treatment?
   A. Alcohol detoxification and repeat PSG
   B. Initiate CPAP at 7 cm/H_2O at home
   C. Start the patient on an autotitrating PAP device
   D. Speak to internist about cutting the doxepin in half

3. He begins using PAP therapy at home but remains hypersomnolent with an ESS of 14. What should be done next?
   A. He should discontinue the doxepin
   B. The dose of doxepin should be titrated and withdrawn while a newer SNRI is introduced
   C. The patient should be counseled on alcohol abuse and educated about the effects of alcohol on OSA
   D. Increase CPAP empirically

4. Hypersomnolence is rarely seen in patients with
   A. MDD
   B. Bipolar disorder
   C. Seasonal affective disorder
   D. Conversion disorders

5. What is characteristic of sleep architecture in patients with depression?
   A. Increase in SWS production
   B. Normal rapid eye movement (REM) cycling sleep
   C. Shortened REM latency
   D. Decreased REM sleep duration and density

ANSWERS

1. A. Cases of OSA with a psychiatric overlay are common and often complex. His wife's lack of observation for apnea should not dissuade a clinician from conducting sleep testing.

2. C. The patient demonstrated significant breathing difficulties during sleep. An autotitrating device for home use would be the proper next step.

3. C. Alcoholism is compounding his problem given the drug is known to increase the number and length of apneas.

4. D. Conversion disorders do not necessarily result in hypersomnolence, but depression bipolar disorder and SADs can have hypersomnolence as a primary symptom.

5. C. Disturbances of sleep are common in depressed patients and belong to the core symptoms of the disorder. Sleep research has demonstrated that besides disturbances of sleep continuity, depression is associated with altered sleep architecture (i.e., a decrease in SWS production and disturbed REM sleep regulation). Shortened REM latency (i.e., the interval between sleep onset and the occurrence of the first REM period), increased REM sleep duration, and increased REM density (i.e., the frequency of rapid eye movements per REM period) have been considered as biological markers of depression.

REFERENCES

Lopez R, Barateau L, Evangelista E, Dauvilliers Y. Depression and hypersomnia: a complex association. *Sleep Med Clin.* 2017;12(3):395–405.
Palagini L, Baglioni C, Ciapparelli A, et al. REM sleep dysregulation in depression: state of the art. *Sleep Med Rev.* 2013;17(5):377–390.

Psychiatric Disease (See Also Section 8 of This Volume)

- MDD
  - Hypersomnia (and/or insomnia) nearly every day are symptoms that are included in the list of diagnostic criteria
  - Hypersomnia can be caused by sedating medications used for treatment
  - Hypersomnia can be caused by medications used to treat the patient and that cause another sleep disorder
    - Antidepressants (an exception is bupropion) can cause a movement disorder
    - Antidepressants (e.g., mirtazapine) can cause weight gain and cause or worsen sleep apnea
      - Mirtazapine has been evaluated as a treatment for sleep apnea. It is not effective and can worsen apnea. (Marshall et al, 2008)
- Other psychiatric disorders
  - Disturbed sleep is a common (but not defining) symptom of several psychiatric conditions
  - Medications used to treat anxiety and psychotic disorders can cause sleepiness
    - Directly owing to a sedating effect
    - Indirectly by further disturbing sleep
- Menstrual-related hypersomnia
  - Epidemiology
    - Rare
    - May be familial (Rocamora et al, 2010)

○ Pathophysiology
- Possibly related to reproductive hormones
○ Clinical features
- Hypersomnia related to menstrual cycle
- Male siblings can have Kleine-Levin syndrome
○ Treatment
- Might respond to oral contraceptives

BONUS QUESTIONS FOR NARCOLEPSY

In comparing two drugs used to treat narcolepsy, choose the *correct* answer for questions 1 through 5.

A. Modafinil
B. Sodium oxybate
C. Both
D. Neither

1. First-line treatment for EDS

2. First-line treatment for cataplexy

3. Recommended to start drug in divided doses

4. Metabolite of GABA

5. Approved for use in children

ANSWERS

1. C

2. B

3. B

4. B

5. B

Summary

Highly Recommended

- *International classification of sleep disorders*, 3rd ed, pp 143-188

Other Disorders That Cause Hypersomnia

From the blueprint, you can expect about 8 to 10 questions covering hypersomnia exclusive of narcolepsy and cataplexy. The topic areas include recurrent hypersomnia (Kleine-Levin syndrome), IH, insufficient sleep, and hypersomnia in psychiatric disease. Of course, hypersomnia is a common symptom of other sleep disorders, such as sleep apnea, and thus the conditions mentioned here would be considered in the differential diagnosis in questions evaluating other areas. In the summary, we use the same sequence as described in the American Board of Internal Medicine blueprint: psychiatric disease, recurrent hypersomnia, IH, insufficient sleep, and post-traumatic hypersomnia.

REFERENCES

American Academy of Sleep Medicine. *International classification of sleep disorders*. 3rd ed. Darien, Ill.: American Academy of Sleep Medicine; 2014.

Kryger MH, Avidan A, Berry R, eds. *Atlas of clinical sleep medicine*. 2nd ed. Philadelphia: Saunders; 2014.

Marshall NS, Yee BJ, Desai AV, et al. Two randomized placebo-controlled trials to evaluate the efficacy and tolerability of mirtazapine for the treatment of obstructive sleep apnea. *Sleep*. 2008;31:824–831.

Rocamora R, Gil-Nagel A, Franch O, Vela-Bueno A. Familial recurrent hypersomnia: two siblings with Kleine-Levin syndrome and menstrual-related hypersomnia. *J Child Neurol*. 2010;25(11):1408–1410.

Parasomnias

| 5.1 | Non–Rapid Eye Movement Parasomnias |

QUESTIONS

Eating Raw Meat at Night

A 31-year-old female business executive is referred to the sleep disorders center for a complaint of sleep-walking. She had many sleepwalking episodes as a child, but they stopped at when she was 12 years old. She was free of any sleep-related problems until the past 4 months. She has been eating every night after going to bed but has no recollection of getting up to go to the kitchen. Yet in the morning, it is evident that she has cooked and eaten some food, and she even appears to have eaten uncooked meat. She has put on 30 lb in the past 4 months.

1. Which statement about this patient's disorder is *true*?
   A. It only occurs during stage N3 sleep
   B. It only occurs in the first third of the night
   C. Episodes are triggered by alcohol consumption
   D. It is not an indication of psychopathology

2. Which statement about management is *most* correct?
   A. A nocturnal polysomnogram (PSG) is indicated
   B. A nocturnal electroencephalograph (EEG) study directed toward capturing seizure activity is indicated
   C. Assessment by a psychiatrist or psychologist is indicated
   D. Further investigations are not needed; clonazepam 0.5 mg at bedtime is usually effective

3. All of the following medications have shown some efficacy *except*:
   A. Zolpidem
   B. Dopaminergic agents
   C. Opiates
   D. Topiramate

4. If the patient is found to have moderate obstructive sleep apnea (OSA) and is treated with continuous positive airway pressure (CPAP), what would you expect about her sleep-eating episodes?
   A. They will increase in frequency because the amount of stage N3 sleep increases
   B. They will decrease in frequency even though the amount of stage N3 sleep might increase
   C. There will be no effect on the frequency of the episodes
   D. The patient will continue to sleepwalk, but she will stop eating at night

The Screamer

A 7-year-old boy lets out bloodcurdling screams while in bed at night. His parents rush into his room, and each time they notice that he is standing up, rocking back and forth, with his eyes open and staring right through them. He is sweating, appears angry, and screams out, "No! No! No!" The boy is otherwise healthy. He sleeps 9 hours a night and plays in a hockey league.

5. Which statement about this disorder is *false*?
   A. The events occur during stage R (rapid eye movement [REM]) sleep
   B. Children with this condition generally have no recollection of the nocturnal events
   C. Episodes most often occur in the first third of the night
   D. The disorder might have a genetic basis

6. The boy's parents are very concerned about the episodes and ask for your diagnosis. The *least* likely disorder would be
   A. Seizure disorder
   B. Psychogenic state
   C. Sleep terrors
   D. Rhythmic movement disorder

An overnight sleep study lasting 10 hours is performed. The child spends 45% of the night with findings similar to those shown in Figure 5.1–1. The patient has some abrupt arousals while in this state. No abnormal motor activity is seen on synchronized digital video monitoring.

7. This fragment shows which of the following?
   A. Hypersynchronous theta
   B. Continuous seizures
   C. Stage N3 sleep
   D. Sweat artifact

8. Based on the data in Figure 5.1–1, what would you recommend?
   A. Carbamazepine to treat the seizure
   B. Clonazepam to be used as needed when he sleeps away from home
   C. Risperidone nightly
   D. Increase in nocturnal sleep time

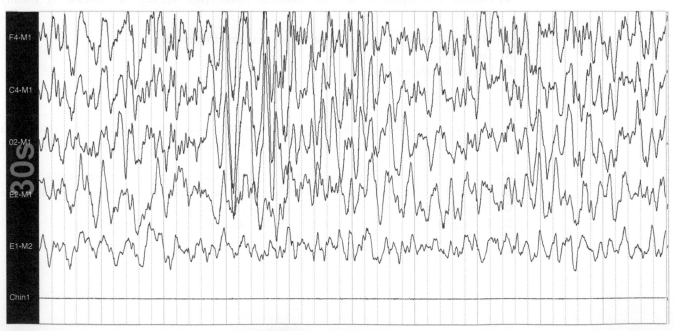

FIGURE 5.1–1 Questions 7 and 8.

Wandering

A 20-year-old female college student is referred for the treatment of insomnia. She has been found wandering around the halls of her dorm at night. She has no recollection of the events and is embarrassed when her roommate mentions this to her in the morning. She has been falling asleep in her morning classes. These nocturnal episodes occur about once a month. She has developed severe insomnia. She requested a medication to reduce the events.

9. What is the likeliest diagnosis?
   A. Psychophysiologic insomnia
   B. Anxiety disorder
   C. Sleepwalking
   D. REM sleep behavior disorder (RBD)

10. What other features are *not* likely to be present?
   A. Positive family history
   B. Sleep deprivation
   C. Hypnagogic hallucinations
   D. History starting in childhood

11. What treatment is *most* likely to be effective?
   A. Low-dose clonazepam taken 1 to 2 hours before bedtime
   B. Topiramate at bedtime
   C. Lithium
   D. Olanzapine
   E. None of the above

ANSWERS

1. **D.** The patient has a sleep-related eating disorder (SRED), a disorder of partial arousal from non–rapid eye movement (NREM) sleep. Although such episodes are more common in stage N3, and they occur more often in the first third of the night, they can occur out of any NREM stage and at any time during the night. Contrary to popular belief, alcohol does *not* trigger these episodes.

2. **A.** In patients with a SRED, PSG is indicated (but not required to make the diagnosis by ICSD3) because often OSA or periodic limb movement disorder (PLMD) is present and may be initiating the partial arousal. There is no indication for EEG to look for seizure disorder, nor is there any indication for referral to a psychologist or psychiatrist. A trial of clonazepam is not indicated at this time.

3. **A.** Zolpidem (and olanzapine) and perhaps other medications can actually cause an SRED. The other three medications listed can improve this condition. This question is an example of how knowing only one fact can yield the correct answer. Simply knowing that zolpidem can cause an SRED allows you to choose that answer without actually knowing whether the other three medications are efficacious.

4. **B.** Disorders of partial arousal from NREM sleep can be exacerbated by conditions that cause arousal, for example, OSA syndrome or periodic limb movements (PLMs). Thus, in disorders in which the arousals are common, such as OSA, treatment of that condition should reduce episodes of partial arousal from NREM sleep. On the other hand, when an OSA patient without a history of sleepwalking is started on CPAP, sleepwalking episodes can begin.

5. **A.** This is a description of classic sleep terrors, an NREM parasomnia. It is a disorder of partial arousal. The patient is asleep, but presumably parts of the nervous system are awake, a type of state overlap. This disorder is not associated with REM sleep. Most of the episodes occur in stage N3 and generally occur in the first third of the night. Parasomnias often run in families, and a specific gene, *HLA-DQB1*, is thought to play a role in sleepwalking.

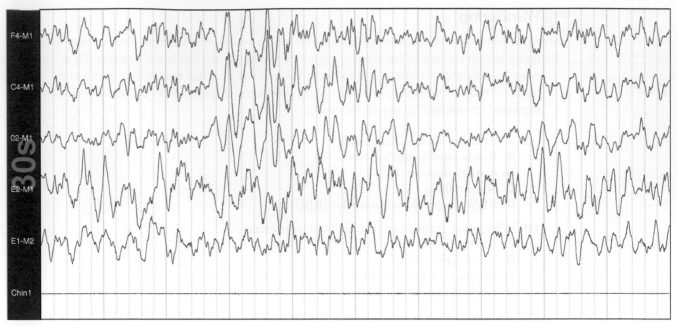

FIGURE 5.1–2 Answer 7: Gain is reduced by half in the top three channels.

6. D.   Not in the differential diagnosis of this case is rhythmic movement disorder (RMD), which most often manifests as head banging or body rocking, typically beginning in early childhood and resolving by adulthood. Although this child did have body rocking, the crying out and autonomic discharge (the "terror") are not part of RMD. The head-banging variety of RMD is also known as *jactatio capitis nocturna*, an imposing name. Both seizures and psychogenic states are in the differential diagnosis of sleep terrors.

7. C.   This is stage N3 sleep in a child. As shown, the waveform amplitude can be huge, and the EEG can be misclassified as seizure or artifact. In Figure 5.1–2, the EEG channels are reduced, making stage N3 more obvious. Conversely, in older adults, EEG amplitude might have to be increased to properly recognize stage N3.

8. D.   Medications are seldom used to treat sleep terrors in children. Sleep deprivation is a common contributor to NREM parasomnias, and three clues suggest that sleep deprivation is present in this child: (1) 9 hours of sleep is not sufficient for a 7-year-old child; (2) the very high percentage of stage N3 is typical for rebound in a patient who has been sleep deprived; and (3) the child plays hockey, and children who play hockey often practice very early in the morning several days a week.

9. C.   This is a description of sleepwalking. The criteria for the disorder are the combination of ambulation or other complex behaviors, in the context of the five features of disorders of arousal: (1) recurrent, (2) absent responsiveness during the episodes, (3) no dream imagery during the event, (4) no memory of the event, and (5) not better explained by anything else (drugs or diseases).   (ICSD3, pp 228-229)

10. C.   Although narcolepsy is common in college students, sleep walking is not a common feature of this disorder.

11. E.   This is an example of a question in which none of the choices (A–D) would be clinically acceptable. Because one has to pick an answer, the best one is E. One would not normally give a patient a nightly dose of a benzodiazepine to prevent sleepwalking that occurs once a month. One would first focus on dealing with environmental safety issues and behavioral management (avoiding sleep deprivation and stress). Medications that have been recommended are benzodiazepines (most often clonazepam), melatonin, and paroxetine, along with avoidance of medications that have been described to cause sleep walking (Table 5.1–1).

TABLE 5.1–1 Treatment Options for Disorders of Arousal

Component	Confusional Arousal	Sexomnias	Somnambulism (Sleepwalking)	SRED	Sleep Terrors
Environmental safety	X	X	X	X	X
Scheduled anticipatory awakening	X		X		X
Behavioral management	• Reassurance of benign nature • Avoid precipitants: • Sleep deprivation • Alcohol • CNS depressants	• Enhancing sleep hygiene, ensuring optimal sleep duration • Psychotherapy and stress management • Comorbid mood disorder or anxiety	• Avoid precipitants: • Sleep deprivation • Lithium • Nonbenzodiazepines receptor agonists		• Reassurance of benign nature • Relaxation therapy • Hypnosis or autogenic training* • Psychotherapy
Pharmacologic management	• Imipramine • Clomipramine • Clonazepam	• Benzodiazepine • Clonazepam • Antidepressant • Sertraline • GABAergic agents • Lamotrigine • Valproic acid • Serotonin reuptake inhibitors	Benzodiazepines • Clonazepam (0.5–1 mg) • Diazepam (10 mg) • Triazolam (0.25 mg) • Imipramine (50–300 mg) • Melatonin • Paroxetine	• Dopamine agonists, SSRIs, and topiramate[†]	• Paroxetine (20–40 mg) • Clonazepam (0.5–1 mg) • Trazodone • Hydroxytryptophan • Imipramine/clomipramine

*Autogenic training is a special relaxation technique similar to meditation.
[†]Side effects include weight loss, cognitive impairment, paresthesias, visual symptoms, and less frequently, renal calculi.
CBT, Cognitive-behavioral therapy; *CNS,* central nervous system; *GABAergic,* gamma-aminobutyric acid–ergic; *SRED,* sleep-related eating disorder; *SSRI,* selective serotonin reuptake inhibitor.
From Avidon AY: Non-rapid eye movement parasomnias: clinical spectrum, diagnostic features, and management. In Kryger M, Roth T, Dement WC (eds): *Principles and Practice of Sleep Medicine,* 6th ed. Philadelphia: Elsevier; 2017.

Summary

Highly Recommended

- *Atlas of Clinical Sleep Medicine,* ed 2, Chapter 12; make sure you can identify stage N3 sleep
- *International Classification of Sleep Disorders,* ed 3, pp 225-280. (See Box 5.1–1)

Parasomnias are disorders in which undesirable behaviors or phenomena occur while the person is asleep. Expect between 15 and 20 questions (out of 240) on the exam.

Definition of a Non-REM Parasomnia

- Undesirable behavior or phenomena that occur during the sleep period related to NREM sleep

Pathogenesis

- Partial arousal from sleep
- State instability
- The human leukocyte antigen (HLA) gene *HLA-DQB1* increases susceptibility

Risk Factors

- Sleep deprivation
- Emotional stress
- Drugs
  ○ There is no direct evidence that alcohol impacts risk, though it may increase slow wave sleep
  ○ Sedative-hypnotics (e.g., zolpidem) increase risk

Box 5.1–1 Parasomnias: General Classification

The ICSD3 classifies *parasomnias* as follows*:

NREM-Related Parasomnias

- Disorders of arousal (from NREM sleep)
- Sleepwalking
- Sleep terrors
- Sleep-related eating disorder

REM-Related Parasomnias

- RBD
- Recurrent isolated sleep paralysis
- Nightmare disorder

Other Parasomnias

- Exploding head syndrome
- Sleep-related hallucinations
- Sleep enuresis
- Parasomnia due to a medical disorder
- Parasomnia due to a medication or substance
- Parasomnia, unspecified

Isolated Symptoms and Normal Variants

- Sleep talking

---

*Appendix A of the ICSD3, "Sleep-related Medical and Neurological Disorders," includes conditions that might also be classified as "secondary parasomnias" because they occur during sleep. The conditions listed include sleep-related epilepsy, headache, laryngospasm, gastroesophageal reflux, and myocardial ischemia. Although some authors classify catathrenia as a parasomnia (see ATLAS2, Ch 12), the ICSD3 places it in a section called "Isolated Symptoms and Normal Variants" under the heading "Sleep-Related Breathing Disorders." Similarly, bruxism has been considered a parasomnia, but the ICSD3 classifies it as a sleep-related movement disorder. Irrespective of how these conditions are classified, they all are fair game for a quiz question.
NREM, Non–rapid eye movement; *REM,* rapid eye movement.

- Sleep disorders that increase arousals
    - Sleep apnea
    - Periodic limb movements
- Treatment of sleep disorders
    - CPAP treatment can induce sleepwalking

NREM Parasomnia Types

- Sleepwalking
    - Epidemiology
        - Common in children: peak age 12 years (17%–22%)
        - Less common in adults (~4%)
    - Genetic influences
        - If neither parent was affected, 22%
        - If one parent was affected, 45%
        - If both parents were affected, 60%
    - Clinical features
        - Behavior may be complex
        - Patient has no recollection

- ○ Variants
  - Confusional arousals
    - ◆ SRED
      - ◆ Often another sleep pathology is present.
      - ◆ OSA
      - ◆ Movement disorder
    - ◆ Sleepsex
  - Sleep terrors
- ○ Epidemiology
  - Up to 6% in children
  - About 2.5% in ages 15 to 64 years
- ○ Genetic factors
  - Runs in families
- ○ Clinical features
  - Dramatic
  - Abrupt
    - ◆ Screaming
    - ◆ Appears to be in panic
    - ◆ Prominent, sometimes injurious motor activity
  - Events may be initiated by diseases that cause arousals
    - ◆ Sleep apnea
    - ◆ Movement disorders

Treatment

- Reduce sleep deprivation
- Ensure a safe environment
- Offer reassurance
- Pharmacologic therapy is helpful in some circumstances
  - ○ Little published data
  - ○ Benzodiazepines
  - ○ Tricyclic antidepressants (TCAs)
  - ○ Dopaminergic agents, topiramate, and opiates for SRED

REFERENCES

American Academy of Sleep Medicine. *International classification of sleep disorders*. 3rd ed. Darien, Ill.: American Academy of Sleep Medicine; 2014.
Kryger MH, Avidan A, Berry R. *Atlas of clinical sleep medicine*. 2nd ed. Philadelphia: Saunders; 2014.

5.2 Rapid Eye Movement Parasomnias

QUESTIONS

An Old Soldier

An 80-year-old man is referred for evaluation of a possible sleep-breathing disorder. He has been noted to snore and stop breathing during sleep, and his wife is concerned about the symptoms. On several occasions over the past 3 months, while her husband is sleeping, he has struck her with his fists. When she wakes him up, he remembers dreaming that he was fighting off animals or soldiers. You learn that he was a POW for 1 year after his aircraft was shot down over North Vietnam in 1968. You also learn that before coming to your clinic, because of the patient's flat affect, his family doctor decided he was depressed and started him on mirtazapine.

1. What is the *likeliest* disorder to explain his abnormal motor activity during sleep?
   A. Psychomotor epilepsy
   B. Posttraumatic stress disorder (PTSD)
   C. Sleep terrors
   D. RBD

2. In which condition does a nocturnal PSG *not* yield diagnostic or pathophysiologic findings?
   A. Psychomotor epilepsy
   B. PTSD
   C. Sleep terrors
   D. RBD

The patient has an overnight sleep study that shows the following on scoring:

Breathing: Apnea-hypopnea index (AHI) = 4.5 events/hr, respiratory disturbance index (RDI) = 6 events/hr
Sleep: Sleep efficiency = 65%; stages of sleep as a percentage of total study time: stage W = 35%, stage N1 = 15%, stage N2 = 45%, stage N3 = 0%, stage REM = 5%, arousal index = 46/hr

PLMs were not scored, but the recently graduated sleep technologist thought the patient might have restless legs syndrome (RLS); she noted a great deal of leg activity throughout the night. On interpreting the study, you come across the epoch in Figure 5.2–1.

3. What does the epoch in Figure 5.2–1 show?
   A. Stage W
   B. Stage N1
   C. Stage N2
   D. Stage R

4. At this point, you would do all of the following *except*
   A. Stop the mirtazapine
   B. Start the patient on clonazepam
   C. Prescribe prazosin and arrange for imagery-rehearsal therapy
   D. Refer the patient to a neurologist

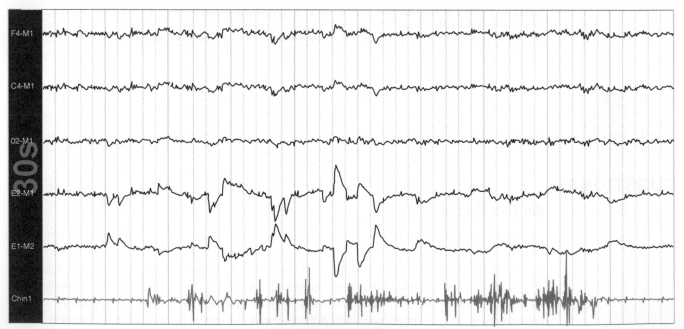

FIGURE 5.2–1 Question 3.

5. Which of the following is the *most* unlikely cause of a chronic form of this disorder?
  A. Narcolepsy
  B. Synucleinopathy
  C. Duchenne muscular dystrophy
  D. Spinocerebellar ataxia type 3

6. Which of the following is the *most* unlikely cause of an acute form of this disorder?
  A. Alcohol withdrawal
  B. TCAs
  C. Selective serotonin reuptake inhibitors (SSRIs)
  D. Caffeine withdrawal

7. The patient mentions that he can no longer taste food. On testing olfactory function, you find he is indeed anosmic. This finding is consistent with which of the following?
  A. Parkinson disease
  B. Cerebrovascular accident
  C. Multiple sclerosis
  D. Polymyalgia rheumatica

8. The patient is started on clonazepam 0.5 mg at bedtime, and this reduces his nocturnal motor activity. However, he complains of severe sleepiness during the daytime. What should you do next?
  A. Start modafinil 200 mg in the morning
  B. Have him take clonazepam 2 hours before bedtime
  C. Perform a PSG to see whether the clonazepam has induced obstructive apnea
  D. Perform a multiple sleep latency test (MSLT) to document his sleepiness and see whether he in fact has narcolepsy

Afraid to Sleep

A 29-year-old female Marine was referred because of severe insomnia. She stated that she awakened almost every night from a nightmare, gasping and short of breath, sweating, heart pounding, and in a state of panic. The dream was always the same—that she was being raped. She admitted that 3 years before she had been raped by a fellow Marine. Fearing that she would have a nightmare, she developed a fear of falling asleep.

9. What best explains her symptoms?
  A. Major depressive disorder
  B. Sleep terror
  C. PTSD
  D. REM behavior disorder

10. Which therapy is *not* likely to be helpful?
  A. Prazosin
  B. Imagery rehearsal therapy
  C. Cognitive behavior therapy for insomnia
  D. Zolpidem

11. Is an overnight sleep study indicated in this patient? Which statement is *correct*?
  A. No. OSA is rare in normal weight female military veterans referred for sleep testing
  B. Yes. OSA in military veterans with PTSD presents more often with insomnia than obesity or increased daytime sleepiness
  C. No. The sleep study is unlikely to show findings that would alter treatment
  D. Yes. The sleep study would confirm the typical findings of the nightmares beginning during REM sleep, which should lead one to prescribe a REM-suppressing agent

ANSWERS

1. **D.** The history is typical for RBD. The other conditions are in the differential diagnosis. With psychomotor epilepsy, the patient would *not* complain about vivid dream imagery; he would likely have no recollection of the events. In PTSD, he would awaken from a disturbing dream reliving the traumatic event. With sleep terrors, there is no vivid dream imagery, and patients usually have no recollection of the event.

2. **B.** Of the disorders listed, PTSD does not have typical PSG findings. Thus, unless you suspect another disorder, PSG is not indicated. The other disorders listed may manifest helpful findings on PSG, which might just be the stage of sleep where the event occurs. (For sleep terrors, however, you would seldom actually order a PSG.)

3. **D.** Figure 5.2–1 shows typical findings in a patient with RBD. The eye channels show rapid eye movements. The chin electromyogram (EMG) has baseline low activity with nonperiodic increases in activity. On examining the corresponding digital video, you would see some motor activity. In the video for this particular epoch, the patient was moving his arm, and in the following epoch, he aggressively punched in the air. Other diagnostic criteria for RBD include REM sleep without atonia, as shown in Figure 5.2–1; a history of sleep-related behavior that can injure the patient or bed partner; documentation of visible motor activity during a PSG; and absence of epileptiform activity. (ICSD3, pp 246-253)

4. **C.** Prazosin and imagery-rehearsal therapy are used to treat patients with PTSD, which this patient does not have. Mirtazapine (and other medications) can cause an acute form of RBD. Clonazepam is generally highly effective in RBD. Finally, you would refer such a patient to a neurologist because in most (if not all) cases, the RBD symptoms are an early manifestation of a neurodegenerative disorder (e.g., Parkinson disease).

5. **C.** Duchenne muscular dystrophy, primarily a muscle disease, does not cause RBD. Whereas a decade ago, most cases of RBD were considered idiopathic, now it is considered an early manifestation of a neurodegenerative disorder; however, RBD symptoms can precede the neurodegenerative disorder by decades. The most common disorders associated with RBD are the synucleinopathies: Parkinson disease, multisystem atrophy (olivopontocerebellar degeneration and Shy-Drager syndrome), and dementia with Lewy bodies.

6. **D.** An acute form of RBD can occur in many situations. Caffeine withdrawal does not cause RBD, but caffeine intoxication can. Even excess chocolate intake has been linked to RBD. The other choices in this question—alcohol withdrawal, TCAs, and SSRIs—have all been linked to the acute form of RBD. In fact, some of these agents can induce RBD symptoms in patients with narcolepsy.

7. **A.** Impaired olfactory and color discrimination are common in both Parkinson disease and RBD. Note that in synucleinopathies, alpha-synuclein accumulates in the olfactory bulbs (see Box 5.2–1).

8. **B.** The patient should take the clonazepam at a dose of 0.5 to 2 mg 2 hours before bedtime. This medication has a long half-life (up to 30 to 40 hours), so a morning hangover can occur. Other options might be to try melatonin at a dose of up to 12 mg or pramipexole at 0.125 to 1.5 mg).

9. **C.** The case is classic for PTSD. It is one of the nightmare disorders. The nightmares may arise out of REM and NREM sleep in these patients. This condition may be comorbid with the other diseases mentioned and also sleep apnea. (St. Louis et al, 2017)

10. **D.** Treatment for PTSD is often problematic. There are positive outcome data for three of the treatment choices but not zolpidem. With respect to the four answers there are no published data that support the use of zolpidem. Studies are emerging on the effect of cannabis on PTSD. (Seda et al, 2015; Lipinska et al, 2016; Lim et al, 2017)

11. **B.** A sleep study is indicated but not to determine the sleep stage from which the nightmare arises. Nearly 50% of active duty females referred for a sleep study have OSA often without the typical signs of obesity or increased age. (Capener et al, 2018) OSA in military veterans

---

Box 5.2–1 What Is a Synucleinopathy?

Synucleins are soluble proteins found primarily in neural tissue and in some tumors. The function of these proteins is unknown, but the three types of synucleins are called *alpha-, beta-,* and *gamma-synucleins.*

Alpha-Synuclein

- Alpha-synuclein is located in
  - Nuclei of cells throughout the brain
  - Presynaptic termini
  - Mitochondria of several regions of the brain, especially the olfactory bulb
- Loss of olfactory function is common in Parkinson disease.
- Normally, soluble alpha-synuclein can aggregate to form insoluble fibrils (possibly leading to amyloid), which are toxic to some neural cells in pathologic conditions characterized by Lewy bodies, which includes:
  - Parkinson disease
  - Dementia with Lewy bodies
  - Multiple system atrophy
  - Olivopontocerebellar atrophy
  - Some cases of Alzheimer disease

Beta-Synuclein

- May be an inhibitor of alpha-synuclein aggregation
- Might protect the CNS from the neurotoxic effects of alpha-synuclein

Gamma-Synuclein

- Found in breast cancer cells
- Marker for tumor progression

CNS, Central nervous system.

---

with comorbid PTSD presents more often with insomnia than obesity or excessive daytime sleepiness, the typical findings in non-PTSD veterans with OSA.   (Rezaeitalab et al, 2018) Posttraumatic nightmares of PTSD occur in both REM and NREM sleep and are commonly associated with other sleep disturbances such as abnormal breathing or movement events, which may require treatment.   (Phelps et al, 2018)

Summary

Highly Recommended

- *Atlas of Clinical Sleep Medicine,* ed 2, Chapter 11.3
- *International Classification of Sleep Disorders,* ed 3, pp 246-253

Although you would expect only a few questions related to the REM parasomnias based on the American Board of Internal Medicine blueprint, questions that encompass this topic are covered in other parts of the exam, including pharmacology, basic science, and movement disorders.

REM Sleep Behavior Disorder (St. Louis et al, 2017)

- Epidemiology
  - Found in 5 in 1000 adults
  - More common in men
  - Patients tend to be older
- Association with neurologic diseases
  - Extrapyramidal diseases
    - Alpha-synucleinopathies (Box 5.2–1)
    - Parkinson disease
    - Dementia with Lewy bodies

- Multiple system atrophy
- Olivopontocerebellar atrophy
- Shy-Drager syndrome
  - ○ Narcolepsy
  - ○ Other neurologic conditions
    - Tourette syndrome
    - Spinocerebellar ataxia type 3
    - Multiple sclerosis
    - Cerebrovascular disease
    - Möbius syndrome (congenital facial paralysis, inability to move eyes)
    - Guillain-Barré syndrome
- ■ Pathophysiology
  - ○ Dysfunction of the system that maintains atonia in REM
- ■ Clinical features
  - ○ Usually, patients present with violent activity during sleep
    - Harmful to patient
    - Harmful to bed partner
  - ○ Symptoms can precede symptoms of neurodegenerative disease by decades
- ■ Diagnosis
  - ○ History
    - Motor activity in response to dream imagery
  - ○ Polysomnography
    - Shows excessive EMG activity of chin, limbs, or both during REM sleep
    - Visual observation can confirm violent or other motor activity
- ■ Treatment
  - ○ Clonazepam 0.5 to 2 mg
  - ○ High-dose melatonin 3 to 12 mg   (Kunz and Mahlberg, 2010)

Other REM Parasomnias

- ■ Nightmares
  - ○ Features
    - Recurrent awakenings from dreams
    - Alert on awakening
    - Difficulty falling asleep after awakenings
  - ○ Differential diagnosis includes awakenings with recurrent dreams in PTSD
- ■ Sinus arrest
  - ○ Occurs in young men
  - ○ Asystole occurs only in REM sleep
- ■ Painful erections
  - ○ Occur in middle-aged and older men

REFERENCES

American Academy of Sleep Medicine. *International classification of sleep disorders*. 3rd ed. Darien, Ill.: American Academy of Sleep Medicine; 2014.

Capener DC, Brock MS, Hansen SL, et al. An initial report of sleep disorders in women in the U.S. Military. *Mil Med*. 2018.

Kunz D, Mahlberg R. A two-part, double-blind, placebo-controlled trial of exogenous melatonin in REM sleep behaviour disorder. *J Sleep Res*. 2010;19(4):591–596.

Lim K, See YM, Lee JA. Systematic review of the effectiveness of medical cannabis for psychiatric, movement and neurodegenerative disorders. *Clin Psychopharmacol Neurosci*. 2017;15(4):301–312.

Lipinska G, Baldwin DS, Thomas KG. Pharmacology for sleep disturbance in PTSD. *Hum Psychopharmacol*. 2016;31(2):156–163.

Phelps AJ, Kanaan RAA, Worsnop C, et al. An ambulatory polysomnography study of the post-traumatic nightmares of post-traumatic stress disorder. *Sleep*. 2018;41(1).

Rezaeitalab F, Mokhber N, Ravanshad Y, et al. Different polysomnographic patterns in military veterans with obstructive sleep apnea in those with and without post-traumatic stress disorder. *Sleep Breath*. 2018.

Seda G, Sanchez-Ortuno MM, Welsh CH, et al. Comparative meta-analysis of prazosin and imagery rehearsal therapy for nightmare frequency, sleep quality, and posttraumatic stress. *J Clin Sleep Med*. 2015;11(1):11–22.

St. Louis EK, Boeve BF. REM sleep behavior disorder: diagnosis, clinical implications, and future directions. *Mayo Clin Proc*. 2017;92(11):1723–1736.

5.4   Name That Stage

QUESTIONS

All the World's a Stage

For each of the following parasomnias, state if it predominantly occurs in

A. REM sleep
B. NREM sleep
C. A and B about equally
D. The transition between wakefulness and sleep

1. Sleep paralysis

2. Hypnagogic hallucinations

3. Hypnopompic hallucinations

4. Sleepwalking

5. Sleep terrors

6. Dream-enactment motor behavior

7. SRED

8. Nightmare disorder

ANSWERS

1.   A

2.   D

3.   D

4.   B

5.   B

6.   A

7.   B

8.   A

This series of questions emphasizes that specific parasomnias tend to occur either in REM sleep or in non-REM sleep but not both. Note that *dream-enactment motor behavior* is another name for RBD. Note also that *hypnagogic* and *hypnopompic* refer, respectively, to the transition between being awake and being asleep and the transition between sleep and becoming awake.

Summary

Highly Recommended

The topic of confusional arousals, although mentioned as a separate entity in the blueprint, is more logically covered as an NREM parasomnia (see Section 5.1). Several other parasomnias are neither REM nor NREM parasomnias, but enuresis is the only one actually mentioned in the blueprint in the parasomnia section. It is covered in the *International Classification of Sleep Disorders*, ed 3, under "Other Parasomnias" (see Box 5.1–1).

Sleep Enuresis in Children

- Definition
  - ○ Occurs in children older than 5 years
  - ○ Involuntary urinary voiding during sleep
  - ○ Occurs at least two times a week
- Epidemiology
  - ○ Common
    - More common in boys than in girls
  - ○ Found in
    - 30% of children aged 3 years
    - 10% of children aged 6 years
    - 3% of children aged 12 years
- Types
  - ○ Primary: Patient has never been consistently dry during sleep
    - Management
      - ◆ Pharmacologic
        - Imipramine is no longer recommended
        - Desmopressin may be useful for temporary relief of symptoms
      - ◆ Behavior modification techniques include
        - Urinating before bedtime
        - Reducing liquid intake at bedtime
        - Bells or buzzers to wake patients when they have voided
  - ○ Secondary: Patient has been previously consistently dry for at least 6 months
    - Management requires, at the very least, urinalysis
    - The patient may need evaluation of kidney, bladder, or metabolic function

Sleep Enuresis in Adults

- Definition
  - ○ Involuntary urinary voiding during sleep
  - ○ Occurs at least two times a week
- Types
  - ○ Primary
    - Patient has never been consistently dry during sleep
    - Primary enuresis is usually caused by congenital abnormalities that involve the nervous system or urinary tract
    - Management requires specialized evaluation and treatment
- Secondary
  - Patient has been consistently dry during sleep, usually for many years
  - Usually caused by
    - ◆ Nervous system disease (e.g., seizure, stroke)
    - ◆ Anatomic lesion that involves the urinary tract (e.g., enlarged prostate, bladder cancer)
    - ◆ Metabolic disease that causes increased nocturnal urinary volume (e.g., diabetes)
    - ◆ Kidney disease (e.g., kidney failure when unable to concentrate urine)
  - Management involves treating the causative disorder

Catathrenia (ICSD3, p 141)

- Features
  - ○ Groaning during sleep
  - ○ Begins in childhood
- Sleep study
  - ○ Can show apnea
  - ○ Can emulate apnea in that the periods of groaning may be misclassified as apnea
- Treatment
  - ○ No satisfactory treatment is available
  - ○ Some patients respond to CPAP

Throughout the ICSD3, under the heading "Isolated Symptoms and Normal Variants," are several conditions that are likely to appear on the board exam in some fashion. One example discussed in this book is catathrenia. Others include snoring, short sleeper, long sleeper, sleep talking, and environmental sleep disorder.

REFERENCE

American Academy of Sleep Medicine. *International classification of sleep disorders*. 3rd ed. Darien, Ill.: American Academy of Sleep Medicine; 2014.

Sleep-Related Movement Disorders

6.1   Limb Movement Disorders

QUESTIONS

The Fidgety General

A 58-year-old Air Force general is referred for management of insomnia. He complains of difficulty falling asleep at bedtime, especially when flying at night from base to base. He worries about the various military operations around the world involving the Air Force, and he cannot turn off his mind. He has participated in military operations and often thinks about the time when his airplane was hit by antiaircraft fire and he was forced to return to base and make an emergency landing. He also finds that when he tries to fall asleep in the passenger section of an airplane, he feels fidgety; to relieve the sensation, he has to get up and walk around the plane. He sometimes has the same sensation when working as a copilot in the cockpit of an aircraft. He has had difficulty with sleep for about 30 years but is seeking help now because his inability to sit in the cockpit has worsened recently. He is concerned there may be a serious neurologic problem. He snores but has never been observed to have apneas. His Epworth Sleepiness Scale (ESS) score is 2 of 24, and his body mass index (BMI) is 25. He had a complete physical examination and screening blood tests 4 months earlier and was told all of his numbers were normal. He takes low-dose aspirin for heart disease prophylaxis.

1. The differential diagnosis of the insomnia includes each of the following *except*
   A. Posttraumatic stress disorder (PTSD)
   B. Psychophysiologic insomnia
   C. Primary restless legs syndrome (RLS)
   D. Secondary RLS

2. Which *one* of the following is required to document the diagnosis of RLS?
   A. Nocturnal polysomnogram (PSG)
   B. Clinical history
   C. Suggested immobilization test (SIT)
   D. Serum ferritin level

3. The patient brought along the results of his prior blood tests. Hemoglobin and hematocrit were 13 g/dL and 39%, respectively. How do you interpret these results, and what would you do next?
   A. Both results are normal. No further blood tests are warranted
   B. The hemoglobin is low, but the hematocrit is normal. Vitamin B_{12} measurement is warranted
   C. Both hemoglobin and hematocrit are borderline low but not abnormal enough to be concerning, and no further blood testing is needed
   D. Both hemoglobin and hematocrit are below the lower limit of normal. The patient is anemic, and thus more testing is required

4. Beyond anemia, other causes of secondary RLS should be evaluated *except*
   A. Renal insufficiency
   B. Neuropathy
   C. Thyroid disease
   D. Hepatic failure

5. Because the blood tests were 4 months old, you decide to order additional tests. Which test would be *least* appropriate at this point?
   A. Serum ferritin
   B. Vitamin B_{12} level
   C. Stool for occult blood
   D. Bilirubin and alkaline phosphatase

6. The results of tests you ordered are as follows:

Test	Result
Serum ferritin	6 ng/mL
Vitamin B_{12}	1200 pg/mL
Stool for occult blood	Positive
Serum bilirubin	Normal
Serum alkaline phosphatase	Normal

What is the next step?
   A. Start the patient on a dopaminergic agent
   B. Start the patient on ferrous sulfate 65 mg/day
   C. Give intramuscular (IM) injections of B_{12}
   D. Arrange for a gastroenterology consultation

Extremely Restless in the Magnetic Resonance Imaging Scanner

A 56-year-old woman was referred to the sleep disorders center with a 25-year history of severe insomnia and restlessness at bedtime. The symptoms first began during her last pregnancy, but she has a history of depression. Zolpidem was not effective in treating the insomnia. Her family doctor recalled an article in a family practice journal that suggested starting insomnia patients on the sedating antidepressant mirtazapine. He did so and also prescribed a sustained-release formulation of levodopa for the restlessness. Both medications were taken at bedtime. For the first 8 nights, the medications were effective; the restlessness resolved, and she fell asleep quickly. To that point, she described the medications as "miraculous." However, on the ninth morning, she felt very restless and complained of a headache. She was sent for a magnetic resonance imaging scan. In the scanner, she was so restless when asked to keep still that she started to scream. She was referred to the sleep clinic.

7. What is the *least* likely explanation of the new symptoms?
   A. Disease progression
   B. Augmentation
   C. Effect of mirtazapine
   D. Dopamine rebound

8. All of the following are appropriate interventions *except*
   A. Checking serum ferritin level
   B. Stopping mirtazapine
   C. Increasing the levodopa dose and having her take it 2 hours earlier
   D. Stopping levodopa and initiating pramipexole or ropinirole

9. After the above interventions are made, her morning symptoms disappear, and she has partially improved. However, she still has significant nighttime restlessness symptoms and daytime sleepiness that she would like treated. Which of the following is the *most* appropriate next step?
   A. Start her on zolpidem at bedtime
   B. Add an opiate such as codeine at bedtime
   C. Start her on modafinil to treat daytime sleepiness
   D. Stop all dopaminergic medications

Jumpy Legs and Depression

A 62-year-old man with a history of mild RLS is referred to you because of a recent intensification in symptoms. The leg symptoms begin about 6 PM and can be so uncomfortable that he soaks in a hot tub for about an hour before bedtime. He recently started taking an antidepressant to help him cope with the death of a close relative.

10. Which of these antidepressants is *least* problematic with regard to increasing RLS symptoms and periodic limb movements?
    A. Bupropion
    B. Mirtazapine
    C. Trazodone
    D. Imipramine

11. The patient's primary care physician originally started him on a dopaminergic agent, but the patient did not tolerate it because of daytime tiredness and nightmares. Given that the RLS symptoms have continued after changing his antidepressant medication, what would the next *best* treatment for RLS be?
    A. Gabapentin enacarbil
    B. Phenytoin
    C. Topiramate
    D. Zonegran

Restless Legs

12. Which of the following side effects are seen with dopaminergic agonists?
    A. Anorexia
    B. Compulsive gambling
    C. Sleep-related eating
    D. Periodic limb movements

13. Which of the following is a nonpharmacologic measure that reduces RLS severity?
    A. Increased chocolate
    B. Reduced caffeine
    C. Increased vitamin C
    D. Decreased simple sugars

14. Pregnant women more commonly have RLS. Which of the following is a known predictor of RLS during pregnancy?
    A. Family history of RLS
    B. Having twins
    C. Age of the woman during pregnancy
    D. Insomnia during early pregnancy

15. Generally, RLS prevalence increases with age. In which age range does RLS prevalence stabilize or decrease slightly?
  A. Preteen to teenage years
  B. Teenage to young adult years
  C. Young adult to middle-age years
  D. Older adult to elderly years

16. A suggested immobilization test is performed on a patient. Which periodic limb movement of wakefulness (PLMW) frequency suggests RLS?
  A. 5 PLMW/hr
  B. 15 PLMW/hr
  C. 20 PLMW/hr
  D. 40 PLMW/hr

Looking for Sleep Apnea; Finding Something Else

A 67-year-old woman presents with symptoms of sleep-onset insomnia, early morning awakenings, and snoring. Her husband states that she moves the entire night and that it is like sleeping with a "twitching fish." She has a BMI of 34 and an ESS score of 9 of 24. A sleep study is ordered by her family doctor because of suspected obstructive sleep apnea (OSA). The study revealed a sleep-onset latency of 90 minutes, a duration typical for this patient. Leg electromyography (EMG) did not show excessive activity during the initial waking period. Total sleep time (TST) was 5 hours. A 5-minute fragment of her study is shown in Figure 6.1–1. She had similar findings during other portions of the sleep study.

17. This fragment is consistent with which of the following?
  A. Obstructive sleep apnea
  B. Restless legs syndrome
  C. Periodic limb movements of sleep (PLMS)
  D. Periodic limb movement disorder (PLMD)

18. Extrapolating from this fragment, what is the patient's periodic limb movement index (PLMI)?
  A. 5 events/hr
  B. 11 events/hr
  C. 55 events/hr
  D. 132 events/hr

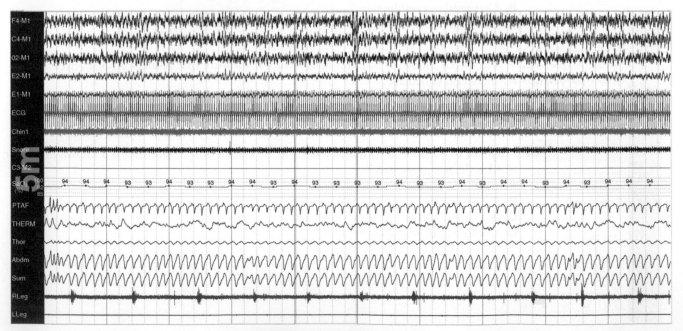

FIGURE 6.1–1 Questions 17 to 19.

19. What is the *most* appropriate first step in treatment of this patient's nighttime and daytime symptoms?
  A. Dopaminergic agent at bedtime
  B. Modafinil in the morning
  C. Clonazepam at bedtime
  D. Cognitive behavioral therapy (CBT)

The Right Test for the Wrong Reason

A 45-year-old woman falls asleep quickly and then wakes up several times during the night. She is unhappy about her difficulty maintaining sleep but is otherwise healthy and does not complain of restless arms or legs. However, her husband has noted she frequently twitches and jerks throughout the night; he has not noted snoring. Her ESS score is 8 of 24. The patient states that her family doctor wanted her to have a sleep study because he thought she had RLS.

20. What should the first step be in your assessment of this patient?
  A. In-laboratory PSG
  B. Home sleep apnea testing
  C. Actigraphy
  D. Suggested immobilization testing

21. The patient has an overnight sleep study; a 2-minute fragment is shown in Figure 6.1–2. What does this fragment show?
  A. Multiple respiratory events
  B. Periodic limb movements without arousals
  C. Periodic limb movements with arousals
  D. Diagnostic features of RLS

22. What is the likelihood of a patient with periodic limb movements having RLS symptoms?
  A. 20%
  B. 40%
  C. 60%
  D. 80%

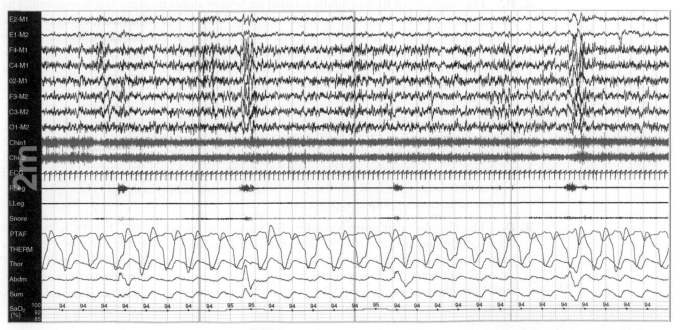

FIGURE 6.1–2 Questions 21 and 22.

23. What is the *most* appropriate first step in the pharmacologic treatment of this patient?
   A. Pramipexole
   B. Zolpidem
   C. Clonazepam
   D. Oxycodone

Periodic Limb Movements of Sleep

24. Which of the following genetic factors has been well correlated with PLMS?
   A. Arylsulfatase A deficiency
   B. *BTBD9*
   C. *CLCN1*
   D. Hexosaminidase A deficiency

25. The *minimum* amplitude of a periodic leg movement when scoring a PSG is
   A. 2 μV
   B. 4 μV
   C. 8 μV
   D. 16 μV

26. Which of the following criteria must be included for the diagnosis of PLMD by the *International Classification of Sleep Disorders*, edition 3 (ICSD3)?
   A. Sleep disturbance or daytime impairment
   B. A mean sleep latency of less than 8 minutes
   C. A PLMI of 12/hr in an adult
   D. A PLMI of 3/hr in a child

ANSWERS

1. A.   There is not enough evidence in the history to make a diagnosis of PTSD, although he does mentally revisit a stressful time in his life. Patients with PTSD might complain of insomnia but are troubled by awakenings with recurrent violent dreams. The patient gives a history consistent with RLS, which often is associated with insomnia. Any disorder that causes difficulty falling asleep can also lead to psychophysiologic insomnia. It is worth emphasizing that RLS is a *syndrome*, and the ICSD3 has a single RLS entry; there is no specific designation for primary and secondary RLS.   (ICSD3, pp 282-291)

2. B.   The diagnosis of RLS in adults is based on history alone; no sleep test is required. The mnemonic *URGE* has been used to help remember the four core characteristics for diagnosis: **u**rge to move limbs, **r**est worsens the sensation, **g**etting up and moving offers temporary relief, and sensations worsen in the **e**vening or at night. A PSG should only be done if there is a high probability of an additional sleep disorder, such as OSA. The SIT has been used in research but is not part of routine clinical assessment.   (ATLAS2, pp 178-185; ICSD3, pp 282-291)

3. D.   In men, normal hemoglobin is 14 to 17.5 g/dL, and normal hematocrit is 40% to 50%. In terms of the relationship between RLS and anemia, it is important to emphasize that nutritional deficiencies can cause secondary RLS (e.g., leading to a reduction in central nervous system [CNS] iron) before actual anemia is documented. For anemia to be caused by iron deficiency, iron stores in the marrow are zero, not simply reduced. Thus, given these results, an anemia workup is appropriate.

4. D.   The disorders that cause secondary RLS generally do not include hepatic failure. The other conditions mentioned have been associated with RLS. Another secondary cause is medication side effects. For example, many antidepressants may be associated with or may cause RLS symptoms (an exception is bupropion). With respect to liver disease, some patients with hemochromatosis develop RLS because they may have low CNS iron levels. However, using iron to treat hemochromatosis can worsen it.   (Haba-Rubio et al, 2005)

5. D. There is no reason to order bilirubin and alkaline phosphatase, abnormalities of which would point to liver disease. Serum ferritin should be ordered because low ferritin levels (typically <50 mg/dL) are consistent with reduced iron stores that are a cause of RLS. Because the patient had anemia in the first blood test, a stool for occult blood is indicated. Vitamin B_{12} deficiency can cause peripheral neuropathy and RLS. In particular, older patients with pernicious anemia can have RLS. (Mold et al, 2004)

6. D. The patient has reduced iron stores, the cause of which must be ascertained. Given the positive stool for occult blood, the next step would be a gastrointestinal (GI) evaluation. Men and women in the military may be blood donors, and a history of repeat blood donation has been associated with RLS. (Arunthari et al, 2010)

7. A. This is not an example of disease progression but rather a classic description of augmentation and rebound to dopaminergic agents in RLS. There is also likely a contribution from the mirtazapine. With augmentation, there is usually an initial therapeutic benefit followed by a worsening of symptoms, and symptoms also occur in other parts of the body not initially affected. Symptoms occur earlier, with rebound movements, and restlessness occurs when the medication wears off (for this patient, in the morning). Inexperienced clinicians sometimes increase the dose of a dopaminergic agent, and the augmentation and rebound simply worsen. Indeed, many family physicians use sedating antidepressants for insomnia based on articles they have read. RLS is a common side effect of second-generation antidepressants; about 25% of patients taking mirtazapine develop this symptom. (ATLAS2, pp 185-188; Kim et al, 2008; Rottach et al, 2008)

8. C. Increasing the dose of levodopa would be the wrong thing to do. In fact, patients with RLS should not be started on levodopa at all because the incidence of augmentation is between 30% and 80%, and the rebound in the morning can be quite distressing. Thus, levodopa should simply be stopped, and the patient should be started on either pramipexole or ropinirole. In a patient with unresponsive RLS, always confirm that the serum ferritin level is normal, and advise the patient to stop medications known to worsen restlessness (in this case, mirtazapine).

9. B. Opiates can be highly effective in patients with severe RLS and may be added as treatment. Codeine is generally effective for up to 6 hours. Oxycodone, methadone, and fentanyl patches last longer but are reserved for when symptoms occur for longer times throughout the day. Common opiate side effects include constipation, daytime sedation, and pruritus. Always remember that such agents may cause or worsen sleep-disordered breathing.

10. A. Bupropion inhibits the uptake of dopamine and norepinephrine. Bupropion is not known to increase periodic limb movements or to exacerbate restless legs symptoms, probably because of its effects on dopamine reuptake.

11. A. All of the options are medications that have been associated with treatment of seizures. However, gabapentin enacarbil is the only agent that has been demonstrated to reduce RLS severity. This medication may be a particularly good choice in patients who cannot tolerate dopamine agonists. Pregabalin is also becoming a commonly used first-line treatment for RLS. (Allen et al, 2014; Lee et al, 2011)

12. B. Dopaminergic agents have many side effects, including nausea, sleepiness, and fatigue. A less common side effect of these medications is impulse control disorders (ICDs), which may include compulsive gambling. In one cross-sectional study, 17% of patients who have Parkinson disease and are treated with dopaminergic drugs have an ICD, including gambling, compulsive sexual behavior, compulsive buying, and binge-eating disorders. (Weintraub et al, 2010)

13. B. Caffeine may exacerbate RLS symptoms, thus physicians commonly recommend that caffeine be reduced to minimize symptoms. (http://www.ninds.nih.gov/disorders/restless_legs/detail_restless_legs.htm)

14. A. Although the strongest predictor of RLS during pregnancy is a prior pregnancy with RLS, another important predictor is family history. Other factors may include RLS in the past and a hemoglobin less than 11 g/dL.   (ICSD3, pp 285-286)

15. D. RLS prevalence generally increases with age. However, in the older adult population, RLS prevalence stabilizes or decreases slightly.   (ICSD3, p 286)

16. D. The correct answer is 40 PLMW/hr. At that level, the test is approximately 80% specific and sensitive.   (ICSD3, p 289; Montplaisir et al, 1998)

17. C. This fragment is consistent with PLMS. There is no evidence for obstructive sleep apnea. RLS is not diagnosed using a PSG but is based on clinical symptoms alone. The term *periodic limb movement disorder* (PLMD) is present when the periodic limb movements are associated with insomnia or hypersomnia without a more evident cause. Thus, the PSG findings of PLMS must be associated with clinical sleep symptoms to make the diagnosis of PLMD.

18. D. This fragment shows 11 PLMS in 5 minutes. The index is calculated per hour of sleep; thus, the hour would contain 12 5-minute epochs. The PLMS index would therefore be 12 × 11, or 132.

19. D. Because the patient did not have increased arousals during sleep, it is unlikely that the sleepiness was caused by the periodic limb movements. Thus, there is no indication here to use a dopaminergic agent or a stimulant. The pharmacokinetics of clonazepam, if used as a hypnotic, often result in a hangover the next morning. When used as a hypnotic, it is best that clonazepam be taken 1 to 2 hours before bedtime. Given the history and the findings on PSG, treating the patient's insomnia to increase total sleep time will likely be the most efficacious way to treat her sleepiness.

20. A. The patient should have an overnight sleep study because a movement disorder other than RLS is likely. PLMS can only be diagnosed by in-laboratory PSG. An immobilization test is used for research on RLS but would not necessarily be helpful to make a clinical diagnosis in this case.

21. C. Even in a compressed epoch, changes can be seen in the electroencephalograph (EEG) associated with the second and fourth leg twitch. These are probably arousals, so the patient has PLMS with arousals.

22. A. About 20% of patients with periodic limb movements have clinical RLS symptoms. However, about 80% of patients with RLS have PLMS with or without arousals. As a side note, by definition, a person with PLMD does not in addition have a diagnosis of RLS.

23. A. Dopaminergic agents are likely the treatment of choice in patients with PLMD.

24. B. *BTBD9* is the gene that has been correlated with PLMS in a 2007 *New England Journal of Medicine* article that looked at patients with RLS and PLMS. The other genes are associated with neurologic disorders but not with periodic limb movements. Arylsulfatase A deficiency causes mucopolysaccharidosis VI, which may result in infiltration of the entire upper airway with abnormal soft tissue, resulting in severe obstructive apnea and hypoventilation. Mutations in the *CLCN1* gene may cause Becker myotonia, which may result in sleep apnea. Hexosaminidase A deficiency causes Tay-Sachs disease.   (Stefansson et al, 2007)

25. C. A periodic limb movement should be 8 μV above resting EMG voltage to be a scorable event; it must then return to less than 2 μV above resting EMG within 10 seconds to complete the scoring of the event.   (MANUAL2, Section VII, Movement Rules)

26. A. PLMD has the following criteria: PLMS are scored based on the American Academy of Sleep Medicine (AASM) scoring manual (MANUAL2) and occur at 15/hr or more in an adult and 5/hr or more in a child; the PLMS cause clinically significant sleep disturbance or impairment in mental, physical, social, occupational, educational, behavioral, or other important areas of functioning; and the symptoms are not better explained by another sleep, medical, neurologic, or psychiatric disorder. There are no criteria for PLMS with arousal or multiple sleep latency test (MSLT) findings.

Summary

Highly Recommended

- *AASM Manual for the Scoring of Sleep and Associated Events: Rules, Terminology, and Technical Specifications*, Version 2.5, 2017, Section VII, Movement Rules
- *Atlas of Clinical Sleep Medicine*, ed 2, Chapter 11.2
- *International Classification of Sleep Disorders*, ed 3, pp 282-291
- *Principles and Practice of Sleep Medicine*, ed 6. Chapter 95

The entire section on movement disorders on the examination, which will also include rhythmic movement disorder and bruxism, only makes up about 19 questions or about 8% of the entire exam. About 70% of the movement disorder questions, about 13 questions, will be specific to RLS and PLMS. Some content related to this topic might also be covered elsewhere, for example, under hypersomnolence, and it is possible that questions related to pediatrics may be presented on this topic. Readers should be aware that because of the increasing concern related to augmentation of symptoms with dopamine there is a trend away from the use of traditional dopamine agonists to either alpha 2 delta ($\alpha2\delta$) ligand agonists or transdermal rotigotine.

Restless Legs Syndrome

- Features
  - Essential: URGE criteria
    - **U**rge to move the limb is unpleasant or uncomfortable
    - **R**est (inactivity) worsens or precipitates symptoms
    - **G**etting up and moving or walking improves symptoms
    - **E**vening (or bedtime) worsens or precipitates symptoms
  - Nonessential
    - Family history
    - Response to dopaminergic therapy
    - Sleep disturbance
    - PLMS or PLMW
  - In children for diagnosis
    - The four URGE criteria
    - Supportive pediatric criteria may include
      - Sleep disturbance
      - Positive immediate family history
      - PLMI greater than 5
      - Strong association with attention-deficit/hyperactivity disorder
- Laboratory testing
  - PSG is not required for diagnosis
  - About 80% have PLMS
  - Blood tests for secondary phenotype (Table 6.1–1)
- Epidemiology
  - 5% to 10% of the population
  - More common in
    - Some groups (e.g., French Canadians)
    - Older people
    - A person whose family member is affected
- Genetics
  - Several genes are implicated in different populations
  - Usually inheritance is autosomal dominant
- Phenotypes
  - Primary (often called *early onset*)
    - Younger than 45 years
    - Slowly progressive

Table 6.1–1 Tests to Consider in Patients With Restless Legs Syndrome[a]

Test	Range Male	Range Female	Comments
Hemoglobin	14.0–17.5 g/dL	12.3–15.3 g/dL	
Hematocrit	40.7%–50.3%	36.1%–44.3%	
Iron	60–170 µg/dL	60–170 µg/dL	Deficiency can occur in patients with GI bleeding, malabsorption (e.g., Crohn disease), or heavy menstrual bleeding, and in strict vegetarians and repeat blood donors.
Total iron-binding capacity (TIBC)	240–450 µg/dL	240–450 µg/dL	
Transferrin saturation	20%–50%	20%–50%	Polypeptide transporter of iron
Ferritin	12–300 ng/mL	12–150 ng/mL	Values <70 ng/mL are considered abnormal in the context of RLS.
B_{12}	200–900 pg/mL	200–900 pg/mL	Deficiency can occur in patients with pernicious anemia or malabsorption (e.g., Crohn disease) and in strict vegetarians.
Folate	2.7–17.0 ng/mL	2.7–17.0 ng/mL	Deficiency can occur in pregnancy, with a poor diet, and with medications such as phenytoin.

[a]Iron deficiency is likely when serum iron is low; TIBC/transferrin is high; TIBC is high and percentage transferrin saturation is low; or ferritin is low.
GI, Gastrointestinal; *RLS,* restless legs syndrome.

- Positive family history
- Idiopathic
  - Secondary (sometimes called *late onset,* but it can occur at any age)
    - Deficiencies
      - Vitamin B_{12}
      - Iron stores
      - Folate
    - Diseases associated with RLS
      - Chronic renal failure
      - Cardiovascular disease
      - Congestive heart failure
      - Peripheral vascular disease
      - Chronic obstructive pulmonary disease (COPD)
      - Parkinson disease
      - Neuropathies
      - Fibromyalgia
      - Hypothyroidism
    - Pregnancy
    - Medications
      - Antidepressants (except bupropion)
      - Centrally acting antihistamines (e.g., diphenhydramine)
      - Lithium
      - Antipsychotics with D_2 receptor–blocking properties
        - Olanzapine
        - Risperidone
        - Metoclopramide
        - Promethazine
        - Prochlorperazine
- Pathophysiology
  - Central dopamine dysfunction; dopamine blockers worsen RLS.
  - Reduced CNS iron stores, reduced CNS dopamine, CNS hypoxia (Connor)
  - Endogenous opiate system dysfunction; opiates improve symptoms.

- Treatment (Iftikhar et al, 2017; Wijemanne and Ondo, 2017)
  - First line
    - α2δ ligands are first-line medications
      - Gabapentin, gabapentin enacarbil, and pregabalin
      - Less likely to produce augmentation
    - Dopaminergic agents are also first-line medications
      - Rotigotine (patch), pramipexole, ropinirole
      - May have side effects of augmentation, sleepiness, compulsive behavior, nausea, vomiting
      - Carbidopa–levodopa is used infrequently because of augmentation
  - Second line
    - Benzodiazepines (e.g., clonazepam)
    - Resistant cases: in addition to those above, μ-receptor–type opioids
      - Examples
        - Codeine
        - Oxycodone
        - Methadone
        - Levorphanol
      - Side effects include constipation and respiratory depression
  - Nutritional deficiencies
    - Iron deficiency
      - Oral replacement (e.g., ferrous sulfate 325 mg three times a day)
      - If indicated, parenteral iron (refer to specialist) (Allen, 2018)
      - Stop donating blood
      - Investigate cause of iron loss
    - B_{12} deficiency
      - For pernicious anemia: IM injections of B_{12}
      - For dietary deficiency: B_{12} tablets
      - For folate deficiency: folic acid tablets

Periodic Limb Movements of Sleep

- Definition
  - Not a disorder without symptoms
  - A laboratory PSG finding
- Criteria to score an individual leg movement
  - Duration
    - Minimum, 0.5 second
    - Maximum, 10 seconds
  - Amplitude change 8 μV above baseline
  - Movements in both legs less than 5 seconds apart count as one movement
- Criteria to score a periodic series
  - Minimum number to define a series is four.
  - Minimum time between leg movements is 5 seconds
  - Maximum time between leg movements is 90 seconds
- Found in about 80% of cases of RLS

Periodic Limb Movement Disorder

- Definition
  - A disorder (PLMS plus symptoms of clinical sleep disturbance or impairment of daytime functioning, not otherwise explained)
  - Documented by PSG
    - In adults: by PLMS index greater than 15 per hour
    - In children: by PLMS index greater than 5 per hour
- Clinical features
  - Sleep disturbance
  - Daytime sleepiness
- Treatment
  - See treatment for PLMS

REFERENCES

Allen RP, Chen C, Garcia-Borreguero D, et al. Comparison of pregabalin with pramipexole for restless legs syndrome. *N Engl J Med.* 2014;370(7):621–631.

Allen RP, Picchietti DL, Auerbach M, et al. Evidence-based and consensus clinical practice guidelines for the iron treatment of restless legs syndrome/Willis-Ekbom disease in adults and children: an IRLSSG task force report. *Sleep Med.* 2018;41:27–44.

American Academy of Sleep Medicine. *International classification of sleep disorders.* ed 3. Darien, Ill.: American Academy of Sleep Medicine; 2014:281–316.

American Academy of Sleep Medicine. *The AASM manual for the scoring of sleep and associated events: rules, terminology and technical specifications.* Version 2.5. Darien, Ill.: American Academy of Sleep Medicine; 2017.

Arunthari V, Kaplan J, Fredrickson PA, et al. Prevalence of restless legs syndrome in blood donors. *Mov Disord.* 2010;25(10):1451–1455.

Connor JR, Patton SM, Oexle K, et al. Iron and restless legs syndrome: treatment, genetics and pathophysiology. *Sleep Med.* 2017;31:61–70.

Haba-Rubio J, Staner L, Petiau C, et al. Restless legs syndrome and low brain iron levels in patients with haemochromatosis. *J Neurol Neurosurg Psychiatry.* 2005;76:1009–1010.

Iftikhar IH, Alghothani L, Trotti LM. Gabapentin enacarbil, pregabalin and rotigotine are equally effective in restless legs syndrome: a comparative meta-analysis. *Eur J Neurol.* 2017;24(12):1446–1456.

Kim SW, Shin IS, Kim JM, et al. Factors potentiating the risk of mirtazapine-associated restless legs syndrome. *Hum Psychopharmacol.* 2008;23(7):615–620. doi:10.1002/hup.965.

Lee DO, Ziman RB, Perkins AT, et al. XP053 study group: a randomized, double-blind, placebo-controlled study to assess the efficacy and tolerability of gabapentin enacarbil in subjects with restless legs syndrome. *J Clin Sleep Med.* 2011;7(3):282–292. doi:10.5664/JCSM.1074.

Mold JW, Vesely SK, Keyl BA, et al. The prevalence, predictors, and consequences of peripheral sensory neuropathy in older patients. *J Am Board Fam Pract.* 2004;17:309–318.

Montplaisir J, Boucher S, Nicholas A, et al. Immobilization tests and periodic leg movements in sleep for the diagnosis of restless legs syndrome. *Mov Disord.* 1998;13:324–329.

Rottach KG, Schaner BM, Kirch MH, et al. Restless legs syndrome as side effect of second-generation antidepressants. *J Psychiatr Res.* 2008;43:70–75.

Stefansson H, Rye DB, Hicks A, et al. A genetic risk factor for periodic limb movements in sleep. *N Engl J Med.* 2007;357(7):639–647.

Weintraub D, Koester J, Potenza MN, et al. Impulse control disorders in Parkinson disease: a cross-sectional study of 3090 patients. *Arch Neurol.* 2010;67(5):589–595.

Wijemanne S, Ondo W. Restless legs syndrome: clinical features, diagnosis and a practical approach to management. *Pract Neurol.* 2017;17(6):444–452.

6.2   Other Movement Disorders

QUESTIONS

Rock and Roll

A 3-year-old boy is brought to a sleep disorder center. His parents relate that for the past 6 months, he has been a restless sleeper. From the time he falls asleep and intermittently during the night, his entire body moves continuously, most often rocking from side to side. The child sleeps 12 hours each night and has a 2-hour nap during the daytime. Snoring and apnea have not been observed. He appears to be developmentally normal, and the physical examination is entirely normal. The parents are concerned that this symptom may represent a serious neurologic condition, and they want their son treated.

1. Which of the following disorders is *most* likely in this case?
   A. PLMS
   B. Alternating leg muscle activation (ALMA)
   C. Excessive fragmentary myoclonus
   D. Rhythmic movement disorder

2. When informed about your clinical diagnosis, the parents insist on a sleep test to confirm the diagnosis. Which is the *most* appropriate next step?
   A. A PSG is indicated but *not* treatment with medication
   B. A PSG is indicated, *and* clonazepam 0.125 mg is recommended
   C. A PSG is *not* indicated, *but* treatment with clonazepam 0.125 mg is recommended
   D. *Neither* PSG nor treatment with medication is indicated for this diagnosis

3. Approximately 60% of infants are reported to display at least one type of rhythmic movement by the age of 9 months. What percentage show rhythmic movements at the age of 5 years?

A. 0%

B. 5%

C. 20%

D. 40%

The Chipmunk

A 45-year-old woman is referred for evaluation of possible sleep apnea. She awakens with headaches, and her husband has told her that she snores and sometimes stops breathing during sleep. What really bothers him is that she often sounds "like a chipmunk" and keeps him awake at night. Her BMI is 22. Physical examination findings are shown in Figure 6.2–1. The patient has an overnight sleep study. A fragment used for scoring sleep stages from the study is shown in Figure 6.2–2.

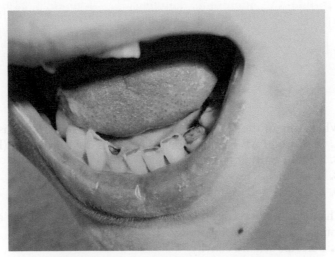

FIGURE 6.2–1 Question 4 (see also Fig. 6.2–2).

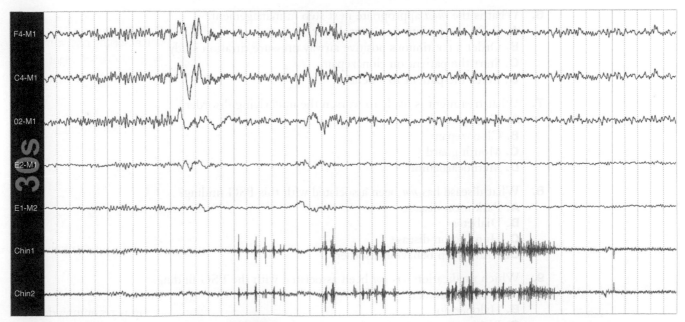

FIGURE 6.2–2 Question 4 (see also Fig. 6.2–1).

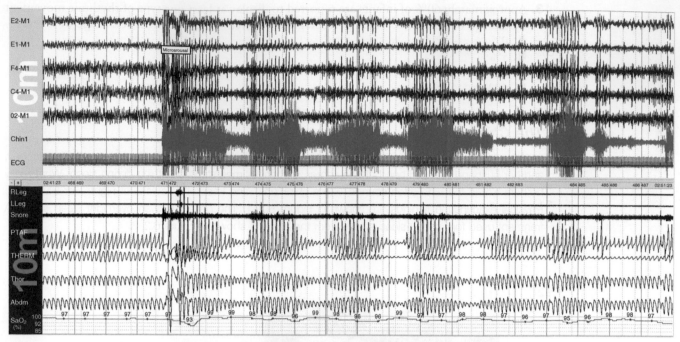

FIGURE 6.2–3 Questions 5 to 9.

4. Which one of the following does this PSG fragment demonstrate?
   A. Increased EMG activity indicating rapid eye movement (REM) sleep behavior disorder
   B. Seizure causing facial twitching
   C. Bruxism
   D. Rhythmic movement disorder

5. The technologist scoring the study believes that the patient also has sleep apnea and shows you the fragment in Figure 6.2–3. What does it show?
   A. Periodic seizure activity
   B. Cheyne-Stokes respiration
   C. Bruxism
   D. Obstructive sleep apnea

6. What is the *most* appropriate next step in management?
   A. Refer the patient to a neurologist
   B. Order a continuous positive airway pressure titration study
   C. Start the patient on clonazepam
   D. Refer the patient to a dentist

7. What treatment is likely to worsen the underlying disorder?
   A. Fluoxetine
   B. Clonazepam
   C. Mouth guard
   D. Methocarbamol

8. What disease has *not* been associated with this PSG finding?
   A. Parkinson disease
   B. Diabetes
   C. Huntington disease
   D. REM sleep behavior disorder

9. Which medication has *not* been associated with the PSG finding?
   A. Methylphenidate
   B. Haloperidol
   C. Lithium
   D. Erythromycin

A Painful Awakening

At her yearly physical examination, a 68-year-old woman complains to her primary care provider about difficulty sleeping. When asked about it, she states that she is often awoken by a pain in one of her legs during the night. The pain is localized to her very tight-feeling calf, has an abrupt onset, and often requires her to massage it in bed. The area is often sore for a few hours when she awakens.

10. What is the appropriate diagnosis?
   A. Hypnagogic foot tremor
   B. Periodic limb movements
   C. Sleep-related leg cramps
   D. Restless legs syndrome

11. This diagnosis will occur nightly in what percentage of 60-year-old adults?
   A. 3%
   B. 6%
   C. 9%
   D. 12%

12. Which of the following medication classes has *not* been commonly associated with leg cramping?
   A. Diuretics
   B. Hypnotics
   C. Oral contraceptives
   D. Statins

ANSWERS

1. D. The condition described is typical for sleep-related rhythmic movement disorder. There are many names for this disorder, including *body rocking, head banging, body rolling, jactatio corporis nocturna*, and *jactatio capitis nocturna*. The movements are continuous and involve large muscle groups. Limb movements are periodic; that is, they occur at a regular interval, for example, every 20 seconds, and they generally only involve the limbs. ALMA is not a disorder but a PSG finding of unclear clinical significance; it bears some similarity to periodic limb movements but differs in that the duration of the burst is shorter (0.1–0.5 second), the events alternate between the legs, and the period of the movements is much shorter (range, 0.5–3.0 Hz). Excessive fragmentary myoclonus is also a PSG finding of unclear clinical significance and not a disorder. There are at least five very brief (less than 0.15 second) muscle bursts per minute, occurring at least for 20 minutes during non-REM (NREM) sleep. (MANUAL2, Section VII, Movement Rules)

2. D. The history is characteristic enough that a PSG is not required for management and is not required by the ICSD3 for diagnosis, unless there is a concern for another disorder. Although disturbing to observers, the phenomenon is generally benign and results in few symptoms. Medication is not generally recommended. In rare cases, when rhythmic movement disorders cause injury, such as in the case of head banging, pharmacologic treatment may be reasonable.

3. B. Whereas rhythmic movements are common in young infants, only 5% of children have reports of rhythmic movements at 5 years of age (Fig. 6.2–4).

4. C. Short twitches in the two chin EMGs suggest that bruxism is present. This example (see Fig. 6.2–4) meets two of the criteria used to score bruxism: brief elevations in chin EMG 0.25 to 2.0 seconds in duration with a train of at least three events in a sequence and sustained elevation of chin EMG at least 2 seconds in duration.

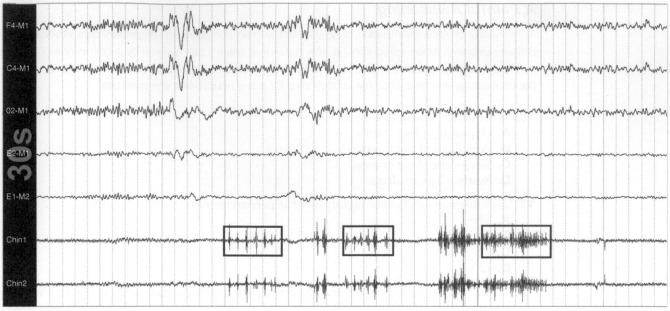

FIGURE 6.2–4 Answers 3 and 4.

5. C. This compressed fragment shows a long stretch of bruxism. The clue is when EEG channels are examined, and the characteristic effect of bruxism is seen in these channels. Superficially, the respiratory channels do resemble Cheyne-Stokes breathing, and when the patient had the episodes of bruxism, it appeared as though there were increases in ventilation followed by decreases in ventilation and small changes in SaO_2.

6. D. This patient should be referred to a dentist; examination showed severe damage to the lower anterior teeth, with some of the teeth possibly infected. This degree of bruxism can be difficult to treat. Treatment is typically with a mouth guard to minimize further damage.

7. A. Fluoxetine and other selective serotonin reuptake inhibitors (SSRIs) should not be considered as treatment for bruxism because they can actually induce bruxism or increase clenching of the jaw. The treatment of choice for bruxism is an oral appliance such as a mouth guard, ideally fit by the dentist. Short-term use of medications such as clonazepam or methocarbamol (a muscle relaxant) may be helpful.

8. B. Several neurologic conditions have been associated with bruxism or jaw clenching. There are no reports of diabetes being associated with sleep bruxism. See the Summary for examples.

9. D. Several medications have been associated with bruxism or jaw clenching, most of them affecting the CNS; no reports exist of antibiotics being associated with the disorder. The most widely encountered drugs associated with bruxism are the SSRIs. See the Summary for examples.

10. C. This description is of sleep-related leg cramps. It is a nearly universal experience in adults older than 50 years of age, although it may occur rarely.   (ICSD3, pp 299-301)

11. B. It has been reported that 6% of adults older than 60 years of age will have nightly leg cramps.   (ICSD3, p 300)

12. B. Hypnotic medications have not been associated with leg cramping. Diuretics, oral contraceptives, statins, intravenous iron sucrose, and long-acting β-agonists all have been associated with leg cramping.   (ICSD3, p 300)

Highly Recommended

■ *International Classification of Sleep Disorders*, ed 3, pp 281-340

As noted earlier, the movement disorders as a total will make up 8% of the exam; of that, about 25% (or four to five questions) will be related to bruxism and rhythmic movement disorders. Although rhythmic movement disorder is common, few patients with this condition are actually referred to a sleep disorders center. Bruxism and the other movement disorders in this section and summary are also not commonly referred but may be found in the course of investigation of other disorders.

Sleep-Related Rhythmic Movement Disorder

■ Features
  ○ Repetitive motor behavior during sleep
  ○ Involves large muscle groups
    • Head banging (jactatio capitis nocturna)
    • Head rolling
    • Body rocking (jactatio corporis nocturna)
■ Epidemiology
  ○ Age 12 months: about 50%
  ○ Age 18 months: about 33%
  ○ Age 5 years: 5%
  ○ Adult prevalence: present but unknown
■ Diagnosis
  ○ Made by history
  ○ Criteria
    • Repetitive stereotypic movements in sleep
    • Involves large muscle groups
    • Disrupts sleep
    • Impaired in daytime
    • Injury
  ○ PSG
    • Done only if another sleep disorder is suspected
    • Should include video recording
    • Shows rolling or banging of the head or rolling or rocking of the body
    • Frequency of about once per second
    • Absent in REM sleep
■ Prognosis
  ○ Benign course typically; is not considered a disorder unless there is a clinical consequence
  ○ Usually improves with age
  ○ Can persist into late adulthood
■ Treatment
  ○ Safety precautions

Bruxism

■ Features
  ○ Clenching of jaw or grinding of teeth during sleep
  ○ Types of abnormal motor activities
    • Tonic
      ◆ Sustained clenching
      ◆ Phasic
      ◆ Periodic grinding

- Symptoms
  - ○ Jaw pain
  - ○ Temporomandibular joint pain
  - ○ Wearing down of teeth
  - ○ Headaches
  - ○ Disturbed sleep
  - ○ Noisy during sleep
- Epidemiology
  - ○ Children: 15%
  - ○ Teenagers: 12%
  - ○ Adults: 8%
  - ○ Older people: 3%
- Diagnosis
  - ○ PSG not required
    - Typical findings (see above)
  - ○ History
    - Report of nocturnal grinding or clenching
    - Discomfort or pain on awakening
      - ◆ Jaw
      - ◆ Head
  - ○ Examination
    - Worn teeth
    - Hypertrophied masseter muscles
- Clinical forms
  - ○ Idiopathic
  - ○ Secondary
    - Associated with diseases
      - ◆ Movement disorders
        - Parkinson disease
        - Huntington disease
      - ◆ Primary sleep disorders
        - Sleep apnea
        - PLMS
        - REM sleep behavior disorder
      - ◆ Neurologic diseases
        - Cerebellar disease
        - Shy-Drager syndrome
        - Associated with drugs or chemicals
      - ◆ Caffeine
      - ◆ Nicotine
      - ◆ Methylphenidate
    - Psychiatric medication examples
      - ◆ Haloperidol
      - ◆ Chlorpromazine
      - ◆ Lithium
      - ◆ Fluoxetine
      - ◆ Sertraline
      - ◆ Citalopram
    - Cardiovascular medication example
      - ◆ Flecainide
- Treatment
  - ○ Oral appliance, ideally a rigid appliance fit by a dentist
  - ○ Withdraw causative medication (see above)
  - ○ Medications
    - None indicated for bruxism by the US Food and Drug Administration
    - Short-term benzodiazepine (e.g., clonazepam)

Sleep-Related Leg Cramps

- Nearly a universal experience in adults older than 50 years old
  - Painful contraction of the muscle
    - Often requires stretching the muscle or massaging it
    - The muscle is often sore afterward
- Diagnosis is by history alone; it does not require a PSG
- Treatment
  - No validated treatment options exist for this disorder

Abnormal Movements or Bursts Seen on Polysomnography (Not Disorders)

- ALMA
  - Bursts
    - Up to 0.5 second in duration
    - Alternates between legs
    - Four bursts needed for scoring
    - Frequency of the alternating burst is 0.5 to 3 Hz
- Hypnagogic foot tremor
  - Bursts
    - 0.25 to 1 second in duration
    - Four bursts needed for scoring
    - Frequency of the burst is 0.3 to 4 Hz
- Excessive fragmentary myoclonus
  - Bursts
    - Less than 0.15 second in duration
    - Five bursts per minute needed for scoring
    - At least 20 minutes in NREM sleep
  - Twitches may be visible

REFERENCES

American Academy of Sleep Medicine: *International classification of sleep disorders: diagnostic and coding manual*, ed 3, Darien, Ill.: American Academy of Sleep Medicine; 2014.

American Academy of Sleep Medicine: *The AASM manual for the scoring of sleep and associated events: rules, terminology and technical specifications*, Version 2.5, Darien, Ill.: American Academy of Sleep Medicine; 2017.

Sleep-Related Breathing Disorders

7.1	Obstructive Sleep Apnea

QUESTIONS

A 38-Year-Old Man With a History of Scrotal Edema

A 38-year-old real estate agent presents in mid-January with a 15-year history of snoring, a 2-year history of witnessed apnea, and excessive daytime sleepiness (EDS). He has an Epworth Sleepiness Scale (ESS) score of 17 of 24. One year ago, he started to notice swelling of his feet and ankles. During the course of the year, he developed severe edema, which peaked on New Year's Eve, when the edema spread to his legs and scrotum. He was admitted to the hospital and was told that he had congestive heart failure (CHF). He was treated for CHF and had lost 60 lb by the time he was discharged 1 week later. He was then sent for a sleep evaluation; a fragment from his sleep study is shown in Figure 7.1–1. The top window is a 30-second epoch, the bottom is a 2-minute epoch.

1. What is the most striking feature noted on the electroencephalogram (EEG)?
   A. Rapid eye movements (REMs)
   B. Vertex sharp waves
   C. Electrocardiography (ECG) artifact
   D. Sawtooth waves

2. Based on this fragment, what do you expect his bed partner to report?
   A. Movements every 20 seconds
   B. Snoring noises separated by long periods of silence
   C. Loud, continuous snoring
   D. Excessive sweating

3. What is the main diagnostic finding?
   A. Hypopneas
   B. Obstructive apneas
   C. Hypoventilation
   D. Cheyne-Stokes breathing (CSB)

4. Considering the findings up to this point, what was the *likeliest* cause of the scrotal edema?
   A. Left ventricular systolic cardiac failure
   B. Systemic arterial hypertension
   C. Pulmonary embolism
   D. Cor pulmonale

5. Based on this diagnostic finding, what should be the next step?
   A. Continuous positive airway pressure (CPAP) titration
   B. Adaptive servoventilation (ASV)
   C. Home oxygen therapy
   D. Referral for fitting of a mandibular advancement device

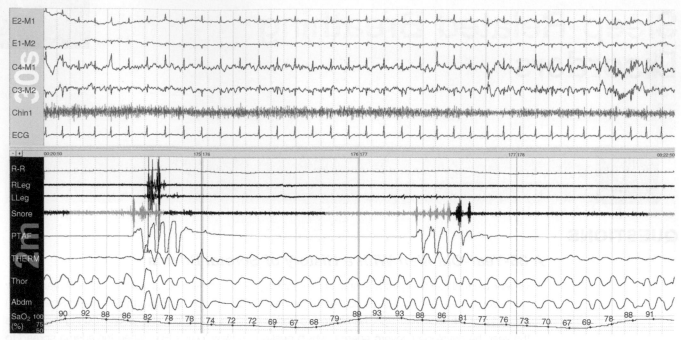

FIGURE 7.1–1 Questions 1 to 5.

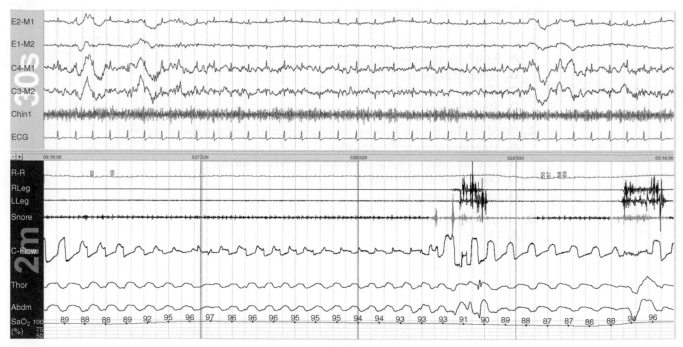

FIGURE 7.1–2 Questions 6 and 7.

6. He is started on positive pressure after 2 hours of monitoring. A fragment from the polysomnogram (PSG) is shown in Figure 7.1–2; C-flow is mask flow measured by the CPAP unit. What does it show?

A. Complete control of the obstructive apnea because the SaO₂ is normal

B. No effect of the CPAP on the patient's physiology

C. Development of complex sleep apnea

D. Flow limitation, indicating incomplete control of the sleep apnea

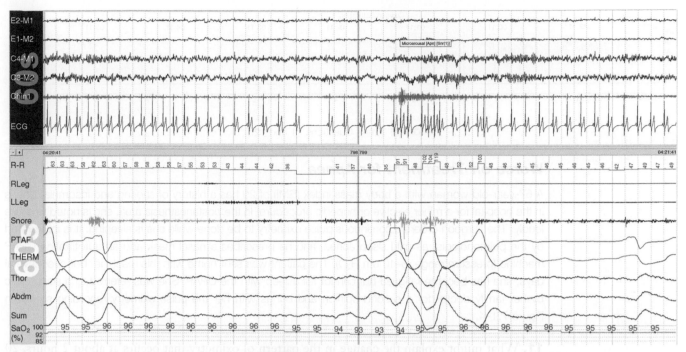

FIGURE 7.1–3 Questions 8 to 10.

7. Given this finding, what is the next step?
   A. Increase CPAP
   B. Decrease CPAP
   C. Change the modality to ASV
   D. Start bilevel pressure with a backup rate

Frantic Call From the Sleep Tech

A 48-year-old patient whose complaint is snoring and daytime sleepiness is in the sleep lab for overnight PSG. He is taking oxycodone for pain. The night tech phones the on-call doctor with concerns that the patient is having a dysrhythmia issue, and the tech does not know how to proceed. The tech captures the PSG screen and sends the image file to the on-call doctor by secure e-mail. The PSG fragment in Figure 7.1–3 shows a 60-second epoch.

8. What is causing the ECG abnormality at the end of the apneic episode?
   A. Hypoxemia
   B. Increased sympathetic tone
   C. Increased vagal tone
   D. Histamine

9. What sleep-breathing abnormality is present in the PSG fragment?
   A. Hypopnea
   B. Obstructive apnea
   C. Central apnea
   D. Mixed apnea

10. What course of action should be taken upon seeing the PSG fragment in this patient with obstructive sleep apnea (OSA)?
   A. Terminate the study and send the patient to the emergency department (ED)
   B. Insert a cardiac pacemaker
   C. Begin CPAP titration
   D. Begin oxygen therapy

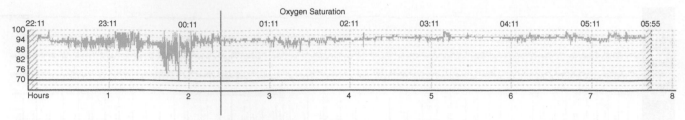

FIGURE 7.1–4 Questions 11 and 12.

Worse on Treatment for Apnea

A 67-year-old woman with a body mass index (BMI) of 29 has a history of snoring and insomnia. She is in the hospital for a minor elective orthopedic procedure. In the postanesthesia area, she is noted to snore loudly. The surgeon orders a continuous pulse oximetry to be done while she is sleeping. It is interpreted by the pulmonologist as mild sleep apnea, and he prescribes a nasal mask and an autotitrating CPAP machine (pressure range, 5–10 cm H_2O). The patient was sent home with this machine, but over several days, she has become fatigued but cannot fall asleep with the CPAP. She was referred to a sleep clinic by her family doctor for a second opinion and brings with her the pulse oximetry recording shown in Figure 7.1–4.

11. What might explain the change in the pattern of oximetry that occurs at about 2 hours, 20 minutes (the *vertical red line* in the figure)?
   A. The patient turned over onto her side
   B. The patient woke up and was awake the rest of the night
   C. The patient did not have any further episodes of REM
   D. All of the above are true

12. What should be the next step?
   A. Increase the range of the autotitrating machine to 5 to 15 cm H_2O
   B. Stop the positive airway pressure (PAP) therapy because the apnea was obviously mild
   C. Start the patient on zolpidem
   D. Order an overnight PSG

Falling Asleep in University Class

A 19-year-old student has been falling asleep repeatedly in class, and his family doctor is concerned he has narcolepsy. The patient has recently started to snore. His BMI is 24. Examination found bilateral enlarged cervical lymph nodes and a large spleen, and chest radiography showed asymmetric hilar soft tissue enlargement.

13. His evaluation by the sleep clinic should include which of the following?
   A. Maintenance of wakefulness test (MWT) without preceding PSG
   B. Home monitoring for seizures
   C. Multiple sleep latency test (MSLT) without preceding PSG
   D. Imaging studies of the pharynx and neck

Obstructive Sleep Apnea Comorbidities

A 38-year-old truck driver with a history of snoring and excessive daytime sleepiness is referred for evaluation of OSA. The patient cannot come for an in-lab sleep study for at least 1 week because he is a long-distance trucker and will be out of town. His ESS score is 24 of 24.

14. What should you advise this patient?
   A. Because he has a long history of snoring, he can delay the test until he is back in town
   B. He cannot drive until his problem is diagnosed and treated
   C. He should start on CPAP with an autotitrating CPAP machine
   D. He can use modafinil until the test can be done

15. A 48-year-old woman with fatigue and insomnia presents to her primary care practitioner. He gives her the Berlin Questionnaire, which is used to calculate the risk of what condition?

A. OSA

B. Depression

C. Bipolar disease

D. Circadian rhythm disorder (advanced or delayed)

16. The term *cor pulmonale* refers to what?

A. Left heart failure caused by a right-to-left cardiac shunt

B. Right heart failure caused by pulmonary hypertension

C. Cardiac rhythm abnormality in asthma

D. Pulmonary hypertension caused by left heart disease

17. Prior to bariatric surgery, a 40-year-old woman with a BMI of 50 and $PacO_2$ of 52 mm Hg is referred to the sleep disorders center to screen for sleep problems. She is noted to have severe ankle swelling. What abnormality *most* likely would explain her peripheral edema?

A. OSA

B. Upper airway resistance syndrome (UARS)

C. Obesity hypoventilation syndrome (OHS)

D. Treatment-emergent apnea

18. A 55-year-old woman with a history of obesity (BMI, 35), hypertension, and snoring was found to have OSA, with an apnea-hypopnea index (AHI) of 15 events/hr. During her titration study (Fig. 7.1–5), the tech notes an episode of ventricular tachycardia and sends her to the ED. Based on the 2-second zoomed window, what is the patient's cardiac rhythm?

A. Ventricular tachycardia

B. Torsades de pointes

C. Not discernible

D. Sinus rhythm

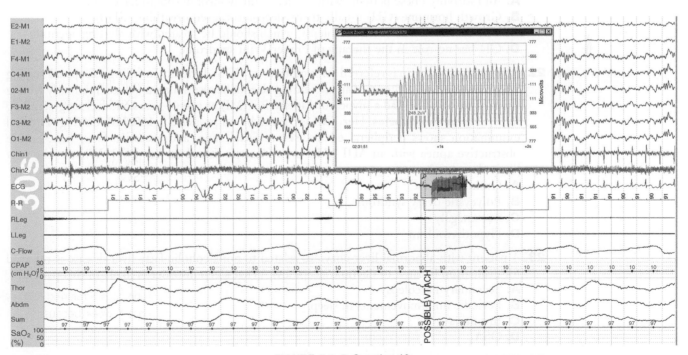

FIGURE 7.1–5 Question 18.

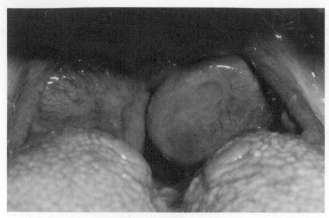

FIGURE 7.1–6 Question 19.

Not Just Middle-Aged Obese Men

19. A thin 6-year-old patient is referred to the sleep disorders center with a history of restless sleep. The patient's pharynx is pictured in Figure 7.1–6. What do you note in the chart?
   A. Enlarged tonsils, grade 4
   B. Mallampati class 4
   C. Hypertrophy of uvula
   D. Normal pharynx

20. Which statement about Prader-Willi syndrome is *true*?
   A. The main symptom is insomnia
   B. There may be sleep-onset REM periods (SOREMPs) on the MSLT
   C. It usually manifests after 20 years of age
   D. Few patients have sleep apnea

21. Which statement is *true* about the management of Prader-Willi syndrome?
   A. All morbidly obese patients with Prader-Willi syndrome should have a PSG
   B. Growth hormone (GH) usually treats sleep-disordered breathing (SDB)
   C. The SOREMPs indicate narcolepsy, which should be treated with alerting agents
   D. GH has no role in the therapy of Prader-Willi syndrome

22. A 48-year-old woman is referred for symptoms of EDS, difficulty in falling asleep and staying asleep, snoring, and witnessed apneas during sleep. She also wakes up quite frequently feeling short of breath. She had a myocardial infarction (MI) at age 44 years and has long-standing hypertension and diabetes. Her BMI is 51 and blood pressure is 160/110 mm Hg. Physical examination shows peripheral edema, severe facial acne, and excessive facial hair. Severe obstructive apnea with an AHI of 70 events/hr was found on her PSG. What is the *most* likely diagnosis?
   A. Cushing disease
   B. Polycystic ovary syndrome
   C. Acromegaly
   D. Hypothyroidism

23. A patient with abnormal liver enzymes related to nonalcoholic fatty liver disease is referred for evaluation because of daytime sleepiness. What sleep disorder is likely in this patient?
   A. Secondary narcolepsy
   B. Periodic limb movements in sleep
   C. Insomnia
   D. OSA

24. Which statement about sleep apnea in menopausal women is *true*?
   A. It is caused by obesity
   B. Prevalence in menopausal women is similar to that in age-matched men
   C. It is more common in women with hot flashes
   D. It seldom responds to CPAP

25. Which statement about sleep in pregnancy is *true?*
  A. The most common reason for nocturnal awakenings is restless legs syndrome
  B. Snoring in pregnancy has been associated with preeclampsia
  C. Snoring in pregnancy has been associated with larger-than-expected babies
  D. Sleep apnea should not be treated with CPAP during pregnancy

26. Compared with men of similar age, apnea severity, and degree of daytime sleepiness, which statement about OSA in women is *true?*
  A. Insomnia is more common
  B. Caffeine consumption is greater
  C. Women are less likely to be on antidepressant medication
  D. Women are less likely to have a history of thyroid disease

27. Comparing OSA in men and women, the *most* significant difference is that women
  A. Are heavier users of alcohol
  B. Tend to have more episodes of central apnea
  C. Tend to have more compliant upper airways
  D. More commonly have apneic episodes clustered in REM sleep

28. What is the *most* common cause of SDB in 10-year-old children?
  A. Enlarged adenoids and tonsils
  B. Obesity
  C. Retrognathia
  D. Congenital malformations

An 8-Year-Old Boy With Attention-Deficit/Hyperactivity Disorder

An 8-year-old boy with a 5-month snoring history is referred for evaluation of restless sleep. His pediatrician has diagnosed attention-deficit/hyperactivity disorder (ADHD), for which he was prescribed methylphenidate. The medication improved his behavior in school but worsened his nighttime sleep.

29. What does his profile photo show (Fig. 7.1–7)?
  A. Maxillary insufficiency
  B. Prognathia
  C. Retrognathia
  D. Normal anatomy

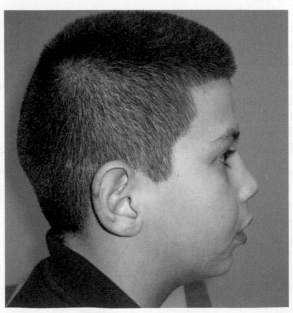

FIGURE 7.1–7 Question 29.

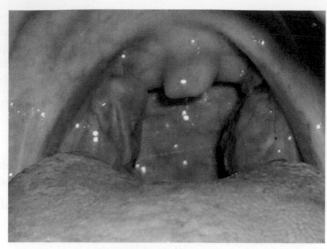

FIGURE 7.1–8 Question 30.

30. Figure 7.1–8 is a photo of this child's tonsils. What does it show?
  A. Grade 4 tonsil enlargement
  B. Grade 3 tonsil enlargement
  C. Mallampati class 3
  D. Mallampati class 4

31. What additional evaluation would be helpful in this patient?
  A. Nasopharyngoscopy
  B. Evaluation of alignment of upper and lower teeth
  C. Neck collar size
  D. BMI

32. What should be done next?
  A. Cephalometrics
  B. Magnetic resonance imaging (MRI) of the upper airway
  C. Tonsillectomy and adenoidectomy
  D. Diagnostic PSG

33. In addition to the standard montage of adult PSGs, what data might be useful to monitor in this patient?
  A. Esophageal pressure
  B. End-tidal PcO_2
  C. End-tidal PO_2
  D. Additional channels are not needed

34. All of the following are true about OSA in children *except*
  A. Sleep architecture is usually normal
  B. Cortical EEG arousals are more common than are movement or autonomic arousals
  C. Obstructive events occur predominantly during REM sleep
  D. Children have a faster respiratory rate and lower functional residual capacity than adults

35. The results from his 8-hour overnight PSG are as follows:
  AHI = 2.1 events/hr (all obstructive); end-tidal PcO_2 >50 mm Hg for 11% of sleep time; low SaO_2 = 93%; mean SaO_2 = 96%
  What is the *best* interpretation of these data?
  A. UARS
  B. OSA
  C. Sleep hypoventilation syndrome
  D. Normal findings

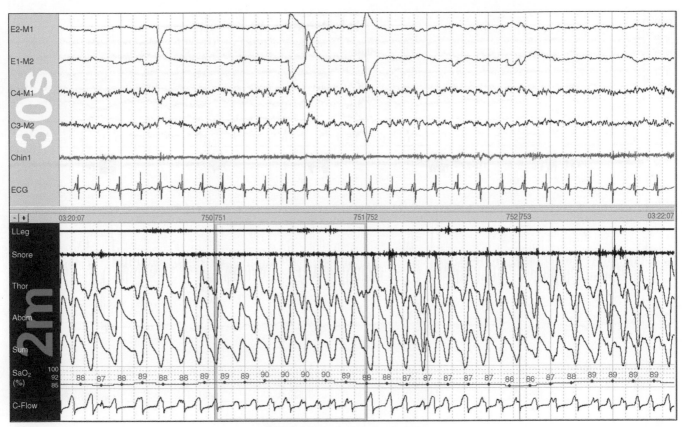

FIGURE 7.1–9 Questions 36 to 38.

36. During CPAP titration, the epoch in Figure 7.1–9 is recorded. Which of the following statements is *correct*?

A. PAP titration is complete because SaO$_2$ is stable and there are no apneas

B. PAP titration is complete but oxygen should be added

C. PAP titration is complete because it is acceptable to have a reduced SaO$_2$ at times

D. The degree of hypoxemia seen here is not acceptable

37. What does the C-flow channel show in Figure 7.1–9?

A. Flow limitation

B. Complete airway occlusions

C. Normal PcO$_2$ trace

D. CSB

38. What is the sleep stage in this epoch, and what effect is it having on the respiratory system?

A. This is REM sleep, and the evident flow limitation is likely caused by reduced tone of the pharyngeal muscles

B. This is stage N3, and the evident flow limitation is caused by increased chemical drive to breathe

C. The K complexes indicate stage N2, and chemical drives to breathe are causing tachypnea

D. The slow eye movements indicate stage N1 sleep, and the increased drive to breathe has resulted in a wide-open upper airway

Lucky to Be Alive

A 56-year-old obese man is in the intensive care unit (ICU) for an MI. The ICU staff has noted episodes of sleep apnea and heavy snoring, and for this reason, his physician ordered a split-night sleep study. When the sleep tech went in to start him on CPAP, she noted frothy fluid on his pillow and that he was

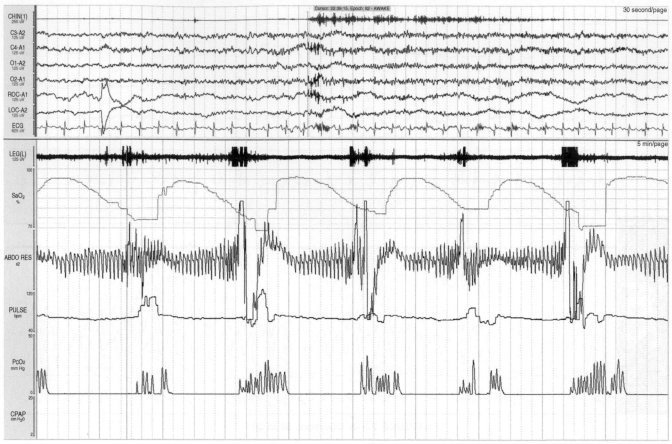

FIGURE 7.1–10 Questions 39 and 40.

coughing. The remainder of the night was uneventful. The patient did beautifully on CPAP. A representative sample of his pretreatment PSG is shown in Figure 7.1–10. Pick the best answer from the next series of questions.

39. The PSG fragment is divided into two windows, the top with an epoch of 30 seconds and the bottom with an epoch length of 5 minutes. Before he was studied on PAP, his EEG continuously had this pattern. What stage of sleep should be scored based on the top window?

  A. Wakefulness

  B. Stage N1

  C. Stage N2

  D. Stage R (REM sleep)

40. Oronasal airflow is being monitored by end-tidal PcO_2. What sleep-breathing abnormality does the bottom window show?

  A. Overlap syndrome

  B. Hypoventilation documented by high end-tidal PcO_2

  C. Central sleep apnea (CSA)

  D. Obstructive apnea

41. Figure 7.1–11 shows a PSG fragment while the patient is being treated. The inset is an enlargement from the CPAP channel. With what is he being treated?

  A. Fixed CPAP

  B. Oxygen

  C. Bilevel with a backup rate

  D. Autotitrating CPAP

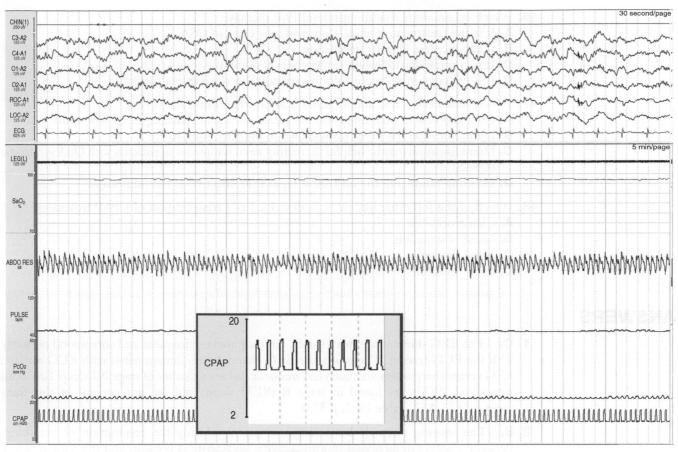

FIGURE 7.1–11 Question 41.

42. How do you put this case together?
   A. The patient had an undiagnosed stroke that caused the abnormal breathing pattern
   B. The patient was in pulmonary edema on a background of OSA
   C. This is sleep apnea in a patient with severe insomnia
   D. This is a straightforward case of chronic right heart failure

BONUS QUESTIONS: SHORT SNAPPERS

43. Which statement about mandibular advancement devices for the treatment of sleep apnea is *true*?
   A. They can be effective in patients with mild to moderate OSA
   B. They have not been evaluated objectively in sleep apnea
   C. They are more effective than CPAP
   D. They are useful in selected patients with CSA

44. Which statement about uvulopharyngopalatoplasty (UPPP) is *true*?
   A. When done with laser, it is much less painful than when performed with a scalpel
   B. The success rate approaches that of CPAP
   C. After surgery, the patient's snoring can be reduced or abolished, but the apnea remains severe
   D. It is particularly effective in patients with retrognathia

45. Which statement about bariatric surgery is *false*?
   A. Postoperative complications are common
   B. If sleep apnea is present, it generally improves
   C. Diabetes control will worsen
   D. Patients who undergo bariatric surgery should be tested for sleep apnea

46. Which statement is *true* about bilevel PAP therapy?
   A. It is the treatment of choice for most new cases of OSA
   B. It can increase alveolar ventilation
   C. It is contraindicated when hypercapnia is present
   D. It is effective in reducing rhinitis symptoms in sleep apnea patients

47. Which statement is *true* about humidification when using CPAP?
   A. Cold and heated humidification has equal efficacy in reducing nasal symptoms
   B. Humidification has never been shown to improve compliance
   C. Humidification may be helpful in treating nasal symptoms in patients with OSA syndrome (OSAS)
   D. Instilling saline into the nostrils at night is as effective as humidification

48. Which of the following has *not* been described as a complication of CPAP treatment?
   A. Claustrophobia
   B. Nasal obstruction
   C. Nasal discharge
   D. Acute tonsillitis

ANSWERS

1. C. The EEG shows some sharp waves, but they are very frequent and correspond perfectly with the ECG tracing. Therefore, the EEG channels are contaminated with ECG artifact. EEG vertex sharp waves are much less frequent and are a marker of stage N1 sleep. Sawtooth waves and REMs are found in stage R (REM sleep) and are not present in this fragment. (ATLAS2, Table 18–2, p 373)

2. B. The snoring channel shows increased activity during the resumption of breathing. Between clusters of increased snoring activity, no activity is present, and the patient is in a quiet state. The leg movements seen in this fragment toward the beginning of the epoch (RLeg, LLeg) correspond to breathing and are not periodic limb movements; no other leg movements are seen.

3. B. This is classic OSA. Airflow is markedly reduced (more than 90% in the thermal channel) for more than 10 seconds and respiratory effort is noted in the thoracic and abdominal belts. Note that both the temperature-sensing channel and nasal pressure channels show markedly reduced (and at times zero) flows. American Academy of Sleep Medicine (AASM) guidelines call for using an oronasal thermal airflow sensor (thermistor, thermocouple, or PVDF sensor) to document apneas and a nasal pressure transducer to document hypopneas. (The AASM manual provides for alternatives when these devices are deemed unreliable.) Note that nasal pressure reads zero when the patient is breathing through the mouth, so nasal pressure is often not a reliable indicator of apnea. (ATLAS2, p 395)

4. D. Cor pulmonale, right heart failure from respiratory disease, is the most likely cause of this patient's peripheral edema. Chronic hypoxemia (which can be only nocturnal) causes pulmonary hypertension that eventually can result in right ventricular failure, increased venous pressure, and peripheral edema. If there had been a CSB pattern, left heart failure would likely have been an important contributor. (ATLAS2, p 268)

5. A. The next step is CPAP titration because OSA was documented. ASV would be used if a CSB pattern or central apnea had been present and if the left ventricular ejection fraction (LVEF) was greater than 40%. Oxygen therapy is not effective in treating OSA, and the patient's apnea and hypoxemia are too severe for treatment with a mandibular advancement device.

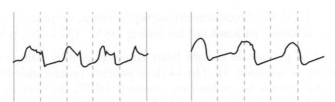

FIGURE 7.1–12 Answer 6.

6. D.   Flattening of the flow trace in the middle of the bottom epoch is evidence for flow limitation; therefore, the airway is still obstructed. Toward the right side, notice that the flow trace now demonstrates a rounded top during unobstructed breathing. Evaluating the shape of the flow trace is very valuable. Figure 7.1–12 is an enlargement of the C-flow trace from the middle of the epoch; it shows flattening of the top of the trace, indicating flow limitation (*left*), and later in the epoch shows a rounded top, indicating unobstructed breathing (*right*). Note that the SaO_2 swings from 97% to 87%, indicating incomplete control of the abnormal breathing events.

7. A.   Because flow limitation has been demonstrated, the next step is to increase the CPAP pressure. Reducing the pressure would increase flow limitation and obstruction. ASV is not indicated at all, and in the absence of central apnea, bilevel pressure with a backup rate is not indicated.

8. C.   Inspiring against an obstructed airway is similar to the Müller maneuver, which increases vagal tone and can cause bradycardia or, as in this example, sinus arrest.   (ATLAS2, Fig. 19–65, p 441)

9. C.   Central apnea is evident from the lack of airflow (monitored by thermal sensor and nasal pressure); there is no breathing effort. Central apnea episodes can occur in patients with primarily obstructive apnea, especially if they are using opiate medications. Snoring noises were present when breathing resumed.

10. C.   Sinus arrest is not a rare finding in patients with OSA. Sinus arrhythmias are usually corrected by CPAP treatment. Inexperienced technologists sometimes send such patients to the ED, and pacemakers have been (inappropriately) placed.

11. D.   All of the answers are possible. The severity of this patient's problem cannot be diagnosed from oximetry alone. Also, if apnea were present, oximetry could not determine the apnea type.

12. D.   Simply changing the pressure range is not going to be helpful because a firm diagnosis has not been established. Stopping the PAP therapy is also the wrong course of action because the patient does show significant hypoxemia. Prescribing a hypnotic at this point is contraindicated. A subsequent in-lab sleep study showed that the patient had very severe obstructive apnea and very severe periodic limb movement disorder (PLMD); the latter obviously could not have been detected with oximetry. Ultimately, both sleep disorders were treated, and the patient has done well.

13. D.   The commonest causes of sleepiness in college students are sleep deprivation (often caused by delayed sleep phase), sleep apnea, depression, medication use, and narcolepsy, in that order. The MWT is not used to diagnose any of those conditions. An MSLT without a preceding PSG cannot rule out abnormalities during sleep that might be the cause of sleepiness. Nothing in the question suggests a diagnosis of epilepsy. The clinical history raises the possibility of Hodgkin lymphoma, which enlarges lymphatic tissue in lymph nodes in the neck and tonsils and can narrow the upper airway and lead to obstructive apnea. Imaging studies would be helpful. The correct sleep evaluations in managing this case would be a PSG followed by MSLT, but this was not one of the choices.   (Espinosa et al, 1996)

14. B.   The maximum ESS score suggests this long-distance truck driver is at high risk for falling asleep at the wheel. For this reason, answer A is incorrect. Answers C and D are incorrect because they would treat the patient without a diagnosis. The patient should be advised not to drive until he has been evaluated and treated.   (ATLAS2, p 132)

15. A.   The Berlin Questionnaire surveys snoring, sleepiness, body weight, and blood pressure to determine a patient's risk for having OSA.   (ATLAS2, p 132)

16. B.   Cor pulmonale is right heart failure caused by pulmonary hypertension (see also the answer to question 4). The likeliest patients to have this in a sleep clinic are those with chronic obstructive pulmonary disease (COPD), the overlap syndrome (COPD plus OSA), and OHS.   (Weitzenblum and Chaouat, 2009)

17. C.   In a patient with morbid obesity, severe ankle swelling, and hypercapnia, it is likely that she has cor pulmonale caused by hypoventilation. When CO_2 is elevated during the daytime, the term *obesity hypoventilation* is used.   (Mokhlesi et al, 2008)

18. C.   Not a single cardiac cycle is clearly visible in the zoomed window. The cycle rate is 20/second, or 1200/min, which is faster than any known tachyarrhythmia. Paroxysmal ventricular tachycardia has a rate up to 250/min, and torsades de pointes and ventricular flutter can be up to 350/min. In this example, the zoomed window is helpful in determining what the rhythm is not. Obviously, sending the patient to the ED was a mistake.

19. A.   The tonsils are markedly enlarged and meet in the midline. Tonsils are graded from 0 (not present) to 4 (meeting in the midline). Mallampati score documents relationship of the tongue to the pharyngeal size and ranges from class 1 (all structures visible) to class 4 (soft palate not visible; Box 7.1–1). Enlarged tonsils are the most common cause of apnea in children.   (ATLAS2, pp 262–265)

20. B.   Children with Prader-Willi syndrome often become morbidly obese. Their main sleep complaint is hypersomnia, often from sleep apnea. SOREMPs may be seen on the MSLT. Elevated ghrelin might explain the hyperphagia of these patients.   (Williams et al, 2008)

21. A.   In one series, all patients with Prader-Willi syndrome had some form of SDB. GH secretion is usually decreased in Prader-Willi syndrome, and GH therapy has been recommended starting in early childhood; it results in height gain and can improve psychomotor development. Obstructive apnea can occur in cases in which there is a rapid increase in the dose of GH. Data are inconsistent on the effect of GH on SDB in Prader-Willi syndrome.   (Castinetti et al, 2008; Goldstone et al, 2008; Miller and Wagner, 2013)

22. B.   Although OSA can occur with each of the conditions, the history and findings are classic for polycystic ovary syndrome (PCOS). The ovaries of these patients have multiple cysts that produce excess androgenic hormone, hence the hirsutism and acne. Patients with PCOS are about seven times more likely than control participants to have OSA (20%–50% of patients have OSA), and those with OSA are more likely to have insulin resistance. The history also includes abnormal or absent menstrual cycle and difficulty in becoming pregnant.   (ATLAS2, p 354; Tasali et al, 2008)

Box 7.1–1 About Mallampati Scores

There is confusion about how to document the Mallampati score. Is it using a class or grade? In 1985, Mallampati and colleagues published classes 1 to 3 to describe the oral findings in an attempt to predict possible difficulty in intubation (Mallampati et al, 1985). What is used currently and called a *Mallampati score* is actually the original score modified by Friedman's group, which described grades 1 through 4 (Friedman et al, 1999).

  This section and the *Atlas* use "class" throughout. Expect inconsistency in whether Roman or Arabic numerals are used for the classes. Whereas this section uses Arabic numbers, the *Atlas* uses Roman numerals.

- Tonsillar hypertrophy documented by grading system
  - Grade 0: absent tonsils
  - Grade 1: tonsils are entirely behind the tonsillar pillars
  - Grade 2: tonsils extend to the pillars
  - Grade 3: tonsils extend beyond the pillars
  - Grade 4: tonsils extend to the midline

23. D. About half of patients with nonalcoholic fatty liver disease (NAFLD; also called nonalcoholic steatohepatitis [NASH]) have features of sleep apnea. Animal research shows that chronic intermittent hypoxia predisposes to liver injury. (Campos et al, 2008; Mishra et al, 2008; Pulixi et al, 2014; Savransky et al, 2007)

24. B. The prevalence of sleep apnea in menopausal women increases compared with premenopausal women and is similar to that of age-matched male control participants. Reasons for the increase in sleep apnea prevalence in women during the menopausal transition are not known. There are many theories, including withdrawal of estrogen and progesterone and a redistribution of fat. Significant obesity might not be an important factor because the weight gain with menopause is usually modest. There is no known relationship of sleep apnea with hot flashes. Sleep apnea responds to treatment as well in women as in men.

25. B. Snoring in pregnancy has been linked statistically with preeclampsia and with smaller-than-expected babies who have lower Apgar scores than children of nonsnoring women. Sleep apnea in pregnant women should be treated because of the potential negative effect on the fetus. The most common cause of nocturnal awakenings in pregnancy is nocturia. (ATLAS2, p 356)

26. A. Given OSA, insomnia is much more common in women than in men. Women are much more likely to also have a history of depression, antidepressant use, and thyroid disease. In men, caffeine consumption is greater. (Shepertycky et al, 2005)

27. D. In premenopausal women, obstructive events often tend to cluster in REM sleep much more so than in men. The reason for this is not well understood. One possible explanation is that the female upper airway is less compliant. (O'Connor et al, 2000)

28. A. Sleep apnea is found in all the conditions, but the most common cause of sleep apnea in children is enlargement of the tonsils and adenoids. Children with sleep apnea present with snoring and observed apnea at times. The presentation is with restless sleep, falling asleep in the classroom, or even with a diagnosis of ADHD.

29. C. This is an example of retrognathia; the lower jaw is too far back (Figs. 7.1–13 to 7.1–15). On lateral inspection, note the relative position of the nasion, anterior nasal spine, and mental protuberance. Sleep-breathing disorders can occur with both retrognathia (an underdeveloped lower mandible, also called *type 2 malocclusion*) or prognathia, which usually occurs with an underdeveloped maxilla.

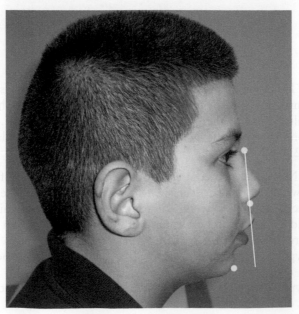

FIGURE 7.1–13 Answer 29.

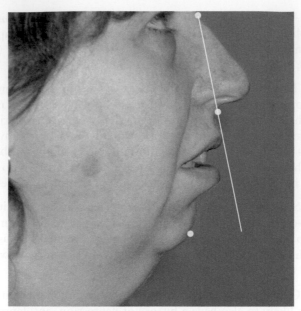

FIGURE 7.1–14 Answer 29.

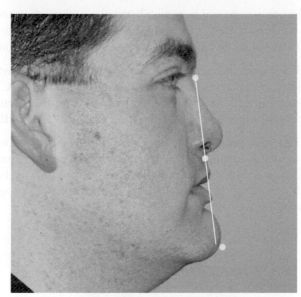

FIGURE 7.1–15 Answer 29.

30. B. This is an example of grade 3 tonsils. In grade 0, tonsils are absent (Fig. 7.1–16). Grade 1 tonsils are hidden behind tonsillar pillars (see the right tonsil in Fig. 7.1–17). Grade 2 tonsils extend to the pillars (see the left tonsil in Fig. 7.1–17). Grade 3 tonsils are visible beyond the pillars (Fig. 7.1–18). Grade 4 tonsils are enlarged to midline (Figs. 7.1–19 to 7.1–21).

31. B. Nasopharyngoscopy is not indicated at this stage of evaluation. BMI and neck collar size would not be particularly helpful in this case since he is clearly not obese. Examination of teeth alignment would confirm the suspected anatomic abnormality (Fig. 7.1–22). One would expect to find crowding of the lower teeth and an overbite (or overjet), as shown in Figure 7.1–22. There are three types of malocclusions:

Type 1: Upper and lower teeth are aligned (bite is normal), but teeth are crowded or malpositioned.

Type 2 (see Fig. 7.1–22): Upper jaw and teeth overlap the lower jaw and teeth. This malocclusion is called *retrognathia*, *overbite*, or *overjet*.

Type 3: The lower jaw protrudes forward, and lower teeth extend over the upper teeth. This is called *prognathia* or *underbite*.

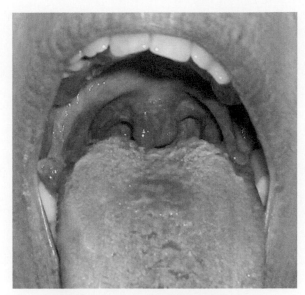

FIGURE 7.1–16 Answer 30. Grade 0 tonsils.

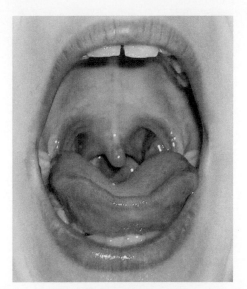

FIGURE 7.1–17 Answer 30. Right tonsil grade 1; left tonsil grade 2.

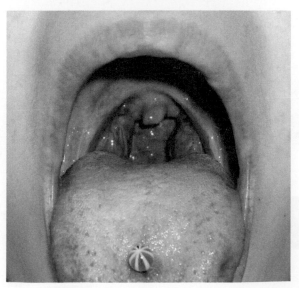

FIGURE 7.1–18 Answer 30. Grade 3 tonsils.

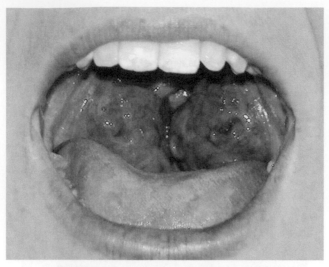

FIGURE 7.1–19 Answer 30. Grade 4 tonsils.

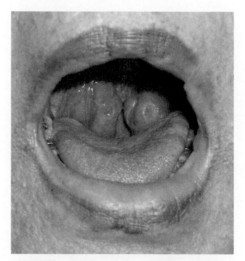

FIGURE 7.1–20 Answer 30. Grade 4 tonsils.

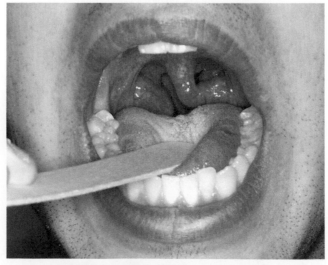

FIGURE 7.1–21 Answer 30. Grade 4 tonsils.

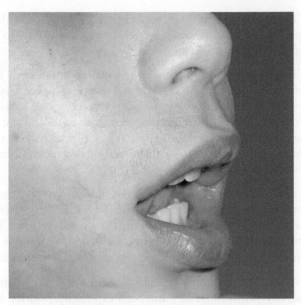

FIGURE 7.1–22 Answer 31. Overjet.

32. D.   Although he likely has OSA, before tonsillectomy, it should be documented with an overnight PSG.

33. B.   In pediatric PSGs, measurement of either end-tidal or transcutaneous PcO_2 is recommended. In ICSD3, criteria for diagnosing pediatric apnea are "obstructive hypoventilation, defined as at least 25% of total sleep time with hypercapnia (PcO_2 >50 mm Hg) in association with one or more of the following: snoring, flattening of the inspiratory nasal pressure waveform, paradoxical thoracoabdominal motion." Note that there is no "end-tidal PO_2" in PSG.

34. B.   In children, movement or autonomic arousals are more common than cortical (EEG) arousals. The other statements are true.

35. B.   No hard and fast criteria exist for diagnosing OSA in children, in part because the range in size from infant to adolescent is so great. One publication   (Lipton and Gozal, 2003) interprets pediatric PSGs as follows:
"Apnea-hypopnea index (AHI) from less than 1 to 4, without a drop in SaO_2: mild OSA. Treat if there are daytime sequelae, such as excessive daytime sleepiness.
"AHI 5 to 10 and/or SaO_2 less than 85%: moderate OSA. Most children should be treated.
"AHI greater than 10 with SaO_2 less than 85% and clinical sequelae: severe OSA. Treatment is strongly recommended."
The ICSD3 criteria for pediatric OSA start at "One or more obstructive apneas, mixed apneas, or hypopneas per hour of sleep," but it also notes other signs that can allow diagnosis (e.g., snoring; labored, paradoxic, or obstructed breathing during the child's sleep; sleepiness, hyperactivity, behavioral problems, or learning problems).   (ICSD3, pp 63–68)
Few normative data are available for hypopneas. This patient qualifies for treatment (tonsillectomy) because his AHI is elevated at 2.1 events/hr and he has clinical sequelae: restless sleep, ADHD (likely from OSA), and need for medication (which only worsened his sleep). Note that he does not meet criteria for diagnosing hypoventilation because his PcO_2 was not elevated more than 25% of the total sleep time.

36. D.   PAP titration is incomplete because the C-flow channel shows flow limitation and the patient still has hypoxemia. Ignoring this degree of hypoxemia is not acceptable.

37. A.   The flattening of the C-flow curve indicates that flow limitation is present. (Note the shape of the C-flow curve in the 30 seconds before the middle of the epoch.) Complete occlusion would show absence of flow. This is not the pattern of CSB.

38. A.   The pattern of the eye channels is classic for REM sleep, in which loss of tone of pharyngeal muscles occurs, and it is likely that this is leading to increased upper airway resistance. The flow limitation is seen in the C-flow channel.

39. A.   The epoch starts off in REM, and REMs occur in the eye channels; there is lack of muscle activity in the chin EMG, and sawtooth waves may appear in the central EEG leads (about one third of the way into the epoch). However, before the halfway point of this epoch, an arousal occurs with an increase in muscle tone, and the patient is awake in the remainder of the epoch. There is the suggestion of alpha activity in the occipital leads and of slow eye movements developing toward the end of the epoch. Thus, for more than half the epoch, the patient is awake.

40. D.   The fragment shows obstructive apnea because there are repetitive apneas (absent airflow documented by the end-tidal PcO_2 channel) throughout in the face of continuous respiratory efforts documented in the abdominal channel. The apneas result in severe oxygen desaturation. End-tidal PcO_2 is never elevated, so there is no hypoventilation. Overlap syndrome is OSA plus COPD, the latter of which is a clinical, not a PSG-based, diagnosis.

41. C.   Notice the very regular deflections in the CPAP channel. Both a high inspiratory positive airway pressure (IPAP) and high expiratory positive airway pressure (EPAP) are being used. The pressure waves generated by the bilevel machine have a clocklike regularity, suggesting that a timed backup rate is being used and that, in essence, the patient is being ventilated by the system. Note that the apnea is completely resolved, hypoxemia is no longer present, and the patient is in slow-wave sleep.

42. B.   Pulmonary edema is suggested by the frothy fluid that was emanating from the patient's mouth when the technologist went into the room to start PAP. The technologist did not appreciate the significance of that finding in this patient with recent MI. Observation of the synchronized digital video confirmed that the stoic patient was wide awake most of the time and struggling to breathe. This bilevel PAP treated both the pulmonary edema and his upper airway obstruction.

BONUS QUESTIONS

43. A.   Mandibular advancement devices can be very effective in OSA, especially in patients with mild to moderate apnea. Several studies have documented this improvement. The devices, however, are not more effective than CPAP, and they might be problematic in patients with severe apnea. They are never useful in patients with CSA.   (ATLAS2, p 295)

44. C.   UPPP involves removing the tonsils, soft palate, uvula, and redundant pharyngeal wall tissue and is much less effective than treatment with CPAP. The success rate is probably about 50%, compared with 70% for CPAP. Patients who have had the surgery can continue to have significant apnea episodes without audible snoring. When the procedure is done with a laser, patients can have a great deal of pain that lasts for weeks. Laser surgery is generally more painful than scalpel surgery. UPPP should not be done in patients with retrognathia because the upper airway obstruction is likely at the base of the tongue and not at the level of the palate.

45. C.   Diabetes control almost always improves after bariatric surgery and significant weight reduction. Postoperative complications are common. Sleep apnea can improve or disappear entirely after surgery and significant weight loss. Patients who are to have bariatric surgery should be assessed for sleep apnea because the risk of sleep apnea is quite high when the BMI exceeds 40.

46. B.   The difference between inspiratory and expiratory pressures makes a bilevel machine function like a ventilator. Bilevel treatment is also used to noninvasively ventilate patients in various clinical settings. Based on clinical trials, there is no scientific reason to start patients on bilevel, rather than fixed, CPAP pressure. However, in specific patient groups, it might be the treatment of choice, for example, in OSA patients with COPD (the overlap syndrome) or in those with kyphoscoliosis.   (ATLAS2, Ch 13.4)

47. C. Patients who use CPAP can develop nasal symptoms, such as nasal obstruction or nasal discharge, as a response to the pressure itself or to dryness. Heated humidification can be effective in relieving such symptoms, much more so than cold humidification. Humidification also improves compliance with using the positive-pressure device.

48. D. Claustrophobia, nasal obstruction, and nasal discharge are all common unwanted effects of CPAP in patients being treated for sleep apnea. Acute tonsillitis has not been described as a consequence of this treatment.

Summary

Highly Recommended

- *AASM Manual for the Scoring of Sleep and Associated Events: Rules, Terminology, and Technical Specifications*, Version 2.5
- *Atlas of Clinical Sleep Medicine*, ed 2, Chapters 13 and 18
- *International Classification of Sleep Disorders*, ed 3
- *Principles and Practice of Pediatric Sleep Medicine*, ed 2, Chapters 27 and 28

Topics You Should Know

The section on SDB will make up about 48 of the 240 questions on the examination (20% of the total questions), so this is an important topic and one that will have a big impact on your overall score. OSA is clearly the most prevalent of these disorders and should be a principal focus when studying sleep medicine. Of the 48 questions in this section on the exam, about 21 will cover OSA. In fact, almost 10% of the exam will be about OSA.

Epidemiology

- Adults
  - OSAS affects about 4% of men and 2% of women
  - The syndrome is present when five or more abnormal obstructed breathing events and sleepiness occur
  - OSA without the daytime sleepiness is much higher in prevalence
  - OSA increases risk of hypertension, coronary artery disease, stroke, and death
- Children   (ATLAS2, Ch 13.3)
  - Overall frequency likely similar to that in adults
  - Found in
    - Enlarged tonsils and adenoids
    - Obesity
    - Laryngomalacia
    - Pierre Robin sequence
    - Down syndrome (see Section 10)
    - Achondroplasia
    - Spinal muscle atrophy
    - Prader-Willi syndrome (see Section 10)
    - Klippel-Feil syndrome (see Section 10)
    - Arnold-Chiari malformation, type II (see Section 10)

Pathophysiology

Upper airway obstruction during sleep leads to the following abnormalities: (ATLAS2, pp 49–52)

- Hypoxemia
- Slowing of heartbeat (vagal effect)

- Cardiac arrhythmias   (ATLAS2, pp 439–449)
- Arterial hypertension
- Arousals
- Reduced REM and slow-wave sleep

Central Nervous System Abnormalities

- Sleepiness
  - Subjective
    - ESS   (ATLAS2, p 130)
  - Objective
    - MSLT   (ATLAS2, p 392)
    - MWT   (ATLAS2, p 392)
- Abnormal cognitive function
  - Poor memory, concentration, and ability to perform tasks that require attention
- Psychiatric symptoms
  - Depressed mood
  - Irritability
- Morning headache
  - May be related to OSA
  - Hypothesized to be due to hypercapnia causing cerebral vasodilation

Cardiorespiratory Symptoms

- Snoring
  - May be benign
  - May be a symptom of OSA
- Gasping, snorting
  - May be a symptom of OSA
- Witnessed apnea
  - Feature of any form of apnea
- Paroxysmal nocturnal dyspnea
  - Symptom of left ventricular failure

Key Findings on Physical Examination in Obstructive Sleep Apnea

- Faces of syndromes associated with OSA
  - Acromegaly
  - Burned-out Graves disease
  - Down syndrome
  - Achondroplasia
  - Pierre Robin syndrome
- Abnormal dental anatomy
  - Mandibular and maxillary structures
    - Type 1: Upper and lower teeth are aligned (bite is normal), but teeth are crowded or malpositioned, and the dental arch is small
    - Type 2: Upper jaw and teeth overlap the lower jaw and teeth (retrognathia, overbite, or overjet)
    - Type 3: Lower jaw protrudes forward, and lower teeth extend over the upper teeth; prognathia or underbite are present
- Arnold-Chiari malformation
  - Type 1 can demonstrate ataxia findings if herniation of cerebellar tonsils is present
  - Patients might also have leg weakness if they also have type 2 with meningomyelocele
- Klippel-Feil anomaly
  - Short neck
  - Can have abnormalities in oral airway
- Crowding of oropharyngeal cavity

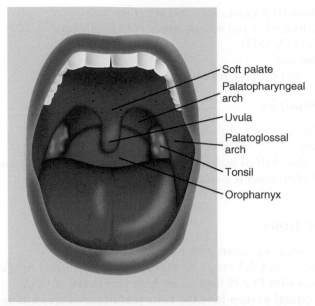

FIGURE 7.1–23 Normal upper airway anatomy. (Modified from Netter F: *Atlas of human anatomy*, ed 5, St. Louis, 2011, Saunders.)

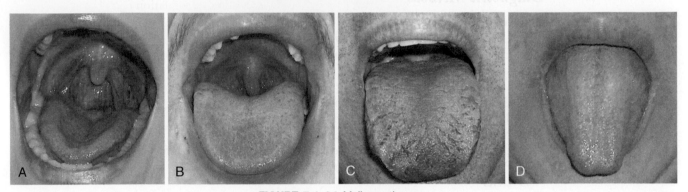

FIGURE 7.1–24 Mallampati score.

- Tongue too large for oral cavity
  - Longitudinal fissure
  - Scalloping of tongue edges
  - Syndromes
    - Down syndrome
- Myxedema
- Modified Mallampati score (Figs. 7.1–23 and 7.1–24)
  - Class 1: All structures are visible: posterior pharyngeal wall, tonsils, uvula, and soft palate (see Fig. 7.1–24, *A*)
  - Class 2: Hard and soft palate, upper portion of tonsils, and uvula are visible (see Fig. 7.1–24, *B*)
  - Class 3: Soft and hard palate and only the base of the uvula are visible (see Fig. 7.1–24, *C*)
  - Class 4: Only the hard palate or tongue is visible (see Fig. 7.1–24, *D*)

Risk Factors

- Obesity   (ATLAS2, pp 266–267)
  - Documented by BMI
    - Neck collar size (≥17 inches in men; ≥15 inches in women)
- Male gender
- Age
  - Much more common in older people
  - Prevalence the same in postmenopausal women as in age-matched men

- Craniofacial abnormalities that affect jaw size
  - Retrognathia and micrognathia   (ATLAS2, pp 257–269)
- NAFLD (NASH)
- Alcohol use
- Drugs that depress drive to breathe (e.g., opiates)

Comorbidities

- Insulin resistance, diabetes
- Obesity
- More than half of patients with treatment-resistant hypertension have OSA
- Atrial fibrillation is common in OSA
- Stroke

Gender Issues

- Apnea often manifests with insomnia in women
- Women with OSA are much more likely to be treated for depression than men with OSA
- Women with PCOS have a very high prevalence of OSA
- Menopausal women have the same prevalence of apnea as age-matched men

Diagnostic Methods

- Levels of sleep tests
  - Level I: attended comprehensive PSG
  - Level II: unattended comprehensive PSG
  - Level III: portable sleep apnea testing, usually four channels
  - Level IV: continuous recording of one variable, usually SaO$_2$
- PSG for sleep apnea: what is recorded   (ATLAS2, p 371)
  - Thermal sensor at the nose and mouth to detect apneas
  - Nasal pressure transducer to detect hypopneas
  - Chest wall and abdominal movement to detect respiratory effort
  - Pulse oximeter with signal averaging of 3 seconds or less
  - ECG
  - Electrooculogram (EOG), chin EMG, EEG
    - End-tidal or transcutaneous PcO$_2$ is added for young children and sometimes if hypoventilation is suspected in adults

Polysomnography for Sleep-Breathing Disorders: Scoring Rules for Adults (ATLAS2, pp 377–379; MANUAL2, Section VIII, Respiratory Rules)

- Apnea
  - Duration 10 seconds or greater
  - 90% or more reduction of nasal or oral airflow using temperature sensors
  - Obstructive type if there is breathing effort during the apnea
  - Central type if there is a cessation of breathing effort during the apnea
  - Mixed type begins with a central apnea and ends with an obstructive apnea
- Hypopnea
  - Definition 1 (recommended per MANUAL2)
    - The peak signal excursions drop by 30% or more of preevent baseline using nasal pressure (diagnostic study), PAP device flow (titration study), or an alternative hypopnea sensor (diagnostic study)
    - The duration of the 30% or more drop in signal excursion is 10 or more seconds
    - A 3% or greater oxygen desaturation is observed from preevent baseline or the event is associated with an arousal

○ Definition 2 (acceptable per MANUAL2)
  • The peak signal excursions drop by 30% or more of preevent baseline using nasal pressure (diagnostic study), PAP device flow (titration study), or an alternative hypopnea sensor (diagnostic study)
  • The duration of the 30% or more drop in signal excursion is 10 or more seconds
  • There is a 4% or greater oxygen desaturation from preevent baseline
■ Respiratory effort–related arousal
  ○ Per the AASM manual: "If electing to score respiratory effort–related arousals, score a respiratory event as a respiratory effort–related arousal (RERA) if there is a sequence of breaths lasting ≥10 seconds characterized by increasing respiratory effort or by flattening of the inspiratory portion of the nasal pressure (diagnostic study) or PAP device flow (titration study) waveform leading to arousal from sleep when the sequence of breaths does not meet criteria for an apnea or hypopnea."
■ Hypoventilation: may use either of the following (MANUAL2)
  ○ An increase in the arterial PcO_2 (or surrogate) to a value greater than 55 mm Hg for 10 or more minutes
  ○ A 10 mm Hg or more increase in arterial PcO_2 (or surrogate) during sleep (in comparison to an awake supine value) to a value exceeding 50 mm Hg for 10 or more minutes
■ Score as CSB if *both* of the following are present:
  ○ Episodes of three or more consecutive central apneas and/or central hypopneas separated by a crescendo and decrescendo change in breathing amplitude with a cycle length of 40 seconds or more
  ○ Five or more central apneas and/or central hypopneas per hour of sleep associated with the crescendo/decrescendo breathing pattern recorded over 2 or more hours of monitoring

Polysomnography for Sleep-Breathing Disorders: Scoring Rules for Children (ATLAS2, pp 300–303; MANUAL2; PEDS2, p 227)

■ Obstructive apnea
  ○ Duration of at least two missed breaths
  ○ 90% or more reduction of nasal/oral airflow using temperature sensors
  ○ Breathing effort during the apnea
■ Central apnea
  ○ Duration of at least 20 seconds
  ○ 90% or more reduction of nasal/oral airflow using temperature sensors if there is a cessation of breathing effort during apnea
■ Mixed apnea
  ○ Duration of at least two missed breaths
  ○ 90% or more reduction of nasal or oral airflow using temperature sensors
  ○ Begins with a central apnea and ends with obstructive features
■ Hypopnea
  ○ Scoring hypopneas as central or obstructive events is optional
  ○ A respiratory event is scored as a hypopnea if *all* of the following criteria are met:
    • The peak signal excursions drop by 30% or more of preevent baseline using nasal pressure (diagnostic study), PAP device flow (titration study), or an alternative hypopnea sensor (diagnostic study)
    • The duration of the 30% or more drop in signal excursion lasts for two or more breaths
    • A 3% or more oxygen desaturation occurs from preevent baseline, or the event is associated with an arousal
  ○ If electing to score obstructive hypopneas, score a hypopnea as *obstructive* if *any* of the following criteria is met
    • Snoring occurs during the event
    • Increased inspiratory flattening of the nasal pressure occurs or PAP device flow signal is evident compared with baseline breathing
    • An associated thoracoabdominal paradox occurs during the event but not during preevent breathing

○ If electing to score central hypopneas, score a hypopnea as *central* if *none* of the following criteria is met:
  • Snoring occurs during the event
  • Increased inspiratory flattening of the nasal pressure or PAP device flow signal is evident compared with baseline breathing
  • An associated thoracoabdominal paradox occurs during the event but not during preevent breathing
■ RERA
  ○ In children, "If electing to score respiratory effort–related arousals, score a respiratory event as a RERA if there is a sequence of breaths lasting ≥2 breaths (or the duration of two breaths during baseline breathing) when the breathing sequence is characterized by increasing respiratory effort, flattening of the inspiratory portion of the nasal pressure (diagnostic study) or PAP device flow (titration study) waveform, snoring, or an elevation in the end-tidal PcO_2 leading to arousal from sleep when the sequence of breaths does not meet criteria for an apnea or hypopnea." (MANUAL2)
■ Hypoventilation
  ○ Score as hypoventilation during sleep when more than 25% of the total sleep time as measured by either the arterial PcO_2 or surrogate is spent with a PcO_2 above 50 mm Hg
■ Periodic breathing
  ○ In children, "Score a respiratory event as periodic breathing if there are ≥3 episodes of central pauses in respiration (absent airflow and inspiratory effort) lasting >3 seconds separated by ≤20 seconds of normal breathing." (MANUAL2)
  ○ Note that in the rules for children, the term *Cheyne-Stokes breathing* is not used in scoring

Treatment

There are many treatments for sleep-breathing disorders, and some of them are controversial and seldom used. It is unlikely that the exam will delve into areas of controversy or newly evolving therapies. It is best to review the standard texts and the published practice parameters mentioned above.
■ PAP therapy
  ○ CPAP (continuous PAP) and variants
  ○ Fixed pressure
  ○ Autotitrating
  ○ Bilevel pressure
    • Spontaneous mode
    • Timed backup
■ Mandibular advancement device
■ Expiratory resistance device
■ Upper airway surgery in selected cases
■ Bariatric surgery for morbid obesity
■ Hypoglossal nerve stimulation in patients with severe OSA, who have failed CPAP, who have BMI <32

REFERENCES

American Academy of Sleep Medicine. *International classification of sleep disorders*, ed 3. Darien, Ill.: American Academy of Sleep Medicine; 2014.
American Academy of Sleep Medicine. *The AASM manual for the scoring of sleep and associated events: rules, terminology and technical specifications, Version 2.5*. Darien, Ill.: American Academy of Sleep Medicine; 2014.
Campos GM, Bambha K, Vittinghoff E, et al. A clinical scoring system for predicting nonalcoholic steatohepatitis in morbidly obese patients. *Hepatology.* 2008;47(6):1916–1923.
Castinetti F, Reynaud R, Brue T. Prader-Willi syndrome and growth hormone treatment. *Ann Endocrinol (Paris).* 2008;69(suppl 1):S6–S10.
Espinosa G, Alarcón A, Morelló A, et al. Obstructive apnea syndrome during sleep secondary to a pharyngeal lymphoma. Improvement with continuous pressure treatment of the upper airway. *Arch Bronconeumol.* 1996;32(10):547–549.
Goldstone AP, Holland AJ, Hauffa BP, et al. Recommendations for the diagnosis and management of Prader-Willi syndrome. *J Clin Endocrinol Metab.* 2008;93(11):4183–4197.
Kryger MH, Avidan A, Berry R. *Atlas of clinical sleep medicine*, ed 2. Philadelphia: Saunders; 2014.

Lipton AJ, Gozal D. Treatment of obstructive sleep apnea in children: do we really know how? *Sleep Med Rev.* 2003;7:61–80.

Miller J, Wagner M. Prader-Willi syndrome and sleep-disordered breathing. *Pediatr Ann.* 2013;42(10):200–204.

Mishra P, Nugent C, Afendy A, et al. Apnoeic–hypopnoeic episodes during obstructive sleep apnoea are associated with histological nonalcoholic steatohepatitis. *Liver Int.* 2008;28(8):1080–1086.

Mokhlesi B, Kryger MH, Grunstein RR. Assessment and management of patients with obesity hypoventilation syndrome. *Proc Am Thorac Soc.* 2008;5(2):218–225.

O'Connor C, Thornley KS, Hanly PJ. Gender differences in the polysomnographic features of obstructive sleep apnea. *Am J Respir Crit Care Med.* 2000;161(5):1465–1472.

Pulixi EA, Tobaldini E, Battezzati PM, et al. Risk of obstructive sleep apnea with daytime sleepiness is associated with liver damage in non–morbidly obese patients with nonalcoholic fatty liver disease. *PLoS ONE.* 2014;9(4):e96349.

Savransky V, Nanayakkara A, Vivero A, et al. Chronic intermittent hypoxia predisposes to liver injury. *Hepatology.* 2007;45(4):1007–1013.

Sheldon SH, Ferber R, Gozal D, Kryger MH, eds. *Principles and practice of pediatric sleep medicine,* ed 2. Philadelphia: Elsevier 2005.

Shepertycky MR, Banno K, Kryger MH. Differences between men and women in the clinical presentation of patients diagnosed with obstructive sleep apnea syndrome. *Sleep.* 2005;28(3):309–314.

Tasali E, Van Cauter E, Hoffman L, Ehrmann DA. Impact of obstructive sleep apnea on insulin resistance and glucose tolerance in women with polycystic ovary syndrome. *J Clin Endocrinol Metab.* 2008;93(10):3878–3884.

Weitzenblum E, Chaouat A. Cor pulmonale. *Chron Respir Dis.* 2009;6(3):177–185.

Williams K, Scheimann A, Sutton V, et al. Sleepiness and sleep disordered breathing in Prader-Willi syndrome: relationship to genotype, growth hormone therapy, and body composition. *J Clin Sleep Med.* 2008;4(2):111–118.

7.2   Central Sleep Apnea

QUESTIONS

The Many Faces of Central Sleep Apnea

1. Central sleep apnea (CSA) with a chaotic irregular breathing pattern is found in
   A. Heart failure
   B. Kidney failure
   C. Opiate use
   D. Obesity

2. Central apnea during wakefulness with a chaotic irregular breathing pattern is found in
   A. Heart failure
   B. COPD
   C. Opiate use
   D. Obesity

3. Cheyne Stokes breathing (CSB) is characterized by
   A. A highly periodic waxing and waning of breathing with central apneas or hypopneas between the hyperpneic phases
   B. An irregular breathing pattern with a slow breathing frequency
   C. A steady, regular breathing pattern with a respiratory rate of more than 20 breaths/min
   D. Continuous obstructed breathing with snorts

4. Which statement about CSB is *false*?
   A. It may be caused by heart failure
   B. It may be caused by stroke
   C. It may be caused by renal failure
   D. It does not respond to oxygen

A Complex Situation

A 53-year-old man is referred for a split-night PSG because his physician believes he might have OSA. He has a BMI of 36.2 and complains of snoring and apneic episodes witnessed by his wife. His ESS score is normal at 4 of 24. He has history of high blood pressure, pulmonary embolism, and heart attack 2 years earlier in addition to remote substance abuse. The sleep technologist observes long periods of hypoxemia during which oscillations in SaO_2 occur (see the fragment in Fig. 7.2–1).

5. What is the *most* likely breathing abnormality evident from this fragment?
   A. Obstructive apneas
   B. Hypopneas
   C. Central apneas
   D. Hypoventilation

6. The technologist started CPAP titration. The interpreting physician reviewed the technologist's notes, which indicated that the titration was difficult. Figure 7.2–2 summarizes the all-night findings. Significant hypoxemia begins about 1 hour and 15 minutes into the study. What are the associated findings?
   A. Episodes of obstructive apnea
   B. Episodes of hypopnea
   C. Central apneas
   D. REM sleep

7. CPAP titration began about 3.5 hours into the study. Was it indicated?
   A. Yes; by that time, the patient had an AHI of 6.1
   B. Yes; the patient had episodes of hypoxemia
   C. No; an accurate apnea type had not been determined
   D. No; there had been insufficient sleep by that time

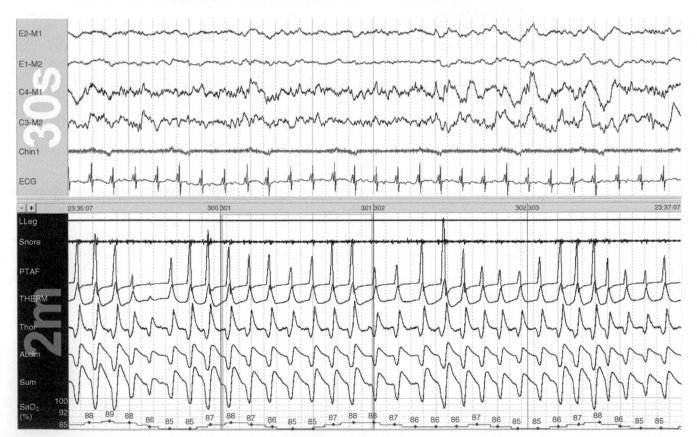

FIGURE 7.2–1 Question 5.

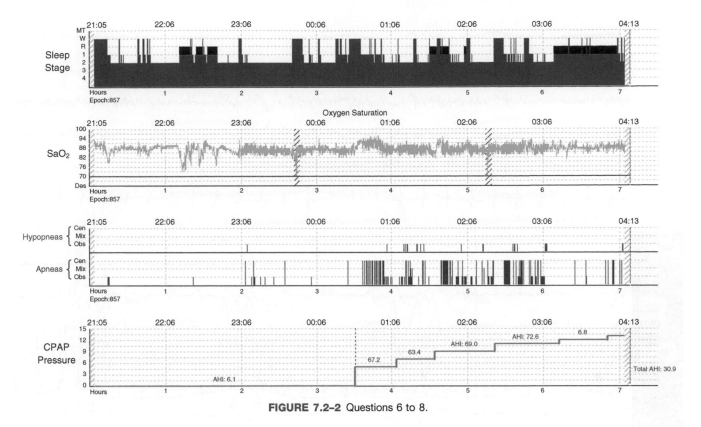

FIGURE 7.2–2 Questions 6 to 8.

8. What effect did CPAP have on the patient's sleep breathing?
   A. CPAP improved it
   B. CPAP worsened his breathing and caused apneas
   C. CPAP had no effect on his breathing
   D. CPAP kept the patient awake

9. Figure 7.2–3 shows a fragment of a PSG taken while the patient was on CPAP. What is the main breathing abnormality?
   A. Obstructive apneas
   B. Hypopneas
   C. Central apneas
   D. Hypoventilation

10. What does the C-flow channel measured by the CPAP machine show?
   A. Episodes of obstruction
   B. Flow limitation
   C. When the patient is breathing, the flow pattern indicates unobstructed flow
   D. CSB

11. The findings in this patient are consistent with which of the following?
   A. Typical OSA
   B. Complex or treatment-emergent sleep apnea
   C. Typical CSB
   D. Biot respiration

12. The interpreting physician believes that one of the patient's medications is responsible for the sleep-breathing abnormality. Which medication would be the *most* likely cause?
   A. Metoprolol
   B. Ramipril
   C. Rosuvastatin
   D. Methadone

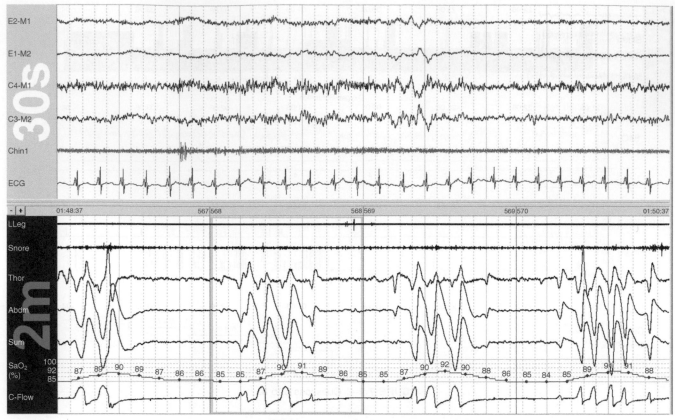

FIGURE 7.2–3 Questions 9 to 12.

Saved From the Knife

Mild OSA was diagnosed in a 46-year-old man after portable home testing ordered by his family doctor. He was referred to an ear, nose, and throat (ENT) physician, who put him on CPAP without a titration study. The patient was not compliant with CPAP and is now being considered for upper airway surgery. Before surgery, an in-lab PSG was done. The patient's main complaint noted in the presleep questionnaire is "loud humming." His BMI is 25, and his ESS score is 5 of 24. A typical 10-minute fragment from the in-lab study is shown in Figure 7.2–4.

13. The sleep technician described the patient "moaning" during sleep. During the night, many clusters were evident, such as the one shown in Figure 7.2–4. The events were scored as central apneas terminating with snores. What should the next step be?
  A. Bilevel titration with backup rate if needed
  B. Titration with ASV
  C. Nocturnal supplemental oxygen
  D. None of the above

14. What does the PSG show?
  A. Obstructive apnea
  B. Central apnea
  C. CSB
  D. Seizure

15. What is the *most* likely diagnosis?
  A. Rhythmic movement disorder
  B. CSA
  C. Catathrenia
  D. Epilepsy

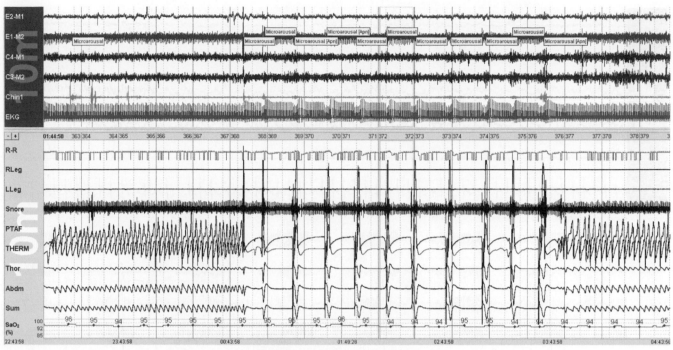

FIGURE 7.2–4 Questions 13 to 15.

Saved by the Knife

A 9-year-old girl is referred for a sleep test by her pediatrician because of insomnia. Her parents describe frequent awakenings, sometimes with shortness of breath. Her past medical history is unremarkable except for streptococcal B tonsillitis 9 months previously. This infection was followed within 1 week by a movement disorder that lasted 3 weeks, characterized by twitches involving some of the muscles of her face and uncoordinated rapid jerking movements affecting all extremities. The fragment shown in Figure 7.2–5 represents what was seen most of the night. The top window is 30 seconds; the bottom is 5 minutes.

16. What is the main and *most* significant finding?
   A. CSA
   B. CSB
   C. OSA
   D. Mixed sleep apnea

17. What is the patient's AHI?
   A. About 80 events/hr
   B. About 40 events/hr
   C. About 20 events/hr
   D. AHI is not reported in this type of breathing pattern abnormality

18. How do you put this case together?
   A. Because the apnea episodes are less than 20 seconds, no diagnosis of central apnea can be made using pediatric rules
   B. The patient has a neurologic disease
   C. The patient likely has cardiac valve disease
   D. The patient has idiopathic central apnea

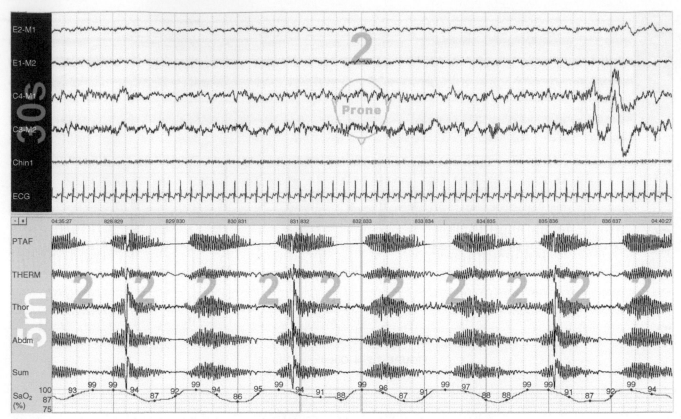

FIGURE 7.2–5 Questions 16 to 18.

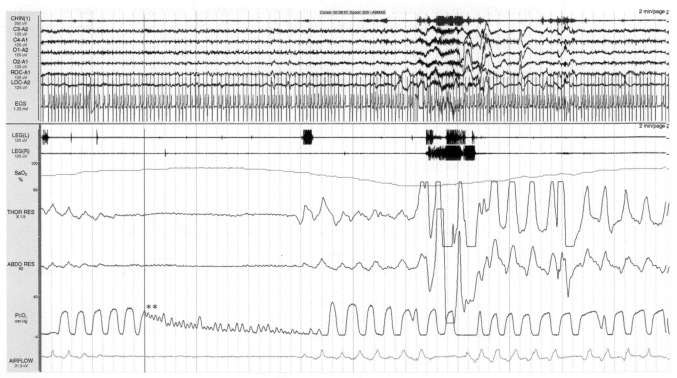

FIGURE 7.2–6 Questions 19 to 22.

Awake Apnea

A 59-year-old man with a combination of insomnia and hypersomnia has a diagnostic PSG, a 2-minute epoch of which is shown Figure 7.2–6. Note that airflow is being monitored by end-tidal PcO_2; the lowest channel is nasal pressure. The technologist scored the entire segment as an awake state without looking at the respiratory data.

19. What is the breathing abnormality shown?
  A. Obstructive apnea
  B. Central apnea
  C. Mixed apnea
  D. Artifact from the patient moving

20. Based on the breathing pattern shown, what can you conclude about this fragment?
  A. The stage cannot be scored as awake because the patient is having abnormal breathing events
  B. The patient is oscillating between wakefulness and sleep
  C. This can definitely be scored as an awake stage
  D. The episode is too long to be called an apnea

21. What condition can lead to this finding?
  A. Stroke
  B. Heart failure
  C. Opiate use
  D. All of the above

22. Describe the finding in the PcO_2 trace beginning at the vertical red line next to the two red asterisks.
  A. 60-Hz artifact
  B. Muscle artifact
  C. Cardiogenic oscillations
  D. Flow limitation

Can't Sleep; Can't Stay Awake

A 55-year-old man presents with severe insomnia and indicates that some nights he does not sleep at all. He has very severe daytime sleepiness and often feels like he is drifting off to sleep, but he does not achieve sleep. His insomnia symptoms began during a hospitalization for left-sided paresis. He does not snore, but his wife states that his breathing becomes very quiet at night. He tried sleeping pills, but they just left him with a severe hangover.

23. What is likely the cause of his insomnia?
  A. Infarction of his suprachiasmatic nucleus (SCN)
  B. Infarction of the ventrolateral preoptic nucleus (VLPO)
  C. Decreased chemical drive to breathe, causing central apnea due to damage of medullary breathing centers
  D. Increased drive to breathe, causing instability of the respiratory control system, leading to central apnea

24. What is the appropriate workup, and what will it likely show?
  A. CO_2 response test; it will be blunted
  B. MRI; it will show infarction in the medulla
  C. PSG; it will show SDB
  D. PSG; it will show alpha-delta sleep but otherwise will be normal

A Nervous New Mother

The mother of a new baby read Dr. Spock's classic *Baby and Child Care* before giving birth. One of Dr. Spock's topics was sleep apnea, and the new mother is concerned about whether her baby might have this condition. When the baby is 1 month old, the mother calls to ask about her child's sleep.

25. She has heard conflicting information about what position her baby should sleep in. What is your advice?
   A. The baby should sleep on the left or right side to lessen the probability of obstructing her upper airway
   B. The baby should sleep on her stomach (face down) to lessen the impact of possible aspiration
   C. The baby should sleep on her back because this has been shown to reduce the prevalence of sudden infant death syndrome (SIDS)
   D. The position the baby sleeps in does not matter

26. The mother has noted that her baby sometimes stops breathing for 2 or 3 seconds and is concerned the baby might die from SIDS. During apneas, the baby's chest and abdomen do not move. What should the mother be told about these breathing pauses?
   A. Episodes of apnea as described are statistically a risk for SIDS, and home monitoring is indicated
   B. The key distinction is length of the pauses; any duration longer than 10 seconds is critical
   C. Central apneas longer than 20 seconds are abnormal and generally require investigation
   D. Duration is not as important as whether a Cheyne-Stokes variation (waxing and waning respiration) is present, which would suggest cardiovascular disease. She should check the baby's breathing pattern before each pause

27. The mother is not reassured by this information and requests that her baby be monitored for possible SIDS. What is the current consensus regarding home monitoring to help prevent SIDS?
   A. Monitoring of respiratory movements alone
   B. Continuous monitoring of an ECG
   C. Monitoring of SaO_2 by pulse oximetry
   D. Home apnea monitoring does not reduce the risk of SIDS

28. The mother asks about disadvantages of the baby's sleeping on her back (supine). What should she be told?
   A. There are no negative effects of sleeping supine
   B. Sleeping supine can result in some negative skeletal changes
   C. The risk of aspiration is increased with sleeping supine
   D. Sleeping supine increases the risk of asthma

Complex Questions

Questions frequently come up from technologists and doctors about central sleep apnea.

29. During PAP titration, a typical patient with OSA develops frequent central apneas as the technologist increases pressure to abolish what he thinks are mild RERAs. What should you advise the technologist?
   A. Increase the CPAP pressure
   B. Reduce the CPAP pressure
   C. Immediately start bilevel PAP with backup
   D. Immediately start ASV

30. During initiation of CPAP titration, a patient with sleep apnea develops long episodes of central apnea. The patient's diagnostic AHI was 24 events/hr, and half the events were mixed apneas. The patient is a thin 34-year-old woman with normal physical examination results; her medical history includes hypothyroidism (on treatment), a history of treated iron deficiency, and maintenance methadone for the treatment of previous heroin addiction. What should you advise the technologist?
    A. Continue to increase the PAP pressure
    B. Reduce the CPAP pressure
    C. Start bilevel without backup
    D. Start ASV

31. A patient's diagnostic AHI was 24 events/hr, and half the events were mixed apneas. The patient is a thin 35-year-old man with normal physical examination results except for hypertension. His medical history includes hypothyroidism (taking medication), and he is taking maintenance oral morphine for the treatment of severe neuropathic pain. His primary care physician asks whether autotitration with CPAP can be done at home. You reply
    A. No. Fixed CPAP pressure of 10 cm H_2O is adequate for most patients and can be prescribed in this case, so an autotitrating CPAP machine is not necessary
    B. Yes. He should be prescribed an autotitration CPAP machine with a wide pressure range (e.g., 5–20 cm H_2O)
    C. No. An in-laboratory CPAP titration study is recommended
    D. It can if the patient uses a full face mask to make sure he gets the full effect of positive pressure

Back From Combat

A 29-year-old combat veteran, a man with a BMI of 26, has a 6-month history of witnessed apneas and severe daytime sleepiness. For the past 2 years, shortly after returning from combat in Iraq, he has awakened frequently yelling and screaming. There is no history of snoring. The awakenings occur during repetitive nightmares. He has phantom lower limb pain and is being treated for mild traumatic brain injury, posttraumatic stress disorder (PTSD), and depression. His medications include oxycodone, mirtazapine, bupropion, and alprazolam.

32. What test should be ordered next?
    A. Out-of-center sleep test (home sleep test)
    B. In-lab PSG
    C. In-lab PSG and MSLT
    D. Hamilton depression scale

33. The patient has an out-of-center sleep test. A representative fragment is shown in Figure 7.2–7. He has 16 such events per hour of recording time. No other abnormalities were seen. What is the diagnosis?
    A. Moderate CSA
    B. Moderate OSA
    C. Postarousal central apnea related to PTSD
    D. Because home sleep tests overestimate apnea severity, the finding is of little clinical significance

34. What should be the next step in management?
    A. Autotitrating CPAP (range, 4–20 cm H_2O)
    B. A clinical trial of prazosin
    C. In-laboratory PAP titration
    D. Comprehensive psychiatric evaluation because the respiratory findings were not significant

35. What is a possible cause of the home study findings?
    A. Obstruction of the upper airway caused by obesity
    B. Oxycodone used for phantom limb pain
    C. Bupropion used for depression
    D. Alprazolam used to treat anxiety disorder

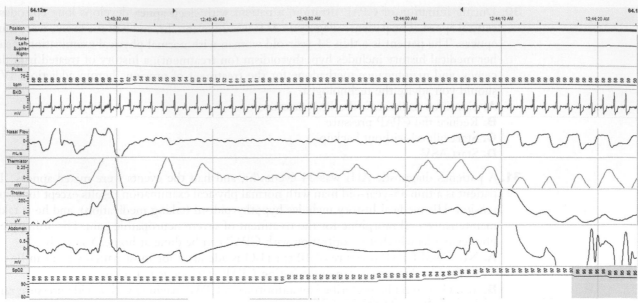

FIGURE 7.2–7 Question 33.

36. The patient is sent home on autotitrating PAP (4 to 20 cm H$_2$O), and the following mean data for 30 days are obtained from his device: AHI = 19 events/hr; central apnea index = 12 events/hr; percent of night with large leak = 2%; percent of nights used = 97%; percent of nights with usage greater than 4 hours = 80%. What is the *best* interpretation of the data?
A. Adherence is acceptable, efficacy is poor with the presence of central apnea, and the leak is acceptable
B. Adherence is unacceptable, efficacy is acceptable, and the mask leak is high
C. Adherence is acceptable, efficacy is acceptable with the persistence of only mild apnea, and the leak is acceptable
D. Adherence is acceptable and efficacy is acceptable with the presence of central apnea, but the leak is high

Bonus Questions Continue From the Case Above

37. Given the above data, what is the *best* next step from the choices below?
A. Evaluate for a possible new PAP interface
B. No change in management is warranted
C. In-lab PAP and possible ASV titration should be initiated
D. A clinical trial of a bilevel PAP device should be initiated using an empiric pressure of 24/12 cm H$_2$O in spontaneous mode

38. After being sent home with a new PAP device, the patient continues to complain of daytime sleepiness. The download indicates good adherence and efficacy. Which is the *best* next step?
A. Clinical trial of methylphenidate
B. Clinical trial of modafinil
C. Clinical reassessment to consider alternate causes of sleepiness
D. No changes in therapy are needed because sleepiness is an acceptable complication of treated apnea and the medications used to treat his PTSD

ANSWERS

1. C. Obesity usually leads to obstructive apneas. The central apneas in heart failure and kidney failure are usually CSB, which is highly regular and repetitive. Opiate-induced central apneas typically manifest as a chaotic, often slow breathing pattern.

2. C. Central apneas are common during wakefulness in heart failure and stroke. In heart failure, CSB is usually present that is typically regular and repetitive. Opiate-induced central apneas usually appear as a chaotic, often slow breathing pattern (<10 breaths/min). Obesity usually leads to obstructive apneas that manifest only during sleep. COPD does not lead to awake apneas.

3. A. CSB is a highly periodic waxing and waning pattern with central apneas or hypopneas between hyperpneic phases. This pattern often occurs when an increased chemical drive to breathe is present.

4. D. The first three conditions may be associated with CSB. Oxygen therapy does improve CSB in acute CHF. The effect of O_2 therapy on CSB in chronic CHF has not been well studied.   (Aldabal and Bahammam, 2010)

5. B. By the process of elimination, the best answer is hypopnea. The events do not meet the criteria for apnea because the thermal signal is never flat. The recommended rules for hypopnea scoring in the AASM manual require a 30% reduction in nasal pressure signal excursion lasting at least 10 seconds and a 3% or more reduction in SaO_2 or an associated arousal. There are five episodes during which nasal pressure excursion is reduced by 30% or more. However, only in the first episode does SaO_2 drop by 3% or more. There are also continuous hypoxemia and small 2% to 3% oscillations in SaO_2. Note that the fragment does not prove hypoventilation; that requires documentation of an elevated PcO_2.

6. D. The episodes of hypoxemia in the second panel coincide with the occurrence of REM sleep in the top panel. The third panel shows episodes of hypopnea and apnea that have been scored and no such scored events correspond to the hypoxemia. Thus, it can be surmised that REM-related hypoventilation is causing the hypoxemia (and not obstructive apneas).

7. C. There really was no indication to start a CPAP titration. The AHI was only 6.1, and the events did not resemble obstructive apnea. Also note that the patient did not have EDS; his ESS score was only 4. Hypoxemia alone is not an indication for CPAP.

8. B. The CPAP actually worsened the patient's breathing and caused apneas. This is apparent in the third panel, which shows a larger number of apneic episodes compared with the pre-treatment baseline. Thus, CPAP can worsen sleep apnea in some patients.

9. C. This fragment shows classic episodes of central apnea with absent or vastly reduced thoracic and abdominal effort during the events.

10. C. The C-flow channel is a display of airflow calculated by the CPAP machine while the patient is breathing. During central apneas, of course, there is no airflow. While the patient is breathing, the C-flow channel shows rounded tops, a normal pattern. In the presence of flow limitation or snoring, a plateau in the trace might be visible. The channel does not show the waxing and waning pattern of CSB.

11. B. The sequence of events, ending with the patient developing more severe apneas of a central type, is described as *treatment-emergent* or *complex sleep apnea*. Complex sleep apnea is most often seen when patients are overtitrated with CPAP.   (ATLAS2, pp 277, 417–421)

12. D. Opiates are well-known risk factors for the development of treatment-emergent or complex sleep apnea. Patients who use opiates chronically often manifest hypoventilation, hypoxemia entering sleep, and central apneas during both wakefulness and sleep. During REM sleep, there may be much less periodicity in their breathing and SaO_2. It is likely that the heightened periodicity of breathing and SaO_2 in NREM sleep is related to opiate depression of a chemical drive to breathe. In REM sleep, nonchemical control of breathing becomes dominant, a response similar to what is seen in CSB.   (ATLAS2, pp 415, 416)

13. D. The next course of action is to actually cancel the operation because the findings do not show anything treatable with surgery.

14. B.   Technically, the episodes seen are scored as central apneas. However, the events have unusual features. The apneas are actually prolonged expirations and seem to be terminated by what look like very deep breaths. The snoring microphones pick up noises that are not typical of snoring. In the absence of a history and with technologist's notes describing other findings, the diagnosis would be central apnea with the cause indeterminate.

15. C.   Catathrenia is a rare and benign condition that has features of SDB, but it may also be a type of parasomnia.   (Guilleminault et al, 2008) It is more common in men and is primarily a social problem for the affected individual.   (ICSD3, p 141) The diagnosis was confirmed by considering the PSG, but much more important, by the interpreting physician contacting the patient's wife, who described the sound as a "humming and groaning" during sleep. Her husband did not have any of the other features of sleep apnea. The lesson from this case is that treatment based only on home sleep testing, without an adequate history, can put the patient at risk for unnecessary treatment (in this case, CPAP) and perhaps inappropriate surgery.

16. B.   This is an example of classic CSB. Simply reporting this as CSA does not sufficiently convey the information obtained in the study. The AASM manual states the rules for determining CSB as follows:

    a. There are episodes of three or more consecutive central apneas and/or central hypopneas separated by a crescendo and decrescendo change in breathing amplitude with a cycle length of 40 or more seconds

    b. There are five or more central apneas and/or central hypopneas per hour of sleep associated with the crescendo/decrescendo breathing pattern recorded over 2 or more hours of monitoring

Not mentioned in the manual is the fact that this pattern is monotonously regular and often disappears during REM sleep. In clinical practice, such a breathing pattern is found most often in congestive heart failure and after a stroke. The cycle length of the periodic breathing pattern seems related to circulatory delay, and the more severe the heart failure and the longer the circulation time between the lungs and the carotid body, the longer the periodic breathing cycle. In most patients with heart failure, the cycle length is about 1 minute. Another situation in which periodic breathing is seen is after acute ascent to high altitude. In this situation, the circulation time between the lungs and the carotid body is much shorter, and the cycle length may be 30 seconds or less. The number of breaths during the hyperpneic phase of the breathing pattern also varies, with a very large number of breaths per cycle with severe heart failure and a small number of breaths in people at high altitude. This type of breathing pattern in heart failure is a predictor of mortality.   (ATLAS2, pp 322–327)

Note that the AASM manual now gives scoring rules to differentiate hypopneas as central or obstructive. Typically, hypopneas are still not differentiated in most scoring reports, but the fact that there are official AASM criteria makes it fair game for a quiz question. The criteria from the AASM manual are as follows. If electing to score obstructive hypopneas, score a hypopnea as *obstructive* if *any* of the following criteria are met:

    a. Snoring occurs during the event

    b. Increased inspiratory flattening of the nasal pressure or PAP device flow signal is evident compared with baseline breathing

    c. Associated thoracoabdominal paradox occurs during the event but not during preevent breathing

If electing to score central hypopneas, score a hypopnea as *central* if *none* of the following criteria is met:

    a. Snoring occurs during the event

    b. Increased inspiratory flattening of the nasal pressure or PAP device flow signal is evident compared with baseline breathing

    c. Associated thoracoabdominal paradox occurs during the event but not during preevent breathing

17. A.   There are seven central apnea events over 5 minutes. Thus, the AHI is 7×12 (the latter being the number of 5-minute epochs per hour), or 84. The best answer is thus 80. The pediatric scoring rules for central apnea are as follows.   (MANUAL2)

Score an apnea as *central* if it meets apnea criteria and is associated with absent inspiratory effort throughout the entire duration of the event *and* at least one of the following is met:

   a. The event lasts 20 or more seconds
   b. The event lasts at least the duration of two breaths during baseline breathing and is associated with an arousal or a 3% or greater arterial oxygen desaturation
   c. The event lasts at least the duration of two breaths during baseline breathing and is associated with a decrease in heart rate to less than 50 beats/min for at least 5 seconds or less than 60 beats/min for 15 seconds (infants younger than 1 year of age only)

18. C.   The CSB pattern is found most often in left ventricular heart failure. The clinical history provides clues to the pathogenesis in this case. The patient had a streptococcus B tonsillar infection followed by bizarre neurologic symptoms indicating Sydenham chorea. This chorea is commonly associated with rheumatic fever, which in turn often causes valvular heart disease. Also called St. Vitus dance, this chorea can appear up to several months after rheumatic fever. The impact of the patient's previous diagnosis of rheumatic fever on the patient's sleep was not appreciated by the pediatrician. After this PSG evaluation, the patient developed acute pulmonary edema and was hospitalized. Mitral insufficiency was diagnosed. She then had an urgent PSG evaluation on CPAP, and positive pressure resolved the apnea episodes. She was treated at home with nasal CPAP and subsequently had a mitral valve replacement. After recovery, the patient's sleep symptoms resolved entirely.

19. B.   This is central apnea because there is no breathing effort noted in the thoracic or abdominal belts at the time of the absent airflow.

20. C.   Abnormal breathing patterns can be present during a waking stage. The most common causes are heart failure and stroke causing CSB and, in some people, taking medications (e.g., opiates) that can suppress breathing.   (ATLAS2, pp 456–457)

21. D.   See the answer to question 20 above. An additional point is that in the first two causes of awake apnea (CHF and stroke), the breathing pattern can be highly periodic, but with opiate use, the pattern is more random, and the baseline breathing frequency can be very low.

22. C.   These are cardiogenic oscillations from the beating heart. Each heartbeat causes a small displacement of air that is picked up by a rapidly responding sensor, in this case a CO_2 sensor. The oscillations are synchronous with the heartbeats and are proof that the airway is open; thus they are only seen in central apneas.   (ATLAS2, p 328)

23. D.   A cerebrovascular accident can result in an increased drive to breathe, leading to breathing instability and the development of central apnea. The fact that his breathing becomes quiet at night suggests central apnea.

24. C.   SDB is very common after a stroke and manifests in 50% to 70% of such patients. Both central and obstructive apneas are common in this setting. All stroke patients should be screened for sleep apnea. Oxygen or ASV may be tried if central apneas are present. CPAP would of course be indicated if the patient has clinically significant obstructive sleep apnea.   (Hermann and Bassetti, 2009)

25. C.   The baby should sleep on her back. Although the mechanisms that cause SIDS are not understood, epidemiologic studies have shown that having the baby sleep supine reduces the risk of SIDS. One hypothesis is that infants sleeping prone might asphyxiate when the upper airway is obstructed by soft pillows or bedding and that they do not arouse in response, or they might arouse but may be too weak to change their head position. The current recommendations include having the child sleep on a firm sleeping surface and avoid soft objects in the crib, bed sharing, and overheating the infant.   (Adams et al, 2009)

26. C.   Brief breathing pauses are common in newborns. Central apneas are generally not a problem unless they are longer than 20 seconds or are associated with cyanosis, pallor, bradycardia, or hypotonia.   (ICSD3, pp 94–98)

27. D.   Studies have not shown that home apnea monitoring reduces SIDS, so it would not be recommended for this infant.   (Adams et al, 2009)

28. B.   The back sleeping position has increased the incidence of flattening of the back of the head (deformational plagiocephaly). The flattening can be prevented by encouraging supervised "tummy time." While awake, infants should spend as much time as possible on their stomachs.   (Adams et al, 2009)

29. B.   The patient has treatment-emergent apnea (or complex apnea). This is often caused by overtitration; thus the first recommendation is to reduce CPAP pressure. In some patients (e.g., those on opiates), ASV or bilevel airway pressure might become necessary.   (Morgenthaler et al, 2014)

30. D.   The patient has treatment-emergent (complex) apnea. When this is caused by opiates (as is the case in this patient on methadone), ASV is often effective treatment. Bilevel PAP without a backup rate will not deal with the central apneas in this case.   (Javaheri et al, 2014)

31. C.   The patient is likely to have complex apnea or develop treatment-emergent apnea with titration. When the apnea is caused by opiate use, as is probable in this patient, ASV is often effective treatment. Unattended autotitrating CPAP is contraindicated in these patients.   (Javaheri et al, 2014)

32. B.   Sometimes the information given in a clinical scenario is used in the immediate or later question. Here it is worth emphasizing that every statement put into a scenario is there to either inform or distract you. Try to determine why a question is being asked. This patient has sleepiness and witnessed apneas but no snoring. You should be suspecting CSA. He also has abnormal behaviors during sleep. There is no indication to do home sleep testing for either of these situations. Narcolepsy is not suspected; therefore, an MSLT is not indicated.

33. A.   The thermal sensor shows almost no airflow; therefore, apnea is present. The slight oscillation in the signal of this channel is synchronous with the ECG, suggesting cardiogenic oscillations and CSA. The lack of respiratory effort (flat line of the thorax and abdominal signals) is diagnostic of central apnea. AHI showing 15 to 30 events/hr indicates that the CSA is of moderate severity. Home sleep tests generally underestimate apnea severity because sleep time is almost always less than recording time. Thus, answer D is incorrect.

34. C.   There is no indication to start a patient with CSA on autotitrating CPAP. In fact, the apnea may worsen with an autotitrating CPAP machine (note that the patient is on an opiate medication). Prazosin might be used for the PTSD nightmares, but it would not affect the apnea.

35. B.   Opiates (oxycodone in this patient) are a common cause of central apneas. The drugs may cause chronic hypoventilation and a low breathing frequency. Bupropion and alprazolam are not described as causing central apneas. Answer A was obviously incorrect because the patient did not have obstructive apnea. Was the patient even obese with a BMI of 26? If you read the question again, you will note that the patient had a phantom lower limb. Is BMI accurate when a limb or part of a limb is missing? The exam-taking lesson is that you must read the question carefully.

36. A.   Adherence of more than 4 hours per night for more than 70% of nights is generally considered acceptable CPAP compliance. The AHI is high with more than 50% of the events central; thus, the apnea is inadequately treated. Such a low mask leak can be ignored. There is an *intentional* leak present whenever the patient is using CPAP. This will wash awake CO_2 in the mask. If there is a poorly fitting mask or holes in the tubing, there will be an *unintentional* leak. Generally, a leak is considered to be large if the unintentional leak is more than 25 L/min. This value will vary somewhat from manufacturer to manufacturer and will also be a function of the specific mask type.

BONUS ANSWERS

37. C.   There is no need for a new interface because the leak is not large. A change in treatment is warranted, however, because the patient continues to have central apneas. Simply switching to a bilevel machine without a backup rate with an empiric pressure is an inadequate answer. He might need a timed backup. It is likely that the patient will require an ASV device, and the most prudent approach is an in-lab positive-pressure titration.

38. C.   The reason for the patient's sleepiness remains unexplained. If this were straightforward OSA and the patient had residual sleepiness on PAP, a clinical trial of modafinil might be indicated. That is not the situation here: This patient's sleepiness could be related to his medications or his psychiatric condition, or he might have posttraumatic brain injury hypersomnia. The trail to the correct answer is always in the question.

Summary

Highly Recommended

- *AASM Manual for the Scoring of Sleep and Associated Events: Rules, Terminology, and Technical Specifications*, Version 2.5
- *International Classification of Sleep Disorders*, ed 3

Topics You Should Know

Although CSA is much less common than OSA, it is a very important topic that sleep specialists will encounter. Expect about 20 of the 240 questions to be on central apnea. Be sure to review the new categories of CSA discussed in the ICSD3.

Epidemiology

- Idiopathic CSA is mostly found in middle-aged or older adults
- CSB is found in patients with a variety of diseases
  - Congestive heart failure (about 50%)   (ATLAS2, pp 322–324)
  - Stroke   (ATLAS2, p 329)
  - Multiple sclerosis   (ATLAS2, pp 226–228)
  - Neuromuscular disorders
  - Drugs that depress the drive to breathe

Pathophysiology

- Central apnea episodes are associated with absent or reduced efforts to breathe caused by various factors
  - Reduced output from the respiratory centers in the central nervous system
  - Unstable or oscillating respiratory control system
    - Prolonged circulation time
  - Increased drive to breathe (high loop gain)
  - Decreased drive to breathe
    - Effect of drugs
    - Central nervous system (CNS) lesions
    - Genetic disorders
  - Weakness of the inspiratory muscles
    - Neuromuscular disorders
- Physiologic changes include
  - Hypoxemia
  - Sleep instability
  - Increased arousals

Risk Factors

- Heart failure
- Cerebrovascular accident
- Use of opiates and other CNS-sedating agents
- Genetic abnormalities (e.g., PHOX2B gene)
- Lesions that affect the brainstem that contain regions that control breathing (e.g., medulla oblongata)
- Findings on physical examination
  - Central sleep apnea
    - Neuromuscular disorder findings
    - Pinpoint pupils (sign of opiate use)
  - CSB
    - May be observed while the patient is awake or asleep
    - A feature of
      - Heart failure
      - Stroke
      - Kidney failure

Diagnostic Methods

See Diagnostic Methods in Obstructive Sleep Apnea located earlier in this section.

Classification of the Central Sleep Apnea Syndromes (ICSD3)

- Adult
  - Central sleep apnea with CSB
  - Central apnea due to a medical disorder without CSB
  - Treatment-emergent central sleep apnea
  - Primary central sleep apnea
  - Central sleep apnea due to high-altitude periodic breathing
  - Central sleep apnea due to a medication or substance
- Pediatric
  - Primary central sleep apnea of infancy
  - Primary central sleep apnea of prematurity

Treatment (Aurora et al, 2012; Javaheri et al, 2014; Morgenthaler et al, 2014)

- For unstable or oscillating respiratory control system
  - Oxygen
  - ASV (to reduce minute ventilation or dampen oscillations) This treatment is contraindicated when LVEF is less than 45%.　(Cowie et al, 2015)
- For depressed CNS control of breathing
  - Bilevel positive airway pressure with backup
  - Noninvasive mechanical ventilation
- For idiopathic cases in which pathophysiology is unclear
  - Trial of CPAP *or*
  - Bilevel with backup *or*
  - ASV

REFERENCES

Adams SM, Good MW, Defranco GM. Sudden infant death syndrome. *Am Fam Physician.* 2009;79(10):870–874.

Aldabal L, Bahammam AS. Cheyne-Stokes respiration in patients with heart failure. *Lung.* 2010;188(1):5–14.

American Academy of Sleep Medicine. *International classification of sleep disorders*, ed 3. Darien, Ill.: American Academy of Sleep Medicine; 2014.

American Academy of Sleep Medicine. *The AASM manual for the scoring of sleep and associated events: rules, terminology and technical specifications, Version 2.5.* Darien, Ill.: American Academy of Sleep Medicine; 2014.

Aurora RN, Chowdhuri S, Ramar K, et al. The treatment of central sleep apnea syndromes in adults: practice parameters with an evidence-based literature review and meta-analyses. *Sleep.* 2012;35(1):17–40.

Cowie MR, Woehrle H, Wegscheider K, et al. Adaptive servo-ventilation for central sleep apnea in systolic heart failure. *N Engl J Med.* 2015;373(12):1095–1105.

Guilleminault C, Hagen CC, Khaja AM. Catathrenia: parasomnia or uncommon feature of sleep disordered breathing? *Sleep.* 2008;31(1):132–139.

Hermann DM, Bassetti CL. Sleep-related breathing and sleep-wake disturbances in ischemic stroke. *Neurology.* 2009;73(16):1313–1322.

Javaheri S, Harris N, Howard J, Chung E. Adaptive servoventilation for treatment of opioid-associated central sleep apnea. *J Clin Sleep Med.* 2014;10(6):637–643.

Kryger MH, Avidan A, Berry R. *Atlas of clinical sleep medicine*, ed 2. Philadelphia: Saunders; 2014.

Morgenthaler TI, Kuzniar TJ, Wolfe LF, et al. The complex sleep apnea resolution study: a prospective randomized controlled trial of continuous positive airway pressure versus adaptive servoventilation therapy. *Sleep.* 2014;37(5): 927–934.

7.3   Sleep-Related Hypoventilation and Hypoxemic Syndromes

QUESTIONS

Sleep Hypoventilation Has Many Faces

1. A man with a BMI of 50 has severe swelling of the ankles and a hematocrit of 58%. What abnormality would *most* likely explain these findings?
  A. OSA
  B. Upper airway resistance syndrome (UARS)
  C. OHS
  D. Treatment-emergent apnea

2. A patient is referred with the diagnosis of pulmonary hypertension. What is the *most* common cause of pulmonary hypertension?
  A. COPD
  B. Idiopathic pulmonary fibrosis
  C. OHS
  D. Asthma

3. Which of the following leads to peripheral edema in hypoventilating (hypercapnic) patients?
  A. Polycythemia caused by a right-to-left cardiac shunt
  B. Pulmonary hypertension leading to right heart failure
  C. Cardiac rhythm abnormality in asthma
  D. Left heart failure causing pulmonary hypertension

4. Which of the following is *not true* about OHS?
  A. It is more common in men
  B. Patients have awake hypoventilation
  C. Patients have sleep hypoventilation
  D. Headache is a common finding

5. What percentage of OSA patients have OHS?
  A. Fewer than 5%
  B. 10% to 20%
  C. 30% to 40%
  D. About 50%

6. Which is *true* about sleep-breathing disorders in kyphoscoliosis?
  A. Sleep-breathing disorders are uncommon in kyphoscoliosis
  B. Hyperventilation is present in severe kyphoscoliosis
  C. CPAP is almost always effective in this population
  D. Nighttime ventilation can improve daytime respiratory failure

7. Which of the following statements about postpolio syndrome is *true*?
   A. Patients with postpolio syndrome almost always develop sleep-breathing disorders within a year of the acute episode of poliomyelitis
   B. Hypoventilation in these patients can be treated with noninvasive ventilation
   C. CPAP is effective in most patients who have sleep-breathing disorders with postpolio syndrome and weakness of the respiratory muscles
   D. OSA is uncommon in this population

8. A patient with OSA is titrated with a bilevel pressure mask in the sleep lab. The technician gives him an EPAP of 10 cm H_2O and a pressure support of 8 cm H_2O, which he tolerates well. What is his IPAP?
   A. 2 cm H_2O
   B. 8 cm H_2O
   C. 14 cm H_2O
   D. 18 cm H_2O

9. Shortly after birth, a newborn develops a distended abdomen, lethargy, and cyanosis. What test will *not* help make the correct diagnosis?
   A. Arterial blood gases
   B. Assay for *PHOX2B* gene
   C. PSG with PcO_2 monitoring
   D. MRI of the upper airway

10. A thin man, age 58 years, has a history of COPD and peripheral edema. A home sleep study shows three prolonged episodes, each about 10 minutes in duration, of hypoxemia (SaO_2 dropped into the 70% range). During hypoxemia episodes, his SaO_2 remained steady without oscillation. What is the likeliest pathogenesis of the hypoxemia?
    A. The patient developed obstructive apnea during REM sleep
    B. Hypotonia of the muscles of respiration, except for the diaphragm, caused hypoventilation in REM sleep
    C. The hypoxemia was probably position dependent and caused by ventilation-perfusion mismatching when the patient was supine
    D. None of the above is true

11. What does the term *overlap syndrome* conventionally refer to?
    A. The combination of sleep apnea and obesity hypoventilation
    B. Any hypoventilation syndrome and narcolepsy
    C. The combination of hypoventilation syndrome, insulin resistance, and high blood pressure
    D. Combination of COPD and OSA

Panic

A father goes to check on his 3-month-old baby boy, who is sleeping in his crib. He notices the child is apparently not breathing and is blue. He screams to his wife to call 911 then lifts the baby. In his arms, the baby feels like a rag doll with no muscle tone. He rocks the baby and yells at him to breathe. Within a minute, the baby awakes and starts crying; his muscle tone and normal color return to normal. Within 5 minutes, the ambulance arrives, and the emergency squad examines the baby. Their only finding is that his abdomen is slightly distended. The ECG shows no rhythm abnormality.

12. The father, still highly anxious, asks the ambulance staff whether the baby should be taken to the hospital.
    A. The baby should not be taken to the hospital because the problem has resolved. No additional follow-up is needed
    B. The baby should be taken to the ED to make sure that long QT syndrome is not present. Then, if the ECG results are normal, the baby can be sent home with an apnea monitor
    C. The baby should be admitted to the hospital and the problem investigated
    D. Because the abdomen is slightly distended, the family should make an appointment with the pediatrician

13. The baby is taken to the ED, where the distended abdomen is confirmed, and he is admitted for further investigation and SaO_2 monitoring. The pediatrician is not concerned with any of the blood tests. Continuous oximetry finds that the SaO_2 hovers around 94% ± 2%. Arterial blood gases reveal PaO_2 of 82 mm Hg and PcO_2 of 51 mm Hg. What should be done next?

A. Discharge the baby and reassure the parents

B. Discharge the baby and arrange for 6 months of home SaO_2 monitoring

C. Schedule comprehensive PSG

D. Discharge the baby with treatment for gastroesophageal reflux

14. There is concern that this child might have congenital central hypoventilation syndrome (CCHS). Which of the following is *not* characteristic of CCHS?

A. CCHS typically manifests after 3 to 4 years of age

B. Most cases are caused by de novo mutations in the *PHOX2B* gene

C. Late diagnosis can result in cognitive deficits

D. Affected children have blunted ventilatory responses to hypoxia and hypercapnia

ANSWERS

1. C. In a patient with morbid obesity and severe ankle edema, it is likely that cor pulmonale caused by hypoventilation is present. Polycythemia is caused by hypoxemia stimulating the kidneys to produce erythropoietin. When elevated PcO_2 is documented in the awake state, the term *obesity hypoventilation syndrome* is used. This condition is also known as *Pickwickian syndrome*, named after a character in Charles Dickens' novel *The Pickwick Papers*. (Mokhlesi et al, 2008)

2. A. COPD is by far the most common cause of pulmonary hypertension. (Weitzenblum et al, 2009, 2013)

3. B. Peripheral edema is a common feature of cor pulmonale and is most often seen in right heart failure caused by pulmonary hypertension. The likeliest conditions to cause cor pulmonale are OHS and the overlap syndrome (a combination of COPD and OSA). Pulmonary hypertension is caused by pulmonary artery constriction in response to hypoxemia and remodeling of the pulmonary vasculature. (Weitzenblum et al, 2009, 2013)

4. A. Surprisingly, most series of OHS show more women than men. This may be because morbid obesity is more common in women. By definition, patients with OHS have awake hypoventilation and, when measured, also show increased PcO_2 during sleep. Headaches are common symptoms in these patients. (Berg et al, 2001; Masa et al, 2001; Mokhlesi et al, 2008)

5. B. OHS is found in about 10% to 20% of patients with OSA. (Mokhlesi et al, 2008)

6. D. Nighttime noninvasive ventilation can significantly improve sleep and daytime blood gases, daytime pulmonary function, and symptoms of hypoventilation. (Ferris et al, 2000)

7. B. Patients with postpolio syndrome often have a history of respiratory failure at the time of an acute poliomyelitis that sometimes required ventilatory support. These patients, usually with bulbar poliomyelitis, often improved and no longer required mechanical ventilation. Then, three or four decades later, they may manifest sleep-breathing problems or hypoventilation. This type of patient may do very well with noninvasive ventilation. If the chest wall muscles are weak, CPAP will not be effective in treating sleep hypoventilation; it might only be effective if the patient also has OSA. Patients with postpolio syndrome have several types of sleep-breathing abnormalities, including OSA. (Dahan et al, 2006; Steljes et al, 1990)

8. D. CPAP gives one pressure above ambient (e.g., 5 cm H_2O). Bilevel PAP gives two pressures above ambient, an EPAP (expiratory positive airway pressure) and a higher IPAP (inspiratory positive airway pressure). The difference between IPAP and EPAP is the level of *pressure support* (PS). Thus, EPAP of 10 and PS of 8 = IPAP of 18 cm H_2O. (Note that the acronym "BiPAP" is often used for "bilevel" but, strictly speaking, BiPAP is a trademark of the Respironics Corporation.)

9. D. The features are those of CCHS. CCHS often occurs in newborns who are found to have hypercapnic respiratory failure (as documented by elevated PcO_2), although in some cases, severe hypoventilation occurs only during sleep. Although this was once considered an isolated defect of the chemical control of breathing, with virtually absent ventilatory response to hypoxemia and hypercapnia, it is now believed to be a disease with more widespread autonomic nervous system abnormalities caused by mutation of the *PHOX2B* gene. The third edition of the *International Classification of Sleep Disorders* establishes two criteria for CCHS: (1) sleep-related hypoventilation is present, and (2) mutation of the *PHOX2B* gene is evident. About 10% to 20% of patients have Hirschsprung disease (caused by an aganglionic colon, leading to bowel distention and constipation), and about 5% ultimately develop neural crest tumors (e.g., neuroblastoma). (ICSD3, pp 113–117)

10. B. Patients with COPD become dependent on their accessory muscles of respiration. REM sleep leads to hypotonia of these muscles, but diaphragm activity is usually preserved. This scenario leads to hypoventilation, causing discrete prolonged oxygen desaturation without the typical cyclic desaturations seen in OSA. (ATLAS2, p 308)

11. D. The term *overlap syndrome* was first coined by the late David Flenley to describe patients who have both COPD and OSA. Overlap syndrome is found in about 1% of the adult population. COPD and OSA share many pathogenic mechanisms involving C-reactive protein (CRP), interleukin 6 and interleukin 8, and tumor necrosis factor-α. (McNicholas, 2009)

12. C. The baby should be taken to the hospital for probable admission because the etiology of the event has not been ascertained. This baby had what is called an *apparent life-threatening event* (ALTE). Some controversy surrounds the acute and long-term management of ALTE; however, all cases should be evaluated in the ED. From there, recommendations are divided between hospital admission if abnormalities are found and releasing the baby on home monitoring if ED evaluation results are negative. One series reported the following findings in children presenting to an ED with ALTE: gastroesophageal reflux, 26%; pertussis, 9%; seizures, 9%; urinary tract infection, factitious illness, brain tumor, atrial tachycardia, patent ductus arteriosus, and opioid-related apnea account for smaller percentages. No etiology could be determined in 23%. Sleep-breathing abnormality was actually a rare finding. It is generally recommended that babies with ALTE be admitted to the hospital for 1 to 3 days of cardiorespiratory monitoring and that they undergo complete blood count, measurement of CRP and glucose levels, evaluation of arterial blood gases, and urinalysis. If no abnormality is found to explain the ALTE, home apnea monitoring is not recommended because it has not been shown to reduce sudden infant death. (Davies et al, 2002; Wijers et al, 2009)

13. C. This baby has two features to suggest the diagnosis may be CCHS. The first clue is that gas exchange is not quite normal. In a healthy infant, SaO_2 should be higher than 94%, PaO_2 should be closer to 90 mm Hg, and $PacO_2$ should be less than 50 mm Hg. The second clue is that the patient has a distended abdomen, suggesting Hirschsprung disease (found in 10%–20% of CCHS patients). Shallow breathing in CCHS is generally present from birth, but it might not be noticeable until apnea episodes or an ALTE occur. About 90% of patients have *PHOX2B* gene mutations. Patients with CCHS often require support with mechanical ventilation.

14. A. Children with CCHS generally present shortly after birth or within the first few months of life. The hypoventilation might not be apparent at first and is found only after the child develops cor pulmonale or erythrocytosis. (ICSD3, pp 113–117)

Summary

Highly Recommended

- *AASM Manual for the Scoring of Sleep and Associated Events: Rules, Terminology, and Technical Specifications*, Version 2.5
- *Atlas of Clinical Sleep Medicine*, ed 2, Chapter 13

Topics You Should Know

The section on SDB will make up about 41 of the 240 questions on the exam. Although patients with hypoventilation/hypoxemic syndromes are uncommon, expect a few questions on this topic because of the therapeutic challenges presented by these patients.

Sleep-Related Hypoventilation and Hypoxemic Syndromes

Epidemiology

- Found in patients with:
  - OHS
  - Congenital central hypoventilation syndrome
  - Overlap syndrome
  - Neuromuscular disorders

Pathophysiology

- Hypoventilation is associated with absent or reduced efforts to breathe
- Hypoventilation is documented by increased PcO_2
- Hypoventilation is inferred with prolonged hypoxemia without breathing pattern abnormalities.
- Reduced efforts to breathe can be caused by:
  - Reduced output from the respiratory centers in the CNS
    - Depression of CNS control of breathing
    - Decreased drive to breathe
      - ◆ Effect of drugs
      - ◆ CNS lesions
      - ◆ Genetic disorders
  - Weakness of the inspiratory muscles
    - Neuromuscular disorders
  - Respiratory diseases
- Physiologic changes include hypoxemia, sleep instability, increased arousals

Risk Factors

- Morbid obesity
- Female gender
- Respiratory disease (COPD)
- Use of opiates and other CNS-sedating agents
- Genetic abnormalities
- Lesions affecting the brainstem

Findings on Examination

- Chronic hypoventilation findings
  - Peripheral edema due to right heart failure
  - Plethoric complexion due to polycythemia
  - Asterixis due to hypercapnia
  - Feature of
    - Morbid obesity
    - Neuromuscular disease my lead to hypoventilation. For example, from
      - ◆ Diffuse muscle atrophy in amyotrophic lateral sclerosis
      - ◆ Progressive weakness or paralysis in postpolio syndrome
- Kyphoscoliosis

Diagnostic Methods

See Diagnostic Methods in Obstructive Sleep Apnea located earlier in this section.

Treatment

- For COPD with nocturnal hypoxemia but without sleep-breathing pattern abnormalities: supplemental oxygen
- For overlap syndrome: CPAP or bilevel PAP
- For depression of CNS control of breathing
  - Bilevel with backup
  - Noninvasive mechanical ventilation
- For neuromuscular disorders
  - Bilevel with backup
  - Noninvasive mechanical ventilation
- For idiopathic cases in which pathophysiology is unclear
  - Trial of CPAP *or*
  - Bilevel with backup *or*
  - ASV

REFERENCES

American Academy of Sleep Medicine. *International classification of sleep disorders*, ed 3. Darien, Ill.: American Academy of Sleep Medicine; 2014.

American Academy of Sleep Medicine. *The AASM manual for the scoring of sleep and associated events: rules, terminology and technical specifications, Version 2.1.* Darien, Ill.: American Academy of Sleep Medicine; 2014.

Berg G, Delaive K, Manfreda J, et al. The use of health-care resources in obesity-hypoventilation syndrome. *Chest.* 2001;120(2):377–383.

Dahan V, Kimoff RJ, Petrof BJ, et al. Sleep-disordered breathing in fatigued postpoliomyelitis clinic patients. *Arch Phys Med Rehabil.* 2006;10:1352–1356.

Davies F, Gupta R. Apparent life threatening events in infants presenting to an emergency department. *Emerg Med J.* 2002;19(1):11–16.

Ferris G, Servera-Pieras E, Vergara P, et al. Kyphoscoliosis ventilatory insufficiency: noninvasive management outcomes. *Am J Phys Med Rehabil.* 2000;79(1):24–29.

Kryger MH, Avidan A, Berry R. *Atlas of clinical sleep medicine*, ed 2. Philadelphia: Saunders; 2014.

Masa JF, Celli BR, Riesco JA, et al. The obesity hypoventilation syndrome can be treated with noninvasive mechanical ventilation. *Chest.* 2001;119(4):1102–1107.

McNicholas WT. Chronic obstructive pulmonary disease and obstructive sleep apnea: overlaps in pathophysiology, systemic inflammation, and cardiovascular disease. *Am J Respir Crit Care Med.* 2009;180(8):692–700.

Mokhlesi B, Kryger MH, Grunstein RR. Assessment and management of patients with obesity hypoventilation syndrome. *Proc Am Thorac Soc.* 2008;5(2):218–225.

Steljes DG, Kryger MH, Kirk BW, Millar TW. Sleep in postpolio syndrome. *Chest.* 1990;98(1):133–140.

Weitzenblum E, Chaouat A. Cor pulmonale. *Chron Respir Dis.* 2009;6(3):177–185.

Weitzenblum E, Chaouat A, Canuet M, Kessler R. Pulmonary hypertension in chronic obstructive pulmonary disease and interstitial lung diseases. *Semin Respir Crit Care Med.* 2009;30:458–470.

Weitzenblum E, Chaouat A, Kessler R. Pulmonary hypertension in chronic obstructive pulmonary disease. *Pneumonol Alergol Pol.* 2013;81:390–398.

Wijers MM, Dutch Paediatric Association, Dutch Institute for Healthcare Improvement (CBO), et al. Multidisciplinary guidelines for "apparent life threatening event." *Ned Tijdschr Geneeskd.* 2009;153:A590.

7.4   Isolated Symptoms and Normal Variants

QUESTIONS

A Sleepy Smoker

A 60-year-old man with a 40-pack-year smoking history complains of shortness of breath, daytime sleepiness, and sleep-maintenance insomnia. He often wakes up gasping for air but denies snoring. His BMI is 32, blood pressure (BP) is 110/80 mm Hg, pulse is 90 beats/min, SaO_2 is 91% by pulse oximetry, and hematocrit is 55%. His venous bicarbonate is elevated at 36 mEq/L. His breath and clothes smell of cigarette smoke. He has peripheral edema and uses sternocleidomastoid muscles while breathing.

1. His oxyhemoglobin dissociation curve is likely flat above
   A. PaO_2 of 40 mm Hg
   B. PaO_2 of 25 mm Hg
   C. SaO_2 of 70%
   D. SaO_2 of 90%

2. What change in SaO_2 would be expected with a 20–mm Hg drop in his PaO_2?
   A. The drop in SaO_2 would be larger than in a subject with normal oxygenation
   B. There would be no change in SaO_2 because his sleep SaO_2 is 91%
   C. A fall in SaO_2 would be less than that in a normal person because he is on the flat portion of the O_2 dissociation curve
   D. His SaO_2 would fall the same amount as in a normal participant

3. What sleep-breathing abnormality would he *most* likely manifest?
   A. Hypoventilation causing hypoxemia
   B. OSA
   C. CSA
   D. Biot respiration

4. Hypoxemia during sleep in this patient would *most* likely occur in
   A. Stage N2
   B. Stage N3
   C. Tonic REM
   D. Phasic REM

Bonus Questions Continue From the Previous Case

5. A variety of stimuli affect breathing via receptors located throughout the body; these receptors include all of the following *except*
   A. Central chemoreceptors
   B. Erythropoietin receptors
   C. Carotid bodies
   D. Pulmonary stretch receptors

6. The patient is admitted to the hospital in hypercapnic respiratory failure. His wife states that he developed a mild upper respiratory infection for which he took a drug that contained 325 mg of acetaminophen and 15 mg of codeine. He took the medication at bedtime, appeared to struggle to breathe a few minutes later, and then became unresponsive. She called 911, and he was intubated by emergency medical services (EMS). What is the likeliest cause of his acute respiratory failure?
   A. Pulmonary embolism
   B. Exacerbation of COPD
   C. Codeine causing bronchoconstriction
   D. Suppression of respiration by the pain medication

Frozen

A 45-year-old obese woman is admitted to a psychiatry ward with acute onset of delirium and hallucinations. After being treated with haloperidol, she became somnolent and could not be aroused. She was transferred to the medical intensive care unit (ICU), where she had a temperature of 34°C and a pulse of 38 beats/min.

7. What is the *likeliest* diagnosis?
   A. Addison disease
   B. Overdosage with haloperidol
   C. Delirium tremens
   D. Hypothyroidism

8. The patient is found to have hypercapnia and is intubated and mechanically ventilated. Blood was taken for testing, and while awaiting results, the ICU team administered 0.15 mg of thyroxine and 100 mg of hydrocortisone. The patient aroused in about 6 hours complaining of chest pain and was noted to have a marked increase in heart rate and many premature ventricular contractions. What is the *likeliest* cause of this clinical course?
  A. Hydrocortisone overdose
  B. Haloperidol withdrawal
  C. Manifest delirium tremens
  D. Too high a thyroxin dose

ANSWERS

1. D. Understanding the oxyhemoglobin dissociation curve is critical in interpreting oximetry data during PSG. The dissociation curve can be thought of as two linear portions, a steep one and a flat one, joined by a shoulder; the latter has an SaO_2 of about 90% (Fig. 7.4–1). On the flat portion above 90% SaO_2, a relatively large decrement in PO_2 is necessary to produce a physiologically significant change in SaO_2. Normally, PaO_2 has to drop by 20 to 30 mm Hg for a physiologically significant drop in SaO_2 to occur. On the steep portion of the curve, which could be the SaO_2 for someone who has COPD or who is hypoventilating, a relatively small drop in PO_2 results in a physiologically significant drop in SaO_2. In this situation, a drop of 20 to 30 mm Hg in PaO_2 results in a much greater drop in SaO_2 compared with a normal baseline PaO_2 (Fig. 7.4–2). This basic physiology shows that a fixed requirement for scoring hypopneas, a 3% or 4% drop in SaO_2, can have very different implications depending on where the subject started from.

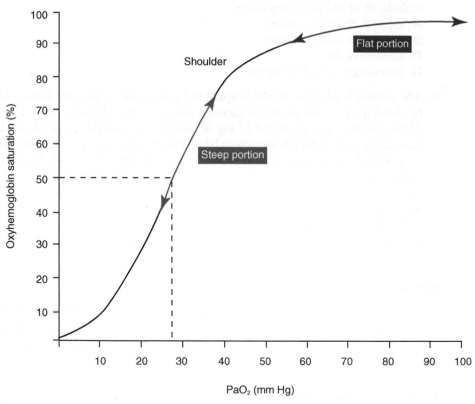

FIGURE 7.4–1 Question 1.

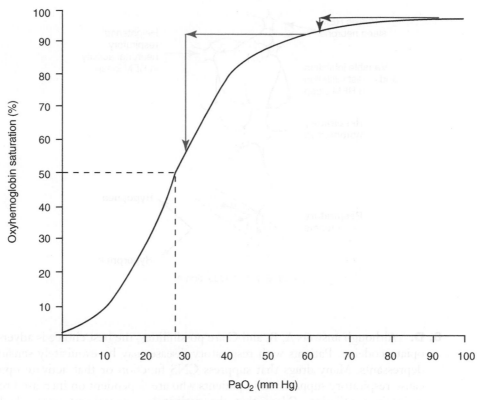

FIGURE 7.4–2 Questions 1 and 2.

2. A. This patient's SaO₂ is on the shoulder of the oxyhemoglobin dissociation curve. There-fore, compared with a normal individual with SaO₂ of 98%, he will manifest a larger drop in SaO₂ for a given drop in PaO₂. Notice in Figure 7.4–2 that a drop of 30 mm Hg in SaO₂ in the patient (*blue arrows*) with baseline SaO₂ of 90% results in a dramatically larger drop in SaO₂ than in a person with a normal SaO₂ (*red arrows*). Also, an elevated blood carbon mon-oxide level (from smoking) is not picked up by the standard pulse oximeter; as result, the pulse oximeter–measured SaO₂ will always be somewhat higher than the patient's true SaO₂.

3. A. Although there is an increased risk of OSA because of obesity, the lack of a snoring history makes OSA less likely. There is no information to indicate CHF or opiate use that might lead to central apnea or that might suggest Biot breathing. The elevated bicarbonate is strongly suggestive of hypercapnia with metabolic compensation, so the best answer is hypoventilation.

4. D. There is a loss of tone of the accessory muscles of respiration just as there is in almost all skeletal muscles during both the tonic and phasic components of REM sleep. The loss of muscle tone seems related to the muscles' spindle density. Muscles with a lower spindle density (e.g., the diaphragm) seem resistant to the tonic reduction in muscle tone; thus, the diaphragm is not paralyzed during REM. However, during the phasic component of REM sleep, there occurs additional inhibition of the respiratory motor neurons, reducing activity of the dia-phragm somewhat and possibly causing hypoventilation. Hypoxemia that occurs in patients with COPD is also related to phasic REM. Thus, both hypoxemia and hypoventilation are most likely to occur in phasic REM sleep (Fig. 7.4–3).

BONUS ANSWERS

5. B. Breathing is controlled by at least three factors: (1) the *state*, either awake or in a stage of sleep; (2) *metabolic factors*, including blood gas changes, with PaO₂ sensed by the carotid bodies and PcO₂ sensed by the carotid bodies and medullary central chemoreceptors; (3) *lung function* (e.g., vagal inputs from pulmonary stretch receptors as might occur in interstitial lung disease). (ATLAS2, pp 46–53)

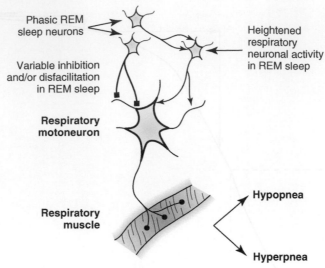

FIGURE 7.4-3 Question 4.

6. D. Although answers A, B, and C are possibilities, the best choice is adverse response to the opiate codeine. Patients with respiratory disease may be exquisitely sensitive to respiratory depressants. Many drugs that suppress CNS function or that activate opioid receptors can cause respiratory suppression in patients who are dependent on increased respiratory drive to maintain ventilation. (Note that the patient had prominent sternocleidomastoid muscle activity.)

7. D. The combination of bradycardia and low body temperature should raise suspicion that the patient has hypothyroidism, although hypothermia related to cold exposure is also a possibility. Patients with "myxedema madness" may have sleep apnea.   (Neal and Yuhico, 2012) About 10% of OSA patients turn out to have subclinical or clinical hypothyroidism.   (Ozcan et al, 2014)

8. D. Treatment of hypothyroidism in this type of patient must be undertaken cautiously; when coexisting sleep apnea is untreated, nocturnal angina and cardiac arrhythmias may occur. Patients should be treated with CPAP and low-dose thyroxine.   (Grunstein and Sullivan, 1988)

Summary

Highly Recommended

■ *Atlas of Clinical Sleep Medicine*, ed 2, Chapter 3.6

Topics You Should Know

The current blueprint for the sleep certification exam has a new subsection section called *Isolated symptoms and normal variants*. This is supposed to cover snoring and catathrenia. However, this topic only makes up fewer than 4 of the 240 questions on the board examination, and the topic is covered in detail earlier in this section. We recommend that the reader focus on the physiology of sleep that has clinical applications.

Control of Breathing

■ Respiratory pacemaker or controller   (ATLAS2, p 45)
  ○ Located in the medulla and pons
  ○ Made up of the dorsal respiratory group (ventrolateral nucleus of tractus solitarius) and ventral respiratory group (pre-Botzinger complex, nucleus ambiguus, nucleus retroambiguus)

- Inputs to pacemaker   (ATLAS2, p 46) about the state of the cerebral cortex
  - Can override homeostatic control
- Inputs about the state of the blood to maintain homeostasis (levels of CO_2, O_2, H^+)
  - Fast-responding peripheral chemoreceptors mainly in carotid bodies
    - ◆ Sense CO_2, O_2, H^+
  - Slow-responding central chemoreceptors in the medulla
    - ◆ Sense CO_2, H^+
- Inputs about the state of the lungs
  - Stretch receptors in the lungs
- Outputs from pacemaker   (ATLAS2, p 46)
  - To diaphragm, upper airway muscles, and accessory muscles of respiration
  - Control hypoxic drive to breathe
    - Curvilinear response with little increase in ventilation until PO_2 falls below 60 mm Hg
    - Decreased with sleep
    - Very blunted in REM
  - Control hypercapnic drive to breathe
    - Linear response
    - Decreased with sleep
    - Very blunted in REM

Upper Airway Control

- Factors that maintain airway patency   (ATLAS2, p 48)
  - Contraction of dilator muscles
  - CNS arousal
  - Lung volume
- Factors leading to airway collapse
  - Loss of muscle tone (e.g., REM sleep hypotonia, alcohol effect)
  - Negative pressure in airway
  - Positive pressure outside airway
  - Anatomic abnormalities
    - Soft tissue (e.g., fat, enlarged tonsils)
    - Skeletal (e.g., retrognathia or micrognathia)

Arousal Responses

- To hypoxia
  - Unreliable (might not arouse at SaO_2 = 70%)
- To hypercapnia
  - Brisk
- To upper airway resistance or occlusion
  - Fastest in REM sleep in normal subjects
- To work of breathing
  - May be most important arousal mechanism in CSB

REFERENCES

Grunstein RR, Sullivan CE. Sleep apnea and hypothyroidism: mechanisms and management. *Am J Med.* 1988;85(6):775–779.

Kryger MH, Avidan A, Berry R. *Atlas of clinical sleep medicine*, ed 2. Philadelphia: Saunders; 2014.

Neal JM, Yuhico RJ. "Myxedema madness" associated with newly diagnosed hypothyroidism and obstructive sleep apnea. *J Clin Sleep Med.* 2012;8(6):717–718.

Ozcan KM, Selcuk A, Ozcan I, et al. Incidence of hypothyroidism and its correlation with polysomnography findings in obstructive sleep apnea. *Eur Arch Otorhinolaryngol.* 2014;271:2937–2941.

Sleep in Other Disorders

8.1 Neurologic Disorders

QUESTIONS

Frightening and Disturbing to Observe

Over the course of a month, a 34-year-old otherwise healthy man without any daytime symptoms displays dystonic posturing and wide-open eyes during sleep that occur at various times in the night. As reported by his wife, each episode lasts 40 to 50 seconds. The patient has no recollection of the events.

1. What is the *most* likely diagnosis?
   A. Nocturnal seizures
   B. Rapid eye movement (REM) sleep behavior disorder
   C. Confusional arousals
   D. Sleep terrors

2. In the *International Classification of Sleep Disorders*, ed 3 (ICSD3), his problem is classified as
   A. REM parasomnia
   B. Non-REM (NREM) parasomnia
   C. Anxiety disorder
   D. Epilepsy disorder

3. Which medication is used to treat this condition?
   A. Pramipexole
   B. A selective serotonin reuptake inhibitor
   C. Carbamazepine
   D. Zolpidem

Shocking

An otherwise healthy 42-year-old patient complains of a single, violent "electric-like" body jerk that occurs at sleep onset. These events, which occur several times a month, have been present as long as he can remember. They tend to be more common when he gets insufficient sleep.

4. What is the likeliest diagnosis?
   A. Fragmentary myoclonus
   B. Persistent benign sleep myoclonus of infancy
   C. Hypnic jerks
   D. Hypnagogic foot tremor

5. How would you manage this patient?
   A. Confirm the diagnosis by polysomnography (PSG), and treat with an anticonvulsant
   B. Reassure the patient about the benign nature of the condition
   C. Start on a dopamine agonist for restless legs syndrome (RLS)
   D. Confirm the diagnosis by a home sleep test (HST), and then treat with positive airway pressure (PAP) therapy

Potpourri

6. Which of the following statements regarding excessive daytime sleepiness (EDS) and myotonic dystrophy 1 (MD1) is *true*?
  A. EDS occurs in 10% of patients with MD1
  B. EDS is exclusively found in MD1 patients with sleep-disordered breathing (SDB)
  C. The severity of EDS does not correlate with the number of nucleotide (CTG) repeats
  D. The presence of sleep-onset REM periods (SOREMPs) on the multiple sleep latency test (MSLT) excludes a diagnosis of MD1

7. A 9-year-old girl presents with REM sleep behavior disorder. This condition is likely to herald the onset of which of the following disorders?
  A. Juvenile Parkinson disease
  B. Narcolepsy
  C. Sleep terrors
  D. Sleepwalking

8. Which of the following neurodegenerative disorders is *most* commonly associated with nocturnal stridor?
  A. Parkinson disease
  B. Multiple system atrophy
  C. Adductor spasmodic dysphonia
  D. Pick disease

ANSWERS

1. A. This is a classic description of nocturnal frontal lobe epilepsy, also known as *nocturnal paroxysmal dystonia*. The other three conditions would be in the differential diagnosis.

2. D. This is classified as a sleep-related epilepsy disorder. Nocturnal paroxysmal dystonia is one of three diseases in the category of nocturnal frontal lobe epilepsy (NFLE): (1) nocturnal paroxysmal arousal, (2) nocturnal paroxysmal dystonia, and (3) episodic nocturnal wanderings. Generally, in these conditions, one parent is affected, and the patient has a mutation in the *CHRNA4, CHRNB2,* or *CHRNA2* gene. (Hirose and Kurahashi, 2012)

3. C. Carbamazepine in small doses leads to remission or improvement in about 70% of patients with nocturnal paroxysmal dystonia. In patients with a specific mutation of the *CHRNA4* gene, zonisamide (Zonegran in the United States) has been found to be more effective than carbamazepine. Genetic counseling should also be offered to the patient and his or her family.

4. C. The patient is describing a hypnic jerk, also known as a *sleep start*. In ICSD3 (p 335), hypnic jerks are described as "sudden, brief, simultaneous contractions of the body or one or more body segments occurring at sleep onset." Hypnic jerks are often associated with a sensation of falling, and three other conditions have a similar manifestation. Benign sleep myoclonus of infancy is manifested by myoclonic jerks that occur during sleep. It typically begins at birth and resolves spontaneously by 6 months. Hypnagogic foot tremor and alternating leg muscle activation can occur at sleep-wake transitions or during light NREM sleep. PSG shows recurrent electromyography (EMG) potentials in one or both feet that are in the myoclonic range (>250 ms). Propriospinal myoclonus at sleep onset is a disorder of recurrent, sudden muscular jerks in the transition from wakefulness to sleep and is often associated with insomnia.

5. B. Because hypnic jerks are common and benign, reassurance is the goal of management. Such patients often worry they have epilepsy. Diagnosis should be made by the history and does not require a PSG.

6. C.   Although the severity of some myotonic dystrophy symptoms directly correlates with the number of abnormal CTG triplet repeats, this is not the case with EDS, which is present in 33% to 39% of patients with MD1. Reduced mean latency and SOREMPs on the MSLT are common findings in patients with MD1. EDS may be found in MD1 in the absence of either obstructive or central sleep apnea syndromes.   (Laberge et al, 2013)

7. B.   REM sleep behavior disorder (RBD) can herald the onset of narcolepsy in the pediatric population. Unlike adult RBD, which can herald a synucleinopathy such as Parkinson disease, pediatric RBD is not associated with juvenile Parkinson disease.   (Nevsimalova et al, 2007)

8. B.   Nocturnal stridor is related to paralysis of the vocal cord abductor muscles. It is seen in some patients with multisystem atrophy and is associated with reduced survival.   (Gaig and Iranzo, 2012)

Summary

Highly Recommended

- *Atlas of Clinical Sleep Medicine*, ed 6, Chapters 11.2 through 11.4
- Kryger M, Roth T, Dement WC, eds. *Principles and Practice of Sleep Medicine*, ed 6, Philadelphia: Elsevier; 2017. Section 12: Neurological Disorders

The sleep medicine certification exam has surprised examinees by an apparent discrepancy between the number of expected and actual neurology questions. The word *neurology* does not appear on the first page of the blueprint, and the examinee might assume that neurologic disorders are covered in other sections, such as with sleep-breathing disorders, hypersomnia, movement disorders, and parasomnias. However, the blueprint reveals that neurology is covered in the section *Sleep in Other Disorders*. There are only 12 questions in that section: neurologic, psychiatric, and other medical disorders.

Sleep in Parkinson disease is not mentioned in the section on movement disorders. It is almost as if neurology were an afterthought to the exam committee. As is apparent in this summary, sleep problems are very common in neurologic disorders, and attempting to broadly cover them in four or five questions seems a stretch.

This summary reviews neurologic disorders not covered elsewhere in this volume. It is unclear whether the exam committee will recalibrate future sleep exams to include more neurology. As you go through the summary, remember that all this content will pertain to only four or five questions. Focus on Parkinson disease, Alzheimer disease, stroke, and epilepsy—in that order—and remember the diseases that can cause RBD.

Narcolepsy and Idiopathic Hypersomnia

- See Section 4 of this volume

REM Sleep Behavior Disorder

- See Section 5 of this volume

Restless Legs Syndrome and Periodic Limb Movements in Sleep

- See Section 6 of this volume

Parkinsonism

- Defined as bradykinesia with one or more of the following:
  - Muscle rigidity
  - 4- to 6-Hz resting tremor
  - Postural instability

- Caused by loss of dopaminergic neurons
- Sleep problems include
  - Insomnia in about 60%
  - Periodic limb movements (PLMs)
  - REM sleep behavior disorder
    - In 30% to 90%, when neuronal destruction is caused by deposits of alpha-synuclein
    - Rare when neuronal destruction is caused by deposits of tau protein
    - May be associated with multisensory hallucinations and delusions that may respond to pimavanserin treatment
  - Excessive daytime sleepiness
    - Can have sleep attacks
    - May be related to dopaminergic medications

Atypical Parkinsonism (Parkinson Plus Syndromes)

- Lesions in other systems lead to worse prognosis
- Nocturnal stridor can develop and can lead to nocturnal death
- Examples include
  - Progressive supranuclear palsy
  - Multiple system atrophy (Shy-Drager syndrome)
  - Olivopontocerebellar degeneration

Stroke (ATLAS2, Chapter 14.2, p 328)

Sleep-Disordered Breathing and Stroke

- Epidemiology
  - SDB increases the risk of stroke
    - Habitual snoring is an independent risk factor for stroke (odds ratio, 1.5)
    - Severe obstructive sleep apnea (OSA) is an independent risk factor for stroke (hazard ratio 3.3)
  - Stroke leads to SDB
    - SDB is present in 50% of patients who have an acute stroke
  - With stroke recovery, SDB improves
  - Central sleep apnea improves more than OSA
- Symptoms
  - Nighttime
    - Sleep-onset insomnia
    - Snoring, stridor
    - Awakening short of breath
    - Orthopnea
  - Daytime
    - Headache
    - Sleepiness
    - Cognitive impairment
- Findings
  - Disordered breathing during sleep
    - OSA (most common)
    - Cheyne-Stokes breathing (CSB)
    - Combination of OSA (most severe in REM) and CSB (most severe in NREM)
    - Central hypoventilation (when stroke affects the brainstem or spinal cord)
  - Abnormal breathing in wakefulness (most often after stroke affecting the brainstem)
    - Neurogenic hyperventilation (indicates poor prognosis)
    - Inspiratory breath holding (apneustic breathing)
    - Irregular rate, rhythm, and tidal volume (Biot breathing)
    - Central hypoventilation (Ondine's curse)
    - Respiratory failure

- Treatment (see also Section 7 of this volume)
  - ○ For OSA: continuous positive airway pressure (CPAP)
  - ○ For CSB and central sleep apnea (CSA)
    - Oxygen
    - Adaptive servoventilation (ASV)
  - ○ For hypoventilation: mechanical ventilation

Sleep-Wake Disturbances in Stroke

- Epidemiology
  - ○ Sleepiness
    - Sleep more than 10 hours (25%)
    - Hypersomnia (25%)
  - ○ Insomnia (~50%)
  - ○ Movement disorder (~10%)
- Symptoms
  - ○ Sleepiness
    - Can improve with modafinil, methylphenidate, and dopaminergic drugs
    - Increased sleep time, EDS
    - Secondary narcolepsy
    - With hyperphagia (secondary Kleine-Levin syndrome)
  - ○ Insomnia
    - Can improve with zolpidem or zopiclone, but side effects are problematic
    - Sleep onset and maintenance
    - Day/night inversion
  - ○ REM sleep behavior disorder (may improve with clonazepam)
  - ○ Especially after strokes that affect the pons
  - ○ RLS (can improve with dopaminergic drugs)
  - ○ Hallucinations and abnormal dreaming
    - Hypnagogic hallucinations
    - Peduncular hallucinosis of Lhermitte (in some strokes that affect the pons and midbrain)
  - ○ Reduction or cessation of dreaming
    - Charcot-Wilbrand syndrome (in some strokes that affect the cerebral cortex, especially deep frontal)

Neuromuscular Diseases

- Poliomyelitis
- Acute poliomyelitis
  - ○ Bulbar
    - Affects respiratory center
    - Central hypoventilation and apnea
  - ○ Spinal
    - Affects motor neurons going to respiratory muscles
    - Respiratory muscle weakness
  - ○ Usually improves with time
- Chronic poliomyelitis
  - ○ Postpolio syndrome
    - Progressive muscle weakness, development of hypoventilation, sleep apnea
    - Sleep-breathing disorders can appear decades after the acute infection
    - Can require nocturnal ventilation or PAP support

Neurodegenerative Diseases

- Anatomic location of pathology
  - ○ Cerebral cortex
    - Alzheimer disease
    - Multiple sclerosis
    - Fatal familial insomnia
  - ○ Basal ganglia
    - Parkinson disease
    - Progressive supranuclear palsy
  - ○ Cerebellum
    - Spinocerebellar ataxia
  - ○ Motor neurons
    - Amyotrophic lateral sclerosis (ALS)
    - Primarily autonomic
    - Multiple system atrophy (Shy-Drager syndrome)
- Sleep disorders
  - ○ SDB
  - ○ Hypersomnia
  - ○ Circadian rhythm disorders
  - ○ Insomnia
  - ○ REM sleep behavior disorder

Polyneuropathy

- Charcot-Marie-Tooth syndrome (hereditary motor and sensory neuropathy)
  - ○ Neuropathy affecting
    - Pharyngeal muscles: upper airway obstruction
    - Diaphragm: hypoventilation
  - ○ Sleep-breathing abnormalities are worse in REM sleep

Neuromuscular Junction Diseases

- Myasthenia gravis
  - ○ Sleep apnea occurs in 60% of cases
  - ○ Obstructive apnea is the most common finding
  - ○ Events are most severe in REM sleep

Muscular Dystrophies

- Myotonic dystrophy
  - ○ Autosomal dominant
  - ○ Peripheral component
    - Involves weakness of facial, sternocleidomastoid, pharyngeal, and diaphragm muscles
  - ○ Central component
    - Loss of serotonin neurons, dysfunction of hypocretin system
    - Sleepiness, REM onsets
    - Abnormal ventilatory control
    - Sleep apnea, hypoventilation
- Duchenne muscular dystrophy
  - ○ Causes lung restriction and chest wall deformity
    - Sleep apnea, hypoventilation
      - ◆ Young children might respond to adenotonsillectomy
      - ◆ Older children with hypoventilation should be treated with noninvasive ventilation
- Rare myopathies that affect control of breathing
  - ○ Sleep apnea and hypoventilation can be seen in
    - Congenital myopathies (e.g., nemaline myopathy)
    - Metabolic myopathies (mitochondrial myopathy, acid maltase deficiency)

- Treatment
  - ○ Guided by PSG results
    - If a sleep-breathing abnormality is found   (Albdewi et al, 2018)
      - ◆ Ventilatory support ranges from CPAP to noninvasive ventilation
      - ◆ Overall clinical status must be considered
    - If no sleep-breathing abnormality is found
      - ◆ A clinical trial of modafinil for daytime sleepiness may be useful
      - ◆ These patients may be very vulnerable to central nervous system (CNS) depressants that worsen breathing during sleep

Alzheimer Disease (ATLAS2, Ch 11.4)

- The *APOE4* genotype increases risk for
  - ○ Alzheimer disease
  - ○ Sleep apnea
- Accumulation of abnormal tau protein in CNS causes sleep problems
  - ○ Suprachiasmatic nucleus
    - Disrupted circadian rhythm
  - ○ Cholinergic neurons in nucleus basalis of Maynert
    - Reduced REM sleep
  - ○ Pedunculopontine tegmental and laterodorsal tegmental nuclei
    - Reduced REM sleep
    - REM behavior disorder
  - ○ Perilocus coeruleus
    - REM behavior disorder
  - ○ Supraspinal autonomic nuclei
    - Autonomic dysfunction
  - ○ Brainstem respiratory centers
    - SDB
- Other factors that contribute to poor sleep and "sundowning"
  - ○ Lack of zeitgebers (e.g., sunlight, clocks)
  - ○ Unfamiliar environment
  - ○ Early bedtime
  - ○ Cognitive impairment
  - ○ Medical problems
  - ○ Sedatives
  - ○ Naps
- PSG findings
  - ○ Increased awakenings
  - ○ Reduced or absent slow-wave sleep (SWS)
  - ○ Poorly formed or absent spindles and K complexes
  - ○ REM is preserved in early Alzheimer disease

Other Dementias

- Dementia with Lewy bodies
  - ○ Lewy bodies in parts of the CNS lead to a syndrome that includes
    - Cognitive decline
    - Parkinsonism
    - Autonomic dysfunction
    - Visual hallucinations
  - ○ Sleep problems more common in Lewy body disease than in Alzheimer disease
    - REM behavior disorder
- Huntington disease
  - ○ Sleep problems include
    - Night/day disruption
    - Disturbed sleep (arousals, less SWS, less REM)
    - Development of apnea

- Creutzfeldt-Jakob disease
  - ○ Encephalopathy caused by prions
    - Neural degeneration
      - ◆ Myoclonic jerks
      - ◆ Progressive cognitive impairment
      - ◆ Death
  - ○ Sleep findings
    - Insomnia (common)
    - Reduced SWS
    - Few or absent spindles and K complexes
    - Reduced REM
    - Periodic sharp-wave complexes
    - Dream reality confusion with aggressive behavior
- Fatal familial insomnia
  - ○ Encephalopathy caused by prions
    - Loss of circadian rhythms
    - Neuroendocrine dysregulation
    - Progressive insomnia
    - Death

Epilepsy (ATLAS2, Ch 11.3)

- Sleep state has an effect on propensity for seizures
  - ○ NREM sleep promotes seizures
    - Cortical synchronization
    - Enhanced interhemispheric impulse transmission
  - ○ REM sleep protects from seizures
    - Inhibition of synchronization
    - Reduced interhemispheric impulse transmission

Sleep-Related Epilepsy Syndromes

- Nocturnal frontal lobe epilepsy (NFLE)
  - ○ The most common form is nocturnal paroxysmal dystonia
  - ○ It is a genetic disorder
    - Mutation in the *CHRNA4, CHRNB2,* or *CHRNA2* genes
    - One parent usually affected
  - ○ Symptoms
    - Nocturnal paroxysmal arousals
    - Nocturnal paroxysmal dystonia
    - Episodic nocturnal wanderings
  - ○ Treatment
    - Carbamazepine
    - Zonisamide for the *CHRNA4* mutation variant
- Temporal lobe epilepsy
  - ○ Awake symptoms
    - Brief periods of impaired consciousness
    - Staring
    - Automatisms
  - ○ Sleep features
    - Seizures can occur during sleep
    - Patient may demonstrate automatisms
- Benign childhood epilepsy with central temporal spikes (BECT; also called *benign rolandic epilepsy*)
  - ○ Seizures occur exclusively in NREM sleep
    - Unilateral

○ Manifestations
- Paresthesias of tongue, lips, gums, and cheek
- Movement of tongue and lips
- Drooling during sleep

Note: There are many other seizure disorders that affect sleep. They are rarely encountered, and it is unlikely that questions about them will appear on the examination. However, you are encouraged to review the PSG features of the more common seizure disorders.   (ATLAS2, Ch 11.3)

Other Neurologic Disorders

Headaches

- Migraine headache
  ○ Onset can occur in either SWS or REM sleep
  ○ Sleep can result in amelioration of headache
- Cluster headache
  ○ Most episodes begin during REM sleep
  ○ Chronic paroxysmal hemicrania is a variant
- Hypnic headache
  ○ Features
    - In older people
    - Occurs only at night
    - One attack per night
    - Lasts 1 to 2 hours
  ○ Prophylaxis
    - Lithium
    - Flunarizine
    - Indomethacin
    - Caffeine
  ○ Treatment
    - Aspirin
- Rare syndromes
  ○ Hemicrania horologia
    - Headaches last 15 minutes
    - Headaches occur every 60 minutes, day and night
  ○ Exploding head syndrome
    - Flashing lights and noises lasting seconds wake the patient from sleep
- Treatment
  ○ Specific treatment of headaches is generally handled by a neurologist

Head Trauma (Traumatic Brain Injury)

- Sleep features
  ○ EDS and hypersomnia
    - May be related to abnormality in hypocretin system
  ○ Insomnia
  ○ Circadian rhythm abnormalities
  ○ Sleep-breathing disorders can occur if the respiratory control system is damaged

Multiple Sclerosis

- Sleep features
  ○ Fatigue and daytime sleepiness (might respond to modafinil)
  ○ Insomnia
  ○ Awakening with leg spasms
  ○ Snoring
  ○ Periodic limb movements common

Brain Tumors

■ Sleep symptoms depend on tumor location
  ○ Tumors that affect the third ventricle can cause narcolepsy
  ○ Tumors that affect the brainstem can cause hypoventilation and respiratory failure

REFERENCES

Albdewi MA, Liistro G, El Tahry R. Sleep-disordered breathing in patients with neuromuscular disease. *Sleep Breath.* 2018;22(2):277–286.

American Academy of Sleep Medicine. *International classification of sleep disorders.* 3rd ed. Darien, Ill.: American Academy of Sleep Medicine; 2014.

Gaig C, Iranzo A. Sleep-disordered breathing in neurodegenerative diseases. *Curr Neurol Neurosci Rep.* 2012;12(2):205–217.

Hirose S, Kurahashi H. Autosomal dominant nocturnal frontal lobe epilepsy; Updated 2012. Available at: <http://www.ncbi.nlm.nih.gov/books/NBK1169/>. Accessed July 4, 2014.

Kryger MH, Avidan A, Berry R. *Atlas of clinical sleep medicine.* 2nd ed. Philadelphia: Saunders; 2014.

Laberge L, Gagnon C, Dauvilliers Y. Daytime sleepiness and myotonic dystrophy. *Curr Neurol Neurosci Rep.* 2013;13(4):340.

Nevsimalova S, Prihodova I, Kemlink D, et al. REM behavior disorder (RBD) can be one of the first symptoms of childhood narcolepsy. *Sleep Med.* 2007;8(7–8):784–786.

8.2   Psychiatric Disorders

QUESTIONS

Diplomatic Insomnia

A senior United Nations (UN) diplomat is referred for severe insomnia. He has trouble falling asleep and staying asleep, and he complains that he is sometimes drenched with sweat during the night. His wife states that he sometimes awakens thrashing his arms. He says, "I can't turn off my mind when I try to fall asleep." He has served in many places around the world during times of crisis. His insomnia began in 1993, when he was working for the UN during the Rwandan Civil War. Daytime episodes occur during which he appears to be hearing and seeing things that he knows are not there but that nonetheless trouble him a great deal.

1. What diagnosis should be considered foremost?
  A. Paranoid schizophrenia
  B. Psychotic depression
  C. Posttraumatic stress disorder
  D. REM sleep behavior disorder

2. The patient describes significant daytime sleepiness and a 45-lb weight gain in the past 6 months since starting a new medication. Which of the following medications *most* likely explains his weight gain?
  A. Modafinil
  B. Propranolol
  C. Methylphenidate
  D. Mirtazapine

3. What medication has the *best* chance of being effective in this patient?
  A. Prazosin
  B. Dilantin
  C. Clonazepam
  D. Risperidone

If Only the Insomnia Could Be Cured

A 45-year-old woman with a body mass index (BMI) of 42 presents with a 5-year history of severe depression, daytime fatigue, and lack of energy. During this period, she has been treated only with psychotherapy and has not improved. Her Epworth Sleepiness Scale (ESS) score is 13 of 24. She lives alone and does not know whether she snores. She was referred to the sleep disorders center by her treating psychologist, who suggested that she be started on a new hypnotic medication, although other hypnotics have been ineffective in the past. The patient was convinced that if her insomnia could be cured, the depression would remit. She has a strong family history of depression. The remainder of her medical history and the physical examination are noncontributory.

4. What is the *most* reasonable next step?
   A. Formal cognitive behavioral therapy (CBT)
   B. In-lab PSG
   C. A selective serotonin reuptake inhibitor (SSRI) to treat her depression
   D. Eszopiclone at bedtime to treat her insomnia

5. The patient undergoes an overnight sleep study, the results of which are given in Table 8.2–1. How would you interpret these findings?
   A. The absence of SWS is the primary reason for her sleep symptoms
   B. The delay in both sleep latency and REM latency are diagnostic of depression
   C. The patient's sleep problem is most likely caused by sleep apnea syndrome
   D. The findings are within normal limits for her age

6. When results of the sleep test are reviewed with the patient, she requests a hypnotic for sleep. What do you recommend as the next step?
   A. CPAP titration study or treatment with empirical AutoPAP
   B. Cognitive behavior therapy
   C. A trial of zolpidem
   D. A trial of trazodone

Cannot Stay Awake

A 24-year-old overweight woman is referred to the sleep disorders center with a complaint of inability to stay awake during the day. She claims to be awake all night, smoking cigarettes, drinking coffee, and feeling agitated and irritable. Lying in bed awake, she often hears voices that tell her what to do. When falling asleep, she often has dreams that are quite vivid, often to the point where she cannot tell whether she is awake or asleep.

Table 8.2–1

Sleep Parameter	Result
Sleep latency	30 min
Arousal index	15/hr
Percentage SWS	0%
Percentage REM sleep	15%
REM latency	180 min
Breathing Parameter	**Result**
AHI	6/hr
REM AHI	25/hr

AHI, Apnea/hypopnea index; *REM,* rapid eye movement; *SWS,* slow-wave sleep.

7. What is the *most* appropriate next step?
   A. The next step should be an overnight sleep study followed by an MSLT to evaluate for narcolepsy
   B. She should be referred to a psychiatrist for treatment of schizophrenia
   C. She should receive CBT to help with insomnia and poor sleep hygiene
   D. Urgent treatment with an anxiolytic such as clonazepam is indicated for her underlying anxiety disorder

8. What findings would likely be seen on this patient's sleep study?
   A. No specific sleep-related abnormalities
   B. A marked increase in SWS
   C. A short REM sleep latency
   D. An above-normal sleep efficiency

ANSWERS

1. **C.**　There are several clues that the patient has posttraumatic stress disorder (PTSD). He had been in a war zone and likely witnessed traumatic events. Such patients often have hallucinations and dissociative flashback episodes. Waking up from a repetitive dream concerning the trauma is also quite common and disturbing. An interesting work on this subject is *Shake Hands with the Devil* by Romeo Dallaire. Dallaire, who was head of the UN mission in Rwanda, describes his own descent into PTSD.

2. **D.**　The patient had been started on mirtazapine, an alpha$_{2A}$ antagonist and mixed 5-HT$_2$/5-HT$_3$ antagonist medication and antidepressant, which is known to cause weight gain. Mirtazapine has been evaluated for the treatment of OSA and was found to be ineffective. It might actually worsen the sleep apnea because of its effect on weight. Sleepiness is also a common side effect of this medication.

3. **A.**　Prazosin is a centrally acting alpha$_1$ adrenergic receptor antagonist. In placebo-controlled studies, it has been shown to be effective in reducing nightmares and sleep disturbances in both combat-related and civilian PTSD. Recent studies have shown less favorable results.

4. **B.**　The next step should be an in-lab PSG because several features suggest OSA. The patient gives a positive response for two of the categories in the Berlin questionnaire (sleepiness and obesity) and therefore is at high risk for OSA. In addition, among patients with sleep apnea, depressive symptoms are much more common in women than in men, as is a history of hypothyroidism. On the other hand, among patients with sleep apnea, alcohol and caffeine use is greater in men than in women.　(ATLAS2, p 154)

5. **C.**　The findings are typical of female patients with sleep apnea. Specifically, although the overall apnea/hypopnea index (AHI) is marginally increased, there is a significant increase in AHI during REM sleep. In depression, you would expect to find a reduction in REM latency; when present, the finding is consistent with, but not diagnostic of, depression. Other findings in depression include a reduction in SWS and often an increase in REM sleep as a percentage of total sleep time.　(ATLAS2, pp 365–367)

6. **A.**　Because the patient has obstructive sleep apnea syndrome (OSAS), the next steps should be CPAP titration followed by treatment with CPAP, if tolerated, or treatment with empiric AutoPAP. CPAP might improve the depressive symptoms or result in total remission. It is possible she never had depression in the first place; perhaps it was a misdiagnosis based on her sleep-related symptoms. The patient might require a hypnotic or even CBT after she has started on CPAP. Although it was once believed that drugs such as trazodone might actually improve sleep apnea, research has not confirmed this.

7. **B.**　The history is most consistent with schizophrenia. Hallucinatory perceptions in patients with schizophrenia can seem similar to what is expected in narcolepsy. Patients with schizophrenia might relate more than one type of hallucination—the type typical of schizophrenia (e.g., hearing voices) and hypnagogic hallucinations related to a primary sleep disorder. The schizophrenic hallucinations are considered by the patient to be "real," and the hypnagogic

hallucinations are thought to be some form of a "dream." An example of a patient with both is shown in Video 20-21, which can be found in the online version of the *Atlas*. Occasionally, a patient is referred for sleep evaluation by a primary care physician who suspects narcolepsy or some other primary sleep disorder, and the diagnosis ends up being schizophrenia. (Conversely, we have encountered patients in whom a psychiatrist incorrectly diagnosed schizophrenia but whose symptoms are typical of narcolepsy.) Sleep specialists not trained in psychiatry should not manage schizophrenia.

8. C. Typical findings in schizophrenia include severe insomnia (at times with day/night inversion), reduced sleep efficiency, reduced amount of SWS, and in about half of the patients, a reduction in REM sleep latency. Many patients with schizophrenia are at risk for OSA, especially if they are being treated with antipsychotic agents that increase weight. An important point to remember about schizophrenics in remission is that worsening of insomnia can signal an impending relapse.   (Jaffe et al, 2006)

Summary

Highly Recommended

- *Atlas of Clinical Sleep Medicine*, ed 2, Chapter 17
- Kryger M, Roth T, Dement WC, eds. *Principles and Practice of Sleep Medicine*, ed 6, Philadelphia: Elsevier; 2017. Section 17: Psychiatric Disorders

The blueprint for the sleep board examination indicates that the entire section incorporating neurology, psychiatry, and other medical conditions totals 12 questions. Thus, expect about four questions of the 240 on the exam to deal specifically with psychiatry disorders and sleep. Questions may also be about psychiatric medications in other parts of the exam. However, the examiners do not expect you to be a psychiatrist if you are not, but they do expect you to be able to recognize patients with mental disorders and advise about their sleep problems.

Anxiety Disorders

Panic Disorder

- Sleep symptoms
  - Sleep initiation and maintenance insomnia
  - Sleep deprivation can worsen daytime anxiety symptoms and can increase panic episodes
  - Half of the patients with panic disorder have sleep panic attacks
    - Awakening in a state of fear that may also manifest shortness of breath, palpitations, or sweating
- Treatment
  - CBT
  - Antianxiety medications

Posttraumatic Stress Disorder

- Awake symptoms
  - Reexperiencing the traumatic event
  - Irritability, outbursts of anger
  - Hypervigilance
  - Exaggerated startle response
- Sleep symptoms
  - Sleep-onset and sleep-maintenance insomnia
  - Awakening from recurrent nightmare, sometimes in a panic-like state
- PSG findings
  - Increased REM density
  - Increased fragmentation of REM sleep
  - Shorter episodes of REM sleep

- Treatment
  - ○ Comorbid conditions might require specific treatment
    - Depression and panic disorder
    - OSA
    - Alcohol or substance abuse
  - ○ Treatment
    - Psychotherapy
    - CBT for sleep and panic symptoms
    - Medications
      - ◆ Prazosin is emerging as an important treatment for sleep abnormalities

Depression (ATLAS2, Ch 17)

- Daytime symptoms
  - ○ Symptoms of depression
  - ○ Daytime fatigue
- Sleep-related symptoms: insomnia
  - ○ Difficulty falling asleep
  - ○ Difficulty staying asleep
  - ○ Restless sleep
  - ○ Early-morning awakening
  - ○ Decreased sleep time
  - ○ Nonrefreshing sleep
  - ○ Nightmares
- PSG findings
  - ○ Overall sleep
    - Long sleep latency
    - Increased wake after sleep onset (WASO)
    - Long awakening in early morning
    - Reduced total sleep time
  - ○ Sleep architecture
    - SWS
    - Decreased percentage of total sleep time
    - REM sleep
      - ◆ Short REM latency
      - ◆ Long first REM episodes
      - ◆ Increased eye density (percentage of REM time in which eyes are moving)
      - ◆ Increased REM as a percentage of total sleep time
- Pharmacotherapy
  - ○ Tricyclic antidepressants (TCAs)
    - TCAs suppress REM sleep
    - All are sedating except protriptyline
  - ○ Monoamine oxidase inhibitors (MAOIs)
    - All MAOIs suppress REM sleep
    - Most can cause insomnia
  - ○ SSRIs
    - All SSRIs suppress REM sleep
    - Most can cause insomnia
    - SSRIs can cause slow eye movements in NREM sleep
  - ○ Selective serotonin-norepinephrine reuptake inhibitors (SSNRIs)
    - Most SSNRIs can cause insomnia
  - ○ Other antidepressants
    - Trazodone
      - ◆ Decreases REM sleep
      - ◆ Increases SWS
      - ◆ Sedative
    - Nefazodone
      - ◆ Increases SWS
      - ◆ Sedative

- Bupropion
  - ◆ Can cause insomnia
  - ◆ Increases REM sleep
- Mirtazapine
  - ◆ Sedative
  - ◆ Weight gain can lead to sleep apnea

Schizophrenia

- Daytime symptoms
  - ○ Delusions, hallucinations, disorganized thoughts
  - ○ Daytime sleepiness when sleep deprivation or sleep apnea is present
- Nighttime symptoms
  - ○ Severe insomnia or no sleep
- PSG findings
  - ○ Sleep efficiency is reduced
  - ○ The amount of SWS is reduced
  - ○ About half of patients have a reduction in REM sleep latency
  - ○ Many have OSA
- Treatment
  - ○ First-generation antipsychotics
    - Reduced sleep latency
    - Improved total sleep time
    - Improved sleep efficiency
    - Inconsistent effects on REM sleep and SWS
  - ○ Second-generation antipsychotics
    - Reduced sleep latency
    - Improved total sleep time
    - Improved sleep efficiency
    - Inconsistent effects on SWS
      - ◆ Clozapine reduces SWS
      - ◆ Risperidone and olanzapine increase SWS

Medication and Substance Abuse

Alcohol

- Sleep problems in people with alcoholism
  - ○ Parasomnias, insomnia, daytime sleepiness
  - ○ Polyphasic sleep during binge drinking
- PSG findings
  - ○ Prolonged sleep latency, REM suppression, increased SWS
  - ○ With acute abstinence: frequent REM episodes, short NREM-REM cycles
  - ○ With recovery and abstinence: increased REM, short REM latency, reduced total sleep time

Stimulants

- Cocaine
  - ○ Use results in prolonged wakefulness
  - ○ Discontinuation results in a crash with an increase in both total sleep and REM sleep time followed by insomnia
- Amphetamines
  - ○ Increase sleep latency and decrease REM sleep
  - ○ Discontinuation results in REM rebound and increase in total sleep time
- MDMA (3,4-methylenedioxymethamphetamine, or ecstasy)
  - ○ Decreases total sleep time
  - ○ Does not affect REM sleep

- Methylphenidate
    - ○ Reduces total sleep time
    - ○ Increases REM latency and time in REM

Central Nervous System Depressant Agents

- Opioids
    - ○ All produce an increase in brief arousals and frequent sleep stage shifts
    - ○ With chronic use, tolerance occurs with suppression of REM sleep and less sleep fragmentation
    - ○ With discontinuation, sleep latency and latency to REM increase
    - ○ Opioids can cause hypoventilation or complex apnea
- Sedative hypnotics
    - ○ Abuse potential of modern hypnotics is low
    - ○ Many patients become dependent on hypnotics and wish to discontinue them
- Tetrahydrocannabinol (THC)
    - ○ In high doses, THC suppresses REM sleep
    - ○ REM rebound can occur with discontinuation

REFERENCES

Jaffe F, Markov D, Doghramji K. Sleep-disordered breathing: in depression and schizophrenia. *Psychiatry (Edgmont).* 2006;3(7):62–68.

Kryger MH, Avidan A, Berry R. *Atlas of clinical sleep medicine.* 2nd ed. Philadelphia: Saunders; 2014.

8.3   Other Disorders

QUESTIONS

Rounds on the Internal Medicine Ward

A pulmonary and sleep medicine fellow is making rounds with interns and residents on an internal medicine ward. He is preparing for the sleep medicine boards and has decided to ask sleep-related questions no matter what case is being presented.

1. The first patient on rounds has a 40-pack-year history of cigarette smoking, chronic productive cough, wheezing, and resting dyspnea. Lung examination reveals hyperresonance to percussion, and forced expiratory volume in 1 second (FEV_1) is 0.7 L. The patient reports poor quality sleep with sleep-onset insomnia and many awakenings during the night. Which of the following would likely have little or no effect on his sleep quality?
- **A.** Oxygen
- **B.** Theophylline
- **C.** Nicotine
- **D.** Nocturnal wheezing

2. The next patient he sees, a 42-year-old man, has been awakening every night with pain and then having trouble falling back to sleep. Pain that occurs 1 to 2 hours after sleep onset suggests which of the following conditions?
- **A.** Bone cancer
- **B.** Duodenal ulcer disease
- **C.** Rheumatoid arthritis
- **D.** Fibromyalgia

3. The third patient on rounds is an obese 57-year-old woman with puffy eyes, somnolence, and a receding hairline. She was admitted to the hospital several days earlier with somnolence. Her thyroid-stimulating hormone (TSH) level was 10 times normal, and a diagnosis of hypothyroidism was made. She has a history of snoring and witnessed apneas. Which statement about hypothyroidism and OSA is *correct*?
A. Thyroid treatment can worsen heart disease in patients with OSA
B. Few hypothyroid patients have OSA
C. Thyroid therapy increases the AHI
D. Hypothyroidism in the setting of OSA presents only with macroglossia

4. The next patient is a 50-year-old man admitted to the hospital with a history of profound weight loss. He has been complaining of night sweats, insomnia, nightmares, and palpitations. Holter monitoring revealed periods of atrial fibrillation (AF) during the night. What is the *most* likely diagnosis?
A. PTSD
B. Tuberculosis
C. Hyperthyroidism
D. Panic disorder

5. The next patient is an older man admitted several days earlier with a history of paroxysmal nocturnal dyspnea and coughing and severe sleep-onset insomnia. Chest radiography confirmed pulmonary edema, and he was treated in the intensive care unit (ICU) with intravenous diuretics. After the pulmonary edema resolved, the ICU nurses noted CSB. He continues to awaken frequently during the night. In patients with heart failure and CSB, when are arousals *most* likely to occur?
A. During the peak of hyperpnea
B. At the end of a central apnea
C. At the onset of a central apnea
D. During hypopneas

6. What treatment has been shown to best improve sleep *and* lessen CSB severity in patients with heart failure?
A. Supplemental oxygen
B. Temazepam
C. Medroxyprogesterone acetate
D. Protriptyline

7. The next patient was admitted with the rather embarrassing symptom of nocturnal diarrhea. Upper and lower endoscopy and tests for malabsorption were entirely negative. The patient complains of numbness in his feet. What is the *most* likely diagnosis?
A. Ulcerative colitis
B. Crohn disease
C. Irritable bowel syndrome
D. Diabetes mellitus

8. The final patient on rounds is a 49-year-old woman admitted for dialysis. She complains of severe daytime sleepiness and disrupted nocturnal sleep. What is the *least* likely finding on a sleep study in this patient?
A. CSB
B. Excessive movements of arms during REM sleep
C. Very high arousal index
D. Increased motor activity during wakefulness at the beginning of the night

ANSWERS

1. A.   The patient has chronic obstructive pulmonary disease by history. Although oxygen improves gas exchange, it has little effect on sleep structure or arousal frequency. The other factors mentioned can worsen sleep. Some hypnotics, such as ramelteon, may be safe in such patients.   (Fleetham et al, 1982; Roth, 2009)

2. B.   Insomnia is common in all the conditions listed. Patients with duodenal ulcers typically awaken with pain, or sometimes with the sensation of hunger, 1 to 2 hours after sleep onset. Or they might awaken at roughly the same time in the early morning. Pain improves with an antacid. Bone cancer pain can be severe and constant, not necessarily at any recurring time. Patients with rheumatoid arthritis have morning stiffness and pain shortly after they awaken. With fibromyalgia the main sleep-related symptom is nonrefreshing sleep.

3. A.   In hypothyroid patients with OSA, the AHI does not decrease significantly when euthyroidism is achieved. Treatment of hypothyroidism with thyroxine in the presence of OSA is potentially hazardous and can lead to cardiovascular complications such as nocturnal angina and cardiac arrhythmias. Management should include CPAP and low-dose thyroxine. (Grunstein and Sullivan, 1988)

4. C.   This is a classic description of hyperthyroidism. Patients with hyperthyroidism often have insomnia, nightmares, and night sweats. All the answers listed can cause night sweats and should be in the differential diagnosis. However, the presence of AF tips the diagnosis in favor of hyperthyroidism.   (ATLAS2, Ch 15.1)

5. A.   Although it seems logical that patients would arouse at the end of a central apnea, that is not the case. The arousals generally occur during the *peak* of a hyperpnea, which is when SaO_2 is at its nadir, and the work of breathing is at its peak. On the other hand, paroxysmal nocturnal dyspnea usually begins at the end of a central apnea. It is worth noting that CSB and heart failure may be present during wakefulness and tend to decrease during REM sleep; the cycle time may be quite long, with many breaths during the hyperpneic phase. Factors that increase sleep instability can trigger CSB.   (ATLAS2, pp 322–326)

6. A.   Oxygen has been shown to both improve CSB and improve sleep quality. Temazepam improves sleep but may have no effect on CSB.   (Biberdorf et al, 1993; Hanly et al, 1989)

7. D.   Patients with diabetes mellitus have many sleep problems, and about 50% complain of insomnia. This patient likely has severe neuropathy, which affects sleep by causing pain and numbness. When the neuropathy affects the gastrointestinal (GI) tract, the patient can develop nocturnal diarrhea. Patients can also have sleep disorders associated with diabetes-related kidney disease.   (ATLAS2, Ch 15.4)

8. B.   Patients in kidney failure have very severe sleep disruption, and about 50% complain of insomnia. RLS is extremely common in this group and is often difficult to treat. In addition, patients with kidney failure often have CSB. Although they have a very high arousal index related to limb movements, they do not have the features of REM sleep behavior disorder.   (ATLAS2, Ch 15.5)

Summary

Must Review

- *Atlas of Clinical Sleep Medicine*, ed 2, Chapter 14
- Kryger M, Roth T, Dement WC, eds. *Principles and Practice of Sleep Medicine*, ed 6, Philadelphia: Elsevier; 2017. Section 16: Other Medical Disorders

The blueprint for the sleep board examination indicates that the entire section on neurology, psychiatry, and other medical disorders totals 12 questions. Thus, expect about four questions of 240 on the exam to deal with the topic of other medical disorders (whatever that means). The examiners know that a sizable minority of test takers are not based in internal medicine but are pediatricians, otolaryngologists, and psychiatrists. In this summary, we focus on the common general medical conditions likely to be seen in a sleep disorders center.

Hyperthyroidism (ATLAS2, Ch 15.1)

- Sleep complaints
  - Insomnia
  - Nightmares
  - Night sweats
  - Palpitations
  - Atrial arrhythmias

Hypothyroidism (ATLAS2, Ch 15.1)

- Causes of sleep-wake abnormalities
  - Reduced metabolic rate
    - Can result in coma
  - OSA related to
    - Obesity
    - Macroglossia
- Sleep findings
  - EDS
  - OSA
  - Can develop respiratory failure
  - Bradycardia

Diabetes Mellitus (ATLAS2, Ch 15.4)

- Abnormalities causing sleep disturbance
  - Glycosuria
    - Nocturia
  - Peripheral neuropathy
    - Numbness
    - RLS
  - Autonomic neuropathy
    - Nocturnal diarrhea
    - Fixed cardiac rate during sleep

Heart Failure (ATLAS2, Ch 14.1)

- Causes of CSB
  - Long circulation time
  - Increased drive to breathe
  - Hypoxemia related to pulmonary edema
- Sleep symptoms
  - Sleep-onset insomnia
  - Restless sleep
  - RLS
  - Paroxysmal nocturnal dyspnea
- Sleep findings
  - CSB (variant of central sleep apnea)
    - Waxing and waning of ventilation
    - Long cycle and many breaths in each cycle of CSB
  - Arousals occur during peak of hyperpnea
  - CSB decreases during REM
  - Periodic limb movements are common
- Treatment
  - Oxygen
  - CPAP (in selected cases)
  - ASV

Acromegaly (ATLAS2, Ch 15.2)

- Hypersecretion of growth hormone
  - Anatomic changes that can lead to OSA
    - Skeletal, involving the face
    - Soft tissue, involving the tongue
    - Obesity

Kidney Failure (ATLAS2, Ch 15.5)

- Causes of insomnia in kidney failure
  - RLS caused by
    - Neuropathy from renal disease
    - Iron deficiency in patients on hemodialysis
  - Periodic movements and sleep
- CSB caused by
  - Acid-base abnormalities

Gastrointestinal Disorders (ATLAS2, Ch 15.3)

- Epigastric pain that awakens the patient can be caused by
  - Gastroesophageal reflux
  - Peptic ulcer disease
  - Pancreatic cancer
- Nocturnal diarrhea can be caused by
  - Inflammatory bowel disease
  - Diabetic neuropathy
  - Neoplasia in the GI tract
- Insomnia can be caused by
  - Any of the above
  - Insulinoma causing hypoglycemia

Fibromyalgia and Chronic Fatigue Syndrome (ATLAS2, Ch 16.4)

- Sleep-wake complaints are common
  - Insomnia
  - Nonrestorative sleep
  - Fatigue
- PSG findings
  - Long sleep latency
  - Low sleep efficiency
  - Increased nocturnal wakefulness
  - Long REM sleep latency
  - Decreased amount of REM sleep
  - Can have alpha-delta sleep pattern
  - Can have a reduction in sleep spindles

REFERENCES

Biberdorf DJ, Steens R, Millar TW, Kryger MH. Benzodiazepines in congestive heart failure: effects of temazepam on arousability and Cheyne-Stokes respiration. *Sleep*. 1993;16(6):529–538.

Fleetham J, West P, Mezon B, et al. Sleep, arousals, and oxygen desaturation in chronic obstructive pulmonary disease: the effect of oxygen therapy. *Am Rev Respir Dis*. 1982;126(3):429–433.

Grunstein RR, Sullivan CE. Sleep apnea and hypothyroidism: mechanisms and management. *Am J Med*. 1988;85:775–779.

Hanly PJ, Millar TW, Steljes DG, et al. The effect of oxygen on respiration and sleep in patients with congestive heart failure. *Ann Intern Med*. 1989;111(10):777–782.

Kryger MH, Avidan A, Berry R, eds. *Atlas of clinical sleep medicine*. 2nd ed. Philadelphia: Saunders; 2014.

Roth T. Hypnotic use for insomnia management in chronic obstructive pulmonary disease. *Sleep Med*. 2009;10(1):19–25.

Instrumentation and Testing in Sleep Medicine

QUESTIONS

New Technologist

1. A new technologist from a sleep clinic in Europe is joining your sleep center. He says that in his old lab, it was difficult to score sleep from the electroencephalogram (EEG). He wonders whether this was because of poor filter settings. You inform him that the proper low-pass and high-pass filters for EEG are:

	Low-Frequency Filter (Hz)	High-Frequency Filter (Hz)
A.	30	3500
B.	3	350
C.	0.3	35
D.	0.03	3.5

2. The technologist shows you a polygraph fragment (Fig. 9–1). He is not satisfied with the recoding. What type of filter do you advise?
   A. 0.3 Hz
   B. 6 Hz
   C. 60 Hz
   D. 300 Hz

3. The technologist needs guidance on the application of electrodes. What are the recommended impedances for EEG, electromyography (EMG), and electrooculography (EOG) for polysomnography (PSG)?
   A. 1 K-Ohm
   B. 5 K-Ohm
   C. 15 K-Ohm
   D. 60 K-Ohm

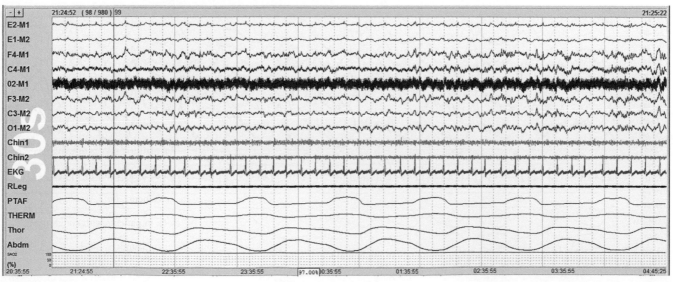

FIGURE 9–1 Question 2.

4. The reason that that E1 is below the L eye and E2 is above the R eye is
   A. To assess the patterns of slow eye movements in determining sleep onset
   B. To better determine rapid eye movements (REMs)
   C. To cause out-of-phase deflections with conjugate eye movements
   D. To help determine spike-wave activity

5. The technologist is tired of placing all the leads on patients undergoing polysomnography. He asks why he has to put 3 chin leads on the patient instead of 2. Your answer is that it is done this way to:
   A. Have a backup EMG in case one fails
   B. Help have a reference for EEG signals
   C. Improve the EMG signal quality
   D. Lateralize the EMG signal

6. Your sleep fellow brings her computer tablet into clinic to read sleep studies in between seeing patients. You comment that
   A. The clinic is too busy to read studies in between patients
   B. The recommended screen size is 15 inches for sleep studies
   C. The suggested Wi-Fi signal is at least 1000 mbps
   D. The tablet may not have enough computing power for sleep study interpretation

7. The M2 electrode is
   A. The right ear mastoid
   B. The mastoid EMG
   C. The middle central
   D. The middle reference

Questions 8 to 10 refer to the following image (Fig. 9–2).

8. What artifact is *most* notable in the above 30-second epoch?
   A. 60 Hz
   B. Blink
   C. Cardioballistic
   D. Sweat

9. What is the *most* effective physical method of managing the above artifact?
   A. Re-reference the electrodes
   B. Replace the electrode box
   C. Cool the room
   D. Replace all the electrodes

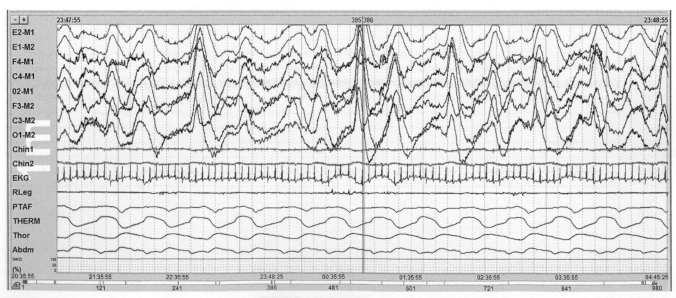

FIGURE 9–2 Questions 8 to 10.

10. If you need to add a filter to limit the artifact, you would *most* likely add a
  A. High-frequency filter
  B. Low-frequency filter
  C. Notch Filter
  D. No filter required

11. EEG recordings for polysomnography require three standard derivation areas, which include
  A. Frontal, central, and occipital
  B. Frontal, parietal, and occipital
  C. Parietal, central, and temporal
  D. Parietal, temporal, and occipital

12. The best EEG location for recording alpha activity (to determine wake vs. sleep) is
  A. Central
  B. Frontal
  C. Occipital
  D. Temporal

13. The best EEG location for recording spindles (to help determine stage N2 sleep) is
  A. Central
  B. Frontal
  C. Occipital
  D. Temporal

14. In order to prevent electrical injury, the polysomnography equipment has
  A. Electrical ground
  B. Copper wires
  C. Patient ground
  D. Silver sensors

Insomnia in a Graduate Student

A 24-year-old graduate student is referred with severe insomnia. It takes her hours to fall asleep, and her performance in school has suffered. The psychologist as part of the assessment before CBTi orders a test. On days 5 to 8, the student had morning classes. The result of the test is shown in Figure 9–3.

15. These data were collected by
  A. Accelerometer
  B. EEG
  C. Electrocardiogram (ECG)
  D. Microphone

16. What do the turquoise boxes likely indicate?
  A. Increased movements suggesting periodic limb movements
  B. Increased activity consistent with being awake
  C. Decreased activity consistent with sleep
  D. Artifact time when the testing device was removed

17. Actigraphy is *most* appropriate to aid in the diagnosis of
  A. Circadian rhythm disturbance
  B. Obstructive sleep apnea
  C. Restless legs syndrome (RLS)
  D. Parasomnias

18. What is the likeliest diagnosis?
  A. Advanced sleep-wake phase disorder
  B. Delayed sleep-wake phase disorder
  C. Irregular sleep-wake rhythm disorder
  D. Non–24-hour sleep-wake rhythm disorder

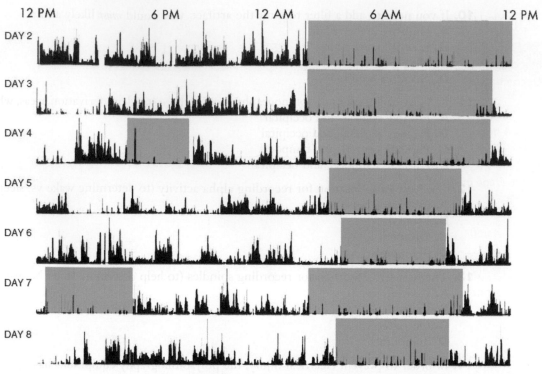

FIGURE 9–3 Questions 15 to 18.

Download. What Now?

A 65-year-old man with a progressive neuromuscular disease came to the sleep clinic because he was awakening with headaches, shortness of breath, and palpitations on his positive airway pressure (PAP) device and removing the mask in the early morning. Before getting his current device, he had been on continuous positive airway pressure (CPAP), which he could not tolerate. The download of his device is shown in Figure 9–4.

19. Does he meet current CMS (Medicare) adherence standards?
  A. Yes
  B. No
  C. Sometimes
  D. CMS does not have adherence standards

20. What type of device is he using?
  A. Standard bilevel
  B. Autotitrating PAP with a range of 8 to 15 cm H_2O pressure
  C. Bilevel spontaneous timed with a backup rate of 10 breaths/min
  D. Adaptive servoventilation (ASV) with pressure support of 8 to 15

21. Is there a clue to the reason for his new symptoms?
  A. There is a large mask leak
  B. He is not using the machine for enough hours each night
  C. The respiratory rate is too high
  D. He has a high apnea/hypopnea index on treatment

22. What is the *most* reasonable next step?
  A. Noninvasive ventilation
  B. Revert to autotitrating CPAP 5–20 cm H_2O
  C. Lower the respiratory rate on his current device to 8 breaths/min
  D. Lower the expiratory positive airway pressure (EPAP) on his current device to 6 cm H_2O

Compliance Report

Usage	03/26/2018 - 04/24/2018
Usage days	**30/30 days (100%)**
>= 4 hours	**15 days (50%)**
< 4 hours	**15 days (50%)**
Usage hours	127 hours 41 minutes
Average usage (total days)	4 hours 15 minutes
Average usage (days used)	4 hours 15 minutes
Median usage (days used)	4 hours 5 minutes

VPAP ST-A	
Serial number	22131590096
Mode	Spont Timed
IPAP	15 cmH2O
EPAP	8 cmH2O
Respiratory rate	10 bpm

Therapy					
Leaks - L/min	Median:	**0.0**	95th percentile:	**0.0**	Maximum:	**0.0**
Events per hour	AI:	**10.6**	HI:	**13.4**	AHI:	**24.0**

Usage - hours

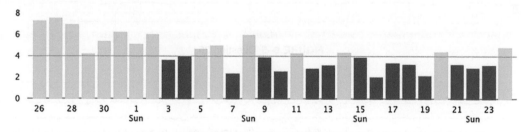

FIGURE 9–4 Questions 19 to 25.

23. What settings are required to prescribe BPAP?
   A. CPAP and inspiratory positive airway pressure (IPAP)
   B. APAP and EPAP
   C. IPAP and EPAP
   D. VPAP and IPAP

24. ASV should be *avoided* in which group of patients with central sleep apnea?
   A. CHF with left ventricular ejection fraction below 45%
   B. Cerebrovascular disease
   C. Opioid use
   D. PAP-emergent central sleep apnea

BONUS QUESTIONS

25. Autotitrating PAP therapy adjusts pressures based on
  A. Airflow resistance
  B. Oxygen saturation
  C. Nasal-oral thermistor
  D. Snoring volume

26. This fragment (Fig. 9–5) shows the required elements to score REM sleep *except*
  A. REMs
  B. Sawtooth waves
  C. Reduced or absent muscle tone
  D. Mixed-frequency EEG

27. What artifact is present in E2-M1 and Chin1 of this epoch (Fig. 9–6)?
  A. Sway artifact
  B. Sweat artifact
  C. Respiration artifact
  D. ECG artifact

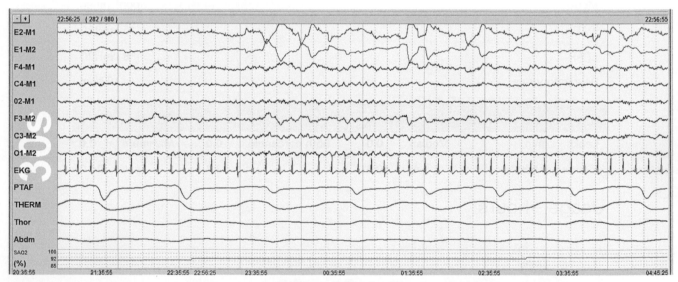

FIGURE 9–5 Question 26.

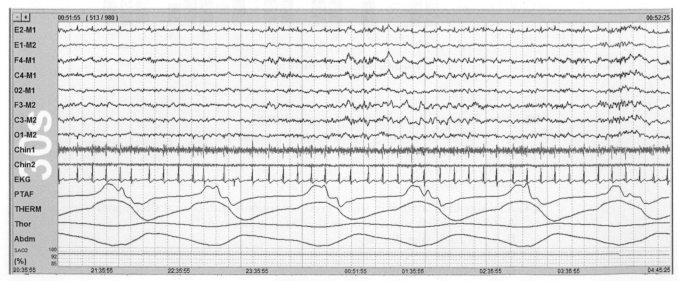

FIGURE 9–6 Question 27.

ANSWERS

1. C.   These are the correct settings for EEG filters. When applying these filters, you are trying to retain most of the activity that you would typically look at in an EEG, from delta waves in the 2-Hz range to beta activity in the midteen Hz, while filtering out much lower activity and much higher activity.   (Scoring Manual 2.5)

2. C.   The correct answer is 60 Hz. The purpose of the notch filter is to eliminate external electrical artifact from the signals. This filter, like all filters beyond the standard, should be applied judiciously so as to not filter out important clinical activity.   (Scoring Manual 2.5)

3. B.   This finding should be verified and documented by the technologist at the beginning of the study.   (Scoring Manual 2.5)

4. C.   The reason to have offset of the eye leads is to better demonstrate when eyes move conjugately. When this pattern occurs, the pattern on the polysomnogram is out of phase to one another. The cornea (front) has a positive polarity. The retina (back) has a negative polarity. EOG placement (LOC and ROC) is on the outer canthus of the eye, offset 1 cm below (LOC) and 1 cm above (ROC) the horizon.   (Scoring Manual 2.5)

5. A.   There are three leads such that if one lead fails, there is a backup so the technologist does not need to wake up the patient to reapply a sensor.   (Scoring Manual 2.5)

6. B.   The recommended screen size for interpretation is 15 inches; smaller screens may not allow the detail required to accurately review data. The recommended screen pixels should be 1600 horizontal and 1050 vertical at a minimum.

7. A.   The M2 is the right mastoid electrode used as a reference for the primary sleep EEG scoring leads (F3-M2, C3-M2, O1-M2). Refer to the 10-20 EEG image below for details of typical sleep electrode placement (Fig. 9–7).

8. D.   This PSG epoch represents sweat artifact (also known as sweat sway). It occurs when electrodes are connected across the head because of the salt contained in sweat. This causes the slow waves seen in the image above.

9. C.   The first step to treat sweat sway would less likely be to add a filter but to try to fix the sweat. One option might be to cool the room to see if the sweat can be lessened (e.g., adding a fan, lowering the temperature).

10. B.   If physical methods fail or are not an option in the situation, a filter should be added. If a filter is added, the correct filter would be a low-frequency filter because the sweat sway is 0.5 to 1 Hz in frequency, and a low-frequency filter would filter out low-frequency signals.

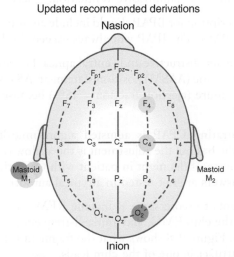

Updated recommended derivations

FIGURE 9–7 Answer 7. (From Hirshkowitz M, Sharafkhaneh A: Diagnostic assessment methods in adults. In Kryger M, Avidan A, Berry R, eds. *Atlas of Clinical Sleep Medicine*. St. Louis, 2014, Elsevier.)

11. A.   The correct derivations are frontal, central, and occipital. These are recorded on the right side of the head with backup recordings on the left side of the head.

12. C.   Alpha activity is generated primarily in the occipital region. Thus, the leads recording over this brain region are most helpful in determining the presence (or absence) of alpha activity.

13. A.   Spindle activity is most effectively captured via the central EEG leads.

14. A.   The relevant safety issue is that the PSG equipment should have an electrical ground to prevent any electrical injury to the patient. The patient ground is part of the EEG sensors and is not for safety but to limit electrical artifact. The wire and sensor compositions do not immediately affect safety.

15. A.   This shows data collected over a week using an accelerometer; the primary sensor in an actigraph. The black lines indicate movements. Actigraphy is often used to assess chronic insomnia and when circadian rhythm disorders are suspected.   (PPSM6, pp 1664)

16. C.   The regions highlighted by the turquoise boxes are periods with decreased movements, and the patient is likely asleep.

17. A.   Actigraphy assesses rest (as a surrogate for sleep) and wake times via measurement of movement. These patterns best assess timing of sleep and thus are best used to understand circadian rhythms. It cannot easily assess sleep apnea or parasomnias. Measurement of RLS can potentially be done via leg-based actigraphy, but it would not be a primary use of actigraphy

18. B.   This is an example of delayed sleep-wake phase disorder. Sleep occurs nightly roughly the same time well after midnight. Note that on day 7, the student is sleeping in the afternoon because of several nights of insufficient sleep.

19. B.   No. To meet CMS standards, the patient must use the device for 4 or more hours for 70% of the nights. He does not meet these standards because he spent only 50% of the nights with 4 or more hours.

20. C.   The reader should understand how to read downloads and be able to determine what type of machine the patient is using and what the settings are. Different companies may use different terms for the same device type. The patient is on a bilevel device with a backup rate of 10 breaths/min. Sleep specialists should be familiar with the types of available machines.

21. D.   The patient has a high AHI of 24 events per hour. His device is not adequately controlling his sleep-disordered breathing.

22. A.   In a patient with a progressive neuromuscular disease affecting the muscles of respiration, failure with CPAP, then bilevel, and then bilevel with a backup rate suggests that the next step should be noninvasive ventilation. There are several such devices on the market.

23. C.   A prescription for BPAP should include an inspiratory pressure (IPAP) and an expiratory pressure (EPAP). The IPAP will always exceed the EPAP, typically by 3 to 4 cm of water.

24. A.   ASV treats obstructive and central apnea. However, based on a 2016 American Academy of Sleep Medicine (AASM) position statement, ASV should not be used in patients with CSA with heart failure (ejection fraction < 45%) because this group had a higher mortality rate (all causes).

25. A.   Autotitrating CPAP is adjusted algorithmically in a manufacturer-specific manner. However, the basis of the adjustment is the airflow resistance. As increasing resistance occurs over the course of the night in patient with OSA, the PAP pressure is increased. The other possible answers are not tested in a typical autotitrating PAP machine.

26. C.   Elements to score stage R include REMs, sawtooth waves, absent or reduced muscle tone from the chin EMG, and a mixed-frequency EEG. This fragment did not include the chin EMG. Figure 9–8 shows what the fragment is like when chin EMG is included. Notice the ECG artifact in one of the chin leads.

27. D.   The two channels are showing an ECG artifact embedded into the traces.

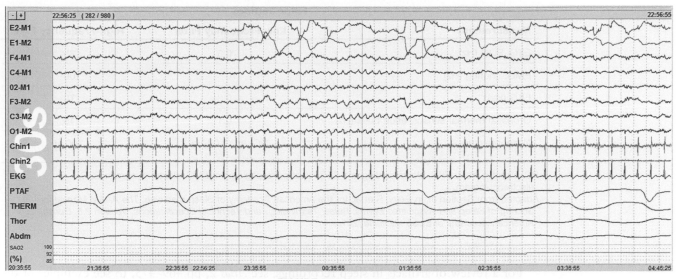

FIGURE 9–8 Answer 26.

Summary

Highly Recommended

- Section III. *AASM Manual for the Scoring of Sleep and Associated Events: Rules, Terminology, and Technical Specifications*, Version 2.5
- Chapter 18. Diagnostic assessment methods in adults. In: Kryger M, Avidan A, Berry R. (eds). *Atlas of Clinical Sleep Medicine*. Philadelphia, 2014, Elsevier

Topics You Should Know

This section was recently added to the last blueprint of the examination. It seems to be an afterthought and seems to be a work in progress. Expect only 12 or 13 questions on this content. The section is made up of questions covering three general topics: *Electrical Components (Sensors, Filters, Analog-Digital Convertors, Display)*

For this content. it is critical that Section III of the *AASM Manual—Technical and Digital Specifications* be reviewed. Key information to be known includes sampling rates and filter settings.

Measurement	Sampling Rates	
	Desirable (Hz)	Minimal (Hz)
High-frequency signals: For scoring of sleep (EEG, EOG, EMG) ECG Snoring	500	200
Medium-frequency signals Airflow (nasal pressure, end-tidal PcO_2, PAP device flow) Effort (ribcage and abdominal movement)	100	25
Low-frequency signals: O_2 (pulse oximetry, transcutaneous PO_2) CO_2 (transcutaneous PcO_2)	25	10

ECG, Electrocardiogram; *EEG,* electroencephalogram; *EMG,* electromyography *EOG,* electrooculography; *PAP,* positive airway pressure.

Adapted from Section III, in Berry, R et al; for the American Academy of Sleep medicine. *The AASM Manual for the Scoring of Sleep and Associated Events: Rules, Terminology and Technical Specifications. Version 2.5. Darien, IL: American Academy of Sleep Medicine. 2018.*

Filter Settings

Measurement	Low-Frequency Filter	High-Frequency Filter
EEG, EOG (Hz)	0.3	35
EMG, snoring (Hz)	10	100
EKG (Hz)	0.3	70
Oronasal thermal sensor, effort belts (Hz)	0.1	15
Nasal pressure	DC, or ≤0.03 Hz	100 Hz

DC, Direct current; *EKG,* electrocardiogram; *EEG,* electroencephalogram; *EMG,* electromyogram; *EOG,* electrooculogram.
Adapted from Section III, in Berry, R et al; for the American Academy of Sleep medicine. *The AASM Manual for the Scoring of Sleep and Associated Events: Rules, Terminology and Technical Specifications. Version 2.5. Darien, IL: American Academy of Sleep Medicine. 2018.*

For a review of artifacts in sleep recordings, see *Atlas 2*, pp 469–475, to see examples of the following: 60-Hz, crosstalk between channels, cardiac artifacts, and sweat artifact.

Technical Aspects of Sleep Devices (Actigraphy, Positive Airway Pressure, and Ventilatory Devices)

Actigraphy is used mainly as a surrogate to determine sleep time. Clinically, it is used to document insomnia and circadian rhythm abnormalities. Read *PPSM 6*, Chapter 171 for a discussion of actigraphy.

PAP devices for sleep apnea are reviewed in Johnson KG, Johnson DC: Treatment of sleep-disordered breathing with positive airway pressure devices: technology update. *Med Devices (Auckl).* 8:425–437, 2015.

Devices used in noninvasive ventilation are reviewed in Selim BJ, Wolfe L, Coleman JM 3rd, Dewan NA: Initiation of noninvasive ventilation for sleep related hypoventilation disorders: advanced modes and devices. *Chest.* 153(1):251–265, 2018.

Types of Positive Airway Pressure Devices

Mode	
CPAP	Constant EPAP = IPAP all night
BiPAP	Constant EPAP, IPAP, PS all night
AutoBiPAP	EPAP and IPAP typically adjust together in response to obstruction maintaining PS
BiPAP ST	Constant EPAP, IPAP, PS all night Backup rate ensures breath within time period Control inspiratory/expiratory lengths
SV	Fixed or auto-EPAP in response to obstruction Variable IPAP and PS targeting recent volumes or ventilation Backup rate and inspiratory and expiratory control
VAPS	Fixed or auto-EPAP in response to obstruction Variable IPAP and PS targeting set goal volume or ventilation Backup rate and inspiratory and expiratory control

BiPAP, Bilevel positive airway pressure; *BiPAP ST,* bilevel, spontaneous timed; *CPAP,* continuous positive airway pressure; *EPAP,* expiratory positive airway pressure; *IPAP,* inspiratory positive airway pressure; *PS,* pressure support; *SV,* servoventilation; *VAPS,* volume-assured pressure support. Data from Johnson KG, Johnson DC: Treatment of sleep-disordered breathing with positive airway pressure devices: technology update. *Med Devices (Auckl),* 8:425–437, 2015.

Using Positive Airway Pressure Devices

Mode	Pressure Adjustments	Patient Population	Limitations or Cautions
CPAP	• EPAP = IPAP, same throughout night	• OSA • CSA worsened by AutoCPAP	• Constant pressure can lead to intolerance or centrals in lateral position and NREM at pressures needed to treat REM or supine events
AutoCPAP	• EPAP = IPAP, changes throughout night in response to events	• OSA or unknown pressure requirements • OSA or unable to tolerate higher pressure all night	• Different devices change in response to different flow or snore changes and at different rates • High leak limits Auto functionality • Setting too low EPAP min can lead to undertreatment
BiPAP	• Constant EPAP, IPAP, PS all night	• OSA requiring high pressures • CPAP intolerance • Hypoventilation or hypoxia despite CPAP • Neuromuscular	• Constant pressure can lead to intolerance or centrals in lateral position and NREM at pressures needed to treat events in REM or supine position
AutoBiPAP	• EPAP and IPAP typically adjust together in response to obstruction • Some devices change EPAP and IPAP independently	• BiPAP need with unknown pressure requirements • BiPAP need: unable to tolerate higher pressure all night	• Respironics EPAP and IPAP can change independently, leading to different pressure support but not to hypoventilation • Setting too low EPAP min can lead to undertreatment
BiPAP ST	• Constant EPAP, IPAP, PS all night • Backup rate ensures breath within time period • Inspiratory and expiratory control	• COPD, obesity hypoventilation with hypoxia, and hypoventilation despite BiPAP • Hypoventilation • Neuromuscular • Narcotic-induced centrals	• Backup rate can worsen periodic centrals by forcing breath when CO_2 low • Respironics inspiration time limits only activated with timed breaths
SV (ASV and BiPAP AutoSV)	• Fixed or auto-EPAP in response to obstruction • Variable IPAP and PS targeting recent volumes or ventilation • Backup rate and +/– inspiratory and expiratory control	• Complex sleep apnea or treatment-emergent CSA • Periodic breathing and Cheyne-Stokes respiration	• Caution if low EF and primarily CSA at baseline • Can worsen hypoventilation because targets are lower than recent average ventilation
VAPS (IVAPS and AVAPS)	• Fixed or auto-EPAP in response to obstruction • Variable IPAP and PS targeting set goal volume or ventilation • Backup rate and +/– inspiratory and expiratory control	• Patients with differing pressure requirements in REM and NREM or supine and nonsupine, causing centrals or intolerance despite BiPAP • Hypoventilation despite BiPAP • COPD • Obesity hypoventilation • Narcotic-induced centrals • Neuromuscular	• Ventilation can vary greatly with AVAPS volume target if respiratory rate changes • IVAPS patient rate drops to second or third set rate during spontaneous breathing

ASV, Adaptive servoventilation; *AVAPS,* average positive airway pressure; *BiPAP,* bilevel positive airway pressure; *BiPAP ST,* Bilevel, spontaneous timed; *COPD,* chronic obstructive pulmonary disease; *CPAP,* continuous positive airway pressure; *CSA,* central sleep apnea; *EF,* left ventricular ejection fraction; *EPAP,* expiratory positive airway pressure; *IPAP,* inspiratory positive airway pressure; *IVAPS,* intelligent volume-assured pressure support; *NREM,* non–rapid eye movement; *OSA,* obstructive sleep apnea; *PS,* pressure support; *REM,* rapid eye movement; *SV,* servoventilation; *VAPS,* volume-assured pressure support. Data from Johnson KG, Johnson DC: Treatment of sleep-disordered breathing with positive airway pressure devices: technology update. *Med Devices (Auckl),* 8:425–437, 2015.

Adaptive Servoventilation

- Continuously changes the inspiratory PS on a breath-by-breath basis and during apneas
- Goal: Even out the breathing variation by targeting recent average ventilation or volume
- Especially for the treatment of periodic breathing or treatment-emergent central apneas; not currently recommended for Cheyne-Stokes respiration in heart failure

	ResMed ASV and Auto ASV	Respironics BiPAP AutoSV Advanced
ASV adjustments	ASV: fixed EPAP ASVAuto: adjusts with AutoSet algorithm	EPAPmin and EPAPmax: pressure testing mode like AutoCPAP (increase 1 every 15 second if at least two obstructive events)
PS adjustments	PS adjusted every 1/50 of a second throughout inspiration based on difference of flow from expected flow to achieve a goal ventilation with smooth waveform. During apneic periods, PS gradually increases with subsequent breaths to a maximum of 10. Limited by PSmin and PSmax.	Current breath's starting PS based on prior breath's PS and how far previous breath was from target volume with gain determined from the PS needed to reach a volume during the last 30 breaths. Intrabreath adjustment of PS based on flow just before halfway point of inspiratory cycle if expected volume differs from target volume. Limited by PSmin and PSmax.

ASV, Adaptive servoventilation; *CPAP*, continuous positive airway pressure; *EPAP*, expiratory positive airway pressure; *PS*, pressure support. Adapted from Johnson KG, Johnson DC: Treatment of sleep-disordered breathing with positive airway pressure devices: technology update. *Med Devices (Auckl)*, 8:425–437, 2015. Tab 4.

Volume-Assured Pressure Support

- Continuously changes the inspiratory PS on a breath-by-breath basis
- Goal: Achieve an average target volume or ventilation over a few breaths to achieve stable ventilation throughout the night
- Average VAPS (Respironics) targets set tidal volume
- Intelligent VAPS (ResMed) targets set estimated alveolar ventilation
- Useful for patients with combined periodic breathing and hypoventilation or patients with REM-related hypoventilation related to conditions such as chronic obstructive pulmonary disease, neuromuscular disorders, or obesity who may need different pressure support levels at different times of the night

	iVAPS	AVAPS
EPAP adjustment	Fixed EPAP	AVAPS: fixed EPAP AVAPS AE: set EPAPmin and EPAPmax with REMstar AutoCPAP-like protocol
PS adjustment	If expected flow differs from target flow, PS adjustments are made every 1/50 second throughout inspiration to achieve goal ventilation with smooth transition.	Determines average PS provided over prior 2 min to achieve volume. If target volume differs from average recent ventilation (6 breaths), PS for next breath is changed at rate of 1/min if recent stable breathing and 0.5/min if unstable breathing. (AE model allows maximum rate of pressure change from 1 to 5/min.)

AE, Auto EPAP; *AVAPS*, average positive airway pressure; *EPAP*, expiratory positive airway pressure; *IVAPS*, intelligent volume-assured pressure support; *PS*, pressure support. Adapted from Johnson KG, Johnson DC: Treatment of sleep-disordered breathing with positive airway pressure devices: technology update. *Med Devices (Auckl)*, 8:425–437, 2015. Tab 5.

Element	Titration Adjustments
Obstruction	▲ Pressures (EPAP)
Hypoventilation	Higher pressure support (▲IPAP/TVa/TV/PSmin) (Higher RR) ▼ Ti and rise time for COPD ▲ Ti, ▼ rise time for OHS
PB, CSR, mixed events	▼ Pressures (EPAP)/▼ PS(IPAP/TVa/TV/PSmin) Increase RR to decrease TV (ASV/IVAPS) Oxygen to stabilize
Irregular centrals (narcotic)	Backup rate
Insufficient effort (Neuro)	Backup rate, high trigger
Baseline hypoxia	Treat obstruction, hypoventilation Oxygen (more with higher pressures caused by FiO_2 dilution)

ASV, Adaptive servoventilation; *COPD,* chronic obstructive pulmonary disease; *EPAP,* expiratory positive airway pressure; *FiO₂,* Fraction of inspired oxygen; *IPAP,* inspiratory positive airway pressure; *IVAPS,* intelligent volume-assured pressure support; *PS,* pressure support; *RR,* respiratory rate; *Ti,* inspiratory time; *TV,* tidal volume; *TVa,* tidal volume assured. Data from Johnson KG, Johnson DC: Treatment of sleep-disordered breathing with positive airway pressure devices: technology update. *Med Devices (Auckl),* 8:425–437, 2015.

Setting	Normal	COPD	Hypoventilation	Restrictive or Neuromuscular
Ti (second)	0.3–2.0	0.3–1.0	0.8–2.0	0.8–1.5
Rise time (msec)	300	150	150–300	300
Trigger	Medium	Medium	Medium to high	High
Cycle	Medium	High	Low to medium	Low

COPD, Chronic obstructive pulmonary disease; *Ti,* inspiratory time. Adapted from Johnson KG, Johnson DC: Treatment of sleep-disordered breathing with positive airway pressure devices: technology update. *Med Devices (Auckl),* 8:425–437, 2015. Tab 3.

Electrical Safety

There is surprisingly little published about electrical safety in sleep medicine. The term "safety" does not appear in the *Manual.* It is recommended that the reader review page 1182 of Patil SP: What every clinician should know about polysomnography. *Respir Care.* 55(9):1179–1195, 2010.

Pediatrics: Not Gone and Not Forgotten

QUESTIONS

Terrified New Parents

A healthy term baby is born and is about to be taken home by the excited parents. It is their first child. A distant cousin had a newborn who died of sudden infant death syndrome (SIDS). They ask the doctor about how to minimize the risk of SIDS in the new baby. Pick the best answer for each of the next three questions.

1. What is the best place for the new baby to sleep?
   A. In the bed with the parents
   B. In a crib in a nearby separate quiet bedroom
   C. In a crib with a soft mattress and comforting stuffed animals near the parents
   D. In a crib with a firm, safe surface in the parents' bedroom for 6 to 12 months

2. What is the best position for the baby to sleep in?
   A. Flat on his or her back
   B. Prone to prevent risk of reflux and aspiration
   C. It doesn't matter
   D. Sleeping on either side

3. What home monitoring device is best to prevent SIDS?
   A. Oximeter
   B. Chest wall sensor
   C. Monitoring has not been shown to reduce SIDS
   D. Auditory monitoring

Insomnia in Youngsters

4. A 10-month-old infant is able to fall asleep quickly and easily on her own while drinking from her bottle of milk in her crib at bedtime. After 2 to 3 hours of sleep, however, she wakes three or four more times at night, and her parents have to come in and give her another bottle to get her back to sleep. What is the likely diagnosis?
   A. Behavioral insomnia of childhood, sleep onset association type
   B. Behavioral insomnia of childhood, limit-setting type
   C. Behavioral insomnia of childhood, dependent type
   D. Behavioral insomnia of childhood, feeding disorder type

5. Jake, an 8-year-old third grader, begins stalling just before bedtime. "I'm not sleepy at all!" Jake will say. Or, "Can I stay up late with you and Dad to watch a movie?" He often asks for several drinks of water and extra hugs after lights out, and it takes a long time to put him to sleep. Jake's parents have begun letting him fall asleep near them on the living room couch each night and moving Jake to his own bed later. What is the likely diagnosis?
   A. Behavioral insomnia of childhood, limit-setting sleep disorder
   B. Behavioral insomnia of childhood, delayed bedtime type
   C. Behavioral insomnia of childhood, sleep onset association type
   D. Behavioral insomnia of childhood, sleep onset association and limit-setting type

6. Behavioral insomnia of childhood, sleep onset association type, means that the child
   A. Requires an extended amount of time and special conditions to fall asleep
   B. Requires conditions that are problematic or demanding
   C. Requires caregiver intervention for the child to return to sleep at night
   D. All of the above

7. What is the earliest age at which you can address sleep onset associations?
   A. Around 6 months
   B. Around 9 months when children begin crawling
   C. Around 18 months when children can use two-word sentences
   D. Around 2 years when children have a vocabulary of about 75 words and can express themselves more fully

8. Positive sleep onset associations include
   A. The use of a security object
   B. Thumb sucking
   C. Bottle feeding and rocking
   D. A and B

9. When giving a parent a consistent bedtime routine to try with an 18-month-old child who has behavioral insomnia of childhood and who currently takes up to 2 hours to fall asleep, the parent should be advised to
   A. Make the bedtime temporarily later to match the time when the child is actually falling asleep
   B. Make the bedtime earlier so that the child falls asleep by the appropriate bedtime even if he or she stalls
   C. Remove the daytime nap temporarily so that the child is very tired at bedtime
   D. Allow the child to fall asleep in the parents' bed to limit stalling behaviors at the end of the routine and then move the child to his or her own bed later

10. If you want to prepare parents for what is likely to happen when they begin teaching a child with behavioral insomnia of childhood to fall asleep independently at bedtime, what should you tell them?
    A. Their child's crying and protesting may get worse before it gets better
    B. Their child's crying and protesting may be worse on the second night than the first night
    C. Their child will sustain no long-term psychological harm if a parent uses a positive, consistent bedtime routine along with extinction or graduated extinction to teach self-soothing
    D. All of the above

Jaundice and Breathing Pauses

A 3-day-old infant is admitted for phototherapy because of jaundice. While under lights, he is noted to have pauses in breathing. Head ultrasound is normal. He undergoes polysomnography (PSG), which showed 3 minutes of the breathing pattern shown in Figure 10–1 (a 2-minute epoch is shown). His total sleep time was 8 hours (480 minutes) during the study.

11. Of the following, the pattern is most consistent with
    A. Cheyne-Stokes breathing (CSB)
    B. Periodic breathing
    C. Obstructive sleep apnea (OSA)
    D. Hypoventilation

12. Which of the following is most characteristic of this finding?
    A. It indicates neurologic dysfunction and requires further workup
    B. It is associated with a higher prevalence of sudden infant death syndrome
    C. It worsens over the first month of life
    D. It is a common finding in infants younger than 2 weeks of age

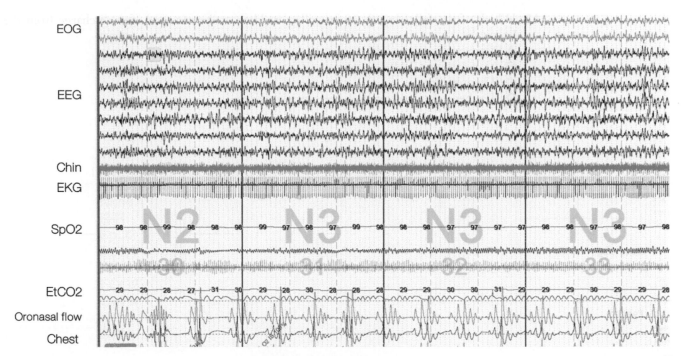

FIGURE 10–1 Questions 11 to 13.

13. Of the following, the next step in management is
   A. Administration of theophylline
   B. Initiation of supplemental oxygen
   C. Intubation and positive-pressure ventilation
   D. Observation and reassurance

Blue Newborn

A 3-day-old full-term infant is transferred to the newborn intensive care unit because he develops hypoxemia with sleep associated with pauses in breathing. When awake, he had no difficulty feeding, and his examination findings were normal. He is initially placed on continuous positive airway pressure (CPAP) but then requires intubation and positive-pressure ventilation. His chest radiograph is clear. A head ultrasound is normal. Attempts to decrease his ventilatory support result in hypercarbia.

14. Of the following, which test will most likely make the diagnosis in this child?
   A. Echocardiography
   B. Head magnetic resonance imaging (MRI)
   C. *PHOX2B* gene mutation testing
   D. Polysomnography

15. Associated sequelae of this disease include all of the following *except*
   A. Autonomic dysregulation
   B. Brain arteriovenous malformations
   C. Hirschsprung disease
   D. Neural crest tumors

16. Of the following, the most likely physiologic abnormality during sleep is
   A. CSB
   B. Decreased tidal volume
   C. Increased ventilatory response to elevated PcO_2
   D. Obstructive apneas

17. Which of the following therapies will most likely to be required after discharge from the hospital?
  A. Nasogastric feeds
  B. Noninvasive CPAP
  C. Theophylline
  D. Tracheostomy and positive-pressure ventilation

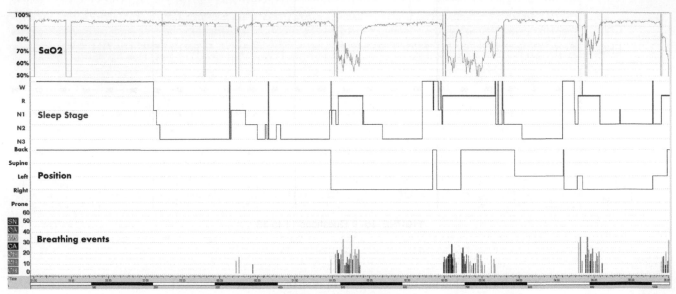

FIGURE 10–2 Question 18.

Failure to Thrive

18. The parents of a 4.5-year-old boy were concerned about his failure to thrive. Although born healthy at term, his weight was only 10 kg at the age of 4.5 years. A 9.5-hour sleep study was done, and the hypnogram (Fig. 10–2) is shown above. What is the main finding?
  A. The apparent oxygen desaturations are probably artifacts
  B. Events only occurred when the child was on his back
  C. Significant apnea occurred whenever he went into rapid eye movement (REM) sleep
  D. The findings are highly suggestive of central hypoventilation syndrome (CCHS)

ASHD?

A 6-year-old obese boy is referred because of snoring and witnessed apneas. He usually sleeps for 11 hours a night. His teachers report inattention and hyperactivity at school. Exam reveals 4+ tonsils. PSG shows an obstructive apnea/hypopnea index (AHI) of 4/hr.

19. Of the following, which is the most likely counsel that should be given to the family?
  A. He does not have OSA because his AHI is normal
  B. He is excessively sleepy because his nocturnal sleep duration is long
  C. CPAP is the first line of therapy for this child
  D. Hyperactivity may be a result of OSA

20. Which of the following is the most likely effect of adenotonsillectomy in this child?
  A. Decrease in AHI
  B. Decrease in body mass index (BMI)
  C. Improvement in attention
  D. Improvement in executive function

21. The most likely reason for persistent OSA after adenotonsillectomy in this child is
   A. White race
   B. Obesity
   C. Severity of OSA
   D. Tonsillar size

Trisomy 21

A 4-year-old boy with Down syndrome is referred from the genetics clinic for evaluation of possible sleep-disordered breathing. According to his parents, he sleeps well at night and snores softly, although he does mouth breathe on occasion. He is well rested in the morning when he wakes up.

22. What is the best next step in the evaluation and management of this child?
   A. An overnight polysomnogram (PSG)
   B. Evaluation by an otolaryngologist
   C. A trial of nasal corticosteroids
   D. Watchful waiting and reassurance
   E. Overnight oximetry

23. This child's PSG shows a severe OSA (AHI of 18.7/hr with SpO_2 of 70%). He is scheduled for adenotonsillectomy. Which is the following is recommended for preoperative care of this patient?
   A. Overnight observation after the study
   B. A follow-up polysomnogram 3 months after surgery
   C. Minimal dosing of opiate-based analgesics
   D. Assessment of the upper airway
   E. All of the above

24. The patient had adenotonsillectomy without complication. After surgery, the patient was sleeping better. However, a postoperative polysomnogram obtained 3 months later showed persistent severe OSA (AHI of 11/hr and SpO_2 nadir of 85%). Treatment options for persistent OSA after adenotonsillectomy include
   A. Evaluation and treatment for hypothyroidism
   B. Craniofacial surgery
   C. Lingual tonsillectomy
   D. Rapid maxillary expansion
   E. All of the above

Mouth Breather

A 5-year-old girl presents to the sleep center for consultation. History is significant for habitual loud snoring, mouth breathing, restless sleep, primary enuresis, frequent morning headaches, difficulty with concentration and attention, and hyperactivity. Sleep-related diaphoresis is also present. On physical examination, her tonsils are only mildly enlarged (2+), and the Mallampati score is 2 sitting and 4 supine. The palate is elongated and highly arched. Answer the next five questions.

25. Which of the following is most characteristic of mouth breathing?
   A. Snoring
   B. Attention and concentration difficulties
   C. Mallampati score of 4 supine
   D. Elongated highly arched palate
   E. Restless sleep

26. Which of the following is true of this patient?

A. Mild tonsillar enlargement (2+) on physical examination rules out pediatric OSA

B. A negative home study result most often rules out pediatric OSA

C. A laboratory-based polysomnogram is indicated before adenotonsillectomy

D. Immediate AutoPap titration is indicated

E. Home pulse oximetry should be done to rule out sleep-related hypoxemia

27. If moderately severe pediatric OSA is diagnosed, which of the following is the first line of treatment?

A. Adenotonsillectomy

B. CPAP

C. Rapid maxillary expansion

D. Uvulopalatal pharyngoplasty

E. An oral appliance

28. A clinically significant obstructive hypopnea in this patient is best defined as a respiratory event that

A. Lasts for at least 2 respiratory efforts

B. Is associated with at least a 50% fall in the thermal signal

C. Is associated with oxygen desaturation greater than or equal to 1% from the baseline

D. Is associated with changes in the peripheral pulse volume

E. Is associated with elevation of carbon dioxide greater than 50 mm Hg for 2 breaths

29. In this patient, a respiratory effort–related arousal (RERA) is present if

A. Airflow measured by pressure transduction falls 50% from the baseline associated with a 3% oxygen desaturation from baseline

B. End-tidal CO_2 rises above 55 mm Hg associated with cardiac deceleration and a 2% desaturation from the oxygen saturation baseline

C. Post-sigh respiratory pauses occur lasting 21 seconds followed by an arousal, awakening, or both

D. Airflow measured by RIP signal falls by 10% from the baseline and is associated with an arousal, awakening, snoring, or increased work of breathing

Low SaO₂ in the Nursery

A 38⅞ weeks' gestation newborn was about to be discharged to home from the normal newborn nursery on day of life 2 when the baby's nurse noted some duskiness of the infant's hands and feet as well as mild perioral cyanosis during sleep. Oxygen saturation monitor revealed an SpO_2 of 80% and heart rate of 95 beats/min. The nurse noted there was no visible respiratory effort at the time. The baby was easily aroused and became pink, and his oxygen saturation rose to 98% while on room air.

30. The next best step in the management of this patient is which of the following?

A. Intubation to assure a patent upper airway

B. Immediately give a loading dose of caffeine to stimulate respiration

C. Order home sleep testing to be done after discharge

D. Send the patient home on an apnea and bradycardia monitor

E. Nocturnal PSG to evaluate the patient's sleep-related respiratory and ventilatory status

31. Which of the following criteria is required for diagnosis of primary central sleep apnea of infancy?

A. Carbon dioxide level greater than 50 mm Hg for more than 25% of the total sleep time

B. Oxygen saturation nadir less than 85% on pulse oximetry

C. Central apneas lasting 12 seconds in length associated with electrocardiogram deceleration of 10% from the baseline on home sleep testing

D. Periodic breathing occurring during 2% of the total sleep time

E. Identification of a prolonged central apnea lasting greater than 20 seconds

32. The infant is diagnosed with primary central apnea of infancy, with carbon dioxide levels staying about 48 mm Hg. Which treatment should be considered?
A. CPAP
B. Oxygen
C. Tracheostomy and mechanical ventilation
D. Acetazolamide

ANSWERS

1. D. Recent recommendations by the American Academy of Pediatrics indicate that the child should sleep on a safe surface in the parents' bedroom for the first 6 to 12 months. Co-sleeping has been associated with increased risk to the newborn. The crib should not contain items such as stuffed animals. (Moon, 2016)

2. A. The back to sleep movement has resulted in a substantial reduction in the prevalence of SIDS. Scientifically poor advice that ignored epidemiologic studies resulted in an epidemic of SIDS around the world. (Obladen, 2017)

3. C. Despite improvements in home monitoring techniques, studies to date have not shown that monitoring reduces the incidence of SIDS. Despite the data, many anxious parents still monitor their newborns. (Adams et al, 2009; Strehle et al, 2012)

4. A. *Behavioral insomnia of childhood, sleep onset association type*, is the correct answer. This diagnosis is made when a child needs a special condition to fall asleep and then requires caregiver interventions to return to sleep during the night. For this and the following two questions, understanding the diagnostic categories is imperative. (ICSD3)

5. D. *Behavioral insomnia of childhood, sleep onset association type and limit-setting type*, is the correct answer. This combined type of behavioral insomnia of childhood is diagnosed when a child both stalls or delays at bedtime and falls asleep in a setting other than his or her own bed.

6. D. *Behavioral insomnia of childhood, sleep onset association type*, involves all three of these.

7. A. Six months is typically the age when almost all healthy babies are physically and neurologically able to sleep 11 to 12 hours without a feeding. Teaching 6-month-old infants to fall asleep independently at bedtime helps to develop good sleep skills from a very young age and often improves sleep significantly for both the child and the other members of the family. (Burnham et al, 2002)

8. D. Positive sleep associations are ones that do not require parental assistance. (Vriend and Corkum, 2011)

9. A. This technique is known as *bedtime fading* and is often very successful at teaching a child to fall asleep quickly and successfully with the improved bedtime routine in his or her own bed. When the new routine is working well, the bedtime can gradually be moved earlier to a more age-appropriate bedtime. Taking away the daytime nap is almost never advisable and almost always worsens nighttime sleep. Allowing a child to fall asleep in a place other than his or her own bed causes sleep onset association–related problems because the child never becomes used to falling asleep in his or her own bed at bedtime. (Piazza et al, 1997)

10. D. Parents should be aware of *all of the above* and should also be prepared for short-term, worst-case scenarios such as some reflux after a period of crying. By teaching children to fall asleep independently, parents will have provided their children with a very important skill. This will also allow children to obtain more sleep at night, which improves growth, development, and daytime functioning. (Hiscock and Wake, 2002; Gradisar et al, 2016)

11. B. The study is consistent with periodic breathing, which is defined as the presence of more than three episodes of central pauses lasting more than 3 seconds separated by less than 20 seconds of normal breathing. The end-tidal CO_2 does not demonstrate hypoventilation; the values are low because of tachypnea. There is absent airflow and inspiratory effort, so it is consistent with central, not obstructive, apnea. CSB is characterized by crescendo and decrescendo change in breathing amplitude with cycle length of greater than 40 seconds.   (MANUAL2)

12. D. Periodic breathing is a common finding in healthy full-term infants, occurring in up to 78% of infants 0 to 2 weeks of age. Periodic breathing usually comprises less than 1% of the total sleep time and resolves by 6 months of life. Higher percentages of periodic breathing or persistence after 6 months of life might indicate underlying disease process and the need for further evaluation.   (Kelly et al, 1985)

13. D. The periodic breathing should resolve over the next few weeks of life.

14. C. The infant has congenital CCHS, which is associated with mutations in the paired-like homeobox 2B (*PHOX2B*) gene. PSG might reveal hypoventilation and central apneas but would not be sufficient to make the diagnosis. Although MRI and cardiac echocardiography are recommended for evaluation, they would likely be normal in this infant.   (Weese-Mayer et al, 2010)

15. B. CCHS is associated with Hirschsprung disease, neural crest tumors, autonomic instability, and cardiac dysrhythmias but not brain arteriovenous malformations.

16. B. CCHS is associated with decreased tidal volume, worse during sleep, particularly non-REM (NREM) sleep. It is associated with *decreased* ventilatory response to hypoxemia and hypercarbia. It is not usually associated with obstructive apneas or CSB.

17. D. This child will most likely need a tracheostomy and positive-pressure ventilation to ensure optimal oxygenation and ventilation to prevent neurologic sequelae. Noninvasive CPAP alone would be insufficient to ensure adequate ventilation and is not recommended for consideration until the child is older. Theophylline is not proven effective therapy for CCHS. Nasogastric feeds are not indicated because there is no history of swallowing or feeding intolerance.

18. C. Severe oxygen desaturation occurred only in REM sleep. There is no reason to suspect that the findings in REM were artifacts. The oxygen desaturations occurred when he was on his back and side. The findings are not suggestive of CCHS because hypoventilation is present from birth in such cases, and the hypoventilation events are actually more common in NREM sleep. This patient was found to have congenital myasthenia gravis and was treated with a bilevel pressure device and pyridostigmine, which resulted in a gain of weight. Two important messages here are that sleep apnea in children can cause failure to thrive and that the cause of the apnea needs to be determined.

19. D. OSA in children can present with hyperactivity and inattention. Pediatric criteria for OSA include obstructive AI of 1/hr or greater or AHI 2/hr or greater, so this child has mild OSA. For a 6-year-old child, a sleep duration of 10 to 13 hours is considered normal. Adenotonsillectomy, not CPAP, is considered first-line treatment for children with OSA.

20. A. Compared with watchful waiting, adenotonsillectomy improves quality of life, symptoms of OSA, and obstructive events on PSG (obstructive AHI and AI). However, there is no evidence that it improves attention or executive function. BMI does not decrease and often increases after treatment.   (Marcus et al, 2013)

21. B. Persistent OSA after adenotonsillectomy has been associated with obesity, black race, and more severe OSA. There is no association with preoperative tonsillar size.

22. A. Children with Down syndrome commonly have OSA, with an incidence of greater than 50% vs. 3% in healthy nonobese children. This is because of a combination of multiple factors, including low tone, midfacial hypoplasia, macroglossia, and narrow nasal passages. A polysomnographic is recommended for all children with Down syndrome in the first four years of life. Evaluation by an otolaryngologist is reasonable but only necessary if the sleep test shows significant OSA. Nasal corticosteroids may be helpful for documented mild OSA. Overnight oximetry can miss occult sleep apnea and is not recommended for screening if PSG is available.   (Alsubie and Rosen, 2017; Bull and Committee on Genetics, 2011)

23. E. Children with severe OSA are at high risk of preoperative complications because of a combination of factors, including narrow airways and antecedent sleep disruption, although the risk of complication in healthy children is low. Thus, all children with severe OSA should be observed after adenotonsillectomy. Research has documented that children with recurrent hypoxemia may have a 10-fold increase in sensitivity to opiates, so dosing most be very cautious. Finally, children with severe OSA may also have other causes of airway obstruction such as turbinate hypertrophy, lingual tonsillar enlargement, or laryngomalacia, so careful evaluation of the upper airway may be helpful. Finally, postoperative PSG is recommended to see if the sleep apnea has resolved because many patients with severe OSA may have persistent OSA after adenotonsillectomy.   (Alsufyani et al, 2017; Brown and Moss, 2007; Brown, 2011; Guilleminault et al, 2007; Konstantinopoulou et al, 2015)

24. E. Children with Down syndrome have multiple risk factors for OSA, and persistent OSA after adenotonsillectomy is common. Risk factors include lingual tonsillectomy, hypothyroidism, maxillary restriction, and craniofacial deficits (including midfacial hypoplasia). Treatment options should be individualized based on each patient's needs, and a multispecialty approach is often best. CPAP is also a treatment option but may be difficult for patients with Down syndrome to tolerate.   (Austeng et al, 2014)

25. D. Snoring, attention and concentration difficulties, restless sleep, and a Mallampati grade 4 airway have all been associated with pediatric OSA. Chronic mouth breathing is also associated with pediatric OSA, but chronic mouth breathing in the absence of other craniofacial abnormalities often results in palatal elongation.

26. C. According to the American Academy of Otolaryngology Head and Neck Surgery guidelines   (Roland et al, 2011) for PSG before adenotonsillectomy, laboratory-based PSG is indicated and recommended before surgery if signs and symptoms are discordant. This patient's signs are consistent with but not diagnostic of pediatric OSA. The patient is otherwise normal, and there is only 2+ tonsillar enlargement. Therefore, a PSG should be done before adenotonsillectomy. Home studies (e.g., ambulatory monitoring, home pulse oximetry) have fairly good specificity (a positive test result at home is likely positive in the laboratory). However, negative predictive value (sensitivity) is quite poor, and a home study does not rule out clinically significant pediatric OSA. AutoPap algorithms are created for adult patients, not pediatric patients. Therefore, erroneous information often results.

27. A. Adenotonsillectomy is the recommended first-line treatment for pediatric OSA, according to current guidelines.   (Marcus et al, 2012; Roland et al, 2011) Although other therapeutic devices may be used, they are typically used as an adjunct treatment or primary treatment if adenotonsillectomy is contraindicated, not considered, or if there is persistent pediatric OSA after adenotonsillectomy.

28. A. An obstructive hypopnea in children is defined as greater than or equal to 30% fall in the pressure signal for at least two respiratory efforts and at least greater than or equal to 3% fall in oxygen saturation, arousal, or awakening.

29. D. An RERA is defined as a notable change in airflow but does not meet the requirements to score the event as an apnea or hypopnea. The event is associated with arousal, evidence of some flow limitation by pressure transduction, snoring, increased work of breathing, or increase in end-tidal CO_2 above the preevent baseline.

30. E.   A diagnosis has not been made; thus, the other courses of action are not appropriate. Home sleep testing is not done in newborns.

31. E.   Primary central sleep apnea of infancy as defined using American Academy of Sleep Medicine criteria as an observed apnea or cyanosis or oxygen desaturation detected by monitoring; the infant is 37 weeks' gestation or greater; PSG shows either recurrent, prolonged (>20 seconds) central apneas or periodic breathing for greater than or equal to 5% of the total sleep time; and the disorder is not better explained by another sleep-related disorder (e.g., OSA), medical disorder, or neurologic disorder or is the effect of medication.

32. B.   Home oxygen is the correct course of action. In most cases, the child "outgrows" the problem.

Summary

Why This Chapter?

The biggest surprise for applicants taking previous sleep medicine board examinations was the discrepancy between the expected and actual number of pediatrics questions. According to previous exam blueprints, only 2% of the exam was to cover "considerations and disorders unique to childhood." Thus, many test takers did not study pediatrics at all, assuming it worthwhile to sacrifice 2% of the test for the benefit of not having to study a large area of sleep medicine. They might also have assumed that a board that deals with adult medicine (the American Board of Internal Medicine) would not have a great deal of pediatrics material in its exam. Unfortunately, they were wrong; past exams have contained many pediatric questions. Even though the current blueprint omits any specific sections devoted to childhood sleep disorders, pediatric cases will be interspersed in various sections of the exam.

Surprisingly, some pediatrics cases that appeared in previous exams often dealt with esoteric conditions seldom actually seen in a typical sleep clinic; for example, in 2009, several questions covered sleep apnea in children with achondroplasia. The message here is that you cannot safely omit a review of pediatric sleep medicine. Thus, you will find pediatric cases dispersed throughout this review book. In this section, we review some areas unique to children.

Highly Recommended

- *International Classification of Sleep Disorders*, ed 3, pp 27–28, 63–68, 94–101, 113–117, and 166–170
- The *AASM Manual for the Scoring of Sleep and Associated Events: Rules, Terminology, and Technical Specifications*, Version 2.5, 2018, pp 62–64
- Sheldon S. Obstructive sleep apnea in children. In: Kryger, Avidan, Berry. *Atlas of Clinical Sleep Medicine*, ed 2, Chapter 13.2. Philadelphia: Elsevier; 2014

Safe Sleep

- SIDS
  - Unexpected death of an infant before the age of 1 year
  - Most cases occur within 4 months of birth
  - The cause is unknown
- Sudden infant death prevention
  - Sleeping supine has reduced prevalence
  - Children should not be exposed to tobacco smoke
  - Home apnea monitoring does not reduce SIDS deaths.   (Adams et al, 2009)
  - Infants should sleep in the parents' room, close to parents' bed, but on a separate safe surface, ideally for first 6 to 12 months.   (Moon et al, 2016)

Behavioral Insomnia of Childhood (ICSD3, pp 27–28)

■ At least two subtypes   (Meltzer, 2010)
  ○ Sleep-association type
    • The child has learned inappropriate sleep associations
    • Insomnia can begin as early as 4 months of age
  ○ Limit-setting type
    • The child resists imposed sleep-wake schedules
    • Inconsistent limit setting by caregivers
    • Usually begins later than the sleep-association type
■ Behavioral treatment is preferred for management
  ○ Treatment includes both child and caregivers   (Meltzer, 2014)
    • Involves unlearning the sleep associations
    • Involves consistency and enforcement of limit setting

Primary Central Sleep Apnea Syndromes in the Newborn (ICSD3, pp 94-101)

■ Definitions
  ○ Apnea is defined as being "significant" if the central events exceed 20 seconds or, if less than 20 seconds, they are accompanied by bradycardia or hypoxemia   (MANUAL2)
  ○ *Primary central sleep apnea of prematurity* occurs in newborns younger than 37 weeks' conceptional age
  ○ *Primary central sleep apnea of infancy* occurs in newborns more than 37 weeks' conceptional age
■ Pathogenesis
  ○ Temporary reduction or absence in effort to breathe caused by abnormal control of ventilation   (Orr et al, 2017)
  ○ Increased or decreased loop gain can lead to central apnea
■ Management might include a sleep study, theophylline, or oxygen, depending on findings.
■ Differential diagnosis
  ○ Normal breathing pauses in newborns
    • Short pauses in breathing are common in healthy newborns
    • More common in active sleep
    • Usually central events
    • Not associated with bradycardia or oxygen desaturation
  ○ Periodic breathing
    • CSB pattern, usually with a cycle length of 10 to 18 seconds and episodes of central apnea 3 or more seconds in duration but fewer than 20 seconds
    • Considered to be a normal variant if unaccompanied by hypoxemia or bradycardia
    • If this occurs on a background of hypoxemia, the required treatment is oxygen, theophylline, and caffeine

Congenital Central Alveolar Hypoventilation Syndrome (ICSD3, pp 113-117)

■ Hypoventilation and its sequelae (cor pulmonale, erythrocytosis) become apparent within months of birth   (Weese-Mayer, 2010)
■ Pathogenesis
  ○ Patients have blunted hypoxic and hypercapnic drives to breathe
  ○ More than 90% of patients have a *PHOX2B* mutation
  ○ About 20% of patients also have Hirschsprung disease. (The combination of Hirschsprung and CCHS is called *Haddad syndrome*.)
    • Sleep study shows apneas and hypopneas or continuous hypoventilation during sleep, documented by hypoxemia and elevated end-tidal PcO_2
■ Management
  ○ Tracheostomy with ventilatory support, diaphragm pacing

- Apparent life-threatening event (Tieder et al, 2013; Wijers et al, 2009)
  - Caregiver finds child with one or more symptoms that may include apnea, pallor or cyanosis, or hypotonia
  - Usually occurs before the age of 6 months
  - The most common cause is gastroesophageal reflux
  - Other causes include seizures and respiratory and other infections
  - Sleep-breathing disorders are not commonly found
  - In 20% to 30% of cases, no cause is determined
  - Admission to a hospital is generally recommended to rule out serious conditions
  - Home apnea monitoring is generally not recommended because it has not been shown to reduce sudden infant death in this population

Obstructive Sleep Apnea in Children (ATLAS2, Ch 13.3; Marcus et al, 2012)

- Symptoms
  - Snoring
  - Gasping
  - Restless sleep
  - Sleepiness
  - Poor school performance
- Causes
  - Enlarged tonsils and adenoids
  - Obesity
  - Craniofacial and other congenital abnormalities
    - Laryngomalacia
    - Pierre Robin sequence
    - Down syndrome (see later)
    - Achondroplasia
    - Spinal muscle atrophy
    - Prader-Willi syndrome (see later)
    - Klippel-Feil syndrome (see later)
    - Arnold-Chiari malformation, type II (see later)
- Sleep study
  - AHI more than 1 event per hour
  - Elevation of end-tidal CO_2
  - Restlessness
  - Movements to reposition the head
- Treatment
  - Surgery (for enlarged tonsils and adenoids) (Marcus et al, 2013; Konstantinopoulou et al, 2015; Brown, 2011)
  - Orthodontic treatment to expand mandible (for small mandible)
  - Weight loss for obesity
  - Positive airway pressure (PAP) therapy
- Syndromes unique to or beginning in childhood
  - Down syndrome (Austeng et al, 2014)
    - OSA can occur because of
      - Enlarged tongue
      - Abnormal skeletal structures of the face
      - Reduced tone of upper airway muscles
      - Enlarged tonsils and adenoids
      - Hypothyroidism
    - Hypoxemia can occur because of right-to-left cardiac shunts.
    - Tonsillectomy effective in about 50% of cases. (Ingram et al, 2017)

○ Prader-Willi syndrome   (Cohen et al, 2014; Ghergan et al, 2017; Williams et al, 2008)
  ● Main features
    ◆ Obesity
    ◆ Hyperphagia caused by increased ghrelin
    ◆ Hypersomnolence
    ◆ May have narcolepsy type 1 with sleep-onset REM periods during a multiple sleep latency test
    ◆ May have narcolepsy type 2
    ◆ Sleep apnea
      ● Infants are more likely to have central apnea
      ● Older children are more likely to have obstructive apnea
  ● Treatment
    ◆ Modafinil for hypersomnolence
    ◆ PAP for obstructive apnea (older children)
    ◆ Oxygen for central apnea (infants)   (Cohen et al, 2014)
    ◆ Growth hormone for small stature (can worsen apnea)
○ Chiari malformation   (Leu, 2015)
  ● Type I: Caudal part of cerebellar tonsils herniate below foramen magnum.
  ● Type II: Caudal part of cerebellar tonsils, brainstem, fourth ventricle herniate below foramen magnum
    ◆ Often have myelomeningocele or spina bifida
    ◆ Compression of respiratory centers in medulla
    ◆ Often develop obstructive and central sleep apnea
    ◆ Responds to PAP therapy
○ Klippel-Feil anomaly   (Rosen et al, 1993)
  ● Congenital abnormal anatomy
    ◆ Fusion of any two of the seven cervical vertebrae
    ◆ Cleft palate may be present
    ◆ Kyphoscoliosis may be present
    ◆ On exam: short neck, low posterior hairline
    ◆ Can develop obstructive or central apnea (or both)
    ◆ Can require surgery to treat anatomic abnormalities
    ◆ PAP treatment is problematic, because the short neck interferes with normal function of PAP headgear.   (ATLAS2, Fig. 13.1–41, p 267; Fig. 13.2–27, B, p 286)
○ Rett syndrome   (Christodoulou and Ho, 2012; Ramirez et al, 2013)
  ● Characterized by severe progressive cognitive impairment that occurs in girls
  ● Patients often have seizures
  ● Pathogenesis
    ◆ Most patients have mutations of the *MECP2* gene
    ◆ Abnormal cortical inputs to the respiratory center cause breathing pattern abnormalities
  ● During wakefulness, hyperventilation is followed by long central apneas with hypoxemia (most common finding)
  ● During sleep, the patient can have central apneas
  ● Night laughing and screaming are common sleep problems

REFERENCES

Adams SM, Good MW, Defranco GM. Sudden infant death syndrome. *Am Fam Physician*. 2009;79(10):870–874.
Alsubie HS, Rosen D. The evaluation and management of respiratory disease in children with Down syndrome (DS). *Paediatr Respir Rev*. 2017. doi:10.1016/j.prrv.2017.07.003.
Alsufyani N, Isaac A, Witmans M, et al. Predictors of failure of DISE-directed adenotonsillectomy in children with sleep disordered breathing. *J Otolaryngol Head Neck Surg*. 2017;46(1):37. doi:10.1186/s40463-017-0213-3.
American Academy of Sleep Medicine. *International classification of sleep disorders*. 3rd ed. Darien, Ill.: American Academy of Sleep Medicine; 2014.
American Academy of Sleep Medicine. *The AASM Manual for the Scoring of Sleep and Associated Events: Rules, Terminology, and Technical Specifications*, Version 2.5. Darien, Ill.: American Academy of Sleep Medicine; 2018.
Austeng ME, Overland B, Kværner KJ, et al. Obstructive sleep apnea in younger school children with Down syndrome. *Int J Pediatr Otorhinolaryngol*. 2014;78(7):1026–1029.

Brown KA, Moss IR. Opiate usage in children with obstructive sleep apnea syndrome. *Anesth Analg.* 2007;105(2): 547–548. doi:10.1213/01.ane.0000268543.56134.c4.

Brown KA. Outcome, risk, and error and the child with obstructive sleep apnea. *Paediatr Anaesth.* 2011;21(7):771–780. doi:10.1111/j.1460-9592.2011.03597.x.

Burnham MM, Goodlin-Jones BL, Gaylor EE. At al. Nighttime sleep-wake patterns and self-soothing from birth to one year of age: a longitudinal intervention study. *J Child Psychol Psychiatry.* 2002;43(6):713–725.

Bull MJ, Committee on Genetics. Health supervision for children with Down syndrome. *Pediatrics.* 2011;128(2): 393–406. doi:10.1542/peds.2011-1605.

Christodoulou J, Ho G. *MECP2*-related disorders (updated 2012). Includes classic Rett syndrome, *MECP2*-related severe neonatal encephalopathy, PPM-X syndrome. Gene Reviews; 2012. Available at: http://www.ncbi.nlm.nih.gov/books/NBK1497/. Accessed March 31, 2018.

Cohen M, Hamilton J, Narang I. Clinically important age-related differences in sleep-related disordered breathing in infants and children with Prader-Willi syndrome. *PLoS ONE.* 2014;9(6):e101012.

Ghergan A, Coupaye M, Leu-Semenescu S, et al. Prevalence and phenotype of sleep disorders in 60 adults with Prader-Willi syndrome. *Sleep.* 2017;40(12).

Gradisar M, Jackson K, Spurrier NJ, et al. Behavioral interventions for infant sleep problems: a randomized controlled trial. *Pediatrics.* 2016;137(6).

Guilleminault C, Huang Y-S, Glamann C, et al. Adenotonsillectomy and obstructive sleep apnea in children: a prospective survey. *Otolaryngol Head Neck Surg.* 2007;136(2):169–175. doi:10.1016/j.otohns.2006.09.021.

Hiscock H, Wake M. Randomised controlled trial of behavioural infant sleep intervention to improve infant sleep and maternal mood. *BMJ.* 2002;324(7345):1062–1065.

Ingram DG, Ruiz AG, Gao D, Friedman NR. Success of tonsillectomy for obstructive sleep apnea in children with Down syndrome. *J Clin Sleep Med.* 2017;13(8):975–980.

Kelly DH, Stellwagen LM, Kaitz E, Shannon DC. Apnea and periodic breathing in normal full-term infants during the first twelve months. *Pediatr Pulmonol.* 1985;1(4):215–219.

Konstantinopoulou S, Gallagher P, Elden L, et al. Complications of adenotonsillectomy for obstructive sleep apnea in school-aged children. *Int J Pediatr Otorhinolaryngol.* 2015;79(2):240–245.

Kryger MH, Avidan A, Berry R. *Atlas of Clinical Sleep Medicine.* 2nd ed. Philadelphia: Saunders; 2014.

Leu RM. Sleep-related breathing disorders and the Chiari 1 malformation. *Chest.* 2015;148(5):1346–1352.

Marcus CL, Brooks LJ, Draper KA, et al. Diagnosis and management of childhood obstructive sleep apnea syndrome. *Pediatrics.* 2012;130(3):576–584.

Marcus CL, Moore RH, Rosen CL, et al. Childhood adenotonsillectomy trial (CHAT). A randomized trial of adenotonsillectomy for childhood sleep apnea. *N Engl J Med.* 2013;368(25):2366–2376.

Meltzer LJ. Clinical management of behavioral insomnia of childhood: treatment of bedtime problems and night wakings in young children. *Behav Sleep Med.* 2010;8(3):172–189.

Meltzer LJ, Mindell JA. Systematic review and meta-analysis of behavioral interventions for pediatric insomnia. *J Pediatr Psychol.* 2014;39(8):932–948.

Moon RY. Task force on sudden infant death syndrome. SIDS and other sleep-related infant deaths: evidence base for 2016 updated recommendations for a safe infant sleeping environment. *Pediatrics.* 2016;138(5).

Obladen M. Cot death: history of an iatrogenic disaster. *Neonatology.* 2017;113(2):162–169.

Orr JE, Malhotra A, Sands SA. Pathogenesis of central and complex sleep apnoea. *Respirology.* 2017;22(1):43–52.

Piazza CC, Fisher WW, Sherer M. Treatment of multiple sleep problems in children with developmental disabilities: faded bedtime with response cost versus bedtime scheduling. *Dev Med Child Neurol.* 1997;39(6):414–418.

Ramirez JM, Ward CS, Neul JL. Breathing challenges in rett syndrome: lessons learned from humans and animal models. *Respir Physiol Neurobiol.* 2013;189(2):280–287.

Roland PS, Rosenfeld RM, Brooks LJ, et al. American Academy of Otolaryngology—head and neck surgery foundation. Clinical practice guideline: polysomnography for sleep-disordered breathing prior to tonsillectomy in children. *Otolaryngol Head Neck Surg.* 2011;145(suppl 1):S1–S15.

Rosen CL, Novotny EJ, D'Andrea LA, Petty EM. Klippel-Feil sequence and sleep-disordered breathing in two children. *Am Rev Respir Dis.* 1993;147(1):202–204.

Strehle EM, Gray WK, Gopisetti S, et al. Can home monitoring reduce mortality in infants at increased risk of sudden infant death syndrome? A systematic review. *Acta Paediatr.* 2012;101(1):8–13.

Tieder JS, Altman RL, Bonkowsky JL, et al. Management of apparent life-threatening events in infants: a systematic review. *J Pediatr.* 2013;163(1):94–99.

Vriend J, Corkum P. Clinical management of behavioral insomnia of childhood. *Psychol Res Behav Manag.* 2011;4:69–79.

Weese-Mayer DE, Berry-Kravis EM, Ceccherini I, et al. ATS congenital central hypoventilation syndrome subcommittee. An official ATS clinical policy statement: congenital central hypoventilation syndrome: genetic basis, diagnosis, and management. *Am J Respir Crit Care Med.* 2010;181(6):626–644.

Wijers MM, Semmekrot BA, de Beer HJ, et al. Multidisciplinary guidelines for "apparent life threatening event" ALTE. *Ned Tijdschr Geneeskd.* 2009;153:A590.

Williams K, Scheimann A, Sutton V, et al. Sleepiness and sleep disordered breathing in Prader-Willi syndrome: relationship to genotype, growth hormone therapy, and body composition. *J Clin Sleep Med.* 2008;4(2):111–118.

Highly Recommended Lists

SECTION 1: NORMAL SLEEP AND ITS VARIANTS

- *Atlas of Clinical Sleep Medicine*, ed 2, Chapters 3.1, 3.3, 3.4, 3.5, 3.8, 3.9, 4.2, 9, and 18
- de Lecea L, Huerta R: Hypocretin (orexin) regulation of sleep-to-wake transitions, *Front Pharmacol.* 5:16, 2014. eCollection 2014. Free full text is available online at http://www.ncbi.nlm.nih.gov/pubmed/24575043
- *Principles and Practice of Pediatric Sleep Medicine*, ed 2, Chapters 1 to 4 and 6
- *Principles and Practice of Sleep Medicine* ed 6, Chapter 20; Abstracts and Clinical Pearls of Chapters 11 to 19
- *AASM Manual for the Scoring of Sleep and Associated Events: Rules, Terminology and Technical Specifications*, Version 2.5
- *Technologist's Handbook for Understanding and Implementing the AASM Manual for the Scoring of Sleep and Associated Events: Rules, Terminology, and Technical Specifications*, 2009

SECTION 2: SLEEP-WAKE TIMING

- *International Classification of Sleep Disorders*, ed 3., pp 199–224
- Morgenthaler TI, Lee-Chiong T, Alessi C, et al: Practice parameters for the clinical evaluation and treatment of circadian rhythm sleep disorders: an American Academy of Sleep Medicine report, *Sleep* 30:1445–1459, 2007
- Quera Salva MA, Hartley S, Léger D, et. al. Non-24-hour sleep-wake rhythm disorder in the totally blind: diagnosis and management. *Front Neurol.* Dec 18;8:686, 2017

SECTION 3: INSOMNIA

- *Atlas of Clinical Sleep Medicine*, ed 2, Chapters 6, 10, and 17
- *International Classification of Sleep Disorders*, ed 3, Insomnia section, pp 19–46
- Atkin T, Comai S, Gobbi G. Drugs for insomnia beyond benzodiazepines: pharmacology, clinical applications, and discovery. *Pharmacol Rev.* Apr; 70(2):197–245, 2018

SECTION 4: CENTRAL DISORDERS OF HYPERSOMNOLENCE

- *Atlas of Clinical Sleep Medicine*, ed 2, Chapter 11.1
- Dauvilliers Y, Barateau L. Narcolepsy and other central hypersomnias. Continuum (Minneap Minn). 2017 Aug;23(4, *Sleep Neurology*):989-1004
- De la Herrán-Arita AK, García-García F: Current and emerging options for the drug treatment of narcolepsy, *Drugs* 73(16):1771–1781, 2013
- *International Classification of Sleep Disorders*, ed 3, pp 143–188

SECTION 5: PARASOMNIAS

- *Atlas of Clinical Sleep Medicine*, ed 2, Chapters 11.3 and 12; make sure you can identify stage N3 sleep
- *International Classification of Sleep Disorders*, ed 3, pp 225–280 (see Box 5.1-1); and pp 246–253

SECTION 6: SLEEP-RELATED MOVEMENT DISORDERS

- *AASM Manual for the Scoring of Sleep and Associated Events: Rules, Terminology, and Technical Specifications*, Version 2.5, 2017, Section VII, Movement Rules
- *Atlas of Clinical Sleep Medicine*, ed 2, Chapter 11.2
- *Principles and Practice of Sleep Medicine*, ed 6. Chapter 95
- *International Classification of Sleep Disorders*, ed 3, pp 281–340

SECTION 7: SLEEP-RELATED BREATHING DISORDERS

- *AASM Manual for the Scoring of Sleep and Associated Events: Rules, Terminology, and Technical Specifications*, Version 2.5
- *Atlas of Clinical Sleep Medicine*, ed 2, Chapters 3.6, 13, and 18
- *International Classification of Sleep Disorders*, ed 3, pp 49–141
- *Principles and Practice of Pediatric Sleep Medicine*, ed 2, Chapters 27 and 28

SECTION 8: SLEEP IN OTHER DISORDERS

- *Atlas of Clinical Sleep Medicine*, ed 6. Chapters 11.2 through 11.4, and 17
- *Principles and Practice of Sleep Medicine*, ed 6. Section 12: Neurological Disorders; Section 16: Other Medical Disorders; and Section 17: Psychiatric Disorders

SECTION 9: INSTRUMENTATION AND TESTING IN SLEEP MEDICINE

- Section III. *AASM Manual for the Scoring of Sleep and Associated Events: Rules, Terminology, and Technical Specifications*, Version 2.5
- *Atlas of Clinical Sleep Medicine*, ed 2, Chapter 18

SECTION 10: PEDIATRICS: NOT GONE AND NOT FORGOTTEN

- *International Classification of Sleep Disorders*, ed 3, pp 27–28, 63–68, 94–101, 113–117, and 166–170
- The *AASM Manual for the Scoring of Sleep and Associated Events: Rules, Terminology, and Technical Specifications*, Version 2.5, 2018, pp 62–64
- *Atlas of Clinical Sleep Medicine*, ed 2. Chapter 13.2

GUIDELINES

- AASM Practice Guidelines (https://aasm.org/clinical-resources/practice-standards/practice-guidelines/)
- AASM Provider fact sheets (https://aasm.org/clinical-resources/provider-fact-sheets/)

Topics Index

Knowledge Base for Sleep Medicine Practitioners in Europe

The Board and the Sleep Medicine Committee of the European Sleep Research Society (ESRS) have compiled the catalog of knowledge that is expected in sleep medicine clinicians in the European Community. This catalog is cross referenced with educational sources and is modified from Penzel T, Pevernagie D, Dogas Z, et al: Sleep Medicine Committee and The European Sleep Research Society. Catalogue of knowledge and skills for sleep medicine, *J Sleep Res.* 23(2):222–238, 2014. (http://onlinelibrary.wiley.com/doi/10.1111/jsr.12095/full). Since the publication of this document, the *International Classification of Sleep Disorders*, ed 3 (ICSD3), has been published, and thus some classification terms have been updated.

The authors have added comments **in blue** to this document. *Text* in blue refers to relevant chapters in *ATLAS2:* Kryger M, Avidan A, Berry R: *Atlas of clinical sleep medicine,* ed 2, Philadelphia, 2014, Saunders.

A. PHYSIOLOGIC BASIS OF SLEEP
(ATLAS2, Chapter 3)

1. The Neurophysiology and Neurobiology of Sleep
   - Macroarchitecture and microarchitecture of sleep
   - Neuroanatomy of sleep
   - Neurochemistry of sleep
   - Sleep-wake functions and consciousness
   - Effects of pharmacologic agents on sleep and wakefulness
2. Regulation of Sleep and Wakefulness
   - Definitions of sleep, sleep transition, wakefulness, sleepiness, and tiredness
   - The two-process model
   - Sleep homeostasis
   - Sleep duration, "core" sleep, and "optional" sleep
   - Chronobiology: The circadian clock and its influence on sleep and circadian rhythms
   - Variation of tiredness (fatigue), sleepiness, and cognitive performance during the day
   - Genetics of sleep regulation
   - Chronotypes and sleep
   - Hormone secretion
   - Thermoregulation

3. Adaptation of Bodily Functions to Sleep
   - Mental and cognitive activities
   - Motor control of skeletal muscles
   - Sensation
   - Activity of the autonomic nervous system
   - Heart and circulatory functions
   - Respiratory functions
   - Metabolic activity
4. Theories on the Functions of Sleep
   - Evolutionary (including phylogeny of sleep)
   - Cerebral restitution
   - Body restitution (including integrity of immune system, recovery, and resilience)
   - Theories on the functions of rapid eye movement (REM) and non-REM (NREM) sleep
   - Sleep, learning, and memory
   - Mental health
5. Effects of Acute and Chronic Sleep Deprivation
   - On emotional state
   - On mood
   - Cognitive function
   - Physical health
   - Immune function
   - Other
6. Sleep and Dreaming
   - Mental processes during NREM and REM sleep, at sleep onset, and upon awakening
   - What is a dream? Neuropsychology and neuroimaging of dreaming
   - Dreaming and brain/medical disorders
   - Dreaming and psychopathologic conditions
7. Aging and Sleep: Sleep in All Stages of Human Development
   - Perinatal sleep
   - Sleep in infancy
   - Sleep in childhood
   - Adolescence and sleep
   - Adult sleep
   - Sleep in later life
8. Gender Differences in Sleep
   - Sleep and the menstrual cycle
   - Sleep and pregnancy
   - Sleep and the menopause/andropause

B. ASSESSMENT OF SLEEP DISORDERS AND DIAGNOSTIC PROCEDURES (ATLAS2, Chapters 13.1, 17, 18, and 19)

1. Classification of Sleep Disorders
   - ICSD2; ICSD3 has been published
   - Other classification systems
2. The Clinical Interview and Clinical Examination
   - Medical history
   - Sleep history
   - Interviewing partner and relatives
   - Semistructured interview techniques
   - General medical examination (including height, weight, body mass index [BMI], collar size, hip/waist ratio, blood pressure measurements)
   - Examination of the upper airway (nasal patency, Friedman-Mallampati scores)
   - Neurologic examination
   - Psychological/psychiatric evaluation
3. Differential Measuring and Monitoring of Sleep and Wakefulness
   - General principles (establishing a differential diagnosis and baseline, quantifying treatment progress, appraising outcome)
   - Sleep questionnaires
   - Questionnaires on mental well-being, daytime function, and so on
   - Sleep diary
   - Measurement of core and surface body temperature
   - Actigraphy (including equipment, handling, interpretation, reporting, advantages, and limitations)
   - Pulse oximetry (including equipment, handling, interpretation, reporting, advantages, and limitations)
   - Cardiorespiratory polygraphy (including equipment, handling, interpretation, advantages, and limitations)
   - Polysomnography (PSG), hookup, montage, and technical aspects (including calibration, recording, sampling, filtering, and displaying)
   - PSG, obligatory and optional sensors
   - PSG, video recording and telemetry
   - PSG, sleep scoring, and reporting (2014 American Association of Sleep Medicine [AASM] scoring guidelines)
   - PSG, event scoring, artifact rejection, and reporting (2014 AASM scoring guidelines)
   - PSG, miscellaneous (split-night recording, full montage, effect of drugs and pathologic conditions on electroencephalogram [EEG])
   - Basic and advanced computer-assisted PSG signal analysis
   - Tests of sleep propensity and alertness: multiple sleep latency test (MSLT), maintenance of wakefulness test (MWT), and other tests (e.g., Osler test)

4. Other Tests and Examinations
   - Cognitive evaluation
   - Psychometric evaluation
   - Neuropsychological tests (including assessment of vigilance, such as psychomotor vigilance task [PVT])
   - Technologies relevant to the cognitive neuroscience of sleep (event-related potentials [ERPs], magnetoencephalogram [MEG], functional magnetic resonance imaging [fMRI])
   - Pulmonary function tests
   - Diagnosis and working hypothesis
   - Analysis of blood and other bodily fluids (e.g., assessment of ferritin, hypocretin, melatonin)
   - Various imaging techniques
5. Miscellaneous Topics (Suitable for Workshops)
   - The clinical interview and further diagnostics management
   - Assessing motivational state
   - Setting up diagnostic tests
   - Scoring, interpretation, and reporting of diagnostic tests
   - Putting all data together to formulate a diagnosis
6. Practical Training in Patient Care (Fellowship in a Sleep Medicine Training Center)
   - ±300 work-hours or 10 European credit transfer and accumulation system (ECTS) credit points

C. INSOMNIA (ATLAS2, Chapter 10)

1. Nosologic Classification, Definitions, Epidemiology
   - Standardized criteria for defining insomnia (ICSD 2; **changed in ICSD3**)
   - Adjustment insomnia (acute insomnia)
   - Psychophysiologic insomnia
   - Paradoxic insomnia
   - Idiopathic insomnia
   - Insomnia due to a mental disorder
   - Inadequate sleep hygiene
   - Behavioral insomnia of childhood
   - Insomnia due to a drug or substance (including alcohol and hypnotic dependence)
   - Insomnia due to a medical condition
   - Insomnia not due to a substance or known physiologic condition, unspecified
   - Physiologic (organic) insomnia, unspecified
   - Definition of insomnia in other classification systems (ICD-10, *Diagnostic and Statistical Manual of Mental Diseases*, ed 4 [DSM-IV], and DSM-V)
2. Pathophysiology
   - Predispositional factors
   - Precipitating factors
   - Perpetuating factors
   - Arousal/hyperarousal models
   - Cognitive-behavioral models
   - Primary versus secondary versus comorbid insomnia

3. Clinical Picture and Diagnosis
   - Daytime and nighttime symptoms of insomnia
   - Clinical evaluation, including psychiatric assessment
   - Questionnaires to assess insomnia complaints
   - Sleep logs and actigraphy
   - Sleep laboratory diagnostics in insomnia (e.g., PSG)
   - Other diagnostic tests in insomnia
4. Special Populations and Comorbidities
   - Mental health (e.g., "comorbid" psychiatric disorders often implicated in differential diagnosis of sleep disorders, such as anxiety and depression, bipolar disorder)
   - Insomnia in older adults
   - Insomnia in children
   - Trauma and chronic stress (e.g., insomnia and life events, posttraumatic stress disorder, burnout)
   - Insomnia and depression
   - Insomnia and personality disorders
   - Insomnia and addiction
   - Insomnia in the physically disabled and in neurologic disorders
   - Insomnia in brain injury
   - Insomnia in medical conditions with bodily discomfort (e.g., pain)
5. Treatment
5.1. Practical Skills for Applying Cognitive Behavioral Therapy (CBT) to Insomnia
   - Sleep information and education
   - Sleep hygiene practice
   - Relaxation and biofeedback methods
   - Establishing routines
   - Sleep-stimulus control
   - Sleep restriction
   - Cognitive restructuring
   - Thought-management methods
   - Paradoxic intention
   - Mindfulness meditation
   - Other novel strategies
5.2. Treatment: Tailoring CBT for Insomnia (CBTi) to Clinical and Service Needs
   - Improving adherence to home practice
   - Working with individuals
   - Working with groups
   - Working with other professionals and services
   - Directed self-help approaches
   - Other cognitive and behavioral treatments (mindfulness, biofeedback, multicomponent CBTi)
   - Behavioral treatment of childhood insomnia; working with parents
5.3. Treatment: Pharmacologic Treatment
   - Overview of hypnotic and other sleep-inducing drugs
   - Indications, choice of drug(s), dose adjustment, (long-term) follow-up
   - Combined treatment (pharmacotherapy and CBTi)
   - Evidence base for CBTi and pharmacotherapy
   - Novel pharmacologic approaches behind firm evidence
6. Miscellaneous Topics (Suitable for Workshops)
   - CBTi (behavioral components, cognitive components, package, adherence)
   - Drug treatment (what works and what does not; efficacy, efficiency, and safety; combining with CBTi)
   - Diagnostic approach to insomniac patients
   - Case records
7. Practical Training in Patient Care (Fellowship in a Sleep Medicine Training Center)
   - See Appendix 1 of the certification guidelines: For MDs
   - ±400 work-hours or 13 ECTS credit points

D. SLEEP-RELATED BREATHING DISORDERS (ATLAS2, Chapter 13)

1. Nosologic Classification, Definitions, Epidemiology
   - (Simple) snoring
   - Obstructive sleep apnea and upper airway resistance syndrome (adult and pediatric)
   - Central sleep apnea (CSA) syndrome and Cheyne-Stokes respiration (primary CSA, CSA due to Cheyne-Stokes breathing pattern, high-altitude periodic breathing, medical condition not Cheyne-Stokes, drug or substance, or primary sleep apnea of infancy)
   - Sleep-related hypoventilation and hypoxemic syndromes (obesity hypoventilation syndrome and others)
   - Other sleep-related breathing disorders
2. Pathophysiology
   - Control of breathing
   - Obstructive sleep–sleep-disordered breathing
   - CSA
   - Cheyne-Stokes respiration in cardiac failure
   - Hypoventilation during sleep
3. Clinical Picture and Diagnosis
   - Obstructive sleep-disordered breathing
   - CSA (including eucapnic and hypercapnic CSA, Cheyne-Stokes respiration, and "complex sleep apnea")
   - Hypoventilation during sleep
   - Differential diagnosis
   - Sleep-disordered breathing in children
   - Diagnostic value of polygraphy and PSG
   - Special conditions (e.g., stroke, hypothyroidism, acromegaly)
4. Comorbidities
   - Hypertension
   - Cardiac failure

- Stroke and other brain disorders
- Respiratory comorbidities (asthma, chronic obstructive pulmonary disease [COPD], other lung diseases, chest wall and neuromuscular diseases)
- Metabolic syndrome
- Proinflammatory condition

5. Treatment
- Conservative measures (including weight reduction and positional therapy)
- Pharmacologic treatment
- Nasal continuous positive airway pressure (CPAP)
- Modifiable PAP (bilevel PAP, auto-CPAP)
- Behavioral sleep medicine (BSM) approaches to improving adherence to treatment
- Surgical procedures
- Dental appliances

6. Miscellaneous Topics (Suitable for Workshops)
- PSG examples
- Nuts and bolts of PAP treatment setup (choice of interfaces and pressure generators, titration algorithms, troubleshooting)
- PAP follow-up: monitoring and improving adherence/compliance
- Behavioral methods to improve patient and service outcomes
- Case records

7. Practical Training in Patient Care (Fellowship in a Sleep Medicine Training Center)
- ±400 work-hours or 13 ECTS credit points

E. HYPERSOMNIAS OF CENTRAL ORIGIN (ATLAS2, Chapter 11.1)

1. Nosologic Classification, Definitions, Epidemiology
- Narcolepsy with cataplexy
- Narcolepsy without cataplexy
- Narcolepsy due to a medical condition
- Narcolepsy, unspecified
- Recurrent hypersomnia/Kleine-Levin syndrome
- Recurrent hypersomnia/menstrual-related hypersomnia
- Idiopathic hypersomnia with long sleep time
- Idiopathic hypersomnia without long sleep time
- Behaviorally induced insufficient sleep syndrome
- Hypersomnia due to a medical condition
- Hypersomnia due to a drug or substance (alcohol)
- Hypersomnia not due to a substance or known physiologic condition
- Physiologic hypersomnia, unspecified

2. Pathophysiology
- Normal regulation of sleep and wakefulness, the "sleep switch"
- Hypothalamic regulation of sleep, especially the role of the hypocretin (orexin) system

- Neurophysiology, neurochemistry, neurogenetics, and neuroimmunology of narcolepsy

3. Clinical Picture and Diagnosis
- Spectrum and differential diagnosis of tiredness (fatigue), sleepiness, and cognitive dysfunction
- Spectrum of narcolepsy (not only the classic tetrad but also fragmented sleep, obesity, psychiatric comorbidity, and so on)
- The role of the MSLT and other techniques in assessing excessive daytime sleepiness (EDS)
- Behaviorally induced insufficient sleep syndrome as an important factor
- Role of actigraphy to determine habitual sleep duration
- The use of hypocretin measurements
- The nondiagnostic value of human leukocyte antigen (HLA) typing for narcolepsy

4. Comorbidities
- Comorbidity in narcolepsy, especially overweight/ obesity
- Mood and anxiety disorders as comorbidity in hypersomnias

5. Treatment
- General aspects: information, acceptance, social guidance
- Behavioral management: sleep-wake timing, sleep extension if necessary, planned naps
- Pharmacologic treatment for EDS
- Pharmacologic treatment for cataplexy, hallucinations, and sleep paralysis
- Pharmacologic treatment for fragmented nighttime sleep

6. Miscellaneous Topics (Suitable for Workshops)
- PSG, MSLT, and MWT examples
- Video session
- Case records, especially regarding diagnosis and treatment of primary hypersomnias

7. Practical Training in Patient Care (Fellowship in a Sleep Medicine Training Center)
- ±100 work-hours or three ECTS credit points

F. CIRCADIAN RHYTHM SLEEP DISORDERS (ATLAS2, Chapter 9)

1. Nosologic Classification, Definitions, Epidemiology
- Delayed sleep phase type
- Advanced sleep phase type
- Irregular sleep-wake type
- Nonentrained type (free running)
- Jet lag type
- Shift-work type
- Due to a medical condition
- Other circadian rhythm sleep disorder
- Due to a drug or substance (including alcohol)

2. Pathophysiology
   - Neuroendocrine pathways and disturbances
   - Blindness
   - Genetics: clock gene polymorphisms
   - Adaptations to shifted work schedules
   - Chronobiotic effect of drugs
3. Clinical Picture and Diagnosis
   - Assessment of circadian phase
4. Comorbidities
   - Psychological and psychiatric issues
5. Health Risks (may overlap with J1)
   - Shift work and other conditions
6. Treatment
   - Behavioral approaches
   - Melatonin
   - Light therapy
   - Other (e.g., stimulants)
7. Miscellaneous Topics (Suitable for Workshops)
   - PSG and actigraphy examples
   - Case records
8. Practical Training in Patient Care (Fellowship in a Sleep Medicine Training Center)
   - ±100 work-hours or three ECTS credit points

G. PARASOMNIAS (ATLAS2, Chapter 12)

1. Nosologic Classification, Definitions, Epidemiology
2. Pathophysiology and Psychopathology
   - State dissociation/activation of central patterns; neurophysiology, genetics, neuroimaging of parasomnias
   - REM sleep behavior disorder (RBD) and neurodegenerative disease
3. Clinical Picture and Diagnosis
   - Differentiation between parasomnias and epileptic seizures
4. Comorbidities
   - Parasomnias and brain disorders, psychiatric disorders
5. Treatment
   - Conservative measures
   - Pharmacologic treatment
   - CBT
6. Miscellaneous Topics (Suitable for Workshops)
   - PSG examples
   - Video PSG
   - Differentiation between epileptic and nonepileptic motor activity during sleep
   - Case records
   - Video session
7. Practical Training in Patient Care (Fellowship in a Sleep Medicine Training Center)
   - ±100 work-hours or three ECTS credit points

H. SLEEP-RELATED MOVEMENT DISORDERS (ATLAS2, Chapter 11.2)

1. Nosologic Classification, Definitions, Epidemiology
   - Restless legs syndrome (RLS)
   - Periodic limb movement disorder
   - Sleep-related leg cramps
   - Sleep-related bruxism and other disorders with orofacial activity
   - Hypnic myoclonus
   - Sleep-related rhythmic movement disorder
   - Propriospinal myoclonus and fragmentary myoclonus
   - Sleep disturbances in Parkinson disease
   - Sleep disturbances in other movement disorders
   - Sleep-related movement disorder, unspecified
   - Sleep-related movement disorder due to a drug or substance
   - Sleep-related movement disorder due to a medical condition
2. Pathophysiology
   - Neurobiologic basis of the control of motor function during sleep
   - Neurophysiology, neuroimaging, genetics of sleep-related movement disorders
   - Neurobiology of RLS/periodic limb movements in sleep (PLMS; should include metabolic factors and basic neurobiology)
3. Clinical Picture and Diagnosis
   - A clinical approach to the patient with sleep-related movement disorders
   - Laboratory evaluation of motor disturbances during sleep
   - Immobilization tests and actimetry in the assessment of sleep-related movement disorders
   - Differential diagnosis in sleep-related movement disorders
4. Comorbidities
   - Sleep-related movement disorders and brain, psychiatric, and medical disorders
5. Treatment
   - Conservative measures
   - Pharmacologic treatment
6. Miscellaneous Topics (Suitable for Workshops)
   - PSG and actigraphy examples
   - Introduction to video PSG
   - Case records
   - Video session
7. Practical Training in Patient Care (Fellowship in a Sleep Medicine Teaching Center)
   - Sleep and brain injury
   - Other psychiatric and behavioral disorders frequently encountered in the differential diagnosis of sleep disorders (mentioned in ICSD2, Appendix B)
   - Mood disorders
   - Anxiety disorders

- Somatoform disorders
- Schizophrenia and other psychotic disorders
- ±100 work-hours or three ECTS credit points

I. MISCELLANEOUS SLEEP-RELATED CONDITIONS AND DISORDERS

1. Nosologic Classification, Definitions, Epidemiology
   - Isolated symptoms, apparently normal variants, and unresolved issues
   - Long sleeper
   - Short sleeper
   - Snoring
   - Sleep talking
   - Sleep starts (hypnic jerks)
   - Benign sleep myoclonus of infancy
   - Hypnagogic foot tremor and alternating leg muscle activation during sleep
   - Propriospinal myoclonus at sleep onset
   - Excessive fragmentary myoclonus
   - Other sleep disorders
   - Other physiologic (organic) sleep disorders
   - Other sleep disorder not due to a substance or known physiologic condition
   - Environmental sleep disorder
   - Sleep disorders associated with conditions classifiable elsewhere (ICSD2, Appendix A; **changed in ICSD3**)
   - Fatal familial insomnia
   - Agrypnia excitata
   - Fibromyalgia
   - Sleep-related epilepsy
   - Sleep-related headaches
   - Sleep-related gastroesophageal reflux disease (GERD)
   - Sleep-related coronary artery ischemia
   - Sleep-related abnormal swallowing, choking, and laryngospasm
   - Sleep disorders associated with conditions classifiable elsewhere (not mentioned in ICSD2, Appendix A; **changed in ICSD3**)
   - Sleep in Parkinson and other neurodegenerative diseases (including dementia)
   - Sleep in disorders associated with chronic pain (e.g., cancer, fibromyalgia)
   - Sleep in disorders associated with chronic fatigue (e.g., chronic fatigue syndrome [CFS], fibromyalgia)
   - Sleep and learning disability
   - Disorders usually first diagnosed in infancy, childhood, or adolescence
   - Personality disorders
2. Pathophysiology and Psychopathology
   - Sleep habits; behaviorally induced insufficient or excessive sleep

- Sleep and social life (relation with family and bed partner, relation with coworkers, co-sleeping, pets)
- Relationship between sleep, analgesia, and fatigue
- Personal remedies for managing sleep (traditional remedies, over-the-counter [OTC] remedies, napping)
- Sleep and substance abuse (alcohol, caffeine, nicotine, recreational drugs, withdrawal, and relapse)
3. Treatment
   - Cognitive-behavioral approaches
   - Pharmacologic treatment
4. Miscellaneous Topics (Suitable for Workshops)
   - PSG examples
   - Examples of other sleep tests
   - Case records
5. Practical Training in Patient Care (Fellowship in a Sleep Medicine Training Center)
   - ±90 work-hours or three ECTS credit points

J. SOCIETAL, ECONOMIC, ORGANIZATIONAL, AND RESEARCH ASPECTS OF SLEEP MEDICINE (ATLAS2, Chapter 5)

1. Demographic and Socioeconomic Aspects of Sleep Disorders
   - Sleep and sleep disorders in the public opinion and lay press
   - Prevalence of sleep disorders
   - Shift work (sleep deprivation and circadian misalignment has a substantial impact on a person's health as well as on society/industry)
   - Absenteeism (due to illness)
   - Traffic and occupational hazards
   - Driver's license
   - Socioeconomic cost
   - Impact of sleep disorders on public health and quality of life
   - Cost-effectiveness and cost/benefits of treating sleep disorders
2. Forensic Aspects of Sleep
   - Sleep and the law
   - Driving and falling asleep
   - Sleepiness and work-related accidents
   - Sleep and crimes of a sexual nature
   - Sleep and murder
   - Clinical assessment and differential diagnosis
   - Expert testimony
3. Organization of a Sleep Medicine Center
   - Human resources, organization chart
   - Professional certification requirements (certified sleep specialists)
   - Facilities, sleep laboratory
   - Quality assurance (including PSG scoring QA: intrascorer and interscorer reproducibility)

4. Training and Consultancy
    - Training practitioners
    - Supervising practitioners
    - Professional intervision
    - Giving advice on service development
5. Research Design and Quantitative Methods (Optional)
    - The research process
    - Hypothesis-driven foundations of quantitative measurements (the process of measuring, psychometric theory, reliability, and validity)

- Introduction to quantitative assessment of sleep
- Foundations of qualitative research
- Self-report methods
- Observation
- Foundations of design
- Sampling and ethics
- Evaluating research
- Analysis, interpretation, and dissemination
- Business case

Knowledge Base for Sleep Medicine Practitioners in Japan

This is a listing of the Certification Examination Guidelines for Japan. The 2018 guidelines can be found at http://jssr.jp/data/recognition.html and the material covered in Japanese at http://jssr.jp/data/pdf/ninteiguideline_2017.pdf. The translation below was provided by the Japanese Sleep Society, and for clarity, some text has been modified by the editors of this review. The disorder entities are from the *International Classification of Sleep Disorders*, 2nd edition (ICSD2). The editors of this Review have added some comments **in blue. Section** in blue font refers to this review book. *ATLAS2* refers to Kryger M, Avidan A, Berry R: *Atlas of Clinical Sleep Medicine*, ed 2, Philadelphia, 2014, Saunders.

1. FUNDAMENTALS OF SLEEP

(Section 1; ATLAS2, Chapter 3)

1.1. Neuroanatomy of Sleep Regulation
1.2. Normal Sleep and Its Variants
1.3. Sleep Development, Aging, and Gender (Including Menopause, the Menstrual Cycle, Pregnancy, and Postpartum)
1.4. Psychophysiology of Dreaming
1.5. Physiology of Sleep (Including Breathing, Circulation, Autonomic Nervous System, Muscle Activity, Body Temperature Regulation, Endocrine System, and Metabolic Function)
1.6. Biologic Rhythms and Mechanisms
  1.6.1. Synchronizing mechanisms and circadian rhythm
  1.6.2. Circadian biologic model of sleep regulation
  1.6.3. Cognitive function and diurnal variation of sleepiness and fatigue
  1.6.4. Work schedules
1.7. The Sleep Environment (Including Climate, Sound, and Light)
1.8. Effects of Acute and Chronic Sleep Deprivation
1.9. Sleep Hygiene
1.10. Sociologic Matters, Including Daylight Savings Time, and Epidemiology Related to Sleep and Sleep Disorders

2. INTERVIEW OF PATIENTS

(Section 1; ATLAS2, Chapters 8 and 20)

2.1. Lifestyle Before Onset of Sleep Symptoms
2.2. Evaluation of Medical Disorders
2.3. Evaluation of Mental Illness
2.4. Evaluation of Use of Medications
  2.4.1. Drugs with alerting or stimulant properties
  2.4.2. Agents that enhance or extend the effects of hypnotics
2.5. Sleep Hygiene
  2.5.1. Naps, bedtime rituals, living and sleeping arrangements
  2.5.2. Dietary history
  2.5.3. Sleep environment
  2.5.4. Use of electronics
  2.5.5. Dietary habits

3. SYMPTOMS OF SLEEP DISORDERS (Section 1; ATLAS2, Chapter 8)

3.1. Evaluation, Diagnosis and Differential Diagnosis of Sleep Disorders (Based on the ICSD2)
  3.1.1. General criteria for insomnia
  3.1.2. Excessive sleepiness during the day
  3.1.3. Snoring, respiratory failure
  3.1.4. Abnormal circadian rhythm and symptoms associated with the timing of sleep
  3.1.5. Motor symptoms related to sleep
  3.1.6. Abnormal behaviors associated with sleep
  3.1.7. Other sleep-related (e.g., bruxism, groaning, gasping, nocturnal enuresis, and snoring)
3.2. Sleep Disorders in Children
3.3. Effect on Health of Sleep Disorders
3.4. Impact of Psychological Factors on Sleep Disorders
3.5. Sleep Disorders in Mental Illness (e.g., Schizophrenia, Dementia, Mood, Anxiety Disorders, and PTSD)

4. THERAPEUTICS (Sections 2-8; ATLAS2, Chapters 6, 10, 13, 17)

4.1. Drug Therapy Overview
  4.1.1. Hypnotics
    4.1.1.1. Effects of hypnotics
    4.1.1.2. Pharmacokinetics of hypnotics
    4.1.1.3. Side effects, dependence, and tolerance
    4.1.1.4. Selection of hypnotics
  4.1.2. Psychostimulants
    4.1.2.1. Mechanisms of action
    4.1.2.2. Pharmacokinetics
    4.1.2.3. Adaptation
    4.1.2.4. Side effects: dependence and tolerance
    4.1.2.5. Selection of psychostimulants
    4.1.2.6. Methylphenidate distribution management committee
    4.1.2.7. Characteristics of a methylphenidate addict
  4.1.3. Dopamine agonists
    4.1.3.1. Antidepressant drugs
    4.1.3.2. Anticonvulsants
    4.1.3.3. Other medications (including Chinese medicines)
4.2. Treatment Overview: Sleep-Disordered Breathing
  4.2.1. Positive airway pressure (CPAP, bilevel, ASV)
    4.2.1.1. Indications
    4.2.1.2. Side effects and mechanisms of action
    4.2.1.3. Understand and manage downloaded (compliance) data
    4.2.1.4. Patient education
  4.2.2. Oral appliances
    4.2.2.1. Indications
    4.2.2.2. Side effects and mechanisms of action
  4.2.3. Surgical therapy
    4.2.3.1. Indications
    4.2.3.2. Side effects and mechanisms of action
  4.2.4. Noninvasive Positive Pressure Ventilation
    4.2.4.1. Indications for the treatment of chronic respiratory failure
    4.2.4.2. Patient education
  4.2.5. When patients do not respond to treatment
4.3. Teaching Sleep Hygiene
4.4. Treatment of Circadian Rhythm Disorders
  4.4.1. Chronotherapy
  4.4.2. High-intensity light therapy
  4.4.3. Strengthening of circadian rhythm by social cues
  4.4.4. Melatonin
4.5. Cognitive Behavioral Therapy

5. TESTS USED FOR SLEEP EVALUATION (Sections 1-8; ATLAS2, Chapters 8 and 18)

5.1. Overnight Polysomnography (PSG)
  5.1.1. Examination environment: Equipment and facilities
  5.1.2. Test preparation (evaluation of referral and patient information)
  5.1.3. Disinfection of equipment
  5.1.4. Data acquisition factors (e.g., filter, sampling, A/D resolution)
  5.1.5. Characteristics of sensors and transducers
  5.1.6. Patient setup (e.g., 10-20 system)
  5.1.7. Calibration
  5.1.8. Observation method (monitoring)
  5.1.9. Troubleshooting artifact processing
  5.1.10. Troubleshooting scoring
  5.1.11. Reporting
  5.1.12. Ancillary variables in sleep-disordered breathing during PSG (e.g., esophageal pressure and $PtCO_2$)
  5.1.13. CPAP titration
  5.1.14. Cyclic alternating pattern (CAP), rapid eye movement (REM) density and power spectrum analysis in secondary analysis of sleep electroencephalography (EEG)
  5.1.15. Normal variants of the sleep EEG
  5.1.16. Data filing system
  5.1.17. Privacy protection
  5.1.18. For children: dealing with caregiver bed sharing
5.2. Detection and Communication of Emergencies During PSG
  5.2.1. Infectious diseases
  5.2.2. Abnormal electrocardiogram
  5.2.3. Response to epilepsy
  5.2.4. Response to hypoxemia
  5.2.5. Response to nervous system and cardiovascular emergencies
  5.2.6. Life-saving first aid
  5.2.7. Falling accident measures (particularly for infants)
5.3. Objective Assessment of Sleepiness
  5.3.1. Multiple sleep latency test (MSLT)
  5.3.2. Maintenance of wakefulness test (MWT)
  5.3.3. Performance tests (e.g., psychomotor vigilance tasks [PVTs])
5.4. Subjective Evaluation Method for Sleep Disorders
  5.4.1. Epworth Sleepiness Scale (ESS)
  5.4.2. Sleep Questionnaires (e.g., Pittsburgh and St. Mary's Hospitals' sleep disorders scales)
  5.4.3. Sleep diary
  5.4.4. Morning/night type scale (e.g., using the Visual Analog Scale)
5.5. Other Devices, Tests, and Data
  5.5.1. Pulse oximeter
  5.5.2. Pulse transit time monitor
  5.5.3. Digital photography
  5.5.4. Core body temperature records (biologic rhythm measurement)
  5.5.5. Biochemical indicators of melatonin rhythm
  5.5.6. Orexin
  5.5.7. Esophageal pressure measurement

5.6. Understanding Upper Airway Anatomy
    5.6.1. Imaging studies
    5.6.2. Fiberscope
    5.6.3. Other

6. SPECIFIC SLEEP DISORDERS

6.1. Insomnia (**Section 3**; ATLAS2, Chapter 10)
    6.1.1. Psychophysiologic insomnia
    6.1.2. Paradoxic insomnia
    6.1.3. Insomnia due to mental illness
    6.1.4. Insomnia due to a substance or drug
    6.1.5. Insomnia due to medical disorders
    6.1.6. Other insomnias (e.g., behavioral insomnia, pediatric idiopathic insomnia)
    6.1.7. Inadequate sleep hygiene

6.2. Sleep-Related Breathing Disorders (**Section 7**; ATLAS2, Chapter 13)
    6.2.1. Central sleep apnea (CSA)
        6.2.1.1. Idiopathic CSA
        6.2.1.2. Cheyne-Stokes respiration: Apnea and CSA related to a medical condition
        6.2.1.3. CSA during early childhood (including newborn)
        6.2.1.4. Sudden infant death syndrome
    6.2.2. Obstructive sleep apnea (OSA)
        6.2.2.1. OSA in adults
        6.2.2.2. OSA in children
    6.2.3. Sleep-related hypoventilation/hypoxemia syndrome (e.g., congenital central alveolar hypoventilation syndrome [CHHS])
    6.2.4. Sleep-related hypoventilation/hypoxemia due to physical disease
    6.2.5. Other sleep-related breathing disorders

6.3. Central Hypersomnias (**Section 4**; ATLAS2, Chapter 11.1)
    6.3.1. Narcolepsy (with and without cataplexy) or due to a medical condition
    6.3.2. Chronic recurrent hypersomnias (Kleine-Levin syndrome, menstruation related)
    6.3.3. Idiopathic hypersomnia
    6.3.4. Sleep deprivation syndrome
    6.3.5. Hypersomnia due to a drug or substance

6.4. Circadian Rhythm Sleep Disorders (**Section 2**; ATLAS2, Chapter 9)
    6.4.1. Delayed sleep phase type (delayed sleep phase disorder)
    6.4.2. Advanced sleep phase type (advanced sleep phase disorder)
    6.4.3. Irregular sleep-wake type (irregular sleep-wake rhythm)
    6.4.4. Free-running type (nontuned)
    6.4.5. Time-zone change type (jet lag)
    6.4.6. Shift-work type (shift-work sleep disorder)

6.5. Parasomnias (**Section 5**; ATLAS2, Chapters 7 and 12)
    6.5.1. Non-REM sleep disorders (those that occur out of NREM sleep), arousal disorders (e.g., sleep starts, sleep walking, confusional arousals)

6.5.2. Parasomnias that occur in conjunction with REM sleep (nightmare disorders, repetitive sporadic sleep paralysis, REM sleep behavior disorder)
6.5.3. Sleep-related disorders: Enuresis, exploding head syndrome, sleep-related head banging, hallucinations, and sleep-eating disorders

6.6. Sleep-Related Movement Disorders (**Section 6**; ATLAS2, Chapter 11.1)
    6.6.1. Restless legs syndrome (RLS)
    6.6.2. Periodic limb movement disorder (PLMD)
    6.6.3. Sleep-related leg cramps
    6.6.4. Sleep-related bruxism
    6.6.5. Sleep-related rhythmic movement disorder

6.7. Sleep Disorders Accompanying Medical Conditions (**Section 8**; ATLAS2, Chapter 15)
    6.7.1. Sleep-related asthma
    6.7.2. Chronic obstructive respiratory disease (COPD)
    6.7.3. Sleep-related gastroesophageal reflux disease (GERD)
    6.7.4. Sleep-related coronary ischemia
    6.7.5. Fibromyalgia syndrome
    6.7.6. Fatal familial insomnia

6.8. Sleep Disorders Accompanying Neurologic Disease (**Sections 4-6, 8**; ATLAS2, Chapter 11)
    6.8.1. Cerebrovascular disease
    6.8.2. Dementia
    6.8.3. Parkinson disease
    6.8.4. Multiple system atrophy
    6.8.5. Amyotrophic lateral sclerosis
    6.8.6. Progressive muscular dystrophy
    6.8.7. Myotonic dystrophy
    6.8.8. Sleep-related headache
        6.8.8.1. Hypnic headache
        6.8.8.2. Sleep apnea headache
        6.8.8.3. Association of headaches with sleep
        6.8.8.4. Sleep disorders and headache
    6.8.9. Sleep-related epilepsy
    6.8.10. Developmental disorders (e.g., intellectual disability, attention deficit/hyperactivity disorder, pervasive developmental disorder)
    6.8.11. Chromosomal abnormalities (Down syndrome, Prader-Willi syndrome, Angelman syndrome, Smith-Magenis syndrome)
    6.8.12. Others (e.g., colic, Tourette syndrome, achondroplasia, congenital malformation syndrome, and chronic fatigue syndrome)

6.9. Isolated Symptoms, Apparently Normal Variants
    6.9.1. Long sleeper
    6.9.2. Short sleeper
    6.9.3. Snoring
    6.9.4. Somniloquy (sleep talking)
    6.9.5. Benign movements during sleep

International Sleep Medicine Board Certification Examinations

WORLD SLEEP SOCIETY

In 2017, there was a merger of the World Sleep Federation (WSF) and the World Association of Sleep Medicine (WASM). There is now a single exam administered by the new world sleep organization. The detailed curriculum on which the exam is based can be downloaded from http://worldsleepsociety.org/wp-content/uploads/2015/08/WASM-Sleep-Medicine-Curriculum-1.2-2012.doc. This is a broad outline of the curriculum.

Examination Category
I. Basic Science
II. Applied Technology
III. Sleep Medicine
IV. Sleep Disorders—Clinical and Laboratory Assessment
V. Safety in the Clinic and Laboratory
VI. Methodology for Sleep Research

The examination is made up of 150 multiple-choice questions organized into three parts as follows:

- *Part 1*—Basic and clinical science (60 questions)
- *Part 2*—Applied methods and standards in sleep medicine (60 questions)
- *Part 3*—Clinical practice (30 questions)

The next exam is scheduled to be provided at the World Sleep 2019 Vancouver meeting, September 20, 2019. Eligibility requirements are in: https://worldsleepcongress.com/scientific-content/exam. The application form can be downloaded from: http://worldsleepsociety.org/programs/examination/application/. For more information, contact info@worldsleepsociety.org.

Knowledge Base for Dental Sleep Medicine Practitioners

The American Board of Dental Sleep Medicine (ABDSM) certification exam is composed of 150 multiple choice questions. Applicants are allowed 3 hours to complete the examination. The examination tests applicants on airway anatomy and physiology, adult and pediatric sleep medicine, oral appliance therapy, alternative treatment modalities, evaluation, treatment and follow-up care.

Information about the ABDSM examination, including the most current version of the certification guidelines, content areas, and recommended reading list, can be obtained at abdsm.org.

AMERICAN BOARD OF DENTAL SLEEP MEDICINE CERTIFICATION EXAMINATION CONTENT AREAS

The list below is provided by the American Board of Dental Sleep Medicine. Although this *Sleep Medicine Review* has content areas that will help in several important parts of the examination, it does not cover all areas of dental sleep medicine. Readers are encouraged to check the ABDSM website at abdsm.org for the latest updates.

Recommended resources: Chapters 57-60, 111-114, and Section 18: Dentistry and Otolaryngology in Sleep Medicine. In: Kryger MH, Roth T, Dement WC, eds. *Principles and practice of sleep medicine.* 6th ed. Philadelphia: Elsevier; 2017.

Chapter in blue refers to this review book. *ATLAS2* refers to Kryger M, Avidan A, Berry R. *Atlas of clinical sleep medicine.* 2nd ed. Philadelphia: Saunders; 2014.

1. Understand the physiology of sleep, medical consequences of sleep-disordered breathing (SDB), and comorbidities. (Chapter 7; ATLAS2, Chapters 3, 13)
   1. Physiology and purpose of sleep, health benefits of normal sleep
   2. Pathophysiology of sleep-related breathing disorders (SRBD) including neurophysiology
   3. SRBD and age including potentiation of disease with age
   4. Signs and symptoms of SRBD
   5. Predisposing factors for SRBD
   6. Prevalence, progression and impact of SRBD in both the treated and untreated patient
   7. SRBD and gender
   8. Understanding sleep deficiency and problematic sleep with impact on cognition, emotional stability, physical performance, vigilance, and society
   9. Deleterious impact of other sleep disorders combined with SRBD
2. Understand SRBD and sleep testing in order to effectively manage patients who have been diagnosed with SRBD. (ATLAS2, Chapters 13, 18)
   1. Normal sleep architecture and respiratory parameters on polysomnography (PSG)
   2. Pathologic sleep architecture and respiratory parameters on PSG
   3. How PSG results predict treatment recommendations (e.g., behavioral therapies, continuous positive airway pressure [CPAP], oral appliance, surgery) and efficacy
   4. Role of portable monitoring devices (HSATs) in dental sleep medicine including data analysis, interpretation and indications (see American Medical Association, AADSM, and American Dental Association statements)
   5. Differences between PSG and HSAT, limitations and advantages, indications for each, and differences among various sleep testing modalities
   6. Various other types of sleep testing (multiple sleep latency test, maintenance of wakefulness test [MWT]), - their purpose, method, and indication
3. Demonstrate knowledge of evidence-based alternatives for treatment of SDB and other common comorbid sleep disorders. (ATLAS2, Chapter 13)
   1. Positive airway pressure (PAP) therapies (CPAP, Autotitrating CPAP [APAP], adaptive servoventilation, bilevel positive airway pressure) advantages and appropriate application of each
   2. Surgical therapeutic options
   3. Behavioral therapeutic methods (positional therapy, sleep hygiene, weight loss, cognitive behavioral therapy)
   4. Other emerging therapies (pharmacology, expiratory positive airway pressure, hypoglossal nerve stimulation [HNS], exercises)
   5. Combining therapies for best outcomes
   6. Oral appliance therapy compared to CPAP
   7. Oral appliance therapy compared to non-PAP interventions
   8. Concept of mean disease alleviation, efficacy, and compliance

4. Completing and interpreting a thorough dental sleep medicine history, examination and appropriate imaging in order to facilitate record keeping and determine the patient's candidacy for therapeutic intervention and to guide treatment planning, treatment goals, treatment expectations, and informed consent. (ATLAS2, Chapters 8, 13.1)
   1. Effects of obesity, drugs and medications, alcohol, smoking, and other factors on the upper airway
   2. Other sleep-related problems (narcolepsy, restless legs syndrome, periodic limb movement disorder and periodic leg movements of sleep, insomnia, insufficient sleep, shift worker syndrome), including the relationship between SDB and concomitant sleep-related issues
   3. Medical comorbidities (hypertension, cardiovascular disease, metabolic syndrome, gastroesophageal reflux disease, depression, anxiety)
   4. Informed consent and ethics
   5. Review of systems
   6. History of present illness including impact on others
   7. Coordinating multidisciplinary care and communication with physicians and dentist of record
   8. Effect of sleep position on sleep-disordered breathing
   9. Self-reported and sleep observer measures using questionnaires (e.g., quality of life measures, Epworth, Berlin, SATED [https://www.ncbi.nlm.nih.gov/pmc/articles/PMC3902880/], and Insomnia Severity Index [ISI])
   10. Temporomandibular joint disorders (TMD) and bruxism assessment, prevalence, as well as their relationship with sleep disorders
   11. Components of a comprehensive examination including oral airway assessment, tongue size and position, hard tissues and tooth alignment, periodontal support, occlusal and skeletal jaw classification, curves of Spee and Wilson, kinetics of jaw motion, muscle palpation, temporomandibular joint evaluation, and so on
   12. Correlating TMD and bruxism assessment with patient symptoms and history
   13. Correlating the findings on history, exam and testing with the proposed therapy
   14. Knowledge of medical record keeping requirements of baseline data and subsequent changes if any
5. Select oral appliances based on matching their design, physical features, and function with the information gathered in the clinical examination and patient interview, as well as apply proper fitting techniques.
   1. American Academy of Sleep Medicine and AADSM clinical practice guidelines for oral appliance therapy in the treatment of obstructive sleep apnea (OSA) and snoring

   2. AADSM protocols and definitions for oral appliance therapy
   3. Mechanism of action and physiologic impact of oral appliance on the upper airway
   4. Indications for oral appliance therapy
   5. Sleep habits, anatomic factors, dexterity, reflexes, range of motion, and other factors that may influence attaining treatment goals
   6. Attributes and limitation of multiple appliance design features
   7. Guiding patient decision making based on history, exam, prospective tests, and patient preferences
   8. Rationale for initial treatment position, including vertical, horizontal and lateral components, and understanding of multiple bite acquisition techniques
   9. Knowledge of practical clinical protocols for acquiring critical impression taking detail in order to deliver a properly retentive device along with assessing fit, comfort, vertical dimension, and protrusion of devices at delivery
6. Assess effectiveness and titrate oral appliance.
   1. Role of patient history in guiding the oral appliance adjustment process
   2. Impact of treatment on signs and symptoms
   3. Monitoring objective measures during follow-up examination
   4. Assessing for optimal timing of objective testing or medical referral
   5. Sleep study protocols for confirming oral appliance efficacy and therapeutic calibration
   6. Oral appliance effectiveness and limitations of therapeutic optimization
   7. Monitoring compliance
7. Management and long-term follow-up of patients in oral appliance therapy.
   1. Impact of weight change, medication change, sleep hygiene and quantity, and so on, with concurrent ongoing oral appliance therapy
   2. Relevance and documentation of changes in patient history, as well as self-reported and sleep-observer measures
   3. Treatment modification related to progressive nature of SDB
   4. Confirming appliance stability and care
8. Understand breathing disorders of sleep in children and adolescents, as well as the diagnostic and treatment options for management of these patients.
   1. Prevalence of snoring and OSA in children
   2. Etiology and physiology of snoring and OSA in children
   3. Signs and symptoms of SDB in children and adolescents
   4. Causes of problematic or insufficient sleep children and impact on development, including neurophysiologic

5. Causes of problematic or insufficient sleep in adolescents and impact on cognition, physical performance, impulse control, and decision making
6. Screening children and adolescents for SDB
7. Referring children and adolescents for medical consultation and diagnosis
8. Treatment of snoring and OSA in children and adolescents, including surgical options, CPAP, rapid palatal expansion, and orthodontic treatment
9. Differences between SDB in children and adults
10. The relationship between SDB and medical and behavior disorders

9. Understanding medical versus dental model of practice.
    1. Diagnosis of SDB by a sleep knowledgeable physician (see standards 2015)
    2. Record keeping for every patient encounter, including subjective, objective, assessment, plan (SOAP) notes and baseline morphologic, functional, and clinical data
    3. Documents required to keep on file
    4. Understand medical insurance requirements and reimbursements
    5. Use of correct and appropriate coding, fraud, and "overuse'
    6. Insurance restrictions on treatment choices (e.g., no preexisting TMD)
    7. Understand Medicare durable medical equipment and Part B, forms, and requirements
    8. Medicare restrictions on treatment choices (e.g., pricing, data analysis, and coding [PDAC] restrictions, 90-day rule)
    9. Record considerations and thought processes for all decisions, including treatment goals, device selection, use of calibration testing, management of side effects, and so on

10. Follow AADSM standards for screening, treating, and managing adult patients with SRBD
11. Medical, legal, and ethical considerations

10. Anticipate and manage side effects of oral appliance therapy (OAT) with proper use of informed consent
    1. Critical parts of informed consent for treatment and dialog with patient
    2. Understand evidence-based expectations of oral appliance (OA) side effects
    3. Understand mandibular protrusion effect on craniofacial muscles
    4. Understand mandibular protrusion effect on TMJ
    5. Understand force vectors OAT on oral hard tissues
    6. Use of occlusal guide and morning exercises for prevention and management of OA side effects
    7. Use of remedies for side effects when they occur
    8. Decision making and responsibilities regarding suspending or abandoning OA treatment

11. Understand evidence available for current practice guidelines and the concept of evidence-based practice
    1. Understanding categories of evidence, filtering, sources, and position or level in the evidence hierarchy
    2. Applying level of evidence in guiding clinical practice and decision making
    3. Techniques for reading articles, including looking for quality and bias
    4. Evaluate specific assigned articles using levels of evidence to assess quality of information
    5. Evaluate areas of dental sleep medicine (DSM) practice where high-quality evidence is lacking
    6. PICO (patient intervention comparison and outcome) use to develop a clinical question and literature search

Normal Sleep and Its Variants

E1.1 Sleep-Wake Mechanisms and Neurophysiology

QUESTIONS

1. Where is the main site of rapid eye movement (REM) sleep generation?
A. Cerebellum
B. Pons
C. Spinal cord
D. Medulla oblongata

ANSWER: **B.**   The pontine tegmentum includes the pedunculopontine nucleus and the laterodorsal tegmental nucleus. These cholinergic neurons (located near the raphe nucleus and the locus coeruleus) are involved in the initiation of REM sleep.   (ATLAS2, p 30)

2. Which statement about REM sleep is TRUE?
A. It is found only in humans
B. It is found in almost all mammals
C. It is absent in birds.
D. It is absent in mammals before birth

ANSWER: **B.**   Although it was once believed that certain species do not have sleep or REM sleep (e.g., sea mammals, the platypus), every mammal that has been studied rigorously sleeps and has REM sleep. Indeed, sleep may be occurring in localized parts of the brain at the same time that parts of the brain are awake.

3. Nuclei in what part of the nervous system are involved in the suppression of muscle tone in stage R?
A. Noradrenergic neurons in the locus coeruleus
B. Histaminergic neurons of the tuberomammillary nucleus
C. Orexin neurons projecting to the basal forebrain
D. Ventral sublaterodorsal nucleus

ANSWER: **D.**   The first three answers describe neurons involved in cortical arousal. Remember that noradrenergic, histaminergic (antihistamines make you sleepy), and orexin (whose deficiency causes sleepiness in narcolepsy) are involved in arousal. The glycinergic and GABAergic neurons of the sublaterodorsal nuclei inhibit the spinal motor nuclei, causing the paralysis of stage R.   (ATLAS2, p 33)

4. Sleep is thought to be associated with an increase in basal forebrain and anterior hypothalamic _____ activity and a decrease in posterior hypothalamic _____ activity.
A. Adenosine/GABAergic
B. GABAergic/adenosine
C. Adenosine/hypocretin
D. Adenosine/acetylcholinergic

ANSWER: **C.**   The correct answer can be deduced by knowing that adenosine accumulates during wakefulness and is thought to lead to sleepiness and that low hypocretin is found in narcolepsy, a disease in which the main symptom is sleepiness.   (ATLAS2, pp 24–25)

5. Arousal, or wakefulness, is associated with a decreased activity in the _____ and an increased activity in the _____.
   A. Anterior hypothalamus/thalamus
   B. Anterior hypothalamus/basal forebrain
   C. Basal forebrain/posterior hypothalamus
   D. Anterior hypothalamus/posterior hypothalamus

ANSWER: **D.**   Because the structures that induce sleep are in the anterior hypothalamus (e.g., the ventrolateral preoptic nucleus [VLPO]), it seems reasonable that decreased activity here would be associated with arousal. Similarly, knowing that mammillary bodies (in the posterior hypothalamus) are histaminergic and that antihistamines cause sleepiness would lead to the inference that increased activity here would be associated with arousal. (ATLAS2, pp 28–30)

6. Arousal is dependent on subcortical activation of cortical pathways and includes all of the following *except*
   A. Posterior hypothalamus
   B. Suprachiasmatic nucleus
   C. Pedunculopontine nucleus
   D. VLPO

ANSWER: **D.**   The VLPO is part of the sleep switch and thus does not play a role in causing arousal. The VLPO inhibits arousal by having projections that inhibit the histaminergic (alerting) neurons of the mammillary bodies.   (ATLAS2, p 28)

7. The reticular activating system (RAS) provides ascending projections to thalamic and cortical areas and includes the following neurotransmitters *except*
   A. Acetylcholine
   B. Serotonin
   C. Norepinephrine
   D. Gamma-aminobutyric acid (GABA)

ANSWER: **D.**   Because GABA is the main inhibitory neurotransmitter in the brain, it is logical that it would *not* be a neurotransmitter involved in arousal.   (ATLAS2, p 24)

8. REM sleep is associated with mixed-frequency, low-amplitude electroencephalogram (EEG) waveforms and rapid eye movements, which are all generated by _____ neurons in the _____.
   A. Acetylcholinergic/substantia nigra
   B. Dopaminergic/substantia nigra
   C. Acetylcholine/pedunculopontine nucleus
   D. Dopamine/laterodorsal nucleus

ANSWER: **C.**   The REM-on cells are cholinergic and are located in the pons. Thus, the correct answer will have both of these facts embedded in them.   (ATLAS2, p 30)

9. Accumulation of which of the following results in sleepiness?
   A. Adenosine
   B. Hypocretin
   C. Leptin
   D. Histamine

ANSWER: **A.**   It is believed that adenosine accumulation during wakefulness results in sleepiness. Adenosine has at least two effects: inhibition of wakefulness-promoting systems in the basal forebrain and activation of sleep-promoting VLPO neurons (Fig. E1.1–1).   (ATLAS2, Fig. 3.1–7)

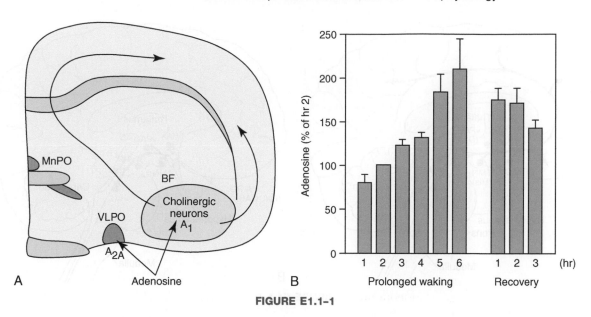

FIGURE E1.1–1

10. The role of caffeine in increasing wakefulness is due to its effect on which of the following?
    A. Hypocretin
    B. Adenosine
    C. Leptin
    D. Histamine

ANSWER: **B.** Caffeine, a xanthine, is an antagonist of adenosine. The basal forebrain, which plays a role in wakefulness, contains cholinergic neurons, which are inhibited by adenosine that accumulates during wakefulness. By antagonizing the effect of adenosine, caffeine reduces the inhibition caused by adenosine and thus increases wakefulness. (ATLAS2, p 116)

11. What is the location of the main sleep switch?
    A. Suprachiasmatic nucleus (SCN)
    B. VLPO
    C. Thalamus
    D. Pineal gland

ANSWER: **B.** Although all these structures are involved in sleep, the VLPO is the main sleep switch. Adenosine activates sleep promotion in VLPO neurons by affecting A_{2A} receptors (see Fig. E1.1–1).

12. Which structures play a role in promoting wakefulness?
    A. Thalamus
    B. Pineal gland
    C. VLPO
    D. Tuberomammillary nucleus (TMN)

ANSWER: **D.** The TMN cells are mainly active during wakefulness, and they release histamine. One way to remember the effect of histamine is to remember that antihistamines can cause sleepiness (Fig. E1.1–2). (ATLAS2, Fig. 3.1–4)

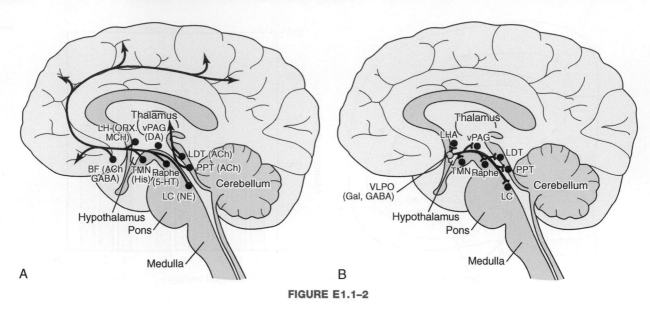

A

B

FIGURE E1.1–2

13. Orexin-releasing cells are located where?
  A. Pineal gland
  B. Thalamus
  C. Lateral hypothalamus
  D. VLPO

ANSWER: **C.**   This is an example of a question in which you may be able to work out the answer by deduction based on understanding the function of the compound. Orexin is reduced or absent in narcolepsy, a disease in which sleepiness is a key symptom. Thus, it is reasonable to deduce that orexin is involved in wakefulness. We should remember that the VLPO is the sleep switch; therefore, VLPO is incorrect. Similarly, we remember that the thalamus is involved in sleep spindle generation; thus, the thalamus is not the correct answer. The pineal gland is involved in melatonin production; therefore, the pineal is not the correct answer.   (ATLAS2, pp 161–164)

14. Which statement about the dorsal raphe is *incorrect*?
  A. It is involved in REM sleep
  B. Cells are active mainly during wakefulness
  C. It releases serotonin
  D. It produces cortical activation via a ventral pathway to the hypothalamus

ANSWER: **A.**   The dorsal raphe is *not* involved in REM sleep generation. It is involved in arousal by releasing serotonin.   (ATLAS2, p 24)

15. What neurotransmitters are released in the VLPO?
  A. Galanin and GABA
  B. Orexin and serotonin
  C. Norepinephrine and histamine
  D. Melatonin and dopamine

ANSWER: **A.**   The correct answer can be deduced because the VLPO is the sleep switch and therefore would not be expected to release neurotransmitters that might cause wakefulness. Thus, answers B and C cannot be correct because orexin (in answer B) and histamine (in answer C) are well known to cause wakefulness. Melatonin is, of course, produced by the pineal gland. Thus, even if you never heard of galanin, you could figure out the answer.   (ATLAS2, pp 29–30)

16. Which brain area is involved in the REM-on process?
    A. VLPO
    B. Thalamus
    C. Pedunculopontine tegmental nuclei
    D. Basal forebrain

ANSWER: **C.**   The pedunculopontine tegmental, laterodorsal tegmental, sublaterodorsal, and precoeruleus/parabrachial nuclei are all involved in REM-on processes. This is hard to remember; however, REM processes begin in the pons, thus structures that are "pontine" should be associated with REM. It is worth remembering that the REM-on neurons of the pedunculopontine tegmental nucleus are cholinergic.

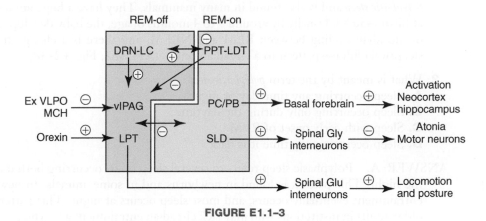

FIGURE E1.1–3

17. What structures play a role in muscle atonia in REM sleep?
    A. Lateral hypothalamic cells
    B. Cells in the VLPO
    C. Cells in the pineal gland
    D. Cell groups in the pons

ANSWER: **D.**   The correct answer can be deduced because none of the first three answers has anything to do with REM. Stimulation of cell groups in the pons can lead to atonia.

| E1.2 | **Circadian Mechanisms and Neurophysiology** |

QUESTIONS

1. In what age group is sleep unaffected by circadian light/dark cycles?
  A. Neonates
  B. Adolescents
  C. Young adults
  D. Normal older people

ANSWER: **A.**   Neonates sleep in short clusters over the 24-hour light/dark cycle. This is called *polyphasic sleep* and is also found in many mammals. They have a huge amount of REM sleep at birth (~50%). Usually by around 3 to 4 months of age, the baby develops a regular pattern of ultradian cycling between REM and NREM, and there is a change from a polyphasic sleep/wakefulness pattern to a circadian one.   (ATLAS2, Fig. 4.2–38)

2. What is meant by the term *polyphasic sleep*?
  A. Sleep occurring any time day or night
  B. Sleep occurring only during the daytime
  C. Sleep with early onset of REM
  D. Sleep occurring any time it is dark

ANSWER: **A.**   Polyphasic sleep refers to several sleep bouts occurring both during the day and the night. This pattern is found in newborns and in some animals. In newborns, circadian entrainment eventually occurs, and most sleep occurs at night. This pattern is also seen in older adults in institutions who may lack circadian entrainment and who may develop irregular sleep-wake disorder.   (ATLAS2, Fig. 4.2–38)

3. Where is the hormone melatonin secreted?
  A. Pineal gland
  B. Adrenal gland
  C. Posterior pituitary gland
  D. Retinohypothalamic tract

ANSWER: **A.**   Pineal gland.   (ATLAS2, Ch 3.3)

4. A patient who is blind from birth has a severe insomnia. What is the likeliest sleep disorder diagnosis?
  A. Advanced sleep phase syndrome
  B. Non–24-hour sleep-wake disorder
  C. Delayed sleep phase syndrome
  D. Depression-related comorbid insomnia

ANSWER: **B.**   The likeliest diagnosis is non–24-hour sleep-wake disorder. It has also been called free-running disorder. Such patients have a free-running sleep-wake rhythm because they are unable to sense light and therefore cannot synchronize their circadian system.   (ATLAS2, p 138; Quera Salva MA, Hartley S, Léger D, Dauvilliers YA. Non-24-Hour Sleep-Wake Rhythm Disorder in the Totally Blind: Diagnosis and Management. Front Neurol.2017 Dec 18;8:686.)

5. Melatonin secretion is inhibited by which of the following? Pick the *best* answer.
  A. Light
  B. Dark
  C. Food
  D. Nonlipophilic beta-blockers

ANSWER: **A.**   Melatonin has been called the hormone of darkness and, at times, the Dracula of hormones. Its secretion is inhibited by light sensed by melanopsin, a photopigment found in the photosensitive ganglion cells of the retina. Tasimelteon, a melatonin receptor 1 and 2 agonist, is used to treat non-24 hour sleep-wake disorder.   (ATLAS2, Ch 3.3)

6. What is the effect of bright light exposure early in the morning (end of the night) on the circadian rhythm of sleep in normal humans?
   A. Causes a phase delay
   B. Causes a phase advance
   C. No effect
   D. Induces sleep right after exposure

ANSWER: **B.** Light exposure (~2500 lux for 2 hours) in the morning causes a phase advance. Light exposure at night causes a phase delay. (ATLAS2, p 92)

7. Melatonin is a hormone produced by the _____ in response to _____.
   A. suprachiasmatic nucleus (SCN)/dark
   B. pineal gland/light
   C. SCN/light
   D. pineal gland/dark

ANSWER: **D.** The hormone melatonin is secreted by the pineal gland. Secretion is inhibited by light and increased by dark. (ATLAS2, p 26)

8. The fact that many biological rhythms will free run in a constant environment implies that
   A. Biological rhythms are passive responses to environmental changes
   B. Biological rhythms are actively produced by internal pacemakers
   C. Biological rhythms are always coupled with environmental changes
   D. None of the above

ANSWER: **B.** The critical observation supporting the concept of an internal pacemaker is the fact that circadian rhythms will continue to regularly oscillate under constant environmental conditions (i.e., without time cues). This condition is referred to as *free running*, in which the rhythm assumes its natural period (τ), the duration for one complete cycle. The free running period is always different from the period of the environmental zeitgeber (T). (ATLAS2, Ch 3.3)

9. Where is the coordinating pacemaker for the mammalian circadian rhythm system?
   A. The pineal gland
   B. The SCN
   C. The ganglion cells in the retina
   D. The raphe nuclei

ANSWER: **B.** Lesions of the SCN in experimental animals produce an arrhythmic organism that is incapable of entraining to a 24-hour environmental rhythm of light and darkness and is without an obvious free-running period in rest-activity cycles. Although major rhythms, such as the sleep-wake cycle, will become chaotic after the SCN is destroyed, other local tissue rhythms, such as liver enzyme levels, may retain a free-running period, which suggests that multiple pacemakers exist within various tissues of an intact organism that are coordinated by a master mechanism within the SCN. (ATLAS2, Ch 3.3)

10. Which of the following is necessary for entrainment of the sleep-wake cycle to the light-dark cycle?
    A. Normal vision
    B. The geniculohypothalamic tract
    C. The retinohypothalamic tract
    D. The retinal rod receptors

ANSWER: **C.** The retinohypothalamic tract contains the axons of melanopsin-containing ganglion cells within the retina. These specialized ganglion cells are the photosensitive receptor elements of the environmental illuminance monitoring system that feeds information about the light-dark cycle into the SCN. Disruption of this information pathway prevents photic entrainment in most diurnal mammals. (ATLAS2, Ch 3.3)

| E1.3 | **Sleep at Different Ages and Stages of Human Life** |

QUESTIONS

1. What is the best tool to diagnose restless legs syndrome (RLS) during pregnancy?
   A. Serum ferritin
   B. Patient history
   C. EMG during sleep
   D. EMG while awake

ANSWER: **B.**   The diagnosis of RLS in pregnant women is made the same as in everyone else: by a detailed history. RLS is a diagnosis based on symptoms, so the following questions are useful:

■ Do you have an urge to move your legs, accompanied by uncomfortable or unpleasant sensations in the legs?

■ Are the symptoms worse at rest and relieved by movement?

■ Are the symptoms worse at night, or do they only occur at that time?

"Yes" answers to all three questions make the diagnosis of RLS. Electromyography (EMG) plays no role in diagnosis (except to rule out some other disorder you might be concerned about), and serum ferritin is used only to determine whether iron deficiency might be playing a role in causation.   (ATLAS2, Ch 11.2)

2. All of the following are true about sleep during pregnancy *except*
   A. RLS appearing for the first time during pregnancy almost always continues after delivery
   B. Treatment of RLS in pregnancy should avoid dopamine agonists and instead focus on iron and folate supplements
   C. Poor sleep quality, as defined by the Pittsburgh Sleep Quality Index (PSQI), becomes significantly more common as pregnancy progresses
   D. The prevalence of RLS increases significantly from the first to third trimester

ANSWER: **A.**   When RLS appears during pregnancy, it often remits after delivery. Treatment with dopamine agonists should be avoided, although it is acceptable to give iron and folate during pregnancy. As for answers C and D, in one study of 189 pregnant woman, the percentage of patients who met diagnostic criteria for RLS increased from 17.5% at recruitment to 31.2% in the third trimester ($P = 0.001$). Also, overall poor sleep quality, as defined by a PSQI score greater than 5, became significantly more common as pregnancy progressed (39.0% compared with 53.5%, $P = 0.001$).   (PPSM6, Chapters 156–157)

3. Falling asleep by first entering REM is *most* typical for which of the following groups?
   A. Neonates
   B. Postmenopausal women
   C. The elderly
   D. Adolescents

ANSWER: **A.**   Neonates spend about 50% of their time in sleep and REM sleep, and in this population, it is common for sleep to be entered via REM. Entering sleep via REM is unusual except in patients with narcolepsy and in some individuals with severe sleep deprivation.   (ATLAS2, p 89)

4. Which statement about quiet sleep in the preterm unborn fetus is *incorrect*?
   A. It appears at about 36 weeks' gestation
   B. It comprises low-voltage delta and theta activity
   C. It is well defined by about 34 weeks' gestation
   D. There is no breathing activity

ANSWER: **D.**   In the fetus, the sleep stages are not as well defined as in children or adults, and sleep is characterized into quiet and active sleep states. There is a great deal of breathing activity during quiet sleep (equivalent to NREM sleep) in a fetus even though no gas exchange actually occurs because the lungs are atelectatic, and the airways are filled with amniotic fluid.   (PEDS2, p 20)

5. Which statement about active sleep in a preterm fetus is *incorrect*?
   A. Low-voltage irregular (LVI) activity is present
   B. REMs are present, and EMG tone is variable
   C. No movements occur, but the fetus grimaces
   D. Respiration and heart rate are variable

ANSWER: **C.**   Although it might be expected that there would be no movements in the fetus during what would be equivalent to REM sleep, in fact, there are movements, grimaces, and twitches.   (PEDS2, p 20)

6. What BEST describes sleep architecture as a percent of total sleep time of a term newborn?
   A. 5% stage 1; 50% stage 2; 25% slow-wave sleep; 20% REM sleep
   B. 5% stage N1; 50% stage N2; 0% stage N3; 50% stage R
   C. 50% to 60% active sleep; 10% to 30% quiet sleep; 20% to 30% indeterminate sleep
   D. Sleep cannot be scored in a newborn

ANSWER: **C.**   There are no formalized scoring rules for newborns younger than the age of 2 months   (MANUAL2). After 2 months of age, the designations are the same as in adults except that an additional stage is defined, called *stage N*, and the specific criteria to define these stages in children are described in the manual. Stage N is used in children older than 2 months, when a child is in NREM sleep, but there are no recognizable K complexes, sleep spindles, or slow waves. In a newborn, sleep structure can be scored as *quiet sleep* (equivalent to NREM); *active sleep* (equivalent to stage R); or *indeterminate sleep*, when neither active nor quiet sleep can be scored. An additional finding, *trace-alternant*, is seen in newborns. The latter is recognized as bursts of high-voltage electrical activity separated by periods of low-voltage activity.

7. What is trace-alternant?
   A. An EEG finding seen in sleeping newborns
   B. An EEG finding seen in patients with multiple system atrophy
   C. The finding of leg movements alternating between the right and left legs
   D. An abnormal breathing pattern in which large breaths alternate with small breaths

ANSWER: **A.**   Trace-alternant is an EEG finding seen in newborns, recognized as bursts of high-voltage electrical activity separated by periods of low-voltage activity.   (PEDS2, p 20)

8. Which statement about sleep in children is *incorrect*?
   A. Sleep spindles appear 2 to 3 months after term birth
   B. K complexes appear by 6 months after term birth
   C. REM-onset sleep continues to 18 months of age
   D. REM as a percent of TST decreases to about 30% by 1 year

ANSWER: **C.**   Many changes occur in sleep structure during the first year, with the appearance of sleep spindles (at 2–3 months) and K complexes (by 6 months) and a reduction in REM sleep. Entering sleep via REM, however, generally ceases between 3 and 6 months.   (PEDS2, p 20)

9. By what age do children generally stop napping during the daytime?
 A. 3 years
 B. 6 years
 C. 9 years
 D. 12 years

ANSWER: **B.**   Children have usually stopped napping when they start grade 1, usually at age 6 years.

10. Adolescents are prone to develop which of the following?
 A. Advanced sleep phase syndrome
 B. Delayed sleep phase syndrome
 C. Irregular sleep-wake syndrome
 D. Free-running circadian pattern

ANSWER: **B.**   Because of changes in their circadian control system, adolescents frequently develop delayed sleep phase syndrome. They fall asleep late and tend to wake up late if given the opportunity to sleep, for example, on weekends. Sleep deprivation is also common because of early school start times and poor sleep hygiene.

11. Which disorder becomes *less* common between the ages of 50 and 60 years?
 A. Sleep disturbance caused by hot flashes
 B. Restless legs syndrome
 C. Insomnia
 D. Obstructive sleep apnea

ANSWER: **A.**   In North America, menopause generally occurs at age 51 years and is defined as 12 months without menstrual cycles. Sleep disturbance can be quite severe because of hot flashes and night sweats. However, these symptoms most often remit or become less severe by age 60 years.

12. When are hot flashes during sleep *least* common?
 A. Stage N2
 B. Stage N3
 C. Stage R
 D. There is no relationship to sleep stage.

ANSWER: **C.**   Hot flashes are least common in REM sleep. It is likely that hot flashes require activity of the thermoregulatory system. It has been hypothesized that hot flashes do not occur in REM because thermoregulation is suppressed.

13. Older people are prone to develop which of the following?
 A. Advanced sleep phase syndrome
 B. Delayed sleep phase syndrome
 C. Irregular sleep-wake syndrome
 D. Free-running circadian pattern

ANSWER: **A.**   Older people frequently develop advanced sleep phase syndrome, going to sleep earlier and awakening earlier.   (ATLAS2, p 97)

14. Which statement about the effect of aging (between ages 40 and 70 years) on the sleep stages as a percent of total sleep time is *incorrect*?
 A. Stage N3 decreases substantially in older men
 B. Stage N3 decreases substantially in women
 C. Stage R sleep is preserved in men
 D. Stage R sleep is preserved in women

ANSWER: **A.**   REM sleep is relatively preserved in both men and women with aging. On the other hand, slow-wave sleep, stage N3, is decreased by about 50% in men but is well preserved in women. Other changes that occur with aging include reduction of spindles and K complexes.

15. Which is the *most* correct statement about arousals in older adults?
   A. The arousal rate in healthy older adults is less than five per hour
   B. The arousal index is increased only when periodic limb movements or sleep-breathing disorders are present
   C. The arousal index is increased in older adults without sleep-disordered breathing
   D. A history of cardiovascular disease is not associated with disturbed sleep

ANSWER: **C.** The arousal index is increased in older people, even in those without a sleep-breathing disorder.

16. Which statement about circadian rhythm of body temperature in older adults is *most* correct?
   A. The circadian phase is advanced, and amplitude is increased
   B. The circadian phase is advanced, and amplitude is decreased
   C. The circadian phase is delayed, and amplitude is increased
   D. The circadian phase is delayed, and amplitude is decreased

ANSWER: **B.** With aging, there occurs a phase advance but a decreased amplitude of circadian rhythm.

E1.4   Sleep Deprivation

QUESTIONS

1. Which statement about selective REM deprivation is TRUE?
   A. It leads to psychopathology
   B. It leads to increased aggression
   C. It leads to hyposexuality
   D. It leads to schizophrenia

ANSWER: **B.** Research done in the 1970s showed that selective REM sleep deprivation results in increased aggression and hypersexuality. (Puca FM, Livrea P, Genco S, et al: REM sleep deprivation in normal humans. Changes in anxiety, depression and aggressiveness, and HVA and 5-HIAA levels in the lumbar cerebrospinal fluid. *Boll Soc Ital Biol Sper* 52:782–787, 1976)

2. In an acutely sleep deprived individual, what is the effect of a 5-minute walk immediately before multiple sleep latency test (MSLT) evaluations?
   A. There is no effect because the MSLT is such a robust test
   B. The MSLT shows even more sleepiness with a 2- to 5-minute reduction in mean sleep latency
   C. The MSLT shows no change in mean latency but shows decreased sleep-onset REM periods (SOREMPs)
   D. The MSLT shows a large impact in mean sleep latency (longer by ~6 minutes)

ANSWER: **D.** Exercise can mitigate the effects of acute sleep deprivation on the MSLT. However, the effect of exercise on performance measures in sleep-deprived individuals is much more modest or nonexistent.

3. During a second night of total sleep deprivation, which is expected to have the longest effect in maintaining alertness: modafinil 200 mg, caffeine 300 mg, or dextroamphetamine 20 mg?
   A. Modafinil
   B. Caffeine
   C. Dextroamphetamine
   D. The three are equivalent

ANSWER: **A.** Modafinil has been shown to have the longest beneficial effect on maintaining alertness. This likely is related to its longer half-life.

4. Which statement about the effect of age on response to sleep deprivation is *correct*?
   A. Younger adults tolerate sleep deprivation much better than older adults
   B. Older adults tolerate sleep deprivation much better than younger adults
   C. There is little difference in performance and alertness decrement related to age, and if anything, the decrement may be less in older than younger men
   D. Because circadian amplitude is greater in older people, decrement from sleep deprivation is greater

ANSWER: **C.** Although it might be expected that older people would not tolerate sleep deprivation compared with younger adults, in fact, if anything, older men might tolerate sleep deprivation better than younger adults. The differences, however, are small.

5. Which statement about the effect of the circadian *CLOCK* gene on tolerance to sleep loss is *correct*?
   A. There is no evidence of any effect of any gene on sleep in humans.
   B. Although variants of the *CLOCK* gene *PER3* predict "morningness" and "eveningness," they have no effect on tolerance of sleep deprivation.
   C. Because the *CLOCK* genes only affect circadian physiology, there is no expected effect on sleep deprivation that affects homeostasis.
   D. Variants of the *CLOCK* gene *PER3* are associated with differing effects on tolerance to sleep deprivation.

ANSWER: **D.** Two groups with variants of the *CLOCK* gene PERIOD3 (*PER3*) have been studied. They have been categorized as PER3(5/5) and PER3(4/4). Whereas PER3(5/5) groups are more likely to show morning preference, PER3(4/4) groups show evening preferences. People with the PER3(5/5) variant have a greater cognitive decline and a greater reduction of brain responses to an executive task in response to total sleep deprivation. These effects are most noticeable during the late night or early morning hours. (Dijk DJ, Archer SN: PERIOD3, circadian phenotypes, and sleep homeostasis, *Sleep Med Rev* 14:151–160, 2010)

6. In normal young adults, after 40 hours of total sleep deprivation, what does the first recovery sleep show?
   A. Increased stage W
   B. Increased stage N2
   C. Increased stage N3
   D. Increased stage R

ANSWER: **C.** In young adults, the main finding in the first night of recovery sleep is a substantial increase in slow-wave sleep. On the second night, slow-wave sleep amounts normalize, and stage R shows an increase. By the third night, values are all normal.

7. "Core" sleep has been defined as the amount of sleep needed to maintain stable neurocognitive function. In adults, this value appears to be which of the following?
  A. 3 to 4 hours
  B. 4 to 5 hours
  C. 5 to 6 hours
  D. 7 to 8 hours

ANSWER: **D.** Some researchers have defined *core sleep* and *optional sleep*, with the former initially defined as about 4 hours. With additional research showing that even with 6 hours of nightly sleep, there may be neurocognitive or performance abnormalities, the value of required or "core" sleep has increased to about 7 to 8 hours.

8. With chronic sleep restriction, what is the *most* consistent sleep architecture finding?
  A. Increased stage N2
  B. Increased stage N3
  C. Increased stage R
  D. Normal sleep architecture

ANSWER: **B.** The most consistent finding with chronic sleep restriction is an increase in slow-wave sleep at the expense of other sleep stages.

9. Progressive nights of sleep restriction to 5 hours are expected to show which of the following?
  A. No effect on psychomotor vigilance task but increased sleep propensity
  B. Abnormal psychomotor vigilance task and increased sleep propensity
  C. No effect on psychomotor vigilance task or sleep propensity
  D. Abnormal psychomotor vigilance task but normal sleep propensity

ANSWER: **B.** Five hours of sleep restriction is expected to show abnormalities in the psychomotor vigilance task (PVT) and an increase in sleep propensity as measured by multiple sleep latency test (MSLT) or maintenance of wakefulness test (MWT).

10. In tests of driving performance on a simulator in subjects restricted to 4 to 6 hours of sleep, which of the following is *correct*?
  A. There is no effect on accident rate
  B. There is an increase in accident rate
  C. There is a decrease in accident rate as subject tries to compensate
  D. Accident rate is increased only when testing is done at night

ANSWER: **B.** Accident rate is increased in sleep-restricted individuals, and the abnormalities are documented both in day and night testing.

11. Chronic sleep restriction to 4 hours is expected to show which effects?
  A. Increased evening cortisol and sympathetic activation
  B. Increased thyrotropin activity and decreased glucose tolerance
  C. Increased leptin and decreased ghrelin levels
  D. All of the above

ANSWER: **A.** This is an important topic. Sleep restriction leads to an increase in cortisol, ghrelin, and sympathetic activity and to a decrease in leptin and thyrotropin, as well as a decreased glucose tolerance result (insulin resistance).

12. What effect does sleep loss (4 hours of sleep for 6 nights) have on response to influenza vaccination?
   A. Sleep deprivation causes a 50% decrease in antibody titers to influenza vaccine at 10 days, which persists for at least 1 year
   B. Sleep deprivation causes a 50% decrease in antibody titers to influenza vaccine at 10 days, which normalizes by 4 weeks
   C. Sleep deprivation causes a 50% increase in antibody titers to influenza vaccine, which persists for at least 1 year
   D. Sleep deprivation has no effect on immune function

ANSWER: **B.**   In addition to the temporary reduction in immune response to influenza vaccination, abnormalities in interleukin-6 and tumor necrosis factor have been reported.

13. Which statement about the effect of sleep deprivation on the cardiovascular system is *incorrect?*
   A. Sleep deprivation is associated with increased C-reactive protein, a marker of cardiovascular risk
   B. Sleep deprivation is associated with increased cardiovascular morbidity
   C. The Nurses' Health Study did not show that sleep deprivation was associated with cardiovasculr events
   D. Shift workers have reduced cardiovascular health

ANSWER: **C.**   The Nurses' Health Study showed that women with inadequate and disrupted sleep had increased cardiovascular events. Gangwisch JE, Rexrode K, Forman JP, et al. Daytime sleepiness and risk of coronary heart disease and stroke: results from the Nurses' Health Study II. Sleep Med. 2014 Jul;15(7):782–8.

14. The purpose of low and high filters is to isolate specific frequency bandwidths relevant to each recording parameter. Which of the following an *incorrect* filter range for the parameter shown?
   A. EEG: 0.3 Hz to 35 Hz
   B. EOG: 0.3 Hz to 35 Hz
   C. EMG: 10 Hz to 100 Hz
   D. ECG: 20 Hz to 100 Hz

ANSWER: **D.**   The recommended low-high frequency filter for electrocardiogram (ECG) is 0.3 to 70 Hz.   (MANUAL2)

15. A *major body movement* (MBM) is defined as
   A. Movement and muscle artifact obscuring the EEG for more than half an epoch to the extent that sleep stage cannot be determined
   B. Movement artifact that manifests for at least 10 seconds in a standard 30-second epoch
   C. Movement or muscle artifact that obscures the entire epoch
   D. Movement artifact that awakens the patient

ANSWER: **A.**   This statement is the definition of *major body movement*.   (MANUAL2)

16. An epoch can be scored as "movement time" when
   A. An MBM occupies more than 50% of any epoch
   B. An MBM occupies at least one third of any epoch
   C. An MBM is at least half of a W epoch
   D. An epoch can never be scored as movement time

ANSWER: **D.**   According to the AASM scoring manual, movement time is no longer scored. Instead, the epoch in which an MBM occurs is scored as W, N1, N2, N3, or REM. The rules are as follows:
   A) If alpha rhythm is seen in any part of the epoch that has an MBM, the score is W
   B) If not A, and the epoch before or after is W, score the epoch with MBM as W
   C) If neither A nor B, score the epoch the same stage as the epoch after the MBM

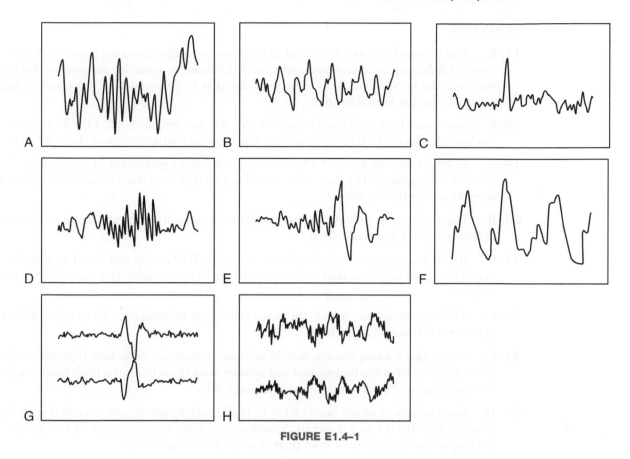

FIGURE E1.4–1

Match the activity given in questions 17 through 24 to the waveforms labeled A through H. The time duration represented by each waveform is 1 second. Six tracings are from an EEG, and two are from an electrooculogram (EOG); each figure is used only once (Fig. E1.4–1).

17. K complex

18. Slow waves

19. Alpha activity

20. Theta activity

21. REM

22. Slow eye movements (SEMs)

23. Vertex sharp waves

24. Sleep spindles
   A. (3.2 to 14)
   B. (3.2 to 15)
   C. (3.2 to 18)
   D. (3.2 to 19)
   E. (3.2 to 12)
   F. (3.2 to 13)
   G. (3.2 to 16)
   H. (3.2 to 17)

ANSWERS:

17. E.   The K complex is an EEG event that consists of well-delineated negative sharp wave (upward deflection by convention) immediately followed by a positive component that stands out from the background EEG. The total duration is 0.5 seconds or more and is usually maximal over the frontal regions.

18. F.   Slow waves have high amplitude (≥75 μV) and low frequency (≤2 Hz). Slow waves are a subset of delta (1–4 Hz) activity and are the defining characteristics of stage N3 sleep.

19. A.   Alpha activity; an 8- to 13-Hz rhythm, usually most prominent in occipital leads and thought to be generated by the cortex, is used as a marker for relaxed wakefulness and central nervous system (CNS) arousals.

20. B.   Theta activity; 4- to 7-Hz waves, typically prominent in central and temporal leads, seen in both stage N1 and REM sleep.

21. G.   REMs are conjugate saccades that occur during REM sleep and correlate with dreaming. They are sharply peaked with an initial deflection usually less than 0.5 second in duration.

22. H.   SEMs are conjugate, usually rhythmic, rolling eye movements with an initial deflection more than 0.5 second in duration.

23. C.   Vertex sharp waves show a sharply contoured, negative deflection (upward on EEG) that stands out from the background and appears most often in central leads placed near the midline; they are characteristically seen in stage N1.

24. D.   Sleep spindle, a phasic burst of 11- to 16-Hz activity prominent in central scalp leads, typically lasts for 0.5 to 1.0 second. Spindles are a scalp representation of thalamocortical discharges; the name derives from their shape, which is spindlelike.

Match one of the following terms, A through Q, to each of the statements numbered 25 through 36. References for the answers are in the AASM scoring manual.

  A. Alpha rhythm
  B. Artifact
  C. Beta
  D. Complex
  E. Delta
  F. Delta sleep
  G. Frequency
  H. K complex
  I. Movement time
  J. Theta
  K. Sawtooth waves
  L. Sleep spindle
  M. Stage N1
  N. Stage N2
  O. Stage N3
  P. REM sleep
  Q. Awake

25. Used to indicate EEG frequencies higher than 13 Hz. Answer: **C**

26. Well-delineated negative sharp wave immediately followed by a positive component, duration of 0.5 or more seconds, usually maximal in amplitude when recorded with frontal derivations. Answer: **H**

27. EEG frequency of 8 to 13 Hz in adults, most prominent in the posterior areas. Characteristic of relaxed wakefulness with the eyes closed. Answer: **A**

28. Moderate amounts (≥20%) of high-amplitude (≥75 μV), slow-wave (≤2 Hz) EEG activity. Answer: **O**

29. Sometimes used as a synonym for stage N3 sleep. Answer: **F**

30. Sleep-scoring epoch during which the record is totally obscured by muscle tone for greater than 15 seconds but less than 1 minute. Answer: **I**

31. A waveform with a frequency of 12 to 14 cps, most prominent in stage N2 sleep. Answer: **L**

32. A stage of relatively low-voltage, mixed-frequency EEG without REMs; SEMs are often present, vertex sharp waves may be seen, and EMG activity is not suppressed. Answer: **M**

33. A nonbiological signal that appears in an EEG of sleep recording and interferes with the signals being recorded. Answer: **B**

34. Notched waveforms in vertex and the frontal regions that sometimes occur in conjunction with bursts of rapid eye movements in REM sleep. Answer: **K**

35. Indicates an EEG frequency of 4 to 7 cps. Answer: **J**

36. 12 to 14 cps sleep spindles and K complexes on a background of relatively low-voltage, mixed-frequency EEG activity. Answer: **N**

For questions 37 through 48, match the electrophysiologic characteristics with the sleep stage(s) where it may be found. Use the terminology W, N1, N2, N3, and R. Note that some characteristics help define a sleep stage, but other characteristics may simply be in a stage defined by something else. Thus, for example, you would not find REMs in stage N2 because they are used to define REM sleep, but you could find alpha rhythm in any stage because it only defines W if it occupies 15 or more seconds of a 30-second epoch.

37. Low-voltage, mixed-frequency activity: stage _____, _____, or _____

38. Vertex sharp waves: stage _____ or _____

39. Sleep spindles: stage _____ or _____

40. K complexes: stage _____ or _____

41. Beta activity: stage _____, _____, or _____

42. Alpha activity (a freebie): stage _____, _____, _____, _____, or _____

43. Theta activity: stage _____, _____, _____, or _____

44. Slow-wave activity: stage _____, _____, _____, or _____

45. Slow eye movements: stage _____ or _____

46. Rapid eye movements: stage _____

47. Atonic electromyogram (EMG) activity: stage _____

48. Low voltage, mixed frequency with sawtooth pattern: stage _____

ANSWERS

37. Low-voltage, mixed-frequency activity. stage N1, N2, or R

38. Vertex sharp waves: stage N1 or N2

39. Sleep spindles: stage N2 or N3

40. K complexes: stage N2 or N3

41. Beta activity: stage W, N1, or R

42. Alpha activity (a freebie): stage W (≥15 seconds), N1 (<15 seconds), N2 (<15 seconds), N3 (<15 seconds), or R (<15 seconds)

43. Theta activity: stage N1, N2, N3, or R (with typical sawtooth pattern)

44. Slow-wave activity: stage N1 (≤6 seconds), N2 (≤6 seconds), N3 (≥6 seconds), or R (≤6 seconds)

45. Slow eye movements: stage W or N1

46. Rapid eye movements: stage R

47. Atonic EMG activity: stage R

48. Low voltage, mixed frequency with sawtooth pattern: stage R

49. Polysomnographic (PSG) waveforms are defined based on four features: (1) amplitude, (2) frequency, (3) waveform shape, and (4) distribution. Below are descriptions of four waveforms, labeled 1 through 4. From letters A through D, pick the *correct* sequence of waveforms corresponding to stages W, N1, N2, N3.
  A. Alpha rhythm, vertex sharp wave, slow wave, K complex
  B. Alpha rhythm, vertex sharp wave, K complex, slow wave
  C. Theta rhythm, eye blink, slow wave, K complex
  D. Sleep spindle, K complex, vertex sharp wave, slow wave

ANSWER: **B.** (MANUAL2)

50. Impedance in PSG is a measure of the contact of the electrode with the skin. All electrode impedances should be below
  A. 5 Ohms
  B. 500 Ohms
  C. 5000 Ohms
  D. 20,000 Ohms

ANSWER: **C.** (MANUAL2)

51. According to the AASM's 2014 recommendations, in a sleep-staging montage, the F4 electrode should be referred to which other electrode?
  A. E1
  B. F3
  C. M2
  D. M1

ANSWER: **D.** (MANUAL2)

52. When the sensitivity control is set at 10 μV/mm, a 100-μV input signal will produce a pen deflection of
  A. 1 mm
  B. 10 mm
  C. 10 cm
  D. 100 mm

ANSWER: **C.** Of course, nobody uses pens anymore!

53. In normal adults, what are the approximate percentages for each sleep stage?

	W	N1	N2	N3	REM
A.	5	5	50	15	25
B.	5	15	40	20	20
C.	5	20	30	20	25
D.	10	10	40	10	30

ANSWER: **A.** (ATLAS2, p 84)

54. In stage R, which of the following findings is *most* characteristic?
  A. Increased muscle tone
  B. Sawtooth waves
  C. Sleep spindles
  D. K complexes

ANSWER: **B.** Sawtooth waves are often seen in the EEG during REM sleep but are not essential to its staging. They look like the teeth of a saw, as shown in the green ovals below in this REM epoch (see Fig. E1.4–2).

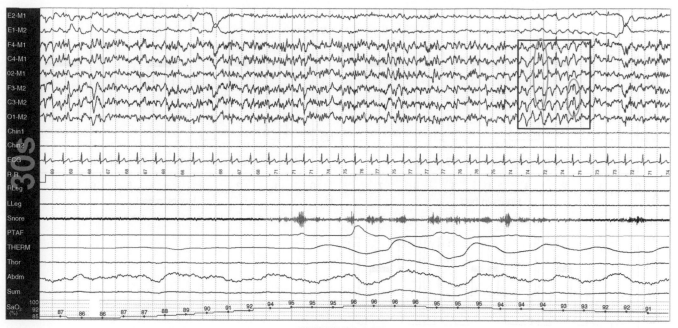

FIGURE E1.4–2

55. Which of the following is a characteristic normal stage N2 sleep?
  A. Absent muscle tone
  B. Delta waves
  C. Sleep spindles
  D. Alpha waves

ANSWER: **C.**

56. Which of the following statements *most* closely characterizes changes in sleep with aging?
  A. Sleep latency increases; percent REM sleep decreases
  B. Slow-wave amplitude increases; percent slow-wave sleep decreases
  C. Stages 1 and 2 increase; slow-wave amplitude increases
  D. Sleep latency decreases; sleep efficiency decreases

ANSWER: **A**

57. Which statement *best* describes the distribution of REM sleep during normal nocturnal sleep?
  A. REM episodes are evenly distributed throughout the night
  B. REM episodes last longer later in the night
  C. REM sleep occurs mainly during the first 120 minutes of the night
  D. REM sleep occurs mainly in the middle third of the night

ANSWER: **B.** Whereas the percentage of REM sleep decreases with aging, in all cases the episodes of REM sleep tend to be longer later in the sleep cycle. Figure E1.4–3 (ATLAS2, Fig. 4.2–25, p 86) shows REM distribution (*horizontal red bars*) in three different ages: A, child; B, young- to-middle-aged adult; C, older adult.

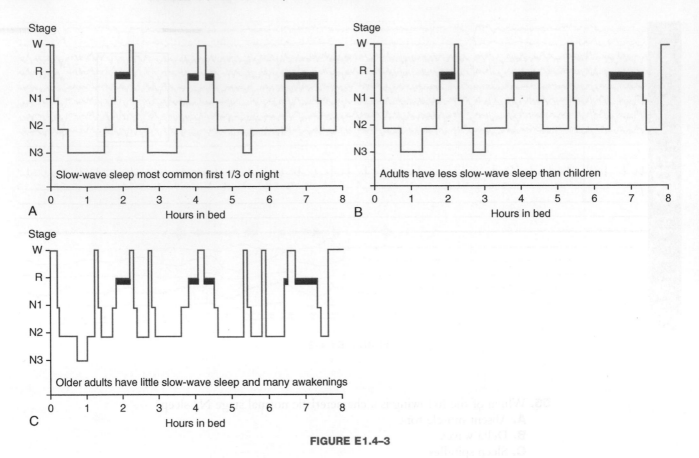

A — Slow-wave sleep most common first 1/3 of night
B — Adults have less slow-wave sleep than children
C — Older adults have little slow-wave sleep and many awakenings

FIGURE E1.4–3

58. *Most* slow-wave sleep typically occurs in what part of the night?
 A. First third of the night
 B. Middle third of the night
 C. Last third of the night
 D. Equally throughout the night

ANSWER: **A.**   This fact is also appreciated in the three hypnograms shown in Figure E1.4–3.

59. Upper limit of normal sleep latency in adults is approximately
 A. Less than 5 minutes
 B. Less than 20 minutes
 C. 20 to 40 minutes
 D. Up to 90 minutes

ANSWER: **B.**

60. According to the AASM practice parameters for use of actigraphy, only two indications are considered standard, including which one of the following?

A. To assist in the evaluation of patients suspected of advanced sleep phase syndrome (ASPS) and delayed sleep phase syndrome (DSPS)

B. To estimate total sleep time in patients with obstructive sleep apnea (OSA) when PSG is not available

C. To determine circadian pattern and estimate average daily sleep time in individuals complaining of hypersomnia

D. For evaluating the response to treatment for patients with insomnia

ANSWER: **B.**   (Morgenthaler T, Alessi C, Friedman L, et al: Practice parameters for the use of actigraphy in the assessment of sleep and sleep disorders: an update for 2007. Sleep 30:519–529, 2007)

  ○ "Actigraphy is a valid way to assist in determining sleep patterns in normal, healthy adult populations." (Standard)

  ○ "When PSG is not available, actigraphy is indicated as a method to estimate total sleep time in patients with obstructive sleep apnea syndrome. Combined with a validated way of monitoring respiratory events, use of actigraphy may improve accuracy in assessing the severity of obstructive sleep apnea compared with using time in bed." (Standard)

61. What stage of sleep is shown on the following PSG fragment in Figure E1.4–4?

A. Stage W

B. Stage N1

C. Stage N2

D. Stage N3

ANSWER: **B.**   This is stage N1. About 10 seconds from the end of this epoch is a vertex sharp wave, and the EEG shows low-amplitude, mixed-frequency waves. This stage frequently also demonstrates slow eye movements.   (MANUAL2)

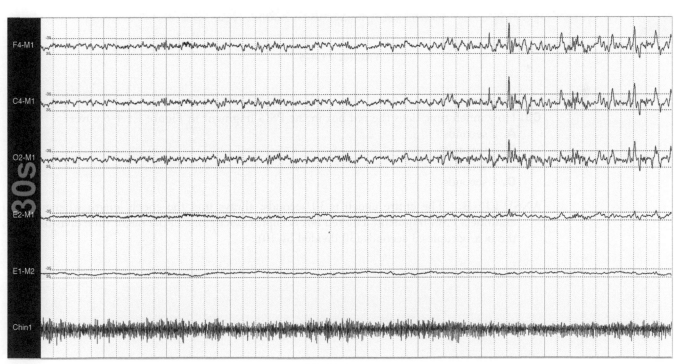

FIGURE E1.4–4

62. What is shown in the red-bordered area in the following PSG (Fig. E1.4–5)?
- **A.** Vertex sharp wave
- **B.** Sawtooth wave
- **C.** Seizure spike
- **D.** K complex

ANSWER: **A.**   This is a vertex sharp wave. Three characteristics of this wave are that it stands out from the background of mixed-frequency, low-amplitude activity; it is maximal over the central region (C4-M1, in this example); and it is of short duration (<0.5 second).   (MANUAL2)

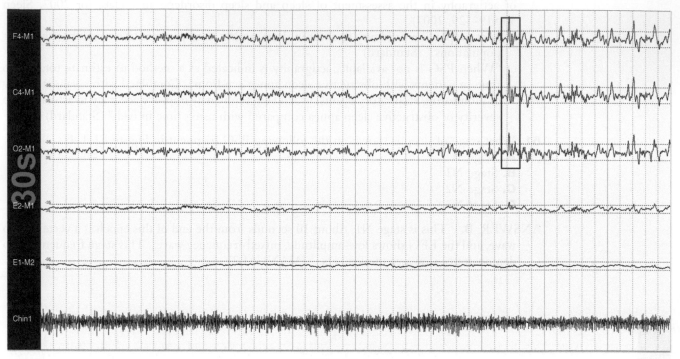

FIGURE E1.4–5

63. How much time does the red box in the PSG fragment in Figure E1.4–6 cover?
- **A.** 2 seconds
- **B.** 3 seconds
- **C.** 4 seconds
- **D.** 5 seconds

ANSWER: **B.**   The entire epoch is 30 seconds; always find the epoch length whenever you examine a PSG fragment. The red box occupies exactly one of the major time divisions, thus the box occupies 3 seconds (30 divided by 10).

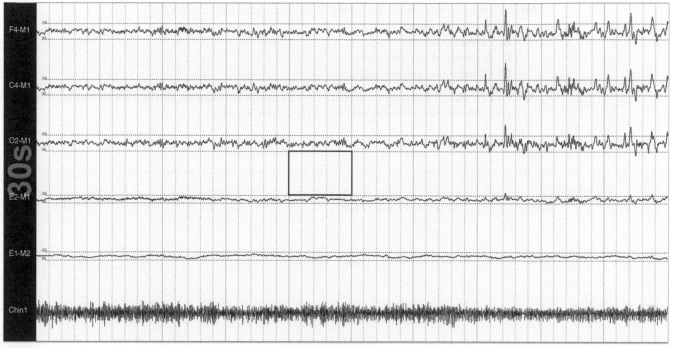

FIGURE E1.4–6

64. How much time does the red box in the PSG fragment in Figure E1.4–7 cover?
- **A.** 0.2 seconds
- **B.** 0.3 seconds
- **C.** 0.5 seconds
- **D.** 0.6 seconds

ANSWER: **D.**   The entire epoch is 30 seconds; always find the epoch length whenever you examine a PSG fragment. There are 10 major time divisions; thus, each major time division occupies 30 divided by 10, or 3 seconds. The red box occupies the minor time division, which is one-fifth of the major time division. Thus, the box covers 3 seconds divided by 5, or 0.6 seconds.

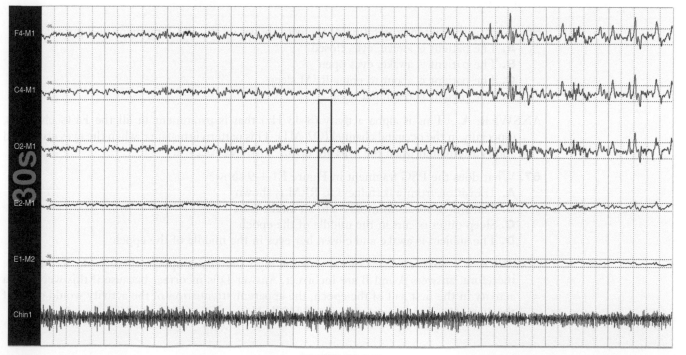

FIGURE E1.4–7

65. What is shown on the following PSG fragment (Fig. E1.4–8)?
  A. Sawtooth waves
  B. Alpha activity
  C. A string of K complexes
  D. Continuous seizure activity

ANSWER: **B.** This is alpha activity (8–13 Hz), prominent in all the EEG channels but especially in the occipital channel O2-M1. (MANUAL2)

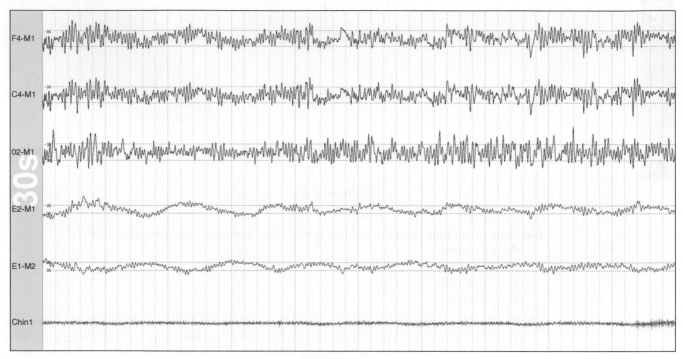

FIGURE E1.4–8

66. What is the *best* interpretation of the data shown on the PSG fragment in Figure E1.4–8?
  A. The patient is awake, eyes closed
  B. The patient is awake, eyes open
  C. The patient is about to enter REM sleep
  D. The patient is reading a book

ANSWER: **A.** This is alpha activity (8–13 Hz) that is prominent in all the EEG channels, especially in the occipital channel (O2-M1). This pattern is maximal when the eyes are closed and is attenuated when the eyes are open. (MANUAL2)

67. What does the PSG fragment in Figure E1.4–9 show?
  A. Transition from wakefulness to REM is shown
  B. Transition occurs from REM to an awake state
  C. Sleep onset occurs in the middle of the epoch
  D. The subject is awake and closed her eyes in the middle of the epoch

ANSWER: **C.** Because EMG tone remains high the entire epoch, there is no REM sleep; therefore, answers A and B are incorrect. Answer D is incorrect because if this were alpha activity in the first half of the epoch, the apparent attenuation of the activity would occur if the eyes were opened, not closed. (MANUAL2)

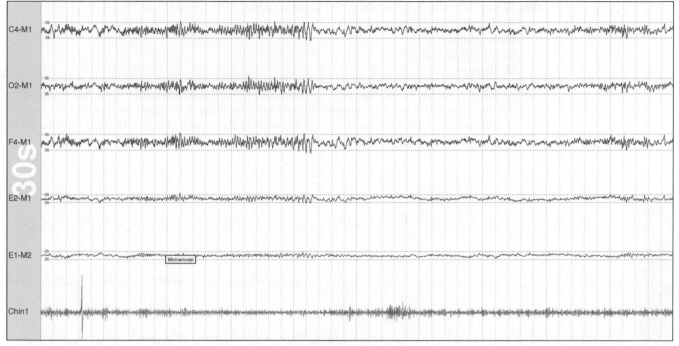

FIGURE E1.4–9

68. What stage of sleep is shown in the PSG fragment in Figure E1.4–10?
   A. Stage R
   B. Stage N1
   C. Stage N2
   D. Stage N3

ANSWER: **C.**   This is stage N2 sleep. A well-developed K complex is evident just before the middle of the epoch. The K complex is a negative sharp wave (in the EEG, negative is an upward deflection) with a duration exceeding 0.5 seconds. The K complex is usually maximal in the frontal derivations and stands out from the background EEG. Spindles (waves usually 12 to 14 Hz) are also characteristic of stage N2 sleep.   (MANUAL2)

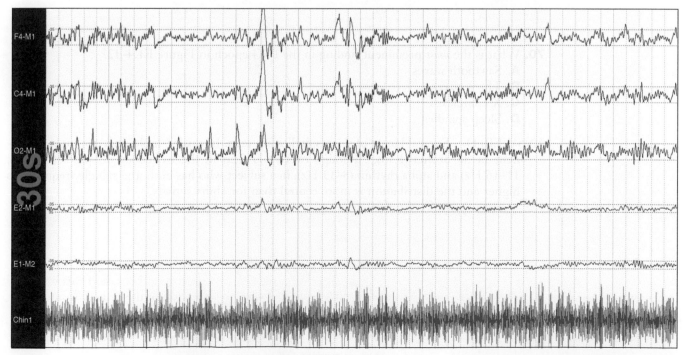

FIGURE E1.4–10

69. What is shown in the highlighted portion of the PSG fragment in Figure E1.4–11?
   A. Vertex sharp wave
   B. K complex
   C. Sawtooth wave
   D. Seizure

ANSWER: **C.**   This is a K complex. A vertex sharp wave is shorter than 1 second in duration. Sawtooth waves have less amplitude and duration than K complexes and in any case are characteristic of REM sleep, not stage N2 seen in this epoch. Finally, there is nothing in the EEG to indicate seizure activity.   (MANUAL2)

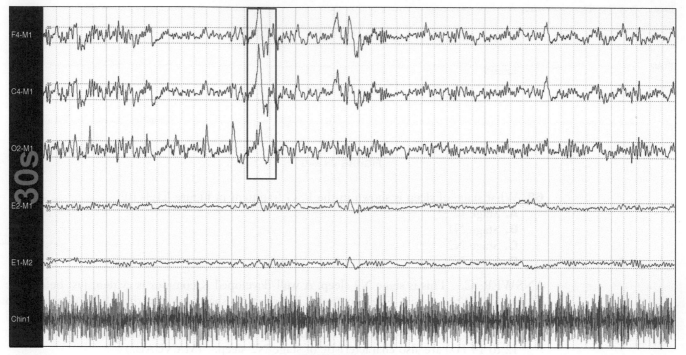

FIGURE E1.4–11

70. What is the *most* prominent finding in the PSG epoch in Figure E1.4–12?
   A. Sawtooth waves
   B. Theta waves
   C. K complexes
   D. Sleep spindles

ANSWER: **D.**   Several bursts of sleep spindles are seen. In this example, they are most prominent in the frontal leads. Although overlap is seen in the frequency of spindles (range, 11–16 Hz) and alpha rhythm (8–13 Hz), in a subject who has both, the spindle frequency is higher and the distribution is more central than for alpha activity.

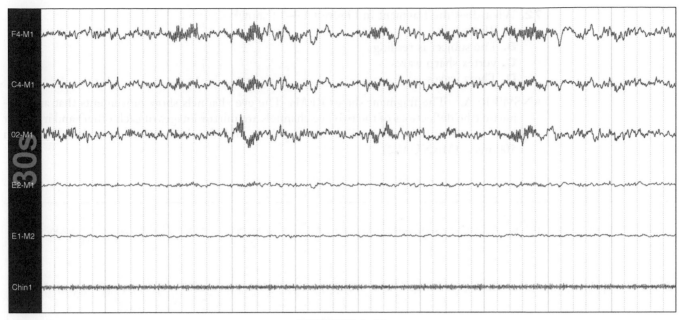

FIGURE E1.4–12

71. The horizontal red dashed lines in Figure E1.4–13 have a vertical distance between them of 70 µV (from +35 to −35). What does the figure show?

A. Status epilepticus
B. Strings of K complexes
C. Stage N3 sleep
D. Stage R sleep

ANSWER: **C.**   This is slow-wave sleep, stage N3. *Slow waves* are defined as having a frequency of 0.5 to 2 Hz. Their peak-to-peak amplitude is greater than 75 µV in the frontal region. More than 20% of the epoch is made up of slow waves. Note that sleep spindles may persist in N3, as seen near the end of the epoch.   (MANUAL2)

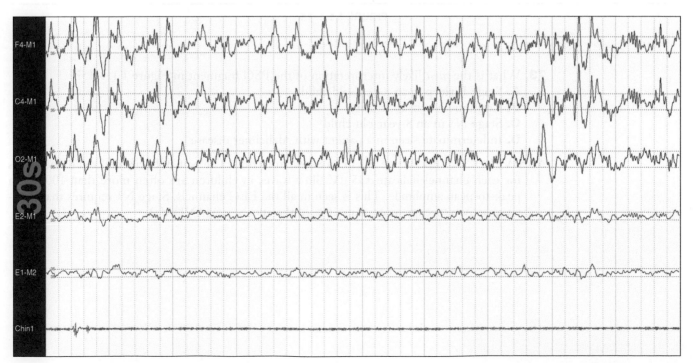

FIGURE E1.4–13

72. What does the fragment in Figure E1.4–14 show?
   A. REMs
   B. The subject is reading
   C. Vertex sharp waves
   D. Theta waves

ANSWER: **A.**   The fragment shows REMs. The eye channels show movements that are conjugate (the deflections of the two eye channels are mirror images of each other) and irregular (eye movements when reading are regular), and the initial deflection lasts less than 500 ms.   (MANUAL2)

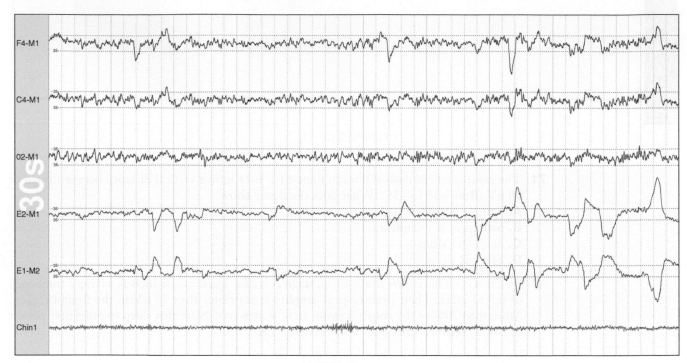

FIGURE E1.4–14

73. What is the *most* likely interpretation of the PSG fragment in Figure E1.4–15?
   A. Stage R sleep in an 8-year-old child
   B. Continuous seizure activity
   C. Stage N3 in an 8-year-old child
   D. Indeterminate sleep in a patient with Alzheimer disease

ANSWER: **C.**   This is stage N3 in an 8-year-old child. The pair of horizontal red dashed lines for each channel indicate ±35 μV. Slow waves in children are often more than 100 μV in peak-to-peak amplitude. This is seen in all the EEG channels. Stage N3 requires that slow-wave activity occupy more than 20% of the epoch.   (MANUAL2)

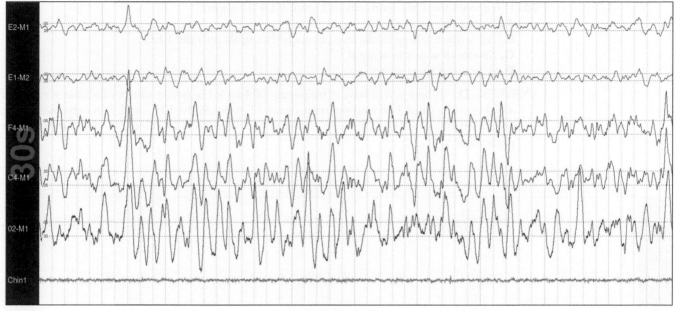

FIGURE E1.4–15

74. How would you interpret the PSG epoch from an 8-year-old patient, shown in Figure E1.4–16?

A. The entire epoch should be scored stage R sleep

B. It shows transition from stage N2 to stage R about 17 seconds into the epoch

C. The epoch should be scored as stage N1 sleep

D. The epoch should be scored as stage N3 sleep

ANSWER: **B.** This epoch should be scored as stage N2 sleep (notice the spindle at 6 seconds into the epoch), because more than half the epoch is stage N2; the transition into stage R begins 17 seconds into the epoch. At that point, there is an abrupt reduction in chin tone, and sawtooth waves appear in the EEG channels. Sawtooth waves have a frequency of 2 to 6 Hz, and they are triangular or serrated in shape. (MANUAL2)

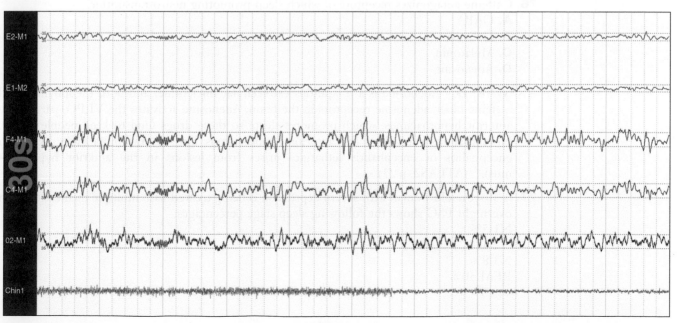

FIGURE E1.4–16

75. What does the PSG fragment in Figure E1.4–17 show?
  A. Seizure activity
  B. An artifact arising in the eye channels that spills into the EEG
  C. Sawtooth waves in stage R
  D. A burst of theta waves

ANSWER: **D.**   Theta waves have a frequency of 4 to 8 Hz (some sources indicate a range of 4–7 Hz). The third 3-second segment shows 12 cycles in the EEG and EOG channels; thus, the frequency is 4 Hz. Theta waves are most often seen in stage N1 sleep and are not pathologic.

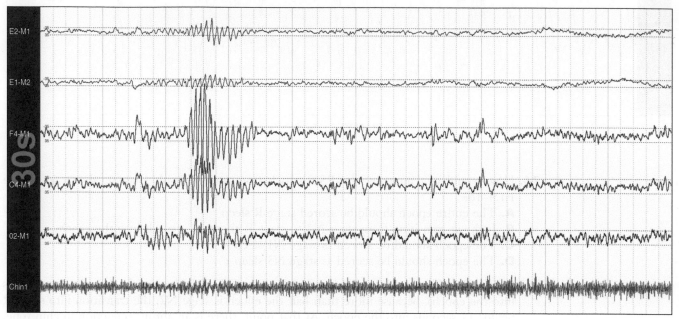

FIGURE E1.4–17

76. Caffeine antagonizes receptors of which sleep-promoting neurotransmitter?
  A. GABA
  B. Galanin
  C. Melatonin
  D. Adenosine

ANSWER: **D.**   Adenosine is a ubiquitous extracellular nucleotide, and both theophylline and caffeine block adenosine receptors in the brain. Adenosine activates the VLPO, part of the anterior hypothalamus, which promotes sleep, so these drugs tend to keep people awake. Note that destruction of the anterior hypothalamus leads to insomnia (Von Economo encephalitis or encephalitis lethargica arises from lesions in the anterior hypothalamus).   (ATLAS2, p 23)

77. A 50-year-old woman with severe depression is being treated with multiple medications. An overnight PSG shows the following sleep stage percentages:
N1 5%
N2 37%
N3 8%
REM 50%

78. Which of the drugs she is taking, listed below, is *most* likely to cause this distribution?

   A. Dextroamphetamine
   B. Bupropion
   C. Citalopram
   D. Trazodone

ANSWER: **B.**   Bupropion (Wellbutrin).   (Nofzinger EA, Reynolds CF 3rd, Thase ME, et al: REM sleep enhancement by bupropion in depressed men, *Am J Psychiatry* 152:274–276, 1995; Mayers AG, Baldwin DS: Antidepressants and their effect on sleep, *Hum Psychopharmacol* 20:533–559, 2005.) Most antidepressants decrease REM sleep, including selective serotonin reuptake inhibitors (SSRIs; e.g., fluoxetine, paroxetine), selective norepinephrine reuptake inhibitors (SNRIs; e.g., venlafaxine, citalopram), tricyclic antidepressants (TCAs; e.g., amitriptyline), and trazodone. Benzodiazepines and nonbenzodiazepine hypnotics (Z drugs) have a mild suppressant effect on REM sleep. (Note: The benzodiazepines suppress slow-wave sleep; Z drugs do not). Two drugs increase REM sleep, bupropion and nefazodone, and the latter is used infrequently. Also associated with increased REM sleep are withdrawal from antidepressants, metabolism of alcohol during sleep, and first use of continuous positive airway pressure in sleep-deprived patients.

79. The PSG can be affected by many drugs typically prescribed in the treatment of sleep disorders. All of the following statements are true *except*

   A. Benzodiazepines tend to suppress slow-wave sleep (SWS) and have no consistent effect on REM sleep
   B. TCAs tend to suppress REM sleep
   C. Fluoxetine is associated with REMs across all sleep stages
   D. Acute presleep alcohol intake produces an increase in SWS and decreased REM sleep early in the night followed by REM rebound and arousals later in the night as the alcohol is metabolized

ANSWER: **D.**   Actually, acute presleep alcohol intake can produce an increase in SWS and REM sleep suppression (i.e., a decreased amount of REM) early in the night. As alcohol is metabolized, there can be REM sleep rebound in the latter portion of the night.

80. Below are four mechanisms of action, labeled 1 through 4, for drugs used to either promote sleep or promote wakefulness. Pick the *correct* sequence of mechanisms, labeled A through D, that matches the sequence shown in 1 through 4.

   (1) Blocks 5-hydroxytryptamine (5-HT) and alpha₁-adrenergic receptors
   (2) Blocks reuptake of serotonin
   (3) Binds to several alpha subunits on the GABA_A receptor
   (4) Enhances dopamine release into the synaptic space
   A. Trazodone, fluoxetine, diazepam, amphetamine
   B. Ramelteon, caffeine, lorazepam, methylphenidate
   C. Zaleplon, paroxetine, trazodone, barbiturates
   D. Modafinil, sodium oxybate, clonazepam, amphetamine

ANSWER: **A.**   Trazodone blocks 5-HT (serotonin) and alpha₁-adrenergic receptors; fluoxetine is an SSRI; diazepam is a benzodiazepine that binds nonselectively to the GABA_A receptor (in contrast to Z drugs, which bind selectively to the GABA_{A1} subunit); and amphetamines, which block the reuptake of dopamine.

81. In addition to shortening sleep latency, drinking alcohol before sleep has all of the following effects *except*

   A. Decreases slow-wave sleep in the first half of the night
   B. Depresses REM sleep in the first half of the night
   C. Causes REM rebound in the second half of the night
   D. Causes reduction in airway dilator muscle tone, increasing airway resistance

ANSWER: **A.**   Alcohol increases SWS in the first half of the night.

82. Antiepileptic drugs have variable effects on sleep. Excessive daytime sleepiness is prominent with all of the following drugs *except*
  A. Lamotrigine
  B. Gabapentin
  C. Tiagabine
  D. Phenobarbital

ANSWER: **A.**   Daytime sleepiness is not a side effect of lamotrigine (Lamictal), whereas it is seen with most antiepileptics, especially gabapentin, tiagabine, and phenobarbital.   (ATLAS2, Table 11.3–3, p 209)

83. Which statement *best* characterizes the sleep pattern of newborns?
  A. Newborns enter REM sleep (called *active sleep*) before quiet sleep (NREM sleep) and have a shorter sleep cycle than adults (~50 minutes)
  B. Newborns enter quiet sleep first and then cycle between REM (active sleep) and quiet sleep about every 30 minutes
  C. About 75% of the sleep cycle is indeterminate sleep; the rest is REM (active) sleep
  D. More than 90% of the sleep cycle is classified as indeterminate sleep, neither REM nor quiet sleep

ANSWER: **A.**   At birth, REM (active sleep) is approximately 50% of total sleep; this percentage declines over the first 2 years to about 20% to 25%. During quiet (NREM) sleep, there are no body movements, breathing is regular, EMG activity is low, and there are no REMs. Indeterminate sleep is also an EEG classification in neonates, when the pattern fits neither active (REM) nor quiet (NREM) sleep. Quiet (NREM) sleep in neonates does not have slow waves or K complexes; slow waves begin to appear at about 3 months, and K complexes appear around 6 months of age.   (PEDS2, p 19)

84. A 7-year-old boy suddenly sits up at night screaming, and during these episodes, he cannot be awakened. These episodes occur at any time during the night. There is no sleepwalking or bedwetting, and during the day, the child seems fine. The *most* likely diagnosis is
  A. Sleep terror
  B. Nightmares
  C. Nocturnal seizures
  D. REM behavior disorder

ANSWER: **A.**   Sleep terror, like sleepwalking, typically begins after an arousal from SWS, most commonly toward the end of the first or second episode of SWS. By contrast, nightmares tend to arise during REM sleep.   (PEDS2, Chapter 39)

85. Which of the following is NOT true about sleep terrors in children?
  A. They are parasomnias that occur almost exclusively during SWS (stage N3)
  B. They do not involve dreaming
  C. They indicate a primary psychological disorder
  D. The child typically has no memory of the event in the morning

ANSWER: **C.**   Sleep terrors do not indicate a primary psychological disorder but rather occur in normal, healthy children. They are distinguished from nightmares in that they are associated with confusion when the child is awakened, and there is no memory of the dream, whereas upon arousal from a nightmare, the child is alert and can recall the dream.   (PEDS2, Chapter 39)

Sleep-Wake Timing

1. A 24-year-old college student has been diagnosed with delayed sleep-wake phase disorder (DSWPD). Which statement about people with this disorder is *true*?
A. They fall asleep when they want to
B. They sleep in late on weekends
C. They seldom have daytime sleepiness
D. They perform best in the morning

ANSWER: **B.** Patients with DSWPD have difficulty falling asleep at normal bedtimes and do not feel sleepy until very late into the night. When awakened at conventional bedtimes, they are very sleepy, and when given the opportunity, they have trouble waking at conventionally early hours, say 7 AM, and they awaken very late on weekends, often past noon. (ATLAS2, p 134; ICSD3, p 191)

2. A 58-year-old retired nurse has been diagnosed by you as having advanced sleep-wake phase disorder (ASWPD). Which statement about this disorder is *true*?
A. Patients with ASWPD do not complain of insomnia
B. Affected individuals cannot sleep until 7 or 8 AM
C. People with this disorder have difficulty waking up
D. Affected individuals perform best in the late evenings

ANSWER: **B.** Patients with ASWPD commonly complain of early morning awakenings. They may routinely wake at 2 to 3 AM. Thus, they have no difficulty waking up, but they have a great deal of difficulty functioning in the late evening. Many individuals with ASWPD self-select careers based on their circadian rhythm. Anesthesiologists, surgeons, and nurses frequently have an advanced sleep phase. (ATLAS2, p 135; ICSD3, p 198)

3. A 28-year-old patient has been diagnosed with DSWPD. Which treatment is effective in patients with this disorder?
A. Bright light exposure in the morning
B. Ramelteon in the morning
C. A tricyclic antidepressant in the morning
D. Wearing wraparound sunglasses in the morning

ANSWER: **A.** Bright light exposure for about 2 hours in the morning has been helpful in phase-advancing patients with DSWPD. Melatonin given 5 to 7 hours before habitual bedtime may also be helpful. (ATLAS2, p 134; ICSD3, p 191)

4. An 84-year-old woman complains of insomnia. After examining her sleep diary, the sleep medicine consultant diagnoses ASWPD. What is typical of people with ASWPD?
A. They often have periodic movements during sleep
B. They have abnormal amounts of rapid eye movement (REM) sleep
C. They wake up early in the morning
D. They respond to morning bright light therapy

ANSWER: **C.** With ASWPD, patients have difficulty staying awake in the evening, and they fall asleep early and awaken early. This is found commonly in older people, but in some cases, it may be familial. Bright light therapy in the morning would tend to advance their phase even more. (ATLAS2, p 135)

5. A woman who has been blind since birth complains of insomnia. The circadian rhythm of sleep in blind humans is always characterized by
- **A.** Phase delay
- **B.** Phase advance
- **C.** Free running sleep-wake cycle
- **D.** None of the above

ANSWER: **D.**   There are many causes of blindness, and not all blind people have circadian rhythm abnormalities such as a free-running sleep-wake cycle or what is known as a *non–24-hour sleep-wake rhythm disorder.* Many blind people maintain normally entrained sleep-wake rhythms despite the absence of conscious light perception. These individuals possess an intact retinal-hypothalamic pathway for monitoring environmental illumination levels. This allows photic input to the circadian timing system to continue to entrain the sleep-wake cycle.   (ATLAS2, p 136; ICSD3, p 209)

6. A 40-year-old patient complains of insomnia that occurs predictably at about 2-week intervals. This patient may have a circadian pacemaker that is
- **A.** Phase delayed
- **B.** Phase advanced
- **C.** Free running
- **D.** Internally desynchronized

ANSWER: **C.**   Free-running blind humans will alternate between sleeping well at night and sleeping poorly at night as their sleep-wake rhythm slowly drifts into and out of synchrony with socially acceptable times of day. Presumably, this is caused by a failure of the luminance monitoring system to provide information about the light-dark cycle to the circadian pacemaker in the SCN.   (ATLAS2, p 136; ICSD3, p 209)

7. An 18-year-old man is diagnosed with DSWPD. Which of the following is likely to have the *greatest* impact on his circadian phase?
- **A.** Full-spectrum light at 750 lux for 24 hours
- **B.** Full-spectrum light exposure for 2 hours before bedtime
- **C.** Full-spectrum light of 2500 lux 6 hours after awakening
- **D.** Blue-green light of 2500 lux exposure for 2 hours after CBTmin

ANSWER: **D.**   This question is really asking about the phase response curve (PRC) to light. The PRC plots circadian time on the x-axis; plotted on the y-axis is whether a stimulus changes (advances or delays) the circadian phase. Minus values on such a plot by convention indicate a delay in circadian time; positive values indicate an advance in circadian time. Supposing a stimulus is shown to have no effect on circadian time, the PRC would be a straight line with a value of zero over the circadian day: For example, a sound pulse given at various times during the day has no effect on circadian time; light, on the other hand, has a profound effect. However, the effect of the light varies depending on when it is applied. Light exposure before the nadir in core body temperature (CBTmin) will delay the circadian phase. Light after the CBTmin will advance the circadian phase. The greatest advance occurs immediately after CBTmin. The melanopsin-containing ganglion cells in the retina may be more sensitive to blue-green light (480-nm wavelength) than full-spectrum light, and 400 lux of blue light may have the same phase-shifting effects as 10,000 lux of full-spectrum light. Thus, answer D, although correct, represents too large a dosage of light than what is needed.   (Lack L, Wright HR: Treating chronobiological components of chronic insomnia. *Sleep Med* 8:637–644, 2007)

8. Chronotherapy has been shown to be effective for
   A. Primary insomnia
   B. ASWPD
   C. Middle of the night insomnia
   D. DSWPD

ANSWER: **D.** Although chronotherapy is often inconvenient, it has been shown to be effective in DSWPD. It has not been shown to be effective in primary insomnia. (ATLAS2, p 134; Barton A, Zee P: A clinical approach to circadian rhythm sleep disorders. *Sleep Med* 8:566–577, 2007)

9. Evening melatonin administration is indicated for
   A. Primary insomnia
   B. Shift-work disorder
   C. DSWPD
   D. Jet lag disorder

ANSWER: **C.** Melatonin taken 5 to 7 hours before bedtime has been used to treat DSWPD. (ATLAS2, p 138, Fig. 9.1–1)

10. The sleep schedule of a patient with non–24-hour sleep-wake disorder
   A. Shows an absence of a circadian rhythm for sleep and wake activity
   B. Is usually characterized by a rhythm that is shorter than 24 hours
   C. Indicates no entrainment to a 24-hour period
   D. Shows a delay of sleep-wake rhythm that occurs every day

ANSWER: **D.** Free-running rhythms are found mostly in blind people. In the absence of synchronization, the period length of the circadian rhythm is just over 24 hours. Thus, the sleep-wake time delays every day by the amount of time that the patient's circadian period exceeds 24 hours. (ICSD3, p 209)

11. If bright light exposure is being used to treat DSWPD, the light should be administered
   A. In the morning, soon after the nadir in core body temperature
   B. In the morning, just before the nadir in core body temperature
   C. In the evening, right before the desired bedtime
   D. In the evening, several hours before the desired bedtime

ANSWER: **A.** Before the nadir in body temperature, light exposure causes a delay in sleep phase, which would worsen a delayed sleep phase. (ATLAS2, p 134; Wyatt JK: Delayed sleep phase syndrome: pathophysiology and treatment options. *Sleep* 27:1195–1203, 2004)

12. You are presenting light therapy using a lamp system to a patient with delayed sleep. Which statement about the use of lamps is *incorrect*?
   A. There is a risk of retinal photoreceptor damage
   B. There is a risk of accelerating age-related macular degeneration
   C. Wavelengths that range from 4500 to 10,000 nm are the most effective at shifting phase
   D. Incandescent lamps are contraindicated

ANSWER: **C.** Wavelengths between 450 and 500 nm have been shown in research studies to be the most effective in phase shifting. About 90% of the light energy of incandescent lamps is infrared, and thus it poses a risk to eyes (e.g., corneal damage).

13. An engineer based in New York City is being sent to Peru to service a computer system. This is his first overseas trip. The flight from New York leaves at noon and arrives in Lima at midnight, and the flight is exactly 12 hours long. The engineer asks what he can do to minimize jet lag. Which do you advise?
   A. Take melatonin on takeoff
   B. Take a 2-hour nap 6 hours into the flight
   C. There is nothing to be done
   D. Try bright light exposure on landing

ANSWER: **C.**   There is nothing to be done. A clinician may not always know what time zone a city is in. The patient gave all the information needed to determine that New York and Lima are in the same time zone. Jet lag can only occur when the destination is in a different time zone than the home time zone. Generally, a difference of two time zones is needed for jet lag to occur.   (ATLAS2, p 137)

14. A recently married couple is going to Paris from New York City on their honeymoon. The flight leaves New York at 5 PM and arrives in Paris at 6 AM. It is a 7-hour flight. What is the time difference between the departure and destination cities?
   A. Paris is 6 hours ahead
   B. Paris is 6 hours behind
   C. Paris is 7 hours ahead
   D. Paris is 8 hours ahead

ANSWER: **A.**   Paris is 6 hours ahead. Generally, knowing the flight duration and the times of departure and arrival allows a calculation. In this example, if the flight leaves New York at 5 PM and flight duration is 7 hours, the flight arrives at midnight New York time. The time of arrival in Paris is 6 AM, so the difference between 12 AM and 6 AM is 6 hours.

15. A software engineer based in New York City is flying to Paris to install a new upgrade to a computer system manufacturing company. He expects to be in France for 1 month and wants to minimize the effects of jet lag. You assume that the patient's lowest temperature (Tmin) occurs at 4 AM. The flight leaves New York at 5 PM and arrives in Paris at 6 AM. It is a 7-hour flight. Which of following suggestions will be *least* helpful?
   A. Minimize light exposure in the 3 hours before Tmin by sleeping or wearing eyeshades
   B. Try bright light exposure in the 3 hours after Tmin
   C. Take melatonin 10 to 12 hours before Tmin
   D. Take a 15-minute nap immediately upon arriving

ANSWER: **D.**   This patient's Tmin at 4 AM New York time will occur at 10 AM Paris time, or 4 hours after arrival in Paris. Light exposure before Tmin leads to phase delay, but light exposure after Tmin would lead to a phase advance. The goal here is to hasten phase advance so that the patient's circadian system alternately catches up to Paris time. Bright light exposure on arrival would tend to phase delay, so the patient should wear sunglasses for at least 4 hours after arrival and then have bright light exposure. Melatonin taken about 10 to 12 hours before Tmin would also have the effect of hastening phase advance.   (ATLAS2, p 137)

16. The patient is referred to the sleep disorder center because of insomnia with the principal complaint that she awakens at 4 AM and cannot fall back to sleep. Early morning awakening is present in the following conditions *except*
   A. DSWPD
   B. Depression
   C. ASWPD
   D. After a resident of Paris flies to Chicago

ANSWER: **A.**   In DSWPD, patients do not have early morning awakening; instead, they wake up in the late morning or sometimes even in the early afternoon, depending on when they finally went to sleep. Early morning awakening is a long-recognized symptom of depression. Early-morning awakening is also very common in ASWPD and after east-west jet travel.   (ATLAS2, pp 134-140)

17. Jet lag disorder in persons living in and traveling eastward from the East Coast of the United States to London, England, with a flight arriving in London at 6 AM after being in the air for 7 hours is *best* treated by
   A. Avoiding bright light upon arrival in London
   B. Taking 10 mg of melatonin on the first night of sleep in London
   C. Taking 50 mg of trazodone for the first two nights after arrival
   D. Avoiding jets that go faster than 400 mph

ANSWER: **A.**   6 AM in London would be 1 AM on the East Coast of the United States. You would expect the core body temperature to not reach its minimal value (CBTmin) until about 2 hours after landing in London. Light exposure immediately upon landing would cause a phase delay based on the PRC.   (ATLAS2, p 137; Barton A, Zee P: A clinical approach to circadian rhythm sleep disorders. *Sleep Med* 8:566–577, 2007; Lack L, Wright HR: Treating chronobiological components of chronic insomnia. *Sleep Med* 8:637–644, 2007)

18. A 30-year-old security guard working the 11 PM to 7 AM shift in a factory complains that he cannot get used to working nights. He is falling asleep doing his rounds in the factory. During the day, he sleeps about 6 to 7 hours. He feels alert in the 1 to 2 hours before his shift begins, but he becomes very fatigued when the shift starts. He works Monday to Friday night and does not try to switch to sleeping nights on weekends. He is concerned that he may be fired. Which treatment might improve his clinical status?
   A. Melatonin at 11 PM before his shift begins
   B. Modafinil at 11 PM before his shift begins
   C. Zolpidem at 8 AM when he gets home after his shift ends
   D. Bright light at 8 AM after his shift ends

ANSWER: **B.**   Modafinil and armodafinil have been approved to improve alertness in shift-work sleep disorder. Preshift caffeine and bright light exposure during the work shift may also be helpful.   (ATLAS2, p 138, Table 9.1-1)

19. A 17-year-old girl comes to the sleep disorders center with daytime sleepiness and an irregular sleep-wake schedule. Medical history is significant for a brain tumor that had been diagnosed 4 four years previously and that had been treated with surgical resection followed by radiation therapy. There is no evidence of tumor at the time that the patient is seen in the sleep clinic. The PSG reveals a sleep efficiency of 94%, 1% stage N1, 59% stage N2, 20% stage N3, and 20% stage R. A multiple sleep latency test (MSLT) revealed a mean sleep latency of 2.5 minutes. There were no sleep-onset REM periods (SOREMPs). Actigraphy revealed five to seven irregular sleep bouts during each 24-hour period without any regularity of the main sleep period. What is the *likeliest* diagnosis?
   A. Secondary narcolepsy
   B. Idiopathic hypersomnia
   C. Non–24-hour sleep-wake rhythm disorder
   D. Irregular sleep-wake rhythm disorder

ANSWER: **D.**   The patient does not have the MSLT features of narcolepsy. With idiopathic hypersomnia, a major sleep episode starts at bedtime. With a free-running sleep disorder, actigraphy demonstrates regularity with a period slightly longer than 24 hours. With an irregular sleep-wake pattern, the possibility of brain pathology should be considered. There is a high incidence of irregular sleep-wake pattern in patients who were treated for brain tumors as children.   (Gapstur R, Gross CR, Ness K: Factors associated with sleep-wake disturbances in child and adult survivors of pediatric brain tumors: a review. *Oncol Nurs Forum* 36:723–731, 2009; ICSD3, p 209)

20. A 22-year-old college senior is referred to the clinic because he is having difficulty getting up for 9 AM classes. Actigraphy was performed and is shown in Figure E2–1. What does the actigraphy show?
  A. Normal results
  B. DSWPD
  C. ASWPD
  D. Irregular sleep-wake rhythm disorder

ANSWER: **B.**   This is an example of DSWPD. When examining actigraphy plots, remind yourself to make sure you understand the time scale and that sleep is inferred from the lack of activity. In this example, on most days, sleep begins after 2 AM.   (ATLAS2, p 134, Fig. 9.1–1)

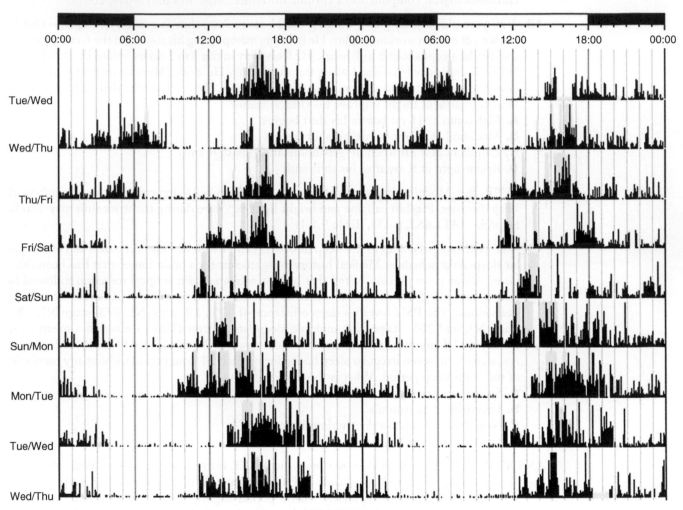

FIGURE E2-1

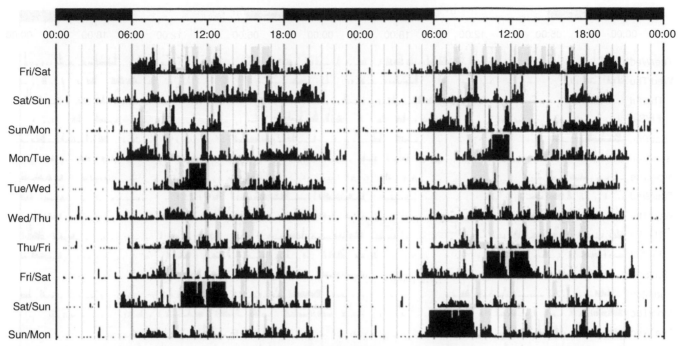

FIGURE E2–2

21. An 84-year-old retired college professor is referred to the clinic because she is having difficulty staying awake at her evening bridge tournaments. Actigraphy was performed and is shown in Figure E2–2. What does the actigraphy show?
  A. Normal results
  B. DSWPD
  C. ASWPD
  D. Irregular sleep-wake rhythm disorder

ANSWER: **C.** The actigraphy shows ASWPD with sleep-onset times between 8 and 9 PM and most awakenings between 4 and 5 AM. (ATLAS2, pp 135-136, Fig. 9.1–4)

22. A 22-year-old blind college senior is referred to the clinic because she is having severe difficulty getting up for 9 AM classes. Actigraphy was performed and is shown in Figure E2–3. What does the actigraphy show?
  A. Non–24-hour sleep-wake disorder
  B. DSWPD
  C. ASWPD
  D. Irregular sleep-wake rhythm disorder

ANSWER: **A.** The actigraphy shows that the patient is going to sleep a bit later and awakens a bit later progressively every day. The circadian rhythm is free running (or nonentrained). This pattern is seen in blind people who have no light perception. In this example, there is no single time when she awakens at a time appropriate for her to make a 9 AM class. Continuation of this pattern for a few more days would have resulted in a few days when she would have awakened at a time appropriate for a 9 AM class. (ATLAS2, pp 136-137, Fig. 9.1–6)

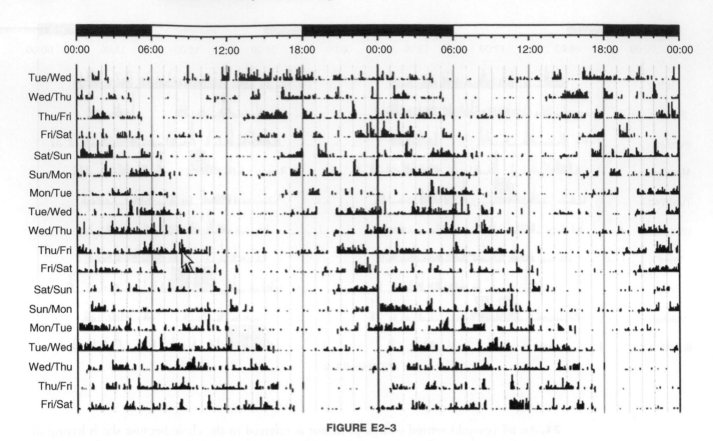

FIGURE E2–3

23. A 66-year-old resident of a nursing home is referred to the clinic because he frequently wanders at night and falls asleep during meals. Actigraphy was performed and is shown here (Fig. E2–4). What does the actigraphy show?
   A. Free-running sleep disorder
   B. DSWPD
   C. ASWPD
   D. Irregular sleep-wake rhythm disorder

ANSWER: **D.**   This is an example of irregular sleep-wake rhythm disorder, found in patients with brain pathology (e.g., tumors or neurodegenerative disorders) and in nursing home residents.   (ATLAS2, pp 136-137, Fig. 9.1–7)

24. A 24-year-old man is referred to clinic because he is having difficulty getting up for work, which starts at 9 AM. He does not become sleepy until 2 AM. He is worried that he will lose his job. A 24-hour melatonin profile was obtained. What dim-light melatonin onset (DLMO) time do you expect to find in him?
   A. Midnight
   B. 2 AM
   C. 4 AM
   D. 6 AM

ANSWER: **A.**   The description is that of DSWPD. DLMO usually occurs about 2 hours before sleep onset. Thus, in this patient, DLMO would be roughly at midnight.   (ATLAS2, p 135, Fig. 9.1–3)

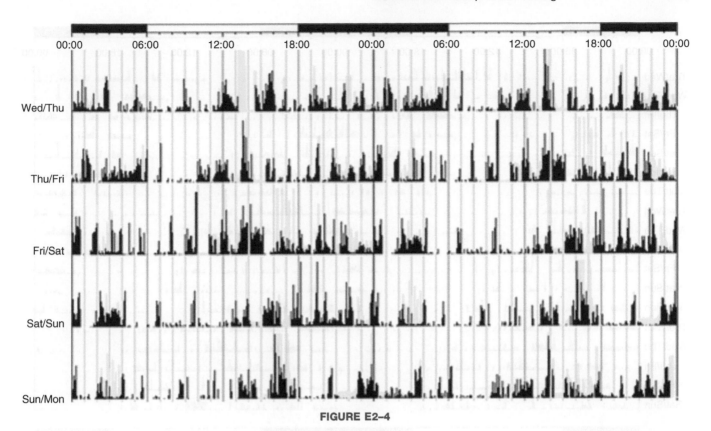

FIGURE E2–4

25. A 24-year-old man complains of fatigue and insomnia. Actigraphy data for 1 month are shown in Figure E2–5. The diagnosis is *most* likely
A. Free-running sleep disorder
B. Progressive DSWPD
C. Progressive ASWPD
D. Irregular sleep-wake rhythm disorder

ANSWER: **A.**   Free-running sleep disorder is characterized by a progressive delay in the circadian clock. The resulting sleep-wake cycle causes insomnia and sleepiness depending on when sleep is attempted in relation to the phase of the circadian clock. This actigraph shows a progressive delay in sleep onset so that, over an approximate 10-day time span, his circadian clock shifts the sleep period 12 hours, and then the cycle repeats. Non–24-hour sleep-wake disorder is most commonly seen in blind individuals but has also been reported after brain injury and in normal-sighted individuals. If the person with this disorder attempts to sleep at night, when the circadian propensity for sleep has shifted to the daytime, he or she may experience insomnia at night and excessive daytime sleepiness. Note that the term "progressive" is not used with DSWPD and ASWPD.   (ATLAS2, p 136)

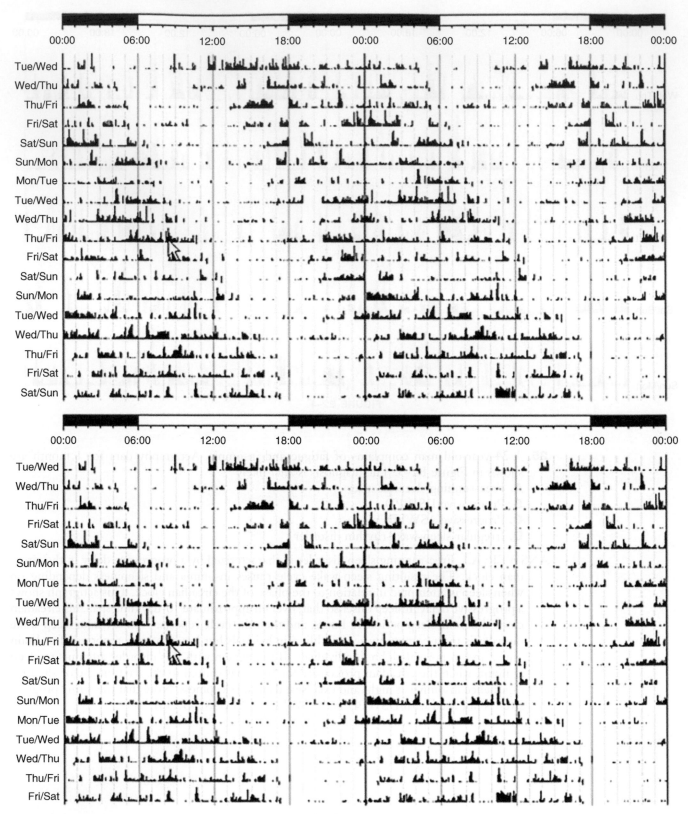

FIGURE E2-5

26. A 75-year-old woman complains of restless sleep. Actigraphy data for a month are shown in Figure E2–6. The diagnosis is *most* likely

    A. Non–24-hour sleep-wake disorder

    B. DSWPD

    C. ASWPD

    D. Irregular sleep-wake rhythm disorder

ANSWER: **D.**   Irregular sleep-wake rhythm disorder. Patients with irregular sleep-wake rhythm disorder have at least three sleep periods across the day and night and lack a single consolidated sleep period. This disorder is most commonly seen in institutionalized older adults and in children with intellectual disabilities. This actigraphy download from Sunday through Thursday shows no consolidated sleep period; instead, multiple short naps occur across the 24-hour period. (ATLAS2, pp 136-137, Fig. 9.1–7)

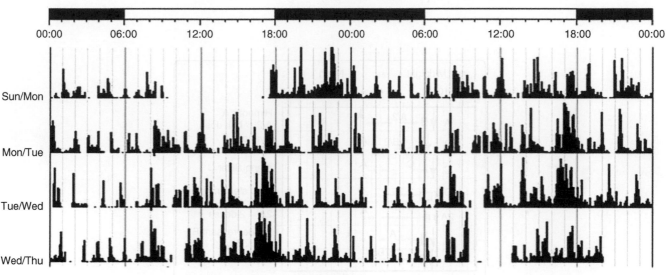

FIGURE E2–6

27. Figure E2–7 is a 1-week sleep diary kept by a 47-year-old man with a 20-year history of trouble falling asleep. He also complains of not being able to sleep without medication. What is the *most* likely explanation for this outcome?

A. Insomnia with hypnotic dependence

B. Chronic pain syndrome

C. DSWPD

D. Non–24-hour sleep-wake rhythm disorder

ANSWER: **A.** It is important for any sleep diary to include all medications that might affect sleep. This case is an extreme example of hypnotic dependence. Because of a decades-long inability to sleep, the patient has come to rely increasingly more on hypnotics. No pain medications are listed, so it is not chronic pain syndrome. He goes to bed at appropriate times, so it is not DSWPD. Although he may awake early when the medications wear off, the real problem is insomnia, and his complaint that he "can't sleep without medication" indicates a dependence on a sleep drug.

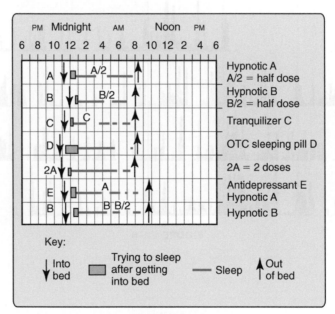

FIGURE E2–7

Insomnia

QUESTIONS

A Case Without Breaks

A 22-year-old woman reports that she has not slept well over the past 2 months. The problem began 2 days after a motor vehicle accident in which her car was "totaled." She did not have any head trauma and sustained only a few minor cuts and contusions. Since the accident, it has taken her an hour or more to initiate sleep every night. She has no difficulty maintaining sleep.

1. What is the *most* likely ICSD3 diagnosis?
   A. Chronic insomnia disorder
   B. Short-term insomnia disorder
   C. Primary insomnia
   D. Psychophysiologic insomnia

ANSWER: **B.**   Chronic insomnia requires at least 3 months' duration. Less than 3 months is short-term insomnia disorder.   (ICSD3, pp 19-48)

2. According to the ICSD3, what is the duration criterion for chronic insomnia disorder?
   A. At least 3 months
   B. At least 1 month
   C. No more than 3 months
   D. At least 6 months

ANSWER: **A.**   The minimum duration criterion for chronic insomnia disorder is 3 months.   (ICSD3, pp 19-48)

3. Assuming her insomnia does not resolve after 90 days, what is the *most* likely ICSD3 diagnosis?
   A. Chronic insomnia disorder
   B. Short-term insomnia disorder
   C. Primary insomnia
   D. Psychophysiologic insomnia

ANSWER: **A.**   The minimum duration criterion for chronic insomnia disorder is 3 months.   (ICSD3, pp 19-48)

4. Which of the following assessments is *most* useful for making the ICSD3 diagnosis of chronic insomnia disorder?
   A. Clinical history
   B. Actigraphy
   C. Polysomnography
   D. Beck Depression Inventory

ANSWER: **A.**   The insomnias can be diagnosed on clinical history alone.   (ICSD3, pp 19-48)

5. Which of the following treatments is *least* likely to be helpful?
   A. Stimulus control
   B. Zolpidem
   C. Eszopiclone
   D. Bupropion

ANSWER: **D.**   Bupropion is an antidepressant with activating qualities and therefore would not be useful for treating insomnia. Both zolpidem and eszopiclone effectively cover sleep-onset problems, as does the behavioral treatment of stimulus control.   (ATLAS2, p 105)

Bad Habits May Lead to Insomnia

A 65-year-old African-American man with a body mass index (BMI) of 32 has had sleep-maintenance insomnia for more than 4 years. Onset of his sleep disturbance cannot be attributed to any specific medical or psychological events. Reportedly, he awakens with worries about his job. He describes mild motor restlessness in his arms before bedtime, and, according to his wife, he snores only when he's consumed one or two alcoholic beverages before bedtime. He smokes two packs of cigarettes per day. He takes Tylenol PM, which has not been of much help. He denies significant daytime sleepiness but does feel "run down."

6. What risk factor(s) does this patient have for insomnia?
   A. Age
   B. Gender
   C. Ethnicity
   D. All of the above

ANSWER: **D.**   Risk factors for insomnia include age (older > younger), gender (females > males), ethnicity (middle-aged blacks > middle-aged whites), socioeconomic status, and genetics.   (ATLAS2, p 149)

7. What is the *most* likely ICSD3 diagnosis?
   A. Obstructive sleep apnea (OSA)
   B. Chronic insomnia disorder
   C. Restless legs syndrome (RLS)
   D. Paradoxical insomnia

ANSWER: **B.**   Chronic insomnia disorder is characterized by the complaint of insomnia lasting at least 3 months. There usually is some evidence for conditioning of the insomnia. No major medical or psychiatric factors play a role. Although this patient does have poor sleep hygiene, that is not one of the choices.   (ICSD3, pp 19-48)

8. You decide sleep hygiene is a problem and provide a handout with the rules for better sleep, with a request that he return in 2 weeks. What should you expect at the next office visit?
   A. Improved sleep hygiene has greatly improved his sleep
   B. He has given up smoking and drinking
   C. His status is for the most part unchanged
   D. He no longer snores

ANSWER: **C.**   Sleep hygiene treatment alone is not considered sufficient treatment for insomnia. Sleep hygiene is usually integrated into an overall treatment plan that includes other behavioral interventions as well as hypnotics in some cases.   (ATLAS2, p 155)

9. His age, BMI, and reports of snoring lead you to recommend an overnight polysomnogram (PSG). The results indicate an apnea-hypopnea index (AHI) of 2 events/hr with oxyhemoglobin desaturation to 89% during three of the apneas. What is the logical next step?
   A. Continuous positive airway pressure (CPAP) titration
   B. Stimulus-control therapy
   C. Ramelteon 8 mg at bedtime
   D. Ropinirole 1.25 mg at bedtime

ANSWER: **B.** There is no rationale for pursuing treatment for OSA given the PSG findings. Of the choices provided, stimulus control makes the most sense because it is an effective treatment for sleep-onset insomnia or sleep-maintenance insomnia. (ATLAS2, p 155)

Wish You Had a Piece of 5-Hour Energy Drink Sales?

A 44-year-old woman with a BMI of 25 comes to see her primary care physician. She has an 8-year history of unrefreshing sleep and early morning awakening. She reports that twice a week, sleep quality and duration are reasonably good, but the other nights are all "horrible." She is worried that she is going to lose her job because of fatigue and decreased memory. She has three energy drinks, each containing 160 mg caffeine, every morning to help her stay awake, and she consumes four or five more before 8 PM.

10. What is the *most* likely ICSD3 diagnosis?
   A. Depression
   B. Psychophysiologic insomnia
   C. Inadequate sleep hygiene
   D. Chronic insomnia disorder

ANSWER: **D.** The latest ICSD (ed. 3, 2014) insomnia diagnoses do not include specific causes. The insomnia duration meets the criteria for chronic insomnia disorder. (ICSD3, pp 19-48)

11. A 2-week sleep diary shows average total sleep time equals 5.8 hours per night. What would you do next?
   A. Ask the patient to withdraw from any caffeine use immediately
   B. Recommend she discontinue use of the energy drinks in a tapered manner over the next few weeks
   C. Prescribe eszopiclone 3 mg at bedtime
   D. Prescribe generic zolpidem 10 mg at bedtime

ANSWER: **B.** She is abusing caffeine to mask daytime fatigue. It is likely that the drink is a perpetuating factor for insomnia. Asking her to abruptly withdraw could be problematic from the standpoint of compliance, and she may get headaches from high-dose caffeine withdrawal. (ATLAS2, p 116)

12. Which of the following therapies will help with her concerns about job loss and decreased memory?
   A. Stimulus control
   B. Sleep restriction
   C. Thought stopping
   D. Cognitive restructuring

ANSWER: **D.** Cognitive therapy addresses dysfunctional beliefs and attitudes related to insomnia. Often people with insomnia catastrophize the potential for disaster, raising anxiety and perpetuating the sleeplessness. (ATLAS2, p 155)

13. On the assumption that she will stop using caffeine, you decide to prescribe a hypnotic. Which of the following is probably the *best* choice?
  A. Generic zolpidem
  B. Brand-name zolpidem (Ambien-CR)
  C. Zaleplon
  D. Eszopiclone

ANSWER: **D.**   Her primary pattern of insomnia is early morning awakening, so she will need a hypnotic that is effective for sleep-maintenance insomnia. Zolpidem has a relatively short half-life and is not the best choice for treating sleep-maintenance problems. Ramelteon is a melatonin agonist approved only for sleep-onset insomnia. Eszopiclone has been demonstrated to reduce time to sleep onset and time awake after sleep onset, and it also increases total sleep time.   (ATLAS2, p 155)

14. Which of the following is *least* likely to cause a parasomnia as an adverse effect?
  A. Generic zolpidem
  B. Brand name zolpidem (Ambien)
  C. Ramelteon
  D. Eszopiclone

ANSWER: **C.**   A warning has been issued for the entire class of hypnotics that a parasomnia may emerge as an unwanted adverse effect. However, there are few reports of sleepwalking, sleep eating, and so on for drugs that are not in the benzodiazepine-receptor agonist (BzRA) class.

There Must Be a Medical Reason for This

An 18-year-old woman is brought to the clinic by her mother, who reports her daughter has had "severe insomnia for over 10 years." They have been to several "specialists," including a neurologist and a psychiatrist. Her medical history is unremarkable. The patient reports that she sleeps about 5 to 6 hours per night and feels alert throughout the day. There is no history of depression.

15. What is the *most* likely ICSD3 diagnosis?
  A. Chronic insomnia disorder
  B. Short sleeper
  C. Primary insomnia
  D. Psychophysiologic insomnia

ANSWER: **B.**   Short sleepers are often identified when they present with insomnia complaints. Their persistent attempts to get 7 to 8 hours of sleep are futile. The key feature is perfectly normal functioning with reduced sleep hours. The reduction in sleep hours is rarely as low as it is for the patients with paradoxical insomnia.   (ICSD3, p 47)

16. Which of the following assessment tools would be *most* valuable for this case?
  A. In-lab PSG
  B. Home PSG
  C. Actigraphy
  D. Retrospective sleep diary

ANSWER: **C.**   Actigraphy is a well-validated methodology for measuring movement and inferring periods of sleep and wakefulness. To assist with the diagnosis, an objective measure of sleep onset and duration is needed. Actigraphy data correlate significantly with PSG total sleep time but not with sleep-onset latency. PSG could be used as an objective measure of total sleep time, but given the expense of the test, it is not as desirable as actigraphy.   (ATLAS2, p 392)

17. Her mother insists that an in-lab PSG be conducted, and you acquiesce. The results indicate a sleep-onset latency of 10 minutes with a total sleep time of 355 minutes. A periodic limb movement index (PLMI) of 15/hr is the only abnormal finding. What should you consider next?

    A. No treatment is warranted at this time

    B. Pramipexole 0.25 mg at bedtime

    C. Zolpidem-CR 12.5 mg at bedtime

    D. Zaleplon 10 mg at bedtime

ANSWER: **A.**   This patient has no complaints of daytime symptoms. The PLMI does not include arousals (that would be the periodic limb movement *arousal* index [PLMAI]), so it adds little value to what we know so far. No pharmacologic intervention is warranted. Short sleepers need to restrict their bedtime to the number of hours of habitual sleep.

18. Before you counsel the patient and her mother, what issue do you want to be sure about?

    A. That she has no daytime fatigue or sleepiness

    B. An absence of depression

    C. Normal cognitive functioning

    D. All of the above

ANSWER: **D.**   You want to tell them that there is no sleep disorder and that the patient should voluntarily restrict bedtime. However, before that advice is given, you want to be absolutely clear that there are no daytime symptoms usually associated with insomnia (e.g., fatigue, cognitive problems, low mood).

19. You later discover that the patient is often tired and irritable with poor mood on days when she has gotten less than 4 hours' sleep the preceding night. Which treatment approach is likely to produce the *best* results?

    A. Cognitive behavioral therapy (CBTi) only

    B. Intermittent use of a hypnotic

    C. Combined CBTi and a hypnotic

    D. Bright light therapy

ANSWER: **C.**   Several studies have attempted to examine the benefits of a combined behavioral and pharmacologic intervention for insomnia. Most studies find either treatment alone to be equally effective in the short run, with CBTi demonstrating longer effects. The benefits of combined therapy are modestly better than either treatment alone.   (ATLAS2, p 155)

Better Sleep in a Hotel

A 32-year-old businessman presents with a 4-year history of difficulty with sleep initiation and maintenance. He has a history of mild depression, diagnosed 2 years earlier, that resolved with 12 weeks of psychotherapy. His only medication is a statin to control cholesterol. There is a family history for depression and cardiovascular disease. His insomnia occurs most nights at home, and the patient sleeps much better on business trips and when staying at his parents' house.

20. What is the *most* likely ICSD3 diagnosis?

    A. Chronic insomnia disorder

    B. Short-term insomnia disorder

    C. Primary insomnia

    D. Psychophysiologic insomnia

ANSWER: **A.**   The insomnia duration meets the criteria for chronic insomnia disorder. The term *psychophysiologic insomnia*, as well as *idiopathic insomnia* and *paradoxical insomnia*, were subtypes of insomnia in previous nosologies.   (ICSD3, pp 19-48)

21. You decide to begin with stimulus-control therapy, and it works well for the patient. The primary goal of this behavioral treatment is to
  A. Take advantage of homeostatic sleep pressure
  B. Associate the bed with sleep
  C. Induce relaxation in bed
  D. Improve general sleep behaviors

ANSWER: **B.**   Classical conditioning is used as a behavioral model for this treatment approach. The goal of stimulus-control therapy is to associate the bed with falling asleep quickly, as opposed to struggling for sleep. The instruction to get out of bed when not sleeping inhibits association of the bed with frustration, anxiety, or worry.   (ATLAS2, p 149)

22. The sleep of people with psychophysiologic insomnia is
  A. Always better away from home
  B. Rarely better away from home
  C. Usually better away from home
  D. Best in the patient's own bed

ANSWER: **C.**   Not all people with psychophysiologic insomnia sleep better away from home. Asking the question about improved sleep in novel environments is useful and may lead to the diagnosis, or it may suggest that the usual sleep environment is not conducive to sleep.

23. Instead of stimulus control, you decide to proceed with a trial of sleep restriction. What mechanism accounts for improved continuity of sleep with this therapy?
  A. Circadian sleep tendency
  B. Conditioning factors
  C. Reduction of anticipatory anxiety
  D. Severe sleep deprivation

ANSWER: **C.**   Sleep restriction utilizes homeostatic sleep pressure and reduced anticipatory anxiety as active components. Asking patients to stay out of bed and engage in an alternative activity for the hours they would usually be trying to sleep helps alleviate the anxiety.   (ATLAS2, p 155)

24. The patient tells you that if he does not get more sleep soon, he will "go crazy and lose his job." These ruminative statements and thoughts are considered to be
  A. Precipitating factors
  B. Predisposing factors
  C. Perpetuating factors
  D. Presumptive factors

ANSWER: **C.**   Spielman's model of the "three P's" suggests that factors perpetuating insomnia can be quite different from precipitating factors. Cognitive arousal and rumination can raise anxiety, leading to increased difficulty with sleep initiation or reinitiation.   (ATLAS2, p 149)

Just Give the Kid a Good Alarm Clock

An 18-year-old young man is referred by his doctor. A senior at the local high school, he is doing quite well with a GPA of 3.7. His parents are concerned that there is "something wrong with his sleep." They report that he has great difficulty getting to sleep before 3 or 4 AM. He is often up late playing video games on his computer with friends. This abnormal sleep pattern began about 1 year ago. The patient also has a history of heroin abuse and depression, and he currently takes escitalopram.

25. What is the *most* likely ICSD3 diagnosis?
A. Insomnia of childhood
B. Chronic insomnia disorder
C. Delayed sleep-wake phase disorder
D. Primary insomnia

ANSWER: **C.** This young man has a delayed sleep-wake phase disorder (DSWPD). The onset of DSWPD is usually during adolescence. DSWPD is characterized by an inability to initiate sleep at the appropriate time needed for school or work followed by difficulty waking up at an appropriate time. Students with DSWPD are often late to school. (ICSD3, p 191)

26. Assuming it is not contraindicated, which treatment has the *best* chance of success?
A. Zolpidem
B. Eszopiclone
C. Olanzapine
D. Bright light therapy

ANSWER: **D.** Bright light therapy is an effective treatment for changing circadian timing. Bright light introduced after the nadir of core body temperature will cause a phase advance, and light given before the nadir will cause a phase delay. Hypnotics have not been effective for treating DSWPD. (ATLAS2, Ch 3.3 and p 134)

27. What secondary factor is common with this disorder?
A. Family discord
B. Chronic tardiness at school
C. Drug abuse
D. All of the above

ANSWER: **D.** Diagnosing and treating DSWPD can be complicated. The patient may be thought of as lazy or oppositional by parents. The patient may abuse drugs or alcohol in attempts to cope with the social impact of the disorder. (ATLAS2, Ch 9)

28. What advice would you give?
A. Avoid morning light after 12 PM
B. Institute stimulus control
C. Get late morning light exposure
D. Institute sleep restriction

ANSWER: **C.** The timing of bright light is critical on school mornings because light before the temperature nadir reinforces the phase delay. Late morning light should be administered no earlier than 3 hours after waking up. The other treatments listed are not effective for circadian disorders. (ATLAS2, p 134)

29. Upon further examination, you find that the patient is clinically depressed. Given his psychiatric state, which therapy is *not* appropriate?
A. Stimulus control
B. Eszopiclone
C. Cognitive behavioral therapy
D. All are appropriate

ANSWER: **D.** Insomnia is often comorbid with mood disorders. Treating insomnia with behavioral or pharmacologic interventions should be undertaken in cases when other medical or psychiatric disorders are present. (ATLAS2, p 151)

A Case of Lifelong Insomnia

A 28-year-old woman comes to your clinic stating that she only sleeps 1 to 2 hours per night. She can never remember being a good sleeper. She tries to initiate sleep at 11 PM most nights and gets out of bed at 6:30 AM. Despite her struggles with sleep, she believes it is important to get rest, so she stays in bed the entire time. She is quite troubled over this problem and believes she has memory impairment and is clumsy because of her sleeplessness. A previous neurologic workup, including magnetic resonance imaging (MRI) of her brain, was unrevealing.

30. What is the *most* likely ICSD3 diagnosis?
    A. Chronic insomnia disorder
    B. Short-term insomnia disorder
    C. Primary insomnia
    D. Paradoxical insomnia

ANSWER: **A.** The insomnia duration meets the criteria for chronic insomnia disorder. In the previous nosology (ICSD2), paradoxical insomnia was also known as *sleep-state misperception*. Individuals usually report sleeping only 1 or 2 hours a night, but their level of daytime function is far better than you would expect given their reported degree of insomnia. They lack a sense of perceptual disengagement; that is, they maintain some awareness of cognitions at night that lead them to perceive little or no sleep.   (ICSD3, pp 26-27)

31. To confirm the diagnosis, what should your next step be?
    A. Have the patient undergo full PSG for 3 nights
    B. Have her keep a sleep diary and wear an actigraph for at least 2 weeks
    C. Treat with a sedating antipsychotic medication
    D. Have her complete the Insomnia Severity Index

ANSWER: **B.** The best course of action is to have the patient keep a sleep diary and wear an actigraph for at least 2 weeks. On follow-up, you can determine whether a mismatch of objective and subjective data is apparent. PSG is neither required nor practical unless you suspect another sleep-fragmenting disorder such as periodic limb movement disorder (PLMD) or OSA.   (ICSD3, pp 26-27)

32. Assuming she undergoes PSG, what would you expect to find?
    A. Normal sleep staging
    B. Perceived sleep-onset latency to be about 1 hour longer than the objective amount
    C. Perceived total sleep time to be 50% of the objective amount or less
    D. An absence of N3 sleep

ANSWER: **C.** Patients with paradoxical insomnia usually overestimate their sleep-onset latency by 1.5 times the objective amount and underestimate their total sleep time by 50% or more.   (ICSD3, pp 26-27)

33. In patients with this diagnosis, the mean sleep latency from an MSLT is usually
    A. Around 3 minutes
    B. Less than 8 minutes
    C. Around 10 minutes
    D. 15 minutes or more

ANSWER: **C.** Paradoxical insomnia patients have levels of functioning far greater than you would expect from their self-reported hours of sleep. Most of these patients score in the mildly sleepy to normal range on the MSLT. Note that this was a subtype in previous nosologies, not the current one.   (ICSD3, pp 26-27)

34. The characteristic feature of short sleepers is
    A. There is no daytime impairment or dysfunction
    B. Sleep times usually are reported to be 2 hours or less
    C. Sleep quality is reported to be poor
    D. There is lack of a circadian rhythm to sleep

ANSWER: **A.** Short sleepers have no impairment in daytime alertness or functioning. This is now characterized as a normal variant.   (ICSD3, p 47)

Hot Woman Cannot Sleep Well and Is Burning for Better Sleep

A 58-year-old woman with a BMI of 34 presents with a complaint of sleep-maintenance insomnia for 6 months. The insomnia occurs about 4 nights per week. She initiates sleep within about 15 minutes, yet she awakens about every hour. Some of the awakenings are due to night sweats, and others are without apparent cause. There is a history of snoring according to her husband; the snoring and weight gain began about 1 year ago. She describes her mood as usually "pretty good," although she has had periods of irritability related to the insomnia.

35. What is the *most* likely ICSD3 diagnosis?
   A. Chronic insomnia disorder
   B. Short-term insomnia disorder
   C. Primary insomnia
   D. Psychophysiologic insomnia

ANSWER: **A.**   She has symptoms of insomnia related to hot flashes, a common clinical condition in midlife women. There can be considerable variability in the intensity and frequency of the hot flashes, and not all result in complete awakening.   (ATLAS2, p 359; ICSD3, pp 19-48)

36. What test should you consider at this point?
   A. Actigraphy
   B. PSG
   C. Sleep diary
   D. Beck Depression Inventory

ANSWER: **B.**   Polysomnography would be appropriate because of the risk factors of high BMI and snoring. Women of this age are almost as likely as men to have OSA, and the complaint of insomnia is more common than in men.

37. If her complaint of insomnia has nothing to do with sleep-disordered breathing, which of the following therapies might be helpful?
   A. Hormone replacement therapy
   B. Eszopiclone
   C. CBTi
   D. All of the above

ANSWER: **D.**   All treatments listed in this question are effective for insomnia. Chronic use of hormone replacement therapy is controversial and may be considered inadvisable in many women because of the increased risk of breast cancer.

A Case of Insomnia Wearing Him Down

A 78-year-old retired man has a complaint of waking too early. He usually goes to bed at about 9 PM and has no trouble getting to sleep but spontaneously awakens at 4 AM every morning and cannot return to sleep. He has periods of reflux for which he takes OTC famotidine. The insomnia makes him feel a bit downhearted, and this limits his motivation to be with friends. His primary care physician gave him a prescription for generic zolpidem, but that did not help him sleep through the night.

38. What is the *most* likely ICSD3 diagnosis?
   A. Insomnia due to a mental disorder
   B. Psychophysiologic insomnia
   C. Advanced sleep-wake phase disorder (ASWPD)
   D. Chronic insomnia disorder

ANSWER: **C.**   This patient has ASWPD, an inability to stay awake late followed by early morning awakening. Older adult patients want to sleep through the night and find waking at 3 to 5 AM both frustrating and unpleasant. They are at risk for being overmedicated because they want to sleep through the night.   (ICSD3, p 198)

39. You are convinced that depression is playing a role and prescribe an antidepressant. What other therapy might be of help to this patient?
   A. 1 mg of melatonin in the evening
   B. Bright light therapy in the morning
   C. Bright light therapy in the evening
   D. Ramelteon 8 mg at bedtime

ANSWER: **C.**   Light therapy can be useful in some cases of depression associated with ASWPD. Melatonin in the evening would reinforce the advanced sleep phase, as would ramelteon, a melatonin agonist.   (ATLAS2, p 35)

40. What pattern of insomnia is the *most* prevalent?
   A. Sleep-onset insomnia
   B. Combined sleep-onset and sleep-maintenance insomnia
   C. Sleep-maintenance insomnia
   D. Early morning awakening

ANSWER: **C.**   Numerous epidemiologic studies have shown sleep-maintenance insomnia to be more prevalent than sleep-onset insomnia or mixed insomnia.   (ATLAS2, p 149)

Potpourri

41. A 46-year-old woman presents with a lifelong history of sleep-onset and sleep-maintenance insomnia. She has used sleeping medications for the past 15 years. She now takes 20 mg zolpidem at bedtime but would like to taper off the drug because it is no longer helping her fall asleep. How should the zolpidem be tapered?
   A. Over a 1-week period
   B. Over several weeks
   C. Over several months
   D. Abrupt withdrawal is preferred

ANSWER: **B.**   It is best to taper hypnotics over several weeks because rapid discontinuation may cause rebound insomnia. Gradual tapering while good sleep habits are put into place (ideally with CBTi) can help build the patient's confidence in sleeping without drugs. A general recommendation is that BzRAs be reduced by one clinical dose per week.

42. A patient with insomnia who has been on zolpidem (10 mg) for 10 years is being weaned from the medication. If she cannot sleep while she is tapering off the drug, she should
   A. Lie in bed quietly and wait for sleep to come
   B. After 20 minutes get up and engage in a quiet, nonarousing activity
   C. After 10 minutes get up and exercise to encourage fatigue
   D. After 40 minutes get up and watch television

ANSWER: **B.**   This is known as *stimulus control*, and it helps to keep the bed associated with sleepiness rather than with wakefulness, worry, and frustration. The quiet activity encourages a return to sleep.   (ATLAS2, p 155)

43. A 48-year-old woman has severe sleep-onset insomnia and complains of severe daytime fatigue. She believes she sleeps only 5 hours a night. She goes to bed at 8 PM but does not fall asleep until midnight and awakens at 5 AM after a fitful sleep. She stays in bed until 7 AM. If it is determined that sleep restriction might be helpful to her, she will be asked to restrict time in bed (TIB) to
   A. 10 hours a night
   B. 8 hours a night
   C. 5 hours a night
   D. 4 hours a night

ANSWER: **C.**   With sleep restriction, the amount of TIB is curtailed to the actual time the patient sleeps. However, to avoid daytime sleepiness, TIB should not be reduced to less than 5 hours. This helps to reassociate the bed with sleep and heightens the sleep drive.   (ATLAS2, p 155)

44. A 50-year-old man has severe insomnia and excessive daytime sleepiness. He goes to bed at 9 PM, falls asleep at 10 PM, and awakens at 3 AM. He is then awake for 2 hours before falling asleep again for 1 hour before he has to get up to go to work. He is treated with sleep restriction, with the TIB restricted to 6 hours starting at midnight. After 1 week, he reports that his sleep has improved, and he is sleeping about 5.5 hours. What do you recommend next?
   A. Advance bedtime by 1 hour and maintain the time he leaves the bed
   B. Advance bedtime by 20 minutes and maintain the time he leaves the bed
   C. Restrict TIB further to 5.5 hours a night by delaying bedtime by 30 minutes
   D. Restrict TIB further to 5 hours a night by delaying bedtime by 60 minutes

ANSWER: **B.**   With sleep restriction, you curtail the amount of TIB to the actual time spent sleeping in an attempt to achieve a sleep efficiency of more than 85%, and then titrate the TIB to achieve this goal. If the patient achieves a sleep efficiency of 85% or more, you would increase TIB by 15 to 20 minutes and reevaluate after a week.   (ATLAS2, p 155)

45. A 30-year-old man has been using zolpidem (10 mg at bedtime) for insomnia for 3 years. Before starting treatment, it took him 2 hours to fall asleep. Initially, he was satisfied with the medication, but then it slowly lost its effectiveness. He stopped the medication and noted that it took him 4 hours to fall asleep, but he otherwise had no additional symptoms. What is the explanation for this?
   A. Rebound insomnia
   B. Augmentation syndrome
   C. Withdrawal syndrome
   D. Paradoxical response

ANSWER: **A.**   The main feature of rebound insomnia is worsening of sleep compared with before treatment, without additional symptoms that suggest drug withdrawal. The term *augmentation* is usually used in sleep medicine to describe worsening of symptoms of RLS with dopamine agonists.

46. A 60-year-old woman has been using flurazepam (15 mg at bedtime) for insomnia for 25 years. Before starting treatment, it took her 2 hours to fall asleep. Initially, she was satisfied with the medication but has noted loss of effectiveness the past few years. You had recommended that she taper the dose by reducing it by half every week. Instead, she stopped the medication entirely. It then took her 4 hours to fall asleep, and she wakened with a severe headache and sweating. She calls the next morning in a panic, worried that she is having a stroke. What do you tell her?
   A. She has rebound insomnia, and her sleep will likely return to baseline in 1 to 3 nights
   B. She has rebound insomnia, and her sleep will likely return to baseline in 1 to 3 weeks
   C. She has a withdrawal syndrome and should restart the medication and follow the tapering schedule
   D. She has an augmentation syndrome and requires an antidepressant

ANSWER: **C.**   This is not rebound insomnia because rebound does not occur with hypnotics with a long half-life. Also, with rebound comes worsening of the insomnia symptoms compared with before the drug but *without* additional symptoms. Her main feature is worsening of sleep compared with before treatment with additional symptoms of headaches and sweating, which are features of drug withdrawal.

47. A 35-year-old woman just started using eszopiclone (3 mg at bedtime) that you have prescribed for insomnia. After the first night, she notices an unpleasant, strong, bitter metallic taste and is concerned that the drug has caused damage to her nervous system. She calls the next morning to report the concern. What do you tell her?

A. This is a well-known and common side effect of eszopiclone and is not clinically dangerous

B. This is a well-known but rare side effect of eszopiclone from damage to the olfactory bulb. She should stop the medication and consult with a neurologist

C. This new symptom is unrelated to the medication, and she should see a neurologist

D. This symptom is caused by material in the capsule touching the tongue. Removing the powder from the capsule and adding it to milk should solve the problem

ANSWER: **A.** A bitter metallic taste is a commonly described side effect of zopiclone and eszopiclone. It is dose dependent and occurs in about 17% of patients using 2 mg and 34% of patients using 3 mg. The symptom is not clinically significant and is not related to the capsule making contact with the tongue. Other side effects of this medication include sleepiness in the morning, dizziness, and dry mouth, each occurring in about 5% of patients. (Najib J: Eszopiclone, a nonbenzodiazepine sedative-hypnotic agent for the treatment of transient and chronic insomnia, *Clin Ther.* 28:491-516, 2006)

48. Which statement about psychophysiologic insomnia is *true*?

A. It does not follow after acute stress

B. This diagnosis cannot be made in a patient with a chronic medical condition

C. The condition responds well to electroshock when the patient has comorbid depression

D. It is also called *conditioned insomnia*

ANSWER: **D.** Psychophysiologic insomnia can complicate and perpetuate insomnia from any cause. The patient has generally adopted (or learned) behaviors that perpetuate the insomnia. The situation becomes conditioned. It is thus also called *conditioned insomnia* or *learned insomnia*. (ICSD3, p 26)

49. A 35-year-old woman can easily fall asleep when visiting friends but cannot fall asleep in her own bed. What is the *likeliest* cause of her insomnia?

A. Münchausen syndrome

B. Psychophysiologic insomnia

C. Paradoxical insomnia

D. Depression

ANSWER: **B.** This is a typical finding in patients with psychophysiologic insomnia: They sleep better in beds other than their own. It occurs because they have made an association between not sleeping and their own bed. In their own bed, they have a heightened anxiety of not being able to fall asleep. (ICSD3, p 26)

50. A 60-year-old woman is referred with the complaint that she sleeps no more than 1 hour a night yet is perfectly wide awake and alert all day. She would like to be treated with hypnotics. What is the *likeliest* finding in the sleep laboratory?

A. About 1 hour of sleep time

B. Sleep within normal limits

C. Periodic movements in sleep

D. Sleep latency exceeding 3 hours

ANSWER: **B.** This patient most likely has sleep-state misperception, called *paradoxical insomnia* in ICSD2. Sleep studies in such patients generally are within normal limits. (ICSD3, p 27)

51. A 35-year-old woman has been using eszopiclone (3 mg at bedtime) for insomnia for 3 years. Before starting treatment, it took her 2 hours to fall asleep. Initially, she was satisfied with the medication but states it slowly has lost its effectiveness. She stopped the drug and noted that it took her 4 hours to fall asleep, but she otherwise had no additional symptoms. She calls the next morning expressing concern about recurrence of insomnia. What should you tell her?

A. She has rebound insomnia, and her sleep will likely return to baseline in 1 to 3 nights
B. She has rebound insomnia, and her sleep will likely return to baseline in 1 to 3 weeks
C. She has a withdrawal syndrome and should restart the medication
D. She has an augmentation syndrome, and the symptoms will progressively worsen

ANSWER: **A.** This is rebound insomnia with the main feature being worsening of sleep compared with before treatment. Rebound insomnia usually lasts 1 to 2 nights. The term *augmentation* is usually used in sleep medicine to describe worsening of symptoms of RLS with dopaminergic medication use.

52. A patient on hemodialysis has severe insomnia. Which statement about insomnia in renal failure is *true*?

A. It is often because of RLS
B. Insomnia is rare in renal failure
C. Insomnia is cured by hemodialysis
D. It is usually the result of central apnea

ANSWER: **A.** At least half of patients on hemodialysis have RLS. The pathophysiology appears to be related to several factors, including reduced iron stores (worse in dialysis patients) and neuropathy (common when renal failure is caused by diabetes). RLS is found in a wide variety of medical conditions, including heart disease, thyroid disease, chronic obstructive pulmonary disease (COPD), neuropathy, and Parkinson disease. It is also common during pregnancy and in any condition in which there is a reduction in iron stores.   (ATLAS2, p 179)

53. A patient with moderate COPD complains of severe insomnia. Which hypnotic medication has been shown to be safe in patients with mild to moderate COPD?

A. Clonazepam
B. Flurazepam
C. Trazodone
D. Ramelteon

ANSWER: **D.** Ramelteon has been shown to not worsen gas exchange in patients with COPD. The other medications listed have not been evaluated. Using hypnotics in COPD patients is problematic because hypnotics can theoretically worsen alveolar ventilation.   (Roth T: Hypnotic use for insomnia management in chronic obstructive pulmonary disease, *Sleep Med.* 10:19-25, 2009)

54. A patient with congestive heart failure (CHF) complains of difficulty falling asleep and staying asleep. Which medication has been shown to improve sleep in heart failure?

A. Amobarbital
B. Clonazepam
C. Flurazepam
D. Temazepam

ANSWER: **D.** Astonishingly, even though insomnia is common in heart failure, no large, randomized clinical trials have examined the effect of hypnotics in patients with CHF. Temazepam was shown to improve sleep structure but not to improve the Cheyne-Stokes breathing pattern in heart failure patients.   (Biberdorf DJ, Steens R, Millar TW, Kryger MH: Benzodiazepines in congestive heart failure: effects of temazepam on arousability and Cheyne-Stokes respiration, *Sleep.* 16:529-538, 1993)

55. A medical student with severe chronic insomnia is concerned about possible long-term effects on her health. Chronic insomnia has been shown to have a very strong association with the development of which condition?
A. Diabetes
B. Alcoholism
C. Central sleep apnea
D. Depression

ANSWER: **D.**   Several important papers have linked insomnia and subsequent depression. The most interesting is the Johns Hopkins precursor study, which followed over 1000 Johns Hopkins medical students for a median of 34 years.   (Chang PP, et al: Insomnia in young men and subsequent depression. The Johns Hopkins Precursor Study, *Am J Epidemiol.* 146:105-114, 1997; Ford DE, Kamerow DB: Epidemiologic study of sleep disturbance and psychiatric disorders: an opportunity for prevention, *JAMA.* 262:1479-1484, 1989; and Li SX, et al: Nocturnal sleep disturbances as a predictor of suicide attempts among psychiatric outpatients: a clinical, epidemiologic, prospective study, *J Clin Psychiatry.* 71:1440-1446, 2010)

56. Use of PSG to evaluate a patient who presents with a complaint of insomnia is indicated when
A. The insomnia has been chronic
B. A primary sleep disorder is suspected
C. Use of hypnotic medication is considered
D. Multiple causes of insomnia are present
E. Total sleep time is less than 5 hours

ANSWER: **B.**   In general, a patient with insomnia should not require polysomnography for diagnosis. However, if another sleep disorder such as OSA or periodic limb movements is suspected, a polysomnogram should be performed.   (Littner M, Hirshkowitz M, Kramer M, et al: Practice parameters for using polysomnography to evaluate insomnia: an update, *Sleep.* 26:754-760, 2003)

57. Which of the following drugs is *not* approved by the Food and Drug Administration (FDA) for the treatment of insomnia?
A. Eszopiclone
B. Zolpidem
C. Zaleplon
D. Trazodone

ANSWER: **D.**   The so-called Z drugs marketed in the United States—eszopiclone, zolpidem, and zaleplon—are all FDA-approved hypnotics and are therefore indicated for insomnia. However, trazodone is a more widely prescribed drug for insomnia, even though it is actually approved only for depression. FDA approval requires that adequate studies have been published to show efficacy and safety for a specific indication, and these studies are not available for trazodone despite its widespread use. The typical dose of trazodone prescribed for sleep is 50 to 150 mg at bedtime; for depression, the typical dosage is 400 to 600 mg every day.   (ATLAS2, Ch 10)

58. Which of the following statements about the Z class of hypnotics is *true*?
A. They act by modulating the function of the GABA$_A$ receptor complex
B. They stimulate hypothalamic melatonin receptors
C. They are a subclass of benzodiazepines
D. They include the drug ramelteon

ANSWER: **A.**   The mechanism of action of the Z drugs—eszopiclone, zolpidem, and zaleplon— is similar to that of the benzodiazepines in that they bind to the GABA$_A$ receptor in some fashion. They are not benzodiazepine molecules and are often referred to as *nonbenzodiazepine hypnotics.* (Eszopiclone is a cyclopyrrolone, zolpidem is an imidazopyridine, and zaleplon is a pyrazolopyrimidine). All of the currently FDA-approved hypnotics, with the exception of ramelteon, act by modulating the function of the GABA$_A$ receptor complex (Fig. E3–1). Ramelteon works as hypnotic by stimulating melatonin receptors in the suprachiasmatic nucleus of the hypothalamus.   (ATLAS2, Ch 10)

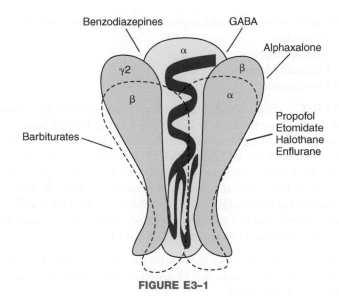

FIGURE E3–1

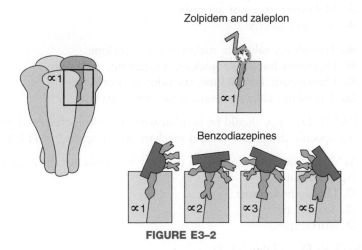

FIGURE E3–2

Figure E3–2 shows that benzodiazepines bind to several alpha units of the GABA$_A$ receptor complex, giving them a wide range of pharmacologic effects in addition to sleep induction (e.g., anxiolysis). In contrast, the Z drugs bind selectively to the alpha$_1$ subunit of the GABA receptor, so they function mainly as sleep inducers without the additional effects of benzodiazepines.

59. Alcohol is a poor hypnotic mainly because
   A. It prolongs sleep latency
   B. Rapid metabolism leads to sleep disturbance and increased arousals in the second half of the night
   C. It causes a hangover the following morning
   D. Its diuretic effect leads to numerous awake periods for urination

ANSWER: **B.**   Alcohol shortens sleep latency. Although answers C and D describe possible effects, alcohol's main drawback as a hypnotic is its rapid metabolism, which causes increased arousals and sleep disturbance in the latter half of the night.

60. The *most* commonly used ingredient in OTC sleep aids is
A. Melatonin
B. Acetaminophen
C. Diphenhydramine
D. Doxylamine

ANSWER: **C.** Diphenhydramine, a first-generation antihistamine, is commonly used as a sleep aid in OTC medications. It is marketed in the United States under the trade name Benadryl. Among OTC drugs that contain diphenhydramine are Nytol, Sleep-Eze, Sominex, Tylenol PM, Simply Sleep, and Advil PM. Doxylamine is another first-generation antihistamine, and it is the active ingredient in Nyquil and Unisom Nighttime. Melatonin is also commonly used to induce sleep, at a dosage of 0.5 to 2 mg/day. The first-generation antihistamines have potential anticholinergic side effects (dry mouth, tachycardia, urinary retention, and constipation), and onset of tolerance is rapid; unlike prescription hypnotics, they are not recommended for long-term treatment of insomnia.

61. Below are four classes of medications commonly prescribed for insomnia, labeled 1 through 4. Pick the *correct* sequence of specific drugs from answers A through D that matches the sequence 1 through 4.
1. Benzodiazepines
2. Nonbenzodiazepine GABA$_A$ agonists
3. Melatonin-receptor agonists
4. Antidepressants

A. Trazodone, zaleplon, melatonin, eszopiclone
B. Diphenhydramine, zopiclone, ramelteon, melatonin
C. Flurazepam, eszopiclone, trazodone, ramelteon
D. Triazolam, zolpidem, ramelteon, amitriptyline

ANSWER: **D.** You should be familiar with these four classes of prescription hypnotics, including specific drugs and general mechanisms of action.   (ATLAS2, Ch 10)

62. Which of the following drugs used for insomnia has the *longest* half-life?
A. Melatonin
B. Diphenhydramine
C. Trazodone
D. Mirtazapine

ANSWER: **D.**   (Table E3–1)

TABLE E3–1 Drugs and Their Half-Lives (Question 62)

Drug	Range of Half-Life
Melatonin	40–60 min
Diphenhydramine	4–8 hr
Trazodone	3–14 hr
Mirtazapine	13–40 hr

63. Which of the following drugs used for sleep is *not* considered to be a sedating antidepressant?

A. Doxepin
B. Mirtazapine
C. Trazodone
D. Triazolam

ANSWER: **D.**   Triazolam is a benzodiazepine and is therefore an anxiolytic. The other drugs are antidepressants. Both benzodiazepines and antidepressants have been used for years as hypnotics to induce sleep. A newer class of drugs for this purpose is the nonbenzodiazepine $GABA_A$ agonists (the so-called Z drugs), of which three are currently marketed in the United States; others are marketed in other countries. Also relatively new is the drug ramelteon, a melatonin receptor agonist.

64. All of the following drugs induce sleep by stimulating the $GABA_A$ receptor *except*

A. Barbiturates
B. Benzodiazepines
C. The Z drugs
D. TCAs

ANSWER: **D.**   Most TCAs act primarily as selective serotonin-norepinephrine reuptake inhibitors (SNRIs) by blocking those serotonin and norepinephrine transporters. Although TCAs have other mechanisms as well (e.g., sodium and calcium channel blockade), they do *not* act by stimulating $GABA_A$ receptors.

65. An increased number of sleep spindles is associated with which of the following drugs?

A. Flurazepam
B. Zopiclone
C. Trazodone
D. Amitriptyline

ANSWER: **A.**   Increased spindle activity can be seen with any of the benzodiazepines, such as flurazepam. Spindles have a frequency of 12 to 14 Hz, are 0.5 to 1.5 second in duration, and can occur in any sleep stage except N1. They are generated from the reticular thalamic nucleus, a thin "peel" of neurons that wrap around the thalamus and modulate sensory activity between the environment and the cortex. These neurons are GABAergic.

66. All of the following PSG effects are common in people taking benzodiazepines *except*

A. Decrease in sleep latency
B. Decrease in wake after sleep onset (WASO)
C. Increased spindle activity
D. Increase in slow-wave sleep

ANSWER: **D.**   The benzodiazepines increase total sleep time and stage N2 sleep, and they also increase spindle density. They are potent suppressors of slow-wave (N3) sleep. However, the clinical significance of suppressing this stage of sleep is uncertain.

67. All psychiatric drugs can affect sleep in some fashion. Each of the following is associated with suppression of rapid eye movement (REM) sleep *except*

A. Trazodone
B. Paroxetine
C. Selegiline
D. Nefazodone

ANSWER: **D.**   Nefazodone, like bupropion, increases REM sleep; the others decrease it. Selegiline is a monoamine oxidase inhibitor; all drugs of this class are potent REM suppressors. It is important to know the effect of drugs on sleep.   (ATLAS2, Ch 6)

68. The half-life of benzodiazepines ranges from hours to days. Among the four drugs of this class listed below, which one has the *longest* half-life?
A. Temazepam
B. Lorazepam
C. Alprazolam
D. Flurazepam

ANSWER: **D.** The half-life of flurazepam is 48 to 120 hours. The others listed have about the same (and a significantly shorter) half-life: 5 to 12 hours for temazepam, 10 to 20 hours for lorazepam, and 9 to 20 hours for alprazolam. (ATLAS2, Ch 6, Table 6–1)

69. Many hypnotics have a short half-life, such as triazolam. The *shortest* half-life among the Z drugs is
A. Zaleplon
B. Zolpidem
C. Zopiclone
D. Eszopiclone

ANSWER: **A.** Zaleplon has a half-life of only 1 to 2 hours, whereas the others are two to three times that amount.

70. The PSG fragment in Figure E3–3 is taken from a patient on multiple medications, including ramelteon for insomnia, theophylline for asthma, paroxetine for depression, and oxycodone for pain. Which medication may be playing a role in the findings?
A. Ramelteon
B. Theophylline
C. Paroxetine
D. Oxycodone

ANSWER: **D.** Opiate medications can cause central apneas, both during wakefulness and sleep. They also may be associated with a slow breathing frequency. The central apneas may be regular, as shown here, or they may be irregular.

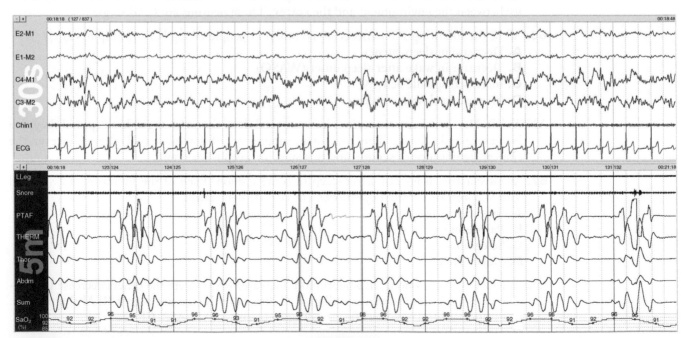

FIGURE E3–3

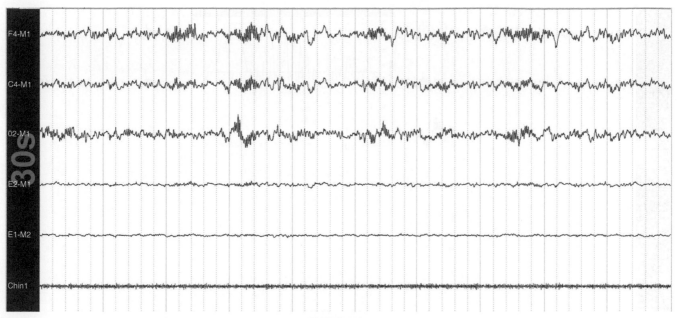

FIGURE E3–4

71. A patient is being treated for depression, insomnia, and asthma. Medications include fluox-
etine, zolpidem, and a fluticasone-salmeterol combination given by inhalation. Which medi-
cation is likely responsible for the findings shown in Figure E3–4?
A. Fluoxetine
B. Zolpidem
C. Fluticasone
D. Salmeterol

ANSWER: **B.**   Of these drugs, the most likely cause of increased spindles is zolpidem. Medications that act on the GABA receptors may increase spindle frequency.   (Lancel M: Role of
GABA-A receptors in the regulation of sleep: initial sleep responses to peripherally administered modulators and agonists, *Sleep.* 22:33-42, 1999)

72. The epoch in Figure E3–5 is from a patient taking multiple medications, including temaze-
pam for sleep induction. The inset window enlarges the yellow highlighted part of the frag-
ment. What is the frequency of the first second of the highlighted part?
A. About 4 Hz
B. About 8 Hz
C. About 13 Hz
D. About 18 Hz

ANSWER: **C.**   The easiest way to answer the question is to simply count the number of peaks
in the first second of the inset window. There are 13 (or arguably 14) peaks. This is a sleep
spindle (normal range, 11–16 Hz). Benzodiazepines, along with other drugs that act on
GABA receptors, increase spindle density and sometimes increase spindle frequency. Although
sleep "lore" suggests that medications such as GABA agonists increase the density of fast or
"pseudospindles" (range more than 16 Hz), empiric support in the literature for this effect
is sparse.

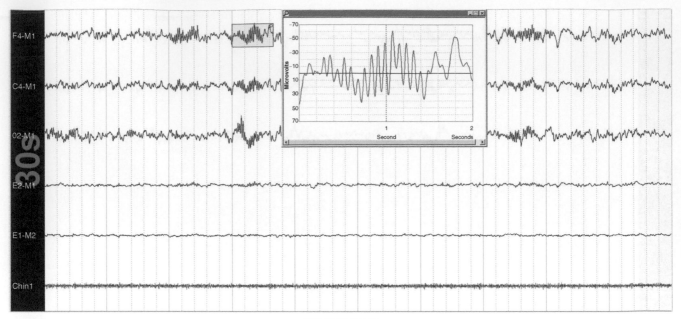

FIGURE E3–5

73. A charming 4-year-old girl does not want to go to sleep at the appointed bedtime. She sleeps in her own bed, but despite a night light and a sound machine, she makes multiple excuses for why she cannot go to sleep: she needs a drink of water; she needs another hug; the ghosts in her closet need to be swept away. Her mother is very accommodating, and often after several glasses of water, four hugs, two closet sweeps, and other demands, she lets the child come into her own bed. There she may watch television with her mother. As result, the child often does not fall asleep until 1 to 2 hours after she was initially put to bed. The disorder characterized by this scenario is called
   A. Behavioral insomnia of childhood, sleep-onset association type
   B. Behavioral insomnia of childhood, limit-setting type
   C. Delayed sleep-wake phase disorder of childhood
   D. Inadequate sleep hygiene of childhood

ANSWER: **B.**   The ICSD3 divides behavioral insomnia of childhood into two distinct disorders. Sleep-onset association type is when the child requires a special condition to fall asleep, such as some stimulation (rocking, watching television), an object (bottle), or a setting (the parents' bed). In the absence of these conditions, the child is unable to fall asleep within a reasonable time. Limit-setting sleep disorder is when the child stalls or refuses to go to sleep, and the caregiver does not enforce limits; the usual cause, as in this case, is the parent's inability to set limits. The child learns what will work with the parent and manipulates the parent to stay awake.   (ICSD3, pp 27-28)

74. A mother brings her 5-year-old son to the doctor's office complaining that he cannot fall asleep without her lying next to him at bedtime. The symptom has been present for 3 years. What is the *most* likely diagnosis?
   A. Behavioral insomnia of childhood, sleep-onset association type
   B. Behavioral insomnia of childhood, limit-setting type
   C. Night terrors
   D. Nightmares

ANSWER: **A.**   This is the typical history of a child with behavioral insomnia of childhood, sleep-onset association type. Falling asleep requires a special condition (sleeping next to mother), and the associations are problematic (disturbing the mother's sleep).   (ICSD3, pp 27-28)

75. A mother brings her 5-year-old son to the doctor's office complaining that he does not fall asleep until 11 PM. He complains about monsters in the room, worrying about nightmares and wanting water. He stalls going to bed even though he is sleepy. The symptom has been present for 3 years. What is the *most* likely diagnosis?
  A. Behavioral insomnia of childhood, sleep-onset association type
  B. Behavioral insomnia of childhood, limit-setting type
  C. Night terrors
  D. Nightmares

ANSWER: **A.**   Typical symptoms are stalling behaviors at bedtime and refusal to return to bed after awakening at night, with the caregiver not setting limits appropriately.   (ICSD3, pp 27-28)

Cannot Go Gently Into a Good Night

A 47-year-old woman with a 5-year history of depression and gastroesophageal reflux disease (GERD) presents to the clinic with a complaint of sleep-onset insomnia and maintenance insomnia, which began about 1 month before the depression. The depression has resolved with pharmacologic intervention, but the insomnia persists. She is not currently taking a hypnotic and is not keen on doing so.

76. What is the *most* likely ICSD3 diagnosis?
  A. Chronic insomnia disorder
  B. Short-term insomnia disorder
  C. Primary insomnia
  D. Paradoxical insomnia

ANSWER: **A.**   Chronic insomnia disorder requires a duration of 3 months or longer. Insomnia is often comorbid with depression and calls for independent evaluation and treatment.   (ICSD3, pp 19-48)

77. What should you do next?
  A. Refer for CBTi
  B. Suggest a referral for GERD evaluation
  C. Increase the antidepressant medication
  D. Request a PSG

ANSWER: **B.**   Whereas CBTi is highly effective, GERD may be the cause of the insomnia. If the GERD is already resolved, CBTi for insomnia would be the next step. PSG is not recommended for routine evaluation of insomnia.

78. Which component of CBTi is *most* likely to reduce her WASO?
  A. Cognitive restructuring
  B. Sleep hygiene
  C. Stimulus control
  D. Relation therapy

ANSWER: **C.**   Sleep hygiene alone is a necessary component of CBTi but is not effective. Stimulus-control therapy can reduce sleep-onset latency and improve sleep maintenance.

79. The patient reconsiders and asks for a prescription for a hypnotic. Which of the following would you choose?
  A. Zolpidem
  B. Eszopiclone
  C. Trazodone
  D. Ramelteon

ANSWER: **B.**   Of the four drugs listed, eszopiclone is more likely to reduce sleep-onset latency and WASO.   (ATLAS2, Ch 6, Table 6–1)

Train, Train

A 22-year-old college student rents an apartment next to railroad tracks. He has trouble initiating sleep almost every night. Sleep onset is usually around 2 AM. He has multiple awakenings at night but can usually get back to sleep within minutes. Interestingly, he denies hearing the train going by at night, even though one passes by at least three times while he is asleep.

80. What is the *most* likely diagnosis?
  A. Chronic insomnia disorder
  B. Advanced sleep-wake phase disorder
  C. Delayed sleep-wake phase disorder
  D. Sleep disruption from environmental circumstances

ANSWER: **C.**   Delayed sleep-wake phase disorder is characterized by sleep onset at 2 AM or later with an inability to sleep at earlier hours. It is a circadian rhythm disorder often overlooked as the cause of sleep-onset difficulties.   (ICDS3, p 191)

81. What initial treatment would you suggest?
  A. Zolpidem 10 mg at bedtime
  B. Improve sleep hygiene
  C. Bright light in the evening 9 to 10 PM
  D. Bright light in the morning 7 to 8 AM

ANSWER: **D.**   Bright light treatment after he reaches core body temperature minimum will cause a phase advance in his sleep schedule, so he can initiate sleep earlier. Bright light exposure late in the day may cause him to fall asleep even later, which is an undesired response.   (ATLAS2, Chs 3.3 and 9.1)

82. Which of the following will be *least* effective for improving his sleep condition?
  A. Improving sleep hygiene
  B. Stimulus control
  C. Melatonin 5 mg taken at 2 AM
  D. Melatonin 5 mg taken at 8 PM

ANSWER: **C.**   Behavioral treatments may be helpful but are unlikely to resolve his sleep difficulties. Melatonin "pulls" the rhythm, so taking it at 2 AM will not help. Melatonin at 8 PM will cause a phase advance.   (ATLAS2, Ch 9.1)

Hypersomnolence

QUESTIONS

1. A 32-year-old Navy helicopter pilot is referred to the sleep clinic with an unusual history. While flying last week, the helicopter's low oil pressure light flashed, and an alarm went off. Instantly, the pilot's head slumped, and he lost strength in his right hand. He recovered quickly and landed safely. You learn that since age 15 years, he's had severe daytime sleepiness; the problem was originally diagnosed as attention-deficit/hyperactivity disorder (ADHD), and he has been on medication for it ever since. He was warned that the pills might increase blood pressure. He never indicated to the Navy he was taking medication, and except for this problem, he has been healthy. What is the *most* likely diagnosis?
A. Epilepsy
B. Cardiac arrhythmia
C. Transient ischemic attack
D. Narcolepsy with cataplexy

ANSWER: **D.** The diagnosis is suggested by severe sleepiness that began as a teenager and the symptom of instant loss of muscle tone in his neck muscles and arm while maintaining consciousness. It is important to remember that there are two forms of narcolepsy: type 1, with cataplexy, (ICSD3, pp 146-155) and type 2, without cataplexy. (ICSD3, pp 155-161) Cerebrospinal fluid (CSF) hypocretin-1 deficiency is characteristic of type 1 narcolepsy. (ICSD3, p 146)

2. A 15-year-old high school student is diagnosed with narcolepsy with cataplexy. She is prescribed a nap to be taken right after lunch and before her 1:00 PM class begins. Her school accommodates this request. Which statement about these midday naps is likely to be *true*?
A. She feels refreshed for 1 to 3 hours after the naps.
B. She dreams infrequently or not at all during naps.
C. She is likely to stop breathing during these naps.
D. She has been noted to twitch during naps.

ANSWER: **A.** Naps are very refreshing for patients with narcolepsy, and strategically timed naps are often helpful. (ATLAS2, p 160) Patients become more alert and energetic for up to several hours after the nap. Students who can take a second nap after school often maintain alertness into the evening. For patients with obstructive sleep apnea (OSA) or idiopathic hypersomnia (IH), the feeling of sleepiness does not improve much with napping.

3. A 16-year-old female student was diagnosed with narcolepsy with cataplexy and started on modafinil, 200 mg in the morning and 200 mg at noon. She responded very well, with relief of daytime sleepiness. Two months after starting treatment, she obtained a learner's permit to drive. Late one night, she violated the permit regulations and drove her friend home. On returning home at 11 PM, her car drifted over to the other lane, and she was hit by an oncoming truck and was killed instantly. She *most* likely had
A. A cataplectic episode
B. A transient ischemic attack
C. A cardiac arrhythmia caused by modafinil
D. A blood modafinil level that was too low

ANSWER: **D.** Although the half-life of modafinil is in the 10- to 15-hour range, clinical experience suggests that it is effective for only about 10 hours after the last dose. The highest concentration is reached 2 to 4 hours after an oral dose. R-modafinil has a longer half-life and is about two times more potent. It is important to know about the medications used to treat the symptoms of narcolepsy. (ATLAS2, pp 113-116 and 173, Table 11.1–1)

4. A 19-year-old student has a 5-month history of severe daytime sleepiness and cataplexy. Overnight polysomnography (PSG) would *most* likely show
   A. Early-onset rapid eye movement (REM) sleep
   B. Late-onset REM sleep
   C. No REM sleep
   D. An increased amount of REM sleep

ANSWER: **A.**   Typical in patients with narcolepsy is early-onset REM sleep. REM sleep normally first appears about 90 minutes after sleep onset. In a patient symptomatic with daytime sleepiness, REM that occurs within 15 minutes of the first electroencephalographic (EEG) sign of any sleep strongly suggests narcolepsy. The ICSD3 now provides for one sleep-onset rapid eye movement period (SOREMP) in the PSG (REM within 15 minutes of sleep onset) to be combined with one SOREMP in the multiple sleep latency test (MSLT) to satisfy the two-SOREMP criterion for diagnosis of narcolepsy.   (ICSD3, p 152)

5. What finding on the MSLT would be *most* confirmatory of narcolepsy?
   A. Mean sleep onset (after lights out) averaging less than 5 minutes for all naps
   B. Hallucinations, sleep paralysis, or both in at least one of the naps in association with REM sleep
   C. Two or more naps in which REM sleep occurs within the first 15 minutes
   D. Average sleep onset of less than 5 minutes and at least one nap on the MSLT showing a SOREMP

ANSWER: **C.**   To help confirm the diagnosis of narcolepsy, the MSLT should show an average sleep latency of 8 minutes or less *and* two or more naps with early-onset REM sleep (SOREMP); this means REM sleep that occurs within 15 minutes of lights out. If there is only one SOREMP in the first four naps of the MSLT, a fifth nap should be done. Also note that the ICSD3 now provides for one SOREMP in the PSG (REM within 15 minutes of sleep onset) to be combined with one SOREMP in the MSLT to satisfy the two-SOREMP criterion for diagnosis of narcolepsy.   (ICSD3, p 152) If there is a short sleep latency (≤8 minutes) and fewer than two SOREMPs by the new criteria, the diagnosis is consistent with IH.

6. A 24-year-old woman was recently diagnosed with narcolepsy. She takes phenytoin for a seizure disorder and oral contraceptives. You are considering starting modafinil. What do you advise her regarding modafinil?
   A. Modafinil has no interactions with her two medications
   B. Modafinil may lower the concentration of the estrogen component of the contraceptive and may increase the level of phenytoin
   C. Modafinil may increase the concentration of both the estrogen component of the contraceptive and the level of phenytoin
   D. Modafinil may lower the concentration of both the estrogen component of the contraceptive and the level of phenytoin

ANSWER: **B.**   Modafinil inhibits the drug-metabolizing enzyme CYP2C19 and thus may increase the blood level of drugs eliminated by that enzyme. Examples of CYP2C19-metabolized drugs include diazepam, phenytoin, and propranolol. Modafinil may also induce the metabolizing enzyme CYP3A4, reducing the levels of medications affected by that enzyme system; drugs that use this metabolic pathway include steroidal contraceptives and cyclosporine.

7. A 22-year-old woman complains of daytime sleepiness. Her overnight PSG shows a REM latency of 30 minutes. The MSLT reveals mean sleep latency of 4 minutes, and two of four naps show REM sleep. She is started on modafinil, 100 mg every morning. One week later, she complains of palpitations and is referred to a cardiologist. After cardiac evaluation, she is diagnosed with Wolff-Parkinson-White syndrome and hypertension. What is your next step?

A. Reassure the patient that modafinil has no effect on the cardiovascular system

B. Discontinue the modafinil and start methylphenidate

C. Discontinue the modafinil and start pemoline

D. Discontinue the modafinil and start sodium oxybate

ANSWER: **D.**   Although modafinil does not cause the severe sympathomimetic effects seen with traditional stimulant medications, increases in blood pressure (both systolic and diastolic) and heart rate have been documented.   (Taneja I, Diedrich A, Black BK, et al: Modafinil elicits sympathomedullary activation, *Hypertension.* 45:612-618, 2005)

8. A 28-year-old man is diagnosed with narcolepsy based on a history that includes severe daytime sleepiness and loss of muscle tone during periods of laughter. He is started on modafinil, 200 mg in the morning, and sodium oxybate, 5 g in equally divided doses (2.5 mg at bedtime and 2.5 mg 4 hours later). The patient calls to report that his wife finds him sleepwalking almost every night. He has no recollection of these events. How would you explain his sleepwalking?

A. It is one of the symptoms of narcolepsy

B. Modafinil is causing it

C. Sodium oxybate is causing it

D. The patient has likely developed temporal lobe epilepsy

ANSWER: **C.**   Sleepwalking has long been recognized as a potential side effect of sodium oxybate.

9. A 35-year-old patient has a 6-year history of daytime sleepiness. He has been treated with Coumadin for 7 years after an episode of severe pulmonary embolism. He also has mild bronchial asthma that is well controlled by inhaled steroids. His overnight sleep study shows frequent arousals and periodic limb movements but is otherwise unremarkable. The MSLT shows mean sleep latency of 3 minutes with REM sleep documented on three of four naps. He is started on modafinil 200 mg in the morning and 200 mg at lunchtime. The medication does not improve his daytime sleepiness, and you consider using methylphenidate. What should you advise the patient?

A. He does not have a disorder that is affected by methylphenidate

B. Methylphenidate may paradoxically improve his asthma

C. Methylphenidate may increase coagulability

D. Methylphenidate increases the level of Coumadin in the blood and may cause bleeding

ANSWER: **D.**   Besides the sympathomimetic side effects of methylphenidate (hypertension and tachyarrhythmias), it may increase the blood level of Coumadin and may also cause thrombocytopenia, increasing the risk of bleeding.   (ATLAS2, p 114)

10. A 27-year-old captain of a fishing vessel has been found asleep at inappropriate times and is referred for a sleep evaluation. His employer asks for a maintenance of wakefulness test (MWT) to indicate that he is fit for duty. The patient gives a history of severe sleepiness and cataplexy for the past 8 years. You order an overnight PSG followed by an MSLT. The decision to order the MSLT instead of the MWT is based on your knowledge of the tests. Regarding these two tests, which of the following statements is *not* true?

A. MSLT is used to measure the physiologic tendency to fall asleep in quiet situations

B. Normal and abnormal ranges of sleep latencies have been established for MSLT and MWT, when administered between 8 AM and 6 PM, and for individuals older than 8 years of age

C. Results of the MWT and MSLT for the same individual correlate well with one another

D. The MSLT should be performed after a preceding PSG with at least 6 hours of recorded sleep, with adequate sleep for the previous 2 weeks documented by a sleep diary or actigraphy

ANSWER: **C.** The MSLT and MWT are not equivalent evaluations of daytime sleepiness. Whereas the MSLT measures the propensity to fall asleep, the MWT measures the ability to stay awake. Surprisingly, the two tests are not highly correlated. There is much greater clinical experience with the MSLT than with the MWT. A mean sleep latency under 8 minutes is considered abnormal for both tests. The MWT has not been validated in the diagnosis of narcolepsy. (ATLAS2, p 392)

11. Which statement about cataplexy is *incorrect*?

A. Loss of both muscle tone and deep tendon reflexes can be triggered by emotion

B. Positive emotional triggers (e.g., laughter, elation) more commonly cause cataplexy than negative emotional triggers (e.g., anger, agitation)

C. Affected areas during cataplexy attacks most commonly include the knees, face, and neck and may range from facial sagging to complete collapse

D. A loss of consciousness occurs with amnesia

ANSWER: **D.** Patients having a cataplexy episode are conscious, and after regaining muscle control, they demonstrate no confusion or neurologic deficits. (ATLAS2, pp 159-160, 162)

12. Which of the following is *not* a clinical feature of patients who have narcolepsy with cataplexy?

A. Daytime sleepiness and possible sleep attacks

B. Respiratory compromise during cataplexy from diaphragm weakness

C. REM-related phenomena such as sleep paralysis and automatic behavior

D. Loss of muscle tone triggered by emotional stimuli

ANSWER: **B.** The diaphragm, the main muscle of inspiration, is spared during cataplexy episodes, and thus there is no respiratory compromise.

13. Which of the following is *not* a feature of cataplexy attacks?

A. Maintenance of consciousness

B. Memory of events

C. Enuresis during most episodes

D. Duration of less than 5 minutes for most episodes

ANSWER: **C.** Enuresis has not been described as a feature of cataplexy. (ATLAS2, pp 159-160, 162)

14. Which statement about sleep paralysis is *incorrect*?
  A. Patients can cry out during the episodes
  B. Patients may have vivid visual hallucinations
  C. Patients may have auditory hallucinations
  D. Patients may have tactile hallucinations

ANSWER: **A.** Patients having an episode of sleep paralysis are conscious but are unable to move their extremities or speak. They may have the perception of impending doom, and even when alone, they may have the sensation that someone else is in the room. They may have vivid visual, auditory, or tactile hallucinations. (ATLAS2, p 119)

15. A patient is brought to the emergency department by his wife because "lately, he's been sleepy all the time." His medication list includes trazodone, quetiapine, methadone, and prn (as needed) alprazolam. You find him arousable but very sleepy; he is oriented to name and date and shows no evidence of respiratory distress. He came in on nasal O_2, and his SaO_2 is 95% by pulse oximetry. The best next step is to
  A. Administer naloxone to reverse any sedating effect of the opiate
  B. Administer flumazenil to reverse any sedating effect of the benzodiazepine
  C. Obtain a stat brain computed tomography scan
  D. Check arterial blood gas

ANSWER: **D.** In patients with recent onset of hypersomnia, you should always consider hypoventilation. This patient is taking several potentially sedating drugs, and methadone is also known to cause hypoventilation. Appropriate treatment would depend on the presence and degree of hypoventilation and hypoxemia. Note that SaO_2 can be normal even in profoundly hypoventilating patients if they are receiving supplemental O_2.

16. A 12-year-old boy has recently developed some bizarre behavior, such as severe daytime sleepiness, and when he awakens, hyperphagia and hypersexual behavior, including masturbation in front of his family. Some days he may sleep up to 18 hours. What is the likely diagnosis?
  A. Paranoid schizophrenia
  B. Narcolepsy secondary to a hypothalamic tumor
  C. Kleine-Levin syndrome (KLS)
  D. Idiopathic hypersomnia with long sleep time

ANSWER: **C.** Patients with KLS are usually male, and they typically have long bouts of sleep. When awake, they often exhibit hyperphagia, hypersexuality, and aggressiveness. This group of symptoms may last one to several weeks followed by remission, and it may recur several times a year. In between these symptomatic periods, the patient is apparently normal. Episodes are typically gone by age 20 years. (ATLAS2, p 161; ICSD3, pp 166-170)

17. The diagnostic criteria for KLS include all of the following *except*
  A. The patient experiences recurrent episodes of excessive sleepiness that can last up to 4 weeks
  B. Episodes recur at least once a year
  C. The patient has normal alertness, cognitive functioning, and behavior between attacks
  D. An MSLT is required for diagnosis and shows a mean sleep latency of less than 8 minutes but no SOREMPs

ANSWER: **D.** KLS, also known as *recurrent hypersomnia*, is a clinical diagnosis, and an MSLT is not required. In fact, an MSLT is difficult to do during a bout of recurrent hypersomnia, because the patient will not cooperate. (ICSD3, pp 166-170)

18. All of the following are true about behaviorally induced insufficient sleep syndrome *except*
   A. The patient persistently fails to obtain the amount of sleep needed to maintain normal levels of alertness and wakefulness
   B. The patient engages in voluntary chronic sleep deprivation
   C. Clinically significant psychopathology is evident
   D. The extent of the sleep deprivation is underappreciated by the patient

ANSWER: **C.**   The problem in behaviorally induced insufficient sleep syndrome is that patients will not get enough sleep when they could do so with effort. Such patients go to sleep too late, wake up too early, or both, a pattern often related to their work. On weekends and during vacations, they typically sleep much longer. Treatment is convincing the patient to get more sleep; with more sleep, their daytime hypersomnolence resolves. (ICSD3, pp 182-186)

19. A 45-year-old man, 186 lb and 5'10" tall, complains of excessive daytime sleepiness. His Epworth Sleepiness Scale (ESS) score is 17 of 24. His wife complains that he snores and stops breathing during sleep. On overnight PSG, his apnea/hypopnea index (AHI) was 20.5 events/hr, and low SaO_2 was 86%. With 8 cm H_2O continuous positive airway pressure (CPAP), his AHI is 0.7 events/hr with a low SaO_2 of 92%. CPAP is prescribed at this pressure, and in follow-up 5 weeks later, he is found to be fully compliant with the mask, wearing it whenever he sleeps. He states that he feels better but still feels sleepy during the day. His ESS score is now 15 of 24. Compliance data show that he uses CPAP an average of 5 hours per night. When asked why only 5 hours, he states, "That's all I sleep; I never get more than 5 or 6 hours a night, and it's been that way since college." The next step is to
   A. Prescribe modafinil for daytime sleepiness along with continued CPAP
   B. Repeat the in-lab CPAP titration to determine whether 8 cm is an adequate pressure
   C. Order an autotitration CPAP study in his home to better determine his correct pressure
   D. Explain that daytime sleepiness is likely a result of insufficient sleep and that he needs more sleep time

ANSWER: **D.**   Three common causes of excessive daytime sleepiness (EDS) are insufficient sleep time, OSA, and medication side effects. This patient was taking no medications. His CPAP was adequately titrated while he slept, but his sleep time was insufficient. Modafinil is indicated as a stimulant for patients treated with CPAP who remain sleepy despite adequate sleep and full compliance with the mask. That is not the situation here.

20. A 50-year-old woman with a history of depression complains of EDS. Her medications include quetiapine, bupropion XL, fluoxetine, and lamotrigine. Which drug is *most* likely responsible for her daytime sleepiness?
   A. Quetiapine
   B. Bupropion XL
   C. Fluoxetine
   D. Lamotrigine

ANSWER: **A.**   Quetiapine is a popular second-generation antipsychotic, and a common side effect is next-day sedation.   (Komossa K, Depping AM, Gaudchau A, et al: Second-generation antipsychotics for major depressive disorder and dysthymia, *Cochrane Database Syst Rev.* 12:CD008121, 2010) Among the drugs listed, quetiapine is much more likely to cause hypersomnia. Medications are a common cause of EDS and should not be overlooked in the history. Drug side effect is often a comorbid cause of hypersomnia, along with sleep apnea or insufficient sleep.

21. A 51-year-old man comes to the sleep clinic with daytime hypersomnolence. His ESS score is 15 of 24. He does factory work from 7 AM to 3 PM 5 days a week. He goes to bed about 9 PM and is up at 5:30 on workdays. He weighs 250 lb, is 5'9" tall, and his Mallampati score is II to III. To help him fall asleep, his doctor prescribed 50 mg trazodone at bedtime. The patient also takes a blood pressure pill and a multivitamin. He thinks he snores, but his wife has not commented on apneas during sleep. The next step should be

   A. Have him stop the trazodone to see if his sleepiness improves

   B. Have him keep a 2-week sleep diary to ensure he is actually getting enough sleep

   C. Start modafinil 200 mg in the morning

   D. Schedule an overnight PSG

ANSWER: **D.** The three most common causes of EDS are insufficient sleep, medication side effects, and OSA. Information is sufficient in this case to suspect OSA, so it should be ruled out as the cause of his hypersomnia. Trazodone is an antidepressant that can cause next-day sleepiness, but 50 mg is a low dose and in any case does not obviate the need to evaluate for OSA.

22. A 62-year-old man has been treated for sleep apnea with CPAP at 13 cm H_2O. He uses the CPAP at least 7 to 8 hours nightly by compliance data, but after 6 months, he still complains of hypersomnolence. In the interim, he has gained 10 lb and now weighs 220 lb (he is 5'8" tall). The next step should be

   A. Check the patient's detailed sleep diary to see how much sleep he is getting

   B. Do an autotitration home study to see if he needs a higher pressure

   C. Send him to the lab for a titration with bilevel pressure

   D. Start a trial of modafinil 200 mg in the morning

ANSWER: **D.** A 10-lb weight gain is unlikely to require a significantly higher pressure, assuming the initial study was adequate. He fits into that subgroup of adequately treated OSA patients with residual hypersomnolence. Modafinil (and armodafinil) are approved by the US Food and Drug Administration (FDA) for treatment of this condition as well as for shift-work sleep disorder. (ATLAS2, pp 113-115)

23. A common cause of hypersomnia in Africa is

   A. Trypanosomiasis

   B. Ebola virus

   C. Acquired immune deficiency syndrome (AIDS)

   D. Malaria

ANSWER: **A.** African trypanosomiasis (sleeping sickness) is caused by transmission of trypanosomes by tsetse flies, and it is a common cause of severe hypersomnia in Western Africa (*Trypanosoma brucei gambiense*) and Eastern Africa (*Trypanosoma brucei rhodesiense*). The possibility of human African trypanosomiasis needs to be assessed in persons with excessive daytime sleepiness who have traveled in or migrated from Africa.

24. In evaluating daytime sleepiness, which of the following is *true* about the ESS and the Stanford Sleepiness Scale (SSS)?

   A. Normative data exist for SSS but not for the ESS

   B. SSS asks how sleepy you are now; ESS asks how sleepy you tend to be in certain situations

   C. Both scales correlate strongly with the MSLT

   D. Both use a seven-part questionnaire

ANSWER: **B.** Normative data exist for ESS but not for SSS. ESS correlates weakly with MSLT; the latter is an objective index of sleep drive. The ESS uses an eight-part questionnaire, and the SSS uses a questionnaire with seven levels of wakefulness, from wide awake to "almost in reverie." (ATLAS2, pp 129, 392)

25. Sleep apnea (SA) in adults is defined as an AHI of 5/hr or greater. *Sleep apnea syndrome* (SAS) is defined as an AHI of 5/hr or greater with daytime *hypersomnolence*. Based on a large epidemiologic PSG study of middle-aged adults, what percent of men and women had SAS?
  A. 2% of women and 4% of men
  B. 9% of women and 24% of men
  C. 6% of both women and men
  D. 5% of both women and men

ANSWER: **A.** In one study, 9% of women and 24% of men had an AHI of 5 or more *without* daytime somnolence. (Young T, Palta M, Dempsey J, et al: The occurrence of sleep-disordered breathing among middle-aged adults, *N Engl J Med.* 328:1230-1235, 1993) In other studies that defined sleep apnea as an AHI of 10 or higher, SAS was found in 3.9% of men and 1.2% of women. (Bixler EO, Vgontzas AN, Lin HM, et al: Prevalence of sleep-disordered breathing in women: effects of gender, *Am J Respir Crit Care Med.* 163:608-613, 2001; and Bixler EO, Vgontzas AN, Ten Have T, et al: Effects of age on sleep apnea in men: I. Prevalence and severity, *Am J Respir Crit Care Med.* 157:144-148, 1998) Sleep apnea by AHI criteria alone is much more prevalent than SAS.

26. Which of the following statements is *most* correct for IH?
  A. IH is about twice as common as narcolepsy.
  B. IH is familial in one third to two thirds of cases.
  C. HLA typing is useful to decide for narcolepsy and against the diagnosis of IH.
  D. Mean sleep latency on MSLT is less than 5 minutes with one or no SOREMPs.

ANSWER: **B.** Whereas there is nothing diagnostically useful about this aspect of IH (many sleep disorders are familial), the other choices are incorrect. IH prevalence is about 60% that of narcolepsy, and HLA typing plays no role in ruling IH in or out. There have been reports of remission. Diagnosis of IH requires a mean sleep latency under 8 minutes with one or no SOREMPs. (ATLAS2, p 160)

27. The hypnogram and actigram in Figure E4–1 are from a 32-year-old man with a history of EDS, prolonged nonrefreshing sleep ranging from 13 to 18 hours, occasional cataplexy-like episodes triggered by both positive and negative emotions, sleep paralysis with hallucinations, and migraine headaches. His ESS score is increased at 19 of 24, affirming EDS. His body mass index is 27, and he has no family history of EDS. PSG over 16 hours shows a sleep efficiency of 92%, sleep latency to stage N2 sleep of 22 minutes, latency to stage R of 55 minutes, and slow-wave sleep (stage N3) makes up 6% of the sleep period. No snoring, apnea, or periodic limb movements in sleep were reported. The MSLT shows a mean sleep latency of 4.3 minutes and no SOREMPs. An MWT shows mean sleep latency of 4.3 minutes and no SOREMPs. Two-week actigraphy shows mean time "asleep" (rest or sleep) over 48% of the recording time. The hypocretin-1 level in his CSF is normal, human leukocyte antigen (HLA)-DQB1*0602 is negative, and psychiatric assessment is normal. No improvement was noted after modafinil, methylphenidate, or melatonin. The diagnosis is *most* likely
  A. Narcolepsy without cataplexy
  B. Narcolepsy with cataplexy
  C. Idiopathic hypersomnolence
  D. Early onset of a neurodegenerative disorder

ANSWER: **C.** This scenario is surprisingly common in clinical practice. By process of exclusion, this is a case of IH, which can rarely present with cataplexy-like episodes. Narcolepsy is not confirmed: MSLT does not show SOREMPs, and the spinal fluid shows a normal hypocretin level. The R latency on the PSG does not meet the threshold for a SOREMP. (ICSD3, p 146) Neurodegenerative diseases are a group of heterogeneous, idiopathic diseases of the central nervous system (e.g., Alzheimer disease, multiple sclerosis, Parkinson disease, and Huntington chorea). They tend to occur in older individuals and may be associated with hypersomnia. (ATLAS2, pp 213-216) There is no evidence in this case of a neurologic disease.

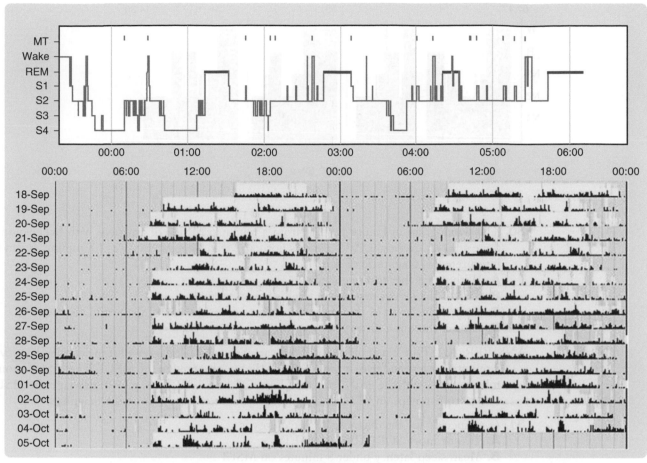

FIGURE E4–1

28. Which statement is *correct* in comparing the definitions of *sleep onset* during an MWT nap and an MSLT nap?

    A. Whereas MWT requires at least three consecutive epochs of any sleep stage, MSLT requires only one epoch with more than 15 seconds of any stage sleep

    B. Whereas MSLT requires at least three consecutive epochs of any sleep stage, MWT requires only one epoch with more than 15 seconds of any stage sleep

    C. In both, sleep onset requires three consecutive epochs of any stage sleep

    D. In both, sleep onset is the first epoch of more than 15 seconds of any stage sleep

ANSWER: **D.** Although both tests assess sleepiness, only the MSLT is useful in documenting narcolepsy. The MWT is often used as an objective way to document "fitness for duty." (ATLAS2, p 392; Littner R, Kushida C, Wise M, et al: Practice parameters for clinical use of the multiple sleep latency test and the maintenance of wakefulness test, *Sleep.* 28:113-121, 2005)

29. Which one of the following is *not* a requirement for the MSLT to be used in the diagnosis of narcolepsy?

    A. The night before the MSLT, a PSG shows at least 6 hours of sleep.

    B. PSG shows no other cause of hypersomnia.

    C. The patient is not on any stimulants or REM-suppressing drugs for 2 weeks before the test.

    D. The patient undergoes a drug screen the day of the test.

ANSWER: **D.** "Stimulants, stimulant-like medications, and REM-suppressing medications should ideally be stopped 2 weeks before the MSLT…. Drug screening may be indicated to ensure that sleepiness on the MSLT is not pharmacologically induced." (Littner MR, Kushida C, Wise M, et al: Practice parameters for clinical use of the multiple sleep latency test and the maintenance of wakefulness test, *Sleep.* 28:119, 2005)

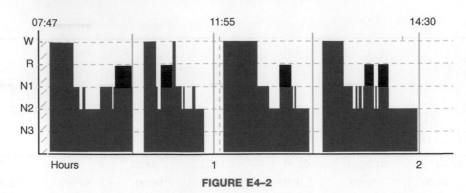

FIGURE E4–2

30. The hypnogram in Figure E4–2 is from a four-nap MSLT of a patient with hypersomnia, done after an overnight PSG that was normal. Mean sleep latency was 1.5 minute. It can be interpreted as diagnostic of narcolepsy
  A. Without further testing
  B. Only if the serum hypocretin level is below normal
  C. Only if the result of the patient's drug screen on the day of the test is negative
  D. Only if there is a history of cataplexy

ANSWER: **A.**   Type 2 narcolepsy (without cataplexy) can be diagnosed if mean sleep latency is 8 minutes or less and two or more SOREMPs are observed in the MSLT. The MSLT should follow a PSG with the goal of at least 7 hours of sleep.   (ICSD3, p 159) Although the MSLT can go to five naps, in this case, a fifth nap would not have altered the diagnosis.

31. *Least* specific for the diagnosis of narcolepsy is
  A. Two or more SOREMPs on MSLT
  B. Mean sleep latency under 8 minutes on MSLT
  C. Low CSF hypocretin level
  D. Presence of cataplexy by history

ANSWER: **B.**   In patients with narcolepsy, the MSLT shows a mean sleep latency of less than 8 minutes and typically less than 5 minutes. However, this single criterion is nonspecific and may be seen in IH as well as in patients who are sleep deprived. The other criteria are much more specific for narcolepsy.   (ICSD3, pp 152, 159)

32. Patients with major depressive disorder may complain of daytime sleepiness. Frequently associated PSG findings in patients with a major depressive episode include all of the following *except*
  A. Sleep continuity disturbances (e.g., prolonged sleep latency, increased wake after sleep onset [WASO], early morning awakening)
  B. Reduced NREM stages 3 and 4
  C. Increased latency to REM sleep
  D. Increased phasic REM activity

ANSWER: **C.**   In untreated major depression, REM latency is shortened.   (ATLAS2, p 365) Note that despite complaints of daytime sleepiness, these patients generally do not demonstrate severe sleepiness on the MSLT.   (ICSD3, pp 179-182)

33. Regarding the diagnosis of IH, which of the following is *correct*?
  A. There is a clear distinction among IH patients "with long sleep time" (≥10 hours) and "without long sleep time" (<10 hours)
  B. The MSLT shows a mean sleep latency of 10 minutes or less
  C. Cataplexy may be present in a small subset of IH patients with a total sleep time greater than 12 hours
  D. Naps are unrefreshing in most patients

ANSWER: **D.**   The *International Classification of Sleep Disorders*, edition 2 (ICSD2, 2005), distinguished between IH with long sleep time and IH without long sleep time. The *International Classification of Sleep Disorders*, edition 3 (ICSD3), states that subsequent studies invalidate such a distinction, and "there are no separate subtypes." To diagnose IH, the MSLT must show a mean sleep latency of 8 minutes or less. The presence of cataplexy would indicate a diagnosis of narcolepsy. In IH, naps are "described as unrefreshing by 46% to 78% of patients." (ICSD3, pp 161-166)

34. To diagnose hypersomnia caused by a medical disorder by ICSD3 criteria, all of the following must be satisfied *except*
  A. EDS almost daily for at least 3 months
  B. An underlying medical or neurologic disorder that can account for the daytime sleepiness
  C. A mean sleep latency of 8 minutes or less on the MSLT
  D. Other possible causes (e.g., sleep apnea, medication side effects) have been ruled out.

ANSWER: **C.**   If the MSLT is performed, the mean sleep latency should be 8 minutes or less with no more than one SOREMP. However, depending on the medical condition, it may not be feasible to do an MSLT. Note that up to 30% of the general population may have a sleep latency of 8 minutes or less on the MSLT, so this finding alone is nonspecific; if present, the patient would also have to meet the criteria listed in answers A, B, and D. (ICSD3, p 171)

35. A 15-year-old high school student has been falling asleep in class. She sleeps about 8 hours each night and reports having vivid hypnagogic hallucinations. The results of her overnight sleep study (PSG) were normal. The PSG was followed by an MSLT, shown in Figure E4–3. Which statement about the MSLT is *correct*?
  A. The study was nondiagnostic because the first nap opportunity was too long.
  B. The findings strongly support a diagnosis of narcolepsy.
  C. The patient does not have pathologic sleepiness because the sleep latency of the first nap is about 15 minutes.
  D. The result is explainable by chronic sleep deprivation.

ANSWER: **B.**   The findings strongly support narcolepsy because three of the naps show REM sleep. Although the first nap shows a sleep latency of 15 minutes, the other naps have a short sleep latency, and the mean sleep latency for all five naps was 6.4 minutes.

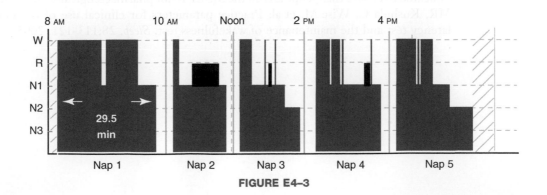

FIGURE E4–3

36. Which of the following features is *more* characteristic of IH than of narcolepsy?
  A. Presence of cataplexy
  B. Naps are often restorative
  C. The condition may remit
  D. Presence of hypnagogic hallucinations

ANSWER: **C.**   Whereas narcolepsy never remits, remission of IH has been reported. Features of narcolepsy include cataplexy, naps that are often restorative, and hypnagogic (preceding sleep) hallucinations.   (ATLAS2, p 160)

37. A principal difference between the ESS and the SSS is
  A. The ESS assesses sleepiness retrospectively, and the SSS assesses it at the moment of the questionnaire
  B. The ESS correlates much better with the MSLT than does the SSS
  C. Whereas the ESS is filled out by the patient, the SSS is filled out by someone close to the patient (e.g., a spouse or significant other)
  D. The nature of the questions in the SSS (e.g., how much sleep do you get in a 24-hour period?) provides for a more objective assessment of sleepiness than the ESS

ANSWER: **A.**   The ESS asks eight questions that rely on subjective assessment of sleepiness over the recent past. The SSS asks how sleepy you are at the time of the questionnaire. Both scales are highly subjective, and neither one correlates very well with the MSLT.

38. Sleep onset during an MWT nap is defined as
  A. First epoch of more than 15 seconds of any stage sleep
  B. Three consecutive epochs of stage 1 sleep
  C. Single epoch of any other stage
  D. Whatever your lab uses for overnight PSG

ANSWER: **A.**   "Sleep onset [for the MWT] is defined as the first epoch of greater than 15 seconds of cumulative sleep. ... Trials are ended after 40 minutes if no sleep occurs, or after unequivocal sleep, defined as three consecutive epochs of stage 1 sleep, or one epoch of any other stage of sleep."   (Littner MR, Kushida C, Wise M, et al: Practice parameters for clinical use of the multiple sleep latency test and the maintenance of wakefulness test, *Sleep*. 28:113-121, 2005)

39. Which one of the following is *not* a requirement for the MSLT to be valid in the diagnosis of hypersomnia?
  A. MSLT is immediately preceded by overnight PSG that shows at least 6 hours of sleep
  B. PSG shows no cause to explain the hypersomnia
  C. The patient is not on any stimulants or REM-suppressing drugs for 2 weeks before the test
  D. The patient undergoes a drug screen on the day of the test

ANSWER: **D.**   Drug screening would be ideal if there is any concern about medication effects, but it is not a requirement. "Stimulants, stimulant-like medications, and REM-suppressing medications should ideally be stopped 2 weeks before MSLT. ... Drug screening may be indicated to ensure that sleepiness on the MSLT is not pharmacologically induced."   (Littner MR, Kushida C, Wise M, et al: Practice parameters for clinical use of the multiple sleep latency test and the maintenance of wakefulness test, *Sleep*. 28:113-121, 2005)

40. All of the following are true about the MSLT *except*

A. Instructions to the patient at the start of each nap are to "lie quietly, keep your eyes closed, and try to fall asleep."

B. Naps are continued for 20 minutes if there is no sleep or for 15 minutes after the first episode of sleep

C. *Sleep latency* is defined as the time from lights out to the first epoch of sleep

D. Early onset of sleep (from average sleep latency of four or five naps) plus early onset of REM sleep in at least one of the naps satisfies criteria for the diagnosis of narcolepsy

ANSWER: **D.** To support a diagnosis of narcolepsy from the MSLT, there must be two naps with early-onset REM sleep, often called a *sleep-onset REM period* (SOREMP). Note that ICSD3 now allows replacement of one SOREMP in the MSLT with one in the PSG that preceded the MSLT, thereby satisfying the two-SOREMP requirement. (ICSD3, p 152)

41. The MSLT is indicated to help diagnose which of the following conditions?

1. Narcolepsy
2. Idiopathic hypersomnia
3. OSA after treatment with positive airway pressure therapy
4. Insomnia
5. Circadian rhythm disorders

A. 1 only
B. 1 and 2
C. 1 and 3
D. 1, 2, and 4
E. All of above

ANSWER: **B.** The MSLT is not indicated for OSA, with or without treatment, or for patients with insomnia or circadian rhythm disorders. (Littner MR, Kushida C, Wise M, et al: Practice parameters for clinical use of the multiple sleep latency test and the maintenance of wakefulness test, *Sleep.* 28:113-121, 2005)

42. What is the *most* potent stimulus that leads to cataplexy in narcolepsy patients?

A. Laughter
B. Anger
C. Sexual activity
D. Bright light

ANSWER: **A.** Laughter is the most common trigger that induces cataplexy. Of patients who have narcolepsy with cataplexy, in 87%, cataplexy is caused by laughter, in 68% by anger, and in 22% during sexual activity. Bright light does not cause cataplexy. (ATLAS2, p 161)

43. A 35-year-old woman has EDS, obesity, hair loss, and hoarseness. What is the *most* likely diagnosis?

A. Acromegaly
B. Stein-Leventhal syndrome
C. Cushing disease
D. Hypothyroidism

ANSWER: **D.** Clues to indicate hypothyroidism include hair loss and hoarseness in an obese woman. Hypothyroidism is a common finding in patients with obstructive OSA. Hypothyroidism can also cause sleepiness without apnea being present. Another common feature of this disease is cold intolerance. (ATLAS2, pp 335-336)

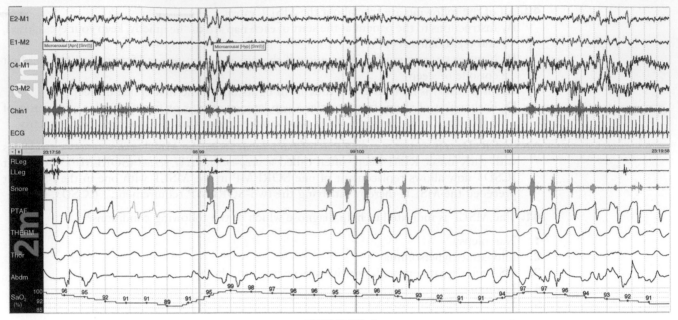

FIGURE E4–4

44. Which statement is *true* about sleep paralysis?
   A. It can occur without another diagnosis
   B. It is the *most* common symptom of narcolepsy
   C. It occurs mainly in non-REM sleep
   D. Breathing stops during paralysis

ANSWER: **A.** Sleep paralysis occurs in many healthy people. It is not the most common symptom in narcolepsy patients (excessive sleepiness is). Sleep paralysis occurs during REM sleep, and breathing does not stop, because the diaphragm is spared the paralysis that affects other skeletal muscles. (ATLAS2, p 160)

45. A 10-minute epoch from an overnight PSG is shown in Figure E4–4. The patient has severe daytime sleepiness. The *most* likely cause for hypoxemia is
   A. OSA
   B. Central sleep apnea
   C. Hypoventilation
   D. Ventilation-perfusion imbalance

ANSWER: **C.** This 10-minute compressed epoch shows SaO_2 consistently in the mid 80s despite excellent airflow. Thus, there is no evidence for obstructive or central sleep apnea. Whereas hypoventilation (increased $PacO_2$) is a possibility, the most common cause of sleep-related hypoxemia is ventilation-perfusion (V-Q) imbalance. Hypoxemia from V-Q imbalance will show an increased alveolar-arterial PO_2 difference if blood gas is obtained. This patient had chronic obstructive pulmonary disease and exercise hypoxemia.

46. In which group would you *most* likely find onset of REM during the first 15 minutes of sleep?
   A. People taking barbiturates
   B. Narcoleptics with cataplexy
   C. Patients with REM sleep behavior disorder
   D. People taking tricyclic antidepressants

ANSWER: **B.** Early REM onset (typically within 15 minutes of sleep onset) during the PSG occurs in about 50% of patients with narcolepsy and cataplexy, and it is very rare in control participants.

47. During an MSLT nap, *sleep onset* is defined as
   A. First epoch of more than 15 seconds of any stage sleep
   B. Three consecutive epochs of stage 1 sleep
   C. Single epoch of any other stage sleep
   D. Whatever your lab uses for overnight PSG

ANSWER: **A.**   Below are two quotes from "Practice parameters for clinical use of the multiple sleep latency test and the maintenance of wakefulness test."   (Littner MR, Kishida C, Wise M, et al: Practice parameters for clinical use of the multiple sleep latency test and the maintenance of wakefulness test, *Sleep.* 28:113-121, 2005)

○   "Sleep onset for the clinical MSLT is determined by the time from lights out to the first epoch of any stage of sleep, including stage 1 sleep. *Sleep onset* is defined as the first epoch of greater than 15 seconds of cumulative sleep in a 30-second epoch. The absence of sleep on a nap opportunity is recorded as a sleep latency of 20 min [and is] included in the calculation of mean sleep latency … the test continues for 15 min from after the first epoch of sleep … duration of 15 min is determined by 'clock time' and is not determined by a sleep time of 15 min."

○   "REM latency is taken as the time of the first epoch of sleep to the beginning of the first epoch of REM sleep regardless of the intervening stages of sleep or wakefulness."

48. MSLT results from a young man with EDS are summarized below. Numbers under each nap refer to the sleep epochs since the beginning of the study; each epoch is 30 seconds (Table E4–1).

Table E4–1				
	Nap 1	**Nap 2**	**Nap 3**	**Nap 4**
Lights out	150	190	250	300
Sleep onset	154	220	None	300
REM onset	170	None	None	None
End nap	184	240	280	340

Which of the following calculations is the *correct* sleep latency for the four naps?

	Nap 1	Nap 2	Nap 3	Nap 4
A.	4 min	30 min	0 min	42 min
B.	4 min	15 min	0 min	21 min
C.	2 min	15 min	0 min	21 min
D.	2 min	15 min	20 min	0 min

ANSWER: **D.**

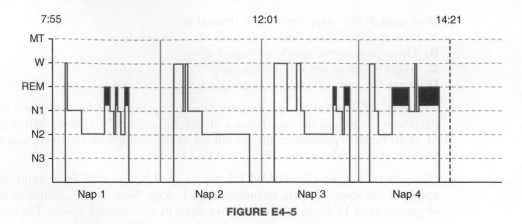

FIGURE E4–5

49. The hypnogram in Figure E4–5 is from a four-nap MSLT of a patient with hypersomnia done after an overnight PSG that was normal. Mean sleep latency was 4.5 minutes. It can be interpreted as diagnostic of narcolepsy
A. Without further testing
B. Only if the patient is also HLA-DQB1*602 positive
C. Only if the serum hypocretin level is below normal
D. Only if result of the patient's drug screen on the day of the test is negative
E. Only if there is a history of cataplexy

ANSWER: **A.**   This histogram shows four naps of an MSLT. Early-onset sleep occurs in each of the naps, and REM occurs in all but the second nap. This is considered diagnostic of narcolepsy.   (ICSD3, pp 146-161)

50. Which of the following drugs would be *least* effective in treating cataplexy?
A. Modafinil
B. Fluoxetine
C. Venlafaxine
D. Clomipramine

ANSWER: **A.**   Fluoxetine, venlafaxine, and clomipramine are all antidepressants and have efficacy in treating cataplexy. Modafinil is a stimulant used to treat hypersomnia, and it has little to no effect on cataplexy.   (ATLAS2, p 173)

51. During an MWT nap, *sleep onset* is defined as
A. First epoch of more than 15 seconds of any stage sleep
B. Three consecutive epochs of stage 1 sleep
C. A single epoch of N2 sleep
D. Whatever your lab uses for the overnight PSG

ANSWER: **A.**   (Littner MR, Kushida C, Wise M, et al: Practice parameters for clinical use of the multiple sleep latency test and the maintenance of wakefulness test, *Sleep.* 28:113-121, 2005)

○ "Sleep onset is defined as the first epoch of greater than 15 seconds of cumulative sleep."
○ "Trials are ended after 40 minutes if no sleep occurs, or after unequivocal sleep, defined as three consecutive epochs of stage 1 sleep, or one epoch of any other stage of sleep."

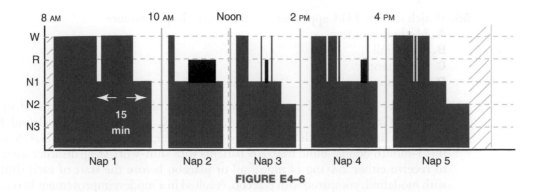

FIGURE E4–6

52. An MSLT is done on a 15-year-old student suspected of having narcolepsy. The results are shown in Figure E4–6. The first nap opportunity occupied about 30 minutes. Which statement about the test is *incorrect*?
    A. The test is diagnostic of narcolepsy
    B. The fifth nap was not necessary
    C. The first nap should have been terminated at 15 minutes
    D. The mean sleep latency is less than 8 minutes

ANSWER: **C.**   In the absence of REM, the clinical MSLT is terminated 15 minutes after the first epoch of any sleep. Thus, it was appropriate for the first nap in this case to be 30 minutes.   (ATLAS2, p 392) The fifth nap was technically not required because the diagnosis of narcolepsy had already been made with the first four naps. Except for the first nap, which had a latency of 15 minutes, the other naps by visual inspection had much shorter latencies. The mean latency was 6.4 minutes.

53. All of the following are true about modafinil *except*
    A. Modafinil is FDA approved for shift-work sleep disorder
    B. It has no appreciable effect on incidence of cataplexy in narcoleptics
    C. Modafinil works through the GABA$_A$ receptor
    D. It is a Schedule IV controlled substance

ANSWER: **C.**   The newer medications to foster sleep (Z drugs) and wakefulness (modafinil and armodafinil) are all Schedule IV controlled substances because of the FDA's concern for addiction potential; they require a Drug Enforcement Agency number to prescribe. Ramelteon (Rozerem) is also a hypnotic but is not a scheduled drug because it does not have addiction potential; no DEA number is required for prescribing ramelteon.

54. All of the following are true about sodium oxybate treatment of narcolepsy *except*
    A. It is effective for cataplexy but not for daytime sleepiness
    B. It can lead to abuse, dependence, and respiratory depression
    C. Because of its short half-life, the drug has to be given in divided doses, with the first dose at bedtime and the next dose a few hours later
    D. It is the sodium salt of gamma-hydroxybutyrate, a rapidly acting sedative-hypnotic medication

ANSWER: **A.**   Sodium oxybate is indicated for both the cataplexy and the daytime sleepiness of narcolepsy.   (ATLAS2, p 113)

55. Which drug is FDA approved for shift-work sleep disorder?
  A. Methylphenidate
  B. Modafinil
  C. Ramelteon
  D. Melatonin

ANSWER: **B.**   Approval of modafinil for shift-work sleep disorder was based in part on the study of Czeisler et al.   (Czeisler CA, Walsh JK, Roth T, et al: Modafinil for excessive sleepiness associated with shift-work sleep disorder, *N Engl J Med.* 353:476-486, 2005) In this 3-month double-blind trial, 209 patients with shift-work sleep disorder were randomized to receive either 200 mg of modafinil or placebo before the start of each shift. Treatment with modafinil, compared with placebo, resulted in a modest improvement in mean nighttime sleep latency. Also, more modafinil-treated patients had improvement in their clinical symptoms (74% vs. 36%, respectively; $P < 0.001$). Modafinil did not adversely affect daytime sleep compared with placebo, and headache was the most common adverse event. The authors concluded that "treatment with 200 mg of modafinil reduced the extreme sleepiness [in] shift-work sleep disorder and resulted in a small but significant improvement in performance as compared with placebo." Armodafinil, an enantiomer of modafinil, is also approved for this disorder.   (ATLAS2, p 113)

56. Which of the following is *not* considered a first-line treatment for sleepiness related to narcolepsy?
  A. Modafinil
  B. Armodafinil
  C. Sodium oxybate
  D. Methylphenidate

ANSWER: **D.**   Modafinil and armodafinil have largely replaced amphetamines as first-line therapy for the sleepiness of narcolepsy. Sodium oxybate is effective for cataplexy and excessive sleepiness and is used when patients have both symptoms. Methylphenidate (Ritalin), long used in this condition, is now relegated to second-line therapy.   (ATLAS2, Table 6–7) The doses for narcolepsy are

Modafinil	100 to 400 mg/day in two doses
Armodafinil	150 to 250 mg in one morning dose
Sodium oxybate	6 to 9 g/night in two doses
Methylphenidate	10 to 60 mg/day

Parasomnias

QUESTIONS

1. Which one of the following is *not* considered a parasomnia?
   A. Rapid eye movement (REM) sleep behavior disorder (RBD)
   B. Sleepwalking
   C. Nocturnal seizure
   D. Periodic limb movements of sleep (PLMS)

ANSWER: **D.**   Parasomnias are "undesirable physical, autonomic or experiential phenomena arising from the sleep period," and they encompass a large number of conditions such as the first three listed.   (ATLAS2, Ch 12) PLMS is an electromyogram (EMG) finding observed during polysomnography (PSG) and is classified as a sleep-related movement disorder.   (ICSD3, p 292)

2. A 4-year-old child awakens 2 hours after being put to bed and is speaking incoherently. His mother finds him confused and disoriented. The episode lasts a few minutes, and he returns to sleep. Which stage of sleep *most* likely occurred just before he awoke?
   A. Non-REM (NREM)
   B. Tonic REM
   C. Phasic REM
   D. Either phasic REM or NREM, each with a 50% probability

ANSWER: **A.**   Arousal disorders, as in this case, are very common in children and occur in up to 4% to 5% of adults. Disorders of arousal are caused by the admixture of wakefulness and NREM sleep. NREM predominates in the first half of the sleep cycle, which explains why confusional arousals are more common in the few hours after sleep onset than later in the night.   (ATLAS2, p 238)

3. Which of the following statements is *most* accurate about confusional arousals in adults?
   A. They are frequently related to underlying psychiatric or psychological problems
   B. Characteristic PSG findings indicate when a person is prone to confusional arousals
   C. People who awake from a confusional arousal often report complete amnesia for any dreaming or mental activity before the event, in contrast to those who awaken from a REM-related nightmare
   D. A PSG is generally recommended to help guide treatment

ANSWER: **C.**   The other statements are false. Polysomnography for assessment of parasomnias is only recommended when behaviors are potentially injurious or disruptive to others in the household.   (ATLAS2, Ch 12)

4. A 21-year-old man referred for evaluation of sleepwalking has a history of intermittent sleepwalking (since age 6 years); on one occasion, he walked outside in the middle of winter. The episodes now occur about once a month. His parents also have a history of sleepwalking. His girlfriend reports that he sometimes talks and acts violently during sleep, and he also kicks, punches, and thrashes. A drug screen was negative, neurologic examination results were normal, and he is asymptomatic while awake. The next step should be
A. Overnight PSG with full electroencephalograph (EEG) montage
B. Psychiatric evaluation
C. Empiric treatment with clonazepam
D. Brain computed tomography (CT) scan

ANSWER: **A.**   Nocturnal seizures need to be ruled out. Disorders of arousal from sleep are not psychiatric disorders, and if there is a psychiatric diagnosis, it would not shed light on his nocturnal problem. Brain CT scan is unlikely to be helpful in a young man with normal neurologic examination results and symptoms only during sleep. Treatment should only be considered after seizures are ruled out. In this case, the overnight PSG was normal, and the diagnosis was simply "disorder of arousal."   (ATLAS2, Ch 12)

5. The 2-minute PSG fragment in Figure E5–1 is from a patient with sleep terrors. It shows
A. A gradual shift into heightened autonomic activity
B. Arousal from obstructive sleep apnea
C. Instantaneous arousal from NREM sleep
D. Seizure activity preceding the arousal

ANSWER: **C.**   This PSG fragment shows a typical arousal from NREM sleep in a patient with sleep terrors. Although these arousals are most common from the deepest stages of NREM sleep (stage N3 or slow-wave sleep [SWS]), they may arise from any stage of NREM sleep or even from relaxed wakefulness. A precipitous and dramatic increase in heart rate occurs, from 75 to 121 beats/min. These arousals are instantaneous and spontaneous and are not caused by the culmination of underlying psychologically or psychiatrically significant sleep-related mentation.   (ATLAS2, pp 238-245)

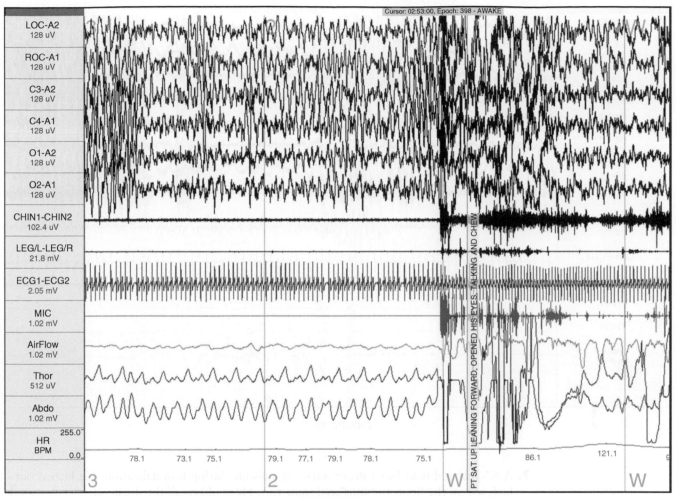

Cursor: 02:53:00, Epoch: 398 - AWAKE

PT SAT UP LEANING FORWARD, OPENED HIS EYES, TALKING AND CHEW

FIGURE E5–1

6. The PSG fragment shown in Figure E5–2 is from a 46-year-old obese man with obstructive sleep apnea (OSA). His apnea-hypopnea index (AHI) was 29 events/hr, and his nadir SaO_2 was 80%. What other diagnosis is suggested by this fragment?

A. Periodic limb movement of sleep

B. Nocturnal seizures

C. Sleep-related eating disorder (SRED)

D. REM sleep behavior disorder (RBD)

ANSWER: **C.** The PSG shows marked chin movements, which indicates chewing during apparent wakefulness. Although awake by EEG, there are periods of sleep seen as well, and the patient had no recollection of "eating Gummi Bears" during this period. SRED is a specialized form of disorder of arousal, like sexsomnia (sleepsex). This disorder is more common in women than in men. PSG evaluations are abnormal in about 80% of cases and show arousals that are usually from SWS. SRED is distinguished from nocturnal eating syndrome (NES) in that patients with NES eat between the evening meal and sleep onset, do not have the propensity to eat bizarre foods, and have full recall of what they eat. Furthermore, unlike most patients with SRED, NES patients do not have a primary sleep disorder (i.e., confusional arousals).   (ATLAS2, p 245; ICSD3, p 240)

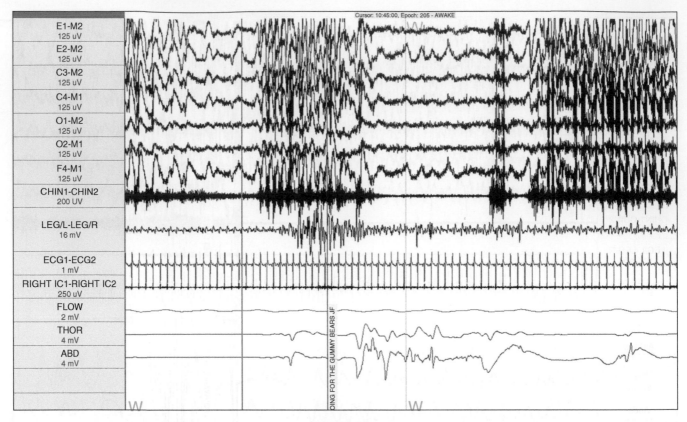

FIGURE E5–2

7. A 67-year-old man had a dream-enacting episode during hospitalization. He leaped out of bed, fell on the floor, and fractured some ribs. He could recall the dream after each episode. There was a reported history of several years of yelling, swearing, and punching his wife while he was sleeping and no evidence on examination of any cognitive problems, tremors, or abnormal daytime movements. The diagnosis is *most* likely

A. RBD

B. Confusional arousal from NREM sleep

C. Nocturnal seizure disorder

D. Lewy body dementia

ANSWER: **A.**   The man has RBD. The PSG manifestation is REM sleep without atonia, as shown in Figure E5–3. A large percentage of patients with RBD later will develop a synucleinopathy, such as Parkinson disease or Lewy body dementia. Patients with confusional arousal from NREM sleep typically have no recall of the event and cannot relate the preceding dream.   (ATLAS2, pp 216-221; ICSD3, p 246)

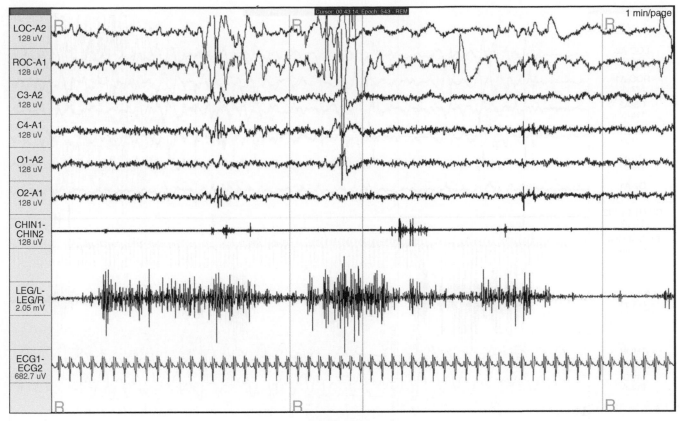

FIGURE E5–3

8. Which of the following statements is *most* accurate about RBD?
  A. Overwhelming male predominance (80%–90%)
  B. About 20% of patients with RBD eventually develop one of the synucleinopathies (Parkinson disease, Lewy body dementia, or multiple system atrophy)
  C. When awakened, patients with RBD remain confused and disoriented, but the next day, they can usually recall the dream
  D. RBD is rarely drug induced

ANSWER: **A.**   When idiopathic, RBD is much more prevalent in men than in women. Actually, a much larger percentage of patients (up to 75%) with RBD eventually develop a synucleinopathy if followed long enough. When awakened, patients with RBD are not confused, and they have good recall of the dream. Finally, RBD is frequently drug induced. Among the medications that have been implicated are tricyclic antidepressants, selective serotonin reuptake inhibitors (SSRIs), and selective serotonin-norepinephrine reuptake inhibitors (SNRIs).   (ATLAS2, pp 216-221; ICSD3, p 246)

9. A 28-year-old patient with narcolepsy was treated with fluoxetine for cataplexy. A PSG fragment is shown in Figure E5–4. The *most* likely diagnosis is
  A. REM sleep without atonia
  B. PLMS
  C. Limb movements associated with hypopneas
  D. Limb movement artifact, because there is no chin activity

ANSWER: **A.**   The fragment in Figure E5–4 shows prominent increased phasic EMG activity from the anterior tibialis muscles. Sparing of the submental muscle is nearly complete. Up to one third of patients with narcolepsy also have RBD as a manifestation of the underlying neurologic disorder. Many drugs prescribed to control cataplexy can cause RBD.   (ATLAS2, pp 216-221; ICSD3, p 246)

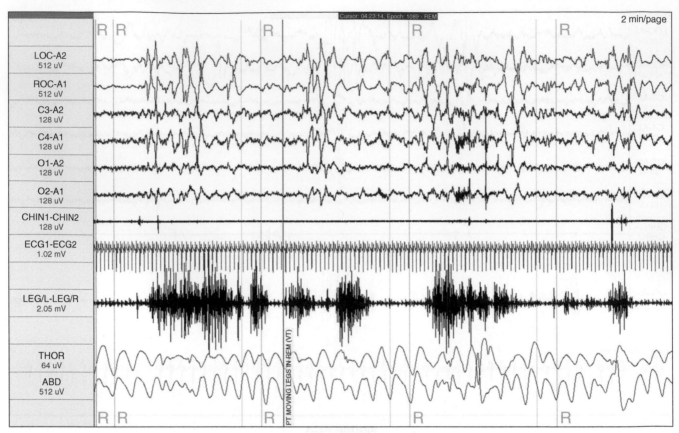

FIGURE E5–4

10. Seizures during sleep are one type of secondary parasomnia, defined as a disease of a specific organ system that mainly manifests during sleep. Of the stages of sleep, what is the *most* accurate sequence of nocturnal seizure frequency, going from *most* to *least*?
   A. NREM, wakefulness after sleep onset (WASO), REM
   B. WASO, NREM, REM
   C. REM, NREM, WASO
   D. There is no significant distinction

ANSWER: **A.**   This frequency sequence is thought to reflect the fact that EEG activity in NREM is highly synchronized, as is seizure activity, but REM has the least synchronized EEG activity.   (ATLAS2, p 195)

11. A 4-year-old girl has a history of nighttime gagging and choking spells for the past 2 years. Because of concern about possible sleep apnea, she has had an adenoidectomy. She also had treatment for esophageal reflux, but the nighttime events continued. Some episodes of tongue biting during the night have also been reported. What should the next step be?
   A. PSG to check for residual sleep apnea
   B. PSG to check for nocturnal seizures (full EEG montage)
   C. Full night video in the child's home to check for seizure activity
   D. Barium swallow

ANSWER: **B.**   Nocturnal seizures can be present without overt generalized tonic-clonic activity. When ordering a PSG in which nocturnal seizures are a possibility, a full EEG montage should be arranged. Such a study was done on this girl, and it revealed electrical seizures without accompanying motor movement (Fig. E5–5). She was treated with carbamazepine with complete relief of the nocturnal choking episodes.

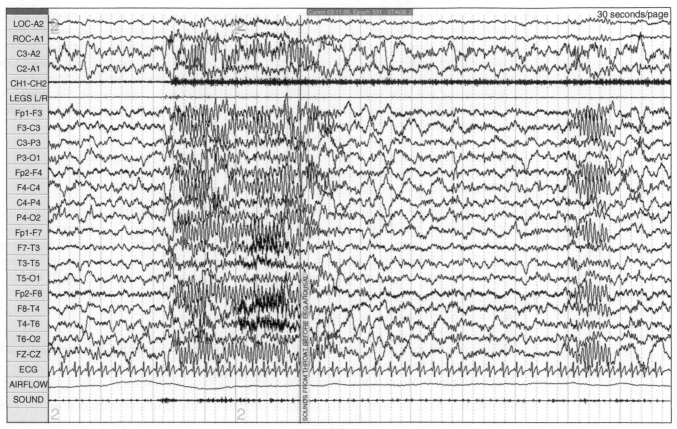

FIGURE E5–5

12. All of the following are correct about enuresis *except*
  A. It can occur during NREM or REM sleep
  B. The sleep of enuretic children is normal
  C. It is confined to children and adolescents and disappears by age 18 years unless a specific urologic problem exists
  D. Enuretic children have no more behavioral or psychological problems than nonenuretic children

ANSWER: **C.**   Enuresis is classified in the category of "other parasomnia" and is in fact more prevalent in adolescence and adulthood than is generally appreciated, occurring in 2.1% of community-dwelling older adults.   (ICSD3, pp 270-275)

13. Homicidal somnambulism, also called *sleep murder*, is a
  A. Form of REM behavior disorder
  B. Phenomenon first described as a side effect from certain hypnotic medications
  C. Successful legal defense when zolpidem is the cause
  D. True parasomnia

ANSWER: **D.**   Homicidal somnambulism occurs during sleepwalking and is thus a parasomnia. The first recorded case was in 1864, long before the use of hypnotics.   (Bonkalo A: Impulsive acts and confusional states during incomplete arousal from sleep: criminological and forensic implications, *Psychiatr Q.* 48:400-409, 1974) The defense in court against a murder charge has been on the order of "The defendant was not in his normal state of mind when he committed the act. Sleepwalking is a parasomnia manifested by automatism; as such, harmful actions committed while in this state cannot be blamed on the perpetrator." This argument has been successful at times. At least two well-known trials for murder while sleepwalking have ended in acquittal.   (Martin L: Can sleepwalking be a murder defense? Available at http://www.lakesidepress.com/pulmonary/Sleep/sleep-murder.htm)

14. A 19-year-old college student consults you because of two episodes about 3 months apart, during which she felt paralyzed during sleep. She described being aware of her surroundings but unable to move even her fingers or to speak. She felt as if she were about to suffocate. Only with great effort, after several minutes, was she "able to break the spell and move." On one of the two occasions, she thought someone else was in the room. She felt fine after each occasion and was able to fall asleep without another episode the same night. She does not drink alcohol and has no significant medical history. She denies having excessive daytime sleepiness (EDS). At this point you would
A. Schedule her for an overnight PSG
B. Schedule an overnight PSG to be followed by a multiple sleep latency test (MSLT)
C. Give a trial of clonazepam, 0.5 mg at bedtime
D. Reassure the patient that this is a normal phenomenon

ANSWER: **D.**   Sleep paralysis is a common REM-related parasomnia that may occur in completely healthy individuals. Absent a concern about narcolepsy or a significant comorbid condition (depression, alcoholism), nothing more needs to be done. No specific treatment is available, although improvement in frequency may be seen with improvement in sleep hygiene if warranted. Reassurance is a key aspect of management.   (ICSD3, pp 254-256)

15. All are true about sleep paralysis *except*
A. It represents persistence of REM atonia into wakefulness
B. It is more common in the setting of excessive sleep time
C. It is one of the classic tetrad of narcolepsy symptoms, along with EDS, cataplexy, and hypnagogic hallucinations
D. In cultural folklore, it was referred to as the "old hag" phenomenon

ANSWER: **B.**   Sleep paralysis is actually more common in the setting of sleep deprivation and supine positioning. The old hag phenomenon came from the belief of people with the condition that a witch, or an old hag, sits or "rides" the chest of the victims, rendering them immobile. Many works of art show this phenomenon, the most famous of which is Henry Fuseli's *Nightmare*, in which an incubus sits on the chest of a young woman, paralyzing her during sleep.   (ATLAS2, p 7) Note that the original meaning of the word *nightmare* referred to a combination of sleep paralysis and hypnagogic hallucinations occurring at sleep onset (Fig. E5–6).

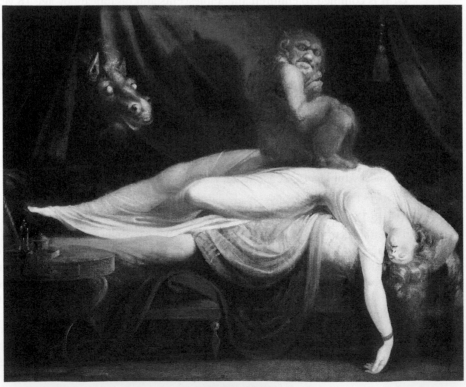

FIGURE E5–6

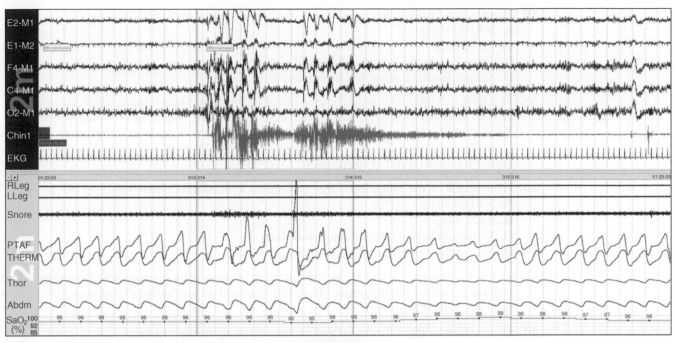

FIGURE E5–7

16. A patient had an overnight PSG with the following finding during an episode of REM sleep (Fig. E5–7). What is the diagnosis?
   A. REM sleep without atonia
   B. Bruxism
   C. Seizures
   D. Movement artifact

ANSWER: **B.**   This patient had complained of severe insomnia. This 2-minute epoch begins in REM sleep (see Fig. E5–7). An abrupt increase in chin EMG occurs with transmitted artifact seen in the EEG and electrooculogram (EOG). These findings are characteristic of sleep bruxism. On digital video, the characteristic chattering noise made by the upper and lower teeth striking against each other was audible. Bruxism is classified either as a sleep-related movement disorder   (ICSD3, p 303) or as a parasomnia.   (ATLAS2, pp 188-189) If indicated, treatment is usually with some type of mouth guard worn during sleep.

17. All of the following distinguish nightmares from sleep terrors *except*
   A. Whereas patients with nightmares typically recall the dream, amnesia is more common in patients with sleep terrors
   B. Whereas arousal from sleep terror is associated with confusion, arousal from nightmare is not
   C. Whereas sleep terrors tend to arise from slow-wave sleep, nightmares tend to arise from REM sleep
   D. In contrast to nightmares, sleep terrors are a common symptom of PTSD

ANSWER: **D.**   Nightmares, an REM parasomnia (but not sleep terrors, an NREM parasomnia), are a common symptom of PSTD. The nightmares are often recurrent, and their content reflects the traumatic event in PTSD. The nightmares in PTSD are disturbing to the patient.   (ICSD3, pp 230, 257)

18. From which of the following do confusional arousals occur?
   A. NREM sleep
   B. REM sleep
   C. Transition between wakefulness and sleep
   D. No predominant stage has been identified

ANSWER: **A.**   Confusional arousals, including sleep terrors and sleepwalking, classically occur in NREM sleep.   (ICSD3, p 229)

19. From which of the following stages of sleep do nightmares occur?
   A. NREM sleep
   B. REM sleep
   C. Transition between wakefulness and sleep
   D. No predominant stage has been identified

ANSWER: **B.**   Nightmares typically arise out of REM sleep. Sleep terrors, which are not nightmares, occur out of NREM sleep. The ICSD3 notes that "nightmares arising either immediately following trauma [acute stress disorder] or one month or more after a trauma [posttraumatic stress disorder] can occur during NREM sleep, especially stage 2, as well as during REM sleep and at sleep onset."   (ICSD3, p 257)

20. From which of the following stages of sleep do sleep starts (hypnic jerks) occur?
   A. NREM sleep
   B. REM sleep
   C. Transition between wakefulness and sleep
   D. No predominant stage has been identified

ANSWER: **C.**   Sleep starts, or *hypnic jerks*, occur in the transition between wakefulness and sleep and are a normal phenomenon. They are classified as an "isolated symptom and normal variant."   (ICSD3, p 335)

21. From which of the following stages of sleep do sleep terrors occur?
   A. NREM sleep
   B. REM sleep
   C. Transition between wakefulness and sleep
   D. No predominant stage has been identified

ANSWER: **A.**   A sleep terror typically begins after an arousal from SWS, most commonly toward the end of the first or second episode of SWS.   (ICSD3, p 230)

22. From which of the following types of sleep does sleepwalking occur?
   A. NREM sleep
   B. REM sleep
   C. Transition between wakefulness and sleep
   D. No predominant stage has been identified

ANSWER: **A.**   Sleepwalking, like a sleep terror, typically begins after an arousal from SWS, most commonly toward the end of the first or second episode of SWS.   (ICSD3, p 229)

23. From which of the following stages of sleep does the paralysis in sleep paralysis originate?
   A. NREM sleep
   B. REM sleep
   C. Transition between wakefulness and sleep
   D. No predominant stage has been identified

ANSWER: **B.**   Sleep paralysis is an intrusion of REM atonia into the awake stage and can be a normal phenomenon. It often occurs during the transition from sleep to wakefulness or from wakefulness to sleep. It is also common in patients with narcolepsy. The five classic symptoms for narcolepsy include (1) EDS, (2) cataplexy, (3) hypnagogic hallucinations, (4) sleep paralysis, and (5) sleep disruption; of the five, only cataplexy is pathognomonic of narcolepsy with hypocretin deficiency.   (ATLAS2, p 127, Fig. 8–13 and Ch 11.1, pp 159-174; ICSD3, p 254)

24. When do hypnagogic hallucinations typically occur? Pick the *best* answer.
   A. NREM sleep
   B. REM sleep
   C. In the transition between wakefulness and sleep
   D. No predominant stage has been identified

ANSWER: **C.**   Hypnagogic hallucinations occur because of the intrusion of REM sleep phenomena outside of REM sleep. They generally occur at sleep onset or offset, in the transition between wakefulness and NREM, and are a classic symptom of narcolepsy.   (ATLAS2, p 127)

25. A patient with the triad of nocturnal enuresis, somniloquy, and somnambulism *most* likely
   A. Has some form of narcolepsy
   B. Has a circadian rhythm disorder
   C. Has central sleep apnea
   D. Is between 5 and 15 years of age

ANSWER: **D.** This is a question in which the patient has three variations of parasomnia. The enuresis makes it likely it is a child.

26. Which is/are *true* regarding SRED?
   A. SRED is often associated with eating peculiar forms or combinations of foods
   B. Medication-induced SRED has been reported with zolpidem, triazolam, lithium carbonate, and anticholinergic medications
   C. Various health side effects are associated, including weight gain, diabetes mellitus, and situational depression
   D. SRED events are typically associated with confusional arousals from NREM sleep but can occasionally occur from REM sleep as well
   E. Answers A, B, and C are correct
   F. Answers A to D are correct

ANSWER: **F.** Answers A to D above describe the clinical features of SRED. (ICSD3, p 240)

27. A patient is referred because his bed partner was concerned that the patient was having upsetting nightmares. The patient moaned quite loudly at times during sleep. The patient undergoes a PSG, a fragment of which is shown in Figure E5–8. What diagnostic entity is shown in the fragment?
   A. RBD
   B. Seizures
   C. Catathrenia
   D. Central sleep apnea

ANSWER: **C.** This is catathrenia, although some features suggestive of the other entities are apparent. The fragment begins in REM (REMs are seen at the beginning), and the characteristic breathing pattern abnormality resembles central apnea. However, noises are also recorded in the snoring channel during what should have been a quiet period, arguing against central apneas. Also, there is no hypoxemia during the events. Catathrenia is classified as an "isolated symptom and normal variant" of breathing during sleep that most often, but not exclusively, occurs during REM sleep. (ATLAS2, pp 251-252; ICSD3, p 141)

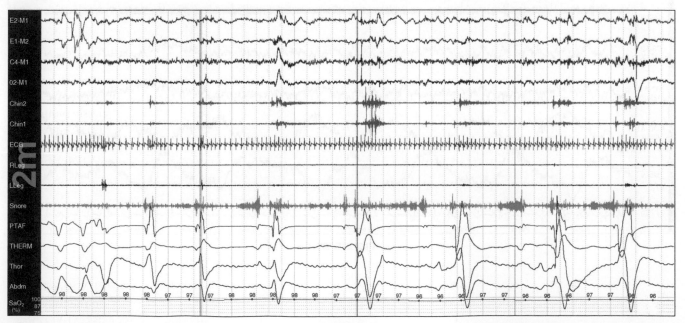

FIGURE E5–8

28. A 65-year-old man has just been diagnosed with RBD. The sleep physician told him to stop one of the drugs he is taking, believing it is likely causing the RBD. The drug is *most* likely
    A. Clonazepam
    B. Fluoxetine
    C. Oxycontin
    D. Eszopiclone

ANSWER: **B.**   Antidepressants have been implicated as a cause of RBD, principally drugs of the SSRI and SNRI class.   (Parish JM: Violent dreaming and antidepressant drugs: or how paroxetine made me dream that I was fighting Saddam Hussein, *J Clin Sleep Med.* 3:529-531, 2007; Schenck CH, Mahowald MW: REM sleep behavior disorder: clinical, developmental, and neuroscience perspectives 16 years after its formal identification in SLEEP, *Sleep.* 25:120-138, 2002) SSRI medications that have caused RBD include fluoxetine (Prozac) and paroxetine (Paxil). A commonly used SNRI that has also caused RBD is venlafaxine (Effexor). Clonazepam is often used to treat patients with RBD. Whereas incidents of confusion, hallucinations, and aggressive behavior may occur with opiates and Z drugs, RBD is not a noted problem.   (ATLAS2, p 221, Fig. 11.3–17)

29. Examine Figure E5–9. What drug is this patient *most* likely taking?
    A. Mirtazapine
    B. Clonazepam
    C. Fluoxetine
    D. Venlafaxine

ANSWER: **C.**   Prominent eye movements during NREM sleep are commonly seen in patients taking fluoxetine (sometimes called "Prozac eyes"). These can be rolling or rapid eye movements.   (Schenck CH, Mahowald MW, Kim SW, et al: Prominent eye movements during REM sleep and REM sleep behavior disorder associated with fluoxetine treatment of depression and obsessive-compulsive disorder, *Sleep.* 15:226-235, 1992) Although first described with fluoxetine, these NREM eye movements are now recognized with other drugs of the SSRI class.   (Geyer JD, Carney PR, Dillard SC, et al: Antidepressant medications, neuroleptics, and prominent eye movements during NREM sleep, *J Clin Neurophysiol.* 26:39-44, 2009) The manifestation may be a mild form of *serotonin syndrome*, which can cause myoclonic jerks, ocular oscillations, and other motor and autonomic signs.

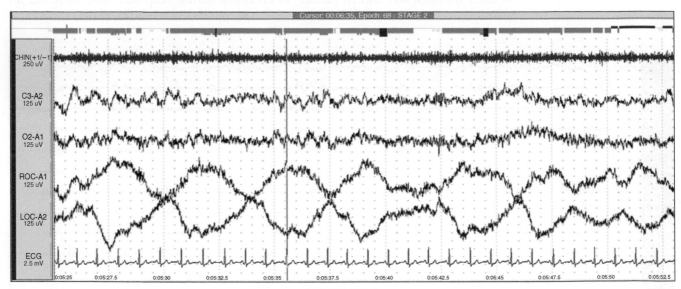

FIGURE E5–9

30. A 51-year-old woman in a nursing home rehab unit is recovering from hip surgery. She has a diagnosis of schizoaffective disorder. She has difficulty sleeping, with nocturnal agitation and a tendency to wander around the ward, responding to chronic auditory hallucinations. Which of the following drugs would you prescribe?
   A. Trazodone
   B. Gabapentin
   C. Clonazepam
   D. Quetiapine

ANSWER: **D.**   Sleep disorders in patients with psychosis are a common problem. Trazodone can be used for simple insomnia, but because psychotic features are present in this case, most clinicians would choose quetiapine (Seroquel), an antipsychotic. Clonazepam is sometimes used for RBD, and gabapentin is used for PLMS and restless legs syndrome.

31. Although such use is technically considered "off label," the one prescription drug that has been *most* used and is reportedly "90% effective" for RBD is
   A. Clonazepam
   B. Melatonin
   C. Pramipexole
   D. Clonidine

ANSWER: **A.**   Clonazepam at a dose of 0.25 to 1 mg before bedtime is effective in 90% of cases. Melatonin, an over-the-counter agent, can also be considered a low-risk, high-yield option.   (ATLAS2, p 220)

32. All of the following are true about sleepwalking in children *except*
   A. The eyes are usually open, but the child may appear confused or agitated
   B. It is more common in children than in adults, and it peaks between 4 and 8 years
   C. Untreated, it may lead to emotional problems in adolescence
   D. It usually begins as an arousal from SWS (stage N3)

ANSWER: **C.**   Sleepwalking is common and is not a sign of psychological problems. It rarely requires any treatment (apart from making the environment safe for the child), and it does not lead to emotional problems in later years.

33. All of the following are true about sleep enuresis *except*
   A. It is present in about 30% of 4-year-old children and in 1% to 2% of 18-year-old young adults
   B. In children of all ages, sleep enuresis is more common in boys than girls by a 3:2 ratio
   C. Secondary sleep enuresis is defined when a child starts bedwetting after being dry for at least 6 consecutive weeks
   D. Sleep enuresis, normal at a certain age, is defined as a problem if it persists beyond 5 years of age

ANSWER: **C.**   Sleep enuresis is considered secondary when the child (older than age 5 years) has been dry for at least 6 consecutive months and now has had enuresis for at least 3 weeks.   (ICSD3, p 270)

Movement Disorders

QUESTIONS

1. A 45-year-old woman with a medical history of severe depression that required hospitalization earlier this year, with comorbid anxiety and thyroid disease, complains of recent difficulty falling asleep because of uncomfortable crawling sensations in her legs. The sensation improves when she moves her legs around or gets up to walk. The sensations occur 4 to 5 nights per week and only after she gets into bed. In the morning, she notes that her sheets and covers are strewn about, and she often finds her pillow on the floor. Physical and neurologic examinations were unremarkable, other than a flat affect. Which of the following is the *most* likely diagnosis?

   A. Psychotic depression
   B. Sleep-related leg cramps
   C. Restless legs syndrome (RLS)
   D. Periodic limb movements during wakefulness
   E. Sleep-related rhythmic movement disorder

   ANSWER: **C.**   The patient presents with the four characteristic features of RLS, and the diagnosis is made on clinical grounds that include (1) uncomfortable or unpleasant sensations often described as "an urge" to move, (2) uncomfortable sensation or urge to move is relieved to some degree by movement, (3) uncomfortable sensation or urge to move occurs during periods of rest or inactivity, and (4) uncomfortable sensation or urge to move occurs more often in the evening or at night. This is unlikely to be sleep-related leg cramps, painful sensations associated with sudden muscle hardness or tightness indicative of a strong contraction. Leg cramps can occur during either wakefulness or sleep, although the description of the patient's symptom is not consistent with sleep-related cramping. Rhythmic movement disorder is characterized by repetitive, stereotyped motor behaviors that generally involve the large muscle groups and usually occur as the patient is transitioning into sleep. Types of rhythmic movement disorders include body rocking, head banging, and head rolling and are more common in children. Periodic limb movements during wakefulness are the motor expression of RLS characterized by periodic limb movements that occur during resting wakefulness. Finally, nothing is provided in the history to suggest psychotic depression.   (ICSD3, pp 282-291; Allen RP, Picchietti D, Hening WA, et al: Restless legs syndrome: diagnostic criteria, special considerations, and epidemiology. A report from the restless legs syndrome diagnosis and epidemiology workshop at the National Institutes of Health, *Sleep Med.* 4:101-119, 2003)

2. A 39-year-old man with a history of chronic loose bowels and abdominal cramps is referred with a 5-year history of sleep-onset insomnia and sleep-maintenance insomnia and restlessness involving his legs at bedtime. Which of the following should *not* be considered in helping determine the cause of the sleep symptoms?

A. Serum ferritin
B. Tissue transglutaminase (TTG) immunoglobulin A (IgA) antibody test
C. Total IgA level
D. Polysomnography
E. Gastrointestinal (GI) endoscopy

ANSWER: **D.** The polysomnogram (PSG) will not be of value in diagnosing this patient's movement disorder, nor will it reveal the cause. The diagnosis of RLS is a clinical one based on history. In terms of etiology, inflammatory bowel diseases (notably Crohn disease and celiac disease) have been associated with RLS. Either current or previous iron deficiency caused by malabsorption may be responsible. Ferritin is elevated in inflammation, and in this state, it may not be an accurate indicator of iron stores. Thus, the test is useful only when it is low, which confirms iron deficiency. Otherwise, examining red blood cell indices and even bone marrow iron may be needed. TTG, an enzyme released by inflamed cells in celiac disease, is elevated in patients with celiac disease. It can be falsely low in patients with genetically reduced IgA levels (who also have an increased incidence of RLS); thus total IgA is usually measured as well. GI endoscopy is useful in confirming inflammatory bowel disease. (Weinstock LB, Bosworth BP, Scherl EJ, et al: Crohn's disease is associated with restless legs syndrome, *Inflamm Bowel Dis.* 16(2):275-279, 2010; Weinstock LB, Walters AS, Mullin GE, Duntley SP: Celiac disease is associated with restless legs syndrome, *Dig Dis Sci.* 55:1667-1673, 2010)

3. A 21-year-old woman with a history of morbid obesity undergoes gastric bypass surgery. In the hospital, she has difficulty falling asleep and staying asleep and complains of an irresistible urge to want to move around before falling asleep. What medication used in the hospital may have led to these symptoms?

A. Morphine
B. Diazepam
C. Metoclopramide
D. Gabapentin
E. Trazodone

ANSWER: **C.** Drugs that antagonize dopamine function are noted to worsen the symptoms of RLS. Metoclopramide, frequently used as an antiemetic after abdominopelvic surgery, is a dopamine antagonist. Antipsychotic medications often have antidopaminergic properties and have also been associated with RLS. Nicotine, alcohol, caffeine, and diphenhydramine have also been noted to worsen RLS symptoms in some patients. Certain anticonvulsants, such as gabapentin and carbamazepine, have been used as therapeutic options for RLS. Carbamazepine has not been found to be useful in clinical practice, so it is not currently recommended for the treatment of patients with RLS. Opioids, more specifically methadone and oxycodone, have been studied for use in patients with RLS and are usually prescribed to patients with refractory or painful RLS and as an aid with nocturnal symptoms. Once the mainstay of RLS therapy, benzodiazepines are now used as an adjunct treatment, especially for patients with coexisting insomnia or augmentation due to dopamine agents. (Oertel WH, Trenkwalder C, Zucconi M, et al: State of the art in restless legs syndrome therapy: practice recommendations for treating restless legs syndrome, *Mov Disord.* 22[suppl 18]:S466-S475, 2007)

4. A patient with a history of heavy blood donation has developed RLS and was found to have iron deficiency. She was started on a regimen of therapeutic iron therapy (ferrous sulfate 325 mg three times a day). At 3-month follow-up, she continues to have these symptoms, they have become more severe, and they occur nightly. Her ferritin level was checked and is 20 ng/mL. What is the next step in therapy?

A. Initiate therapy with levodopa

B. Instruct the patient to have a drink of wine before falling asleep

C. Instruct the patient to walk a mile before going to bed

D. Recommend intravenous (IV) iron infusion

E. Initiate therapy with carbamazepine

ANSWER: **D.**   Treatment of iron deficiency anemia can completely resolve all RLS symptoms for a few patients. Studies of iron repletion and RLS symptom remission vary in outcome and recommendations. One double-blind placebo-controlled trial in 2009 demonstrated the benefits of oral iron therapy in 18 patients with low-normal ferritin RLS.   (Wang J, O'Reilly B, Venkataraman R, et al. Efficacy of oral iron in patients with restless legs syndrome and a low-normal ferritin: A randomized, double-blind, placebo-controlled study, *Sleep Med.* 10(9):973-975, 2009.) A recent study by Ondo (2010) using high-molecular-weight IV iron dextran demonstrated that 18 of 23 participants with refractory RLS had resolution (2), marked reduction (11), moderate reduction (2), and mild reduction (3) of RLS symptoms with this treatment. Low ferritin levels are correlated with higher augmentation rates while on levodopa therapy. Alcohol and vigorous exercise in the evening have been associated with worsening RLS symptoms. Carbamazepine has not been found to be clinically useful for RLS and is not currently recommended for the treatment of RLS.   (Frauscher B, Gschliesser V, Brandauer E, et al: The severity range of restless legs syndrome (RLS) and augmentation in a prospective patient cohort: association with ferritin levels, *Sleep Med.* 10:611-615, 2009; Ondo WG: Intravenous iron dextran for severe refractory restless legs syndrome, *Sleep Med.* 11:494-496, 2010; Wang J, O'Reilly B, Venkataraman R, et al: Efficacy of oral iron in patients with restless legs syndrome and a low-normal ferritin: a randomized, double-blind, placebo-controlled study, *Sleep Med.* 10:973-975, 2009)

5. A patient with RLS starts therapy with carbidopa–levodopa 25/100 mg; he takes 1 tablet at 10 PM and then wakes up at 4 AM with RLS symptoms and has been told by his wife that he looks like he is "running a marathon" in his sleep in the early morning hours. What clinical phenomenon does this represent?

A. Augmentation

B. Rebound

C. Withdrawal

D. Tolerance

E. Dose response

ANSWER: **B.**   Dopaminergic agents (e.g., pramipexole, ropinirole) and carbidopa–levodopa are often used to treat both RLS and periodic limb movements of sleep (PLMS). Once-nightly treatments with carbidopa–levodopa may result in morning end-of-dose rebound, and increases in leg movements are reported to occur in about one fourth of the patients. With rebound, the reappearance of symptoms is compatible with the timing of withdrawal from the medication. Augmentation is a worsening of RLS symptoms during treatment with a dopaminergic medication defined by the persistence or enhancement of symptoms related to dopamine therapy or the shifting of symptoms to a period of 2 to 4 hours earlier than is typical.   (Garcia-Borreguero D, Williams A: Dopaminergic augmentation of restless legs syndrome, *Sleep Med Rev.* 14;339-346, 2010)

6. A 63-year-old patient is started on ropinirole for RLS. What is the mechanism of action of this medication? (D indicates dopamine receptor.)
   A. D1 receptor agonist
   B. D1 receptor antagonist
   C. D3 receptor agonist
   D. D3 receptor antagonist
   E. Dopamine reuptake inhibitor

ANSWER: **C.**   Dopamine receptor agonists have become the treatment of choice for RLS. Pramipexole and ropinirole are both non–ergot derivative agonists with a high affinity for D3-type receptors. An older medication, pergolide, had its major affinity for the D2-type receptor. The latter had many more unwanted effects than the D3 agonists.   (Clemens S, Rye D, Hochman S: Restless legs syndrome: revisiting the dopamine hypothesis from the spinal cord perspective, *Neurology.* 67:125-130, 2006)

7. A 75-year-old man with RLS volunteers to have a specialized brain magnetic resonance imaging (MRI) that can determine localization of iron in the brain. This demonstrates a reduction of iron content in RLS patients compared with age-matched control participants in what region of the brain?
   A. Caudate
   B. Pons
   C. Substantia nigra (SN), pars reticulata
   D. SN, pars compacta
   E. Thalamus

ANSWER: **D.**   Autopsy analysis of the SN, pars compacta, tissue from patients with RLS compared with age-matched control participants without RLS has revealed a complex pattern of iron-related abnormalities. Iron, H-ferritin, and two primary iron transporters are reduced, and transferrin is notably increased. MRI for regional brain iron content also shows reduced brain iron in the SN of patients with RLS compared with age-matched control participants. The SN, pars reticulata, is a largely GABAergic subnucleus of the SN.   (Allen RP, Barker PB, Wehrl F, et al: MRI measurement of brain iron in patients with restless legs syndrome, *Neurology.* 56:263-265, 2001; Connor JR, Boyer PJ, Menzies SL, et al: Neuropathological examination suggests impaired brain iron acquisition in restless legs syndrome, *Neurology.* 61:304-309 2003; ATLAS2, p 180)

8. A 25-year-old man presents with complaints of bilateral temporalis region headaches, difficulty with jaw opening, and snoring. A PSG is performed, a representative fragment of which is presented in Figure E6–1. What is the cause for the rhythmic pattern seen on the tracing?
   A. Obstructive sleep apnea
   B. Periodic limb movements during sleep
   C. Sleep-related rhythmic movement disorder
   D. Muscle artifact
   E. Sleep-related bruxism

ANSWER: **E.**   Figure E6–1 shows rhythmic movement in the chin electromyogram (EMG) channel that is also prominent in the central electroencephalograph (EEG) and electrooculogram (EOG) leads. This is most consistent with the diagnosis of bruxism. The rhythmic movement is not snoring artifact because it does not align with the respiratory signals. Bruxism is a movement disorder characterized by grinding and clenching of the teeth during sleep. Bruxism becomes a pathologic condition when the patient presents with either abnormal wear on the teeth or nonrestorative sleep. It is estimated that approximately 15% of children and 5% of adults exhibit frequent bruxism that leads to a dental or sleep disorder. Patients can present with a variety of symptoms including oral or facial pain, headache, unpleasant oral sensations, limitation of jaw movements, and temporomandibular joint (TMJ) pain. The grinding can be loud enough to be bothersome to bed partners in some cases. Finally, some patients are identified only because of dental evaluations that show tooth wear. PSG features include either typical EMG phasic pattern with a frequency of 1 Hz lasting 0.25 to 2 seconds or sustained tonic activity, or both. Bruxism can be seen in rapid eye movement (REM) sleep but is most common in non–rapid eye movement (NREM) stages 1 and 2. If bruxism is suspected, masseter muscle EMGs should be included in the montage (not shown in the example). EEG is most often reported as continuous and not fragmented in the majority of patients, but frequent stage shifting to lighter stages have also been reported.   (ATLAS2, p 188)

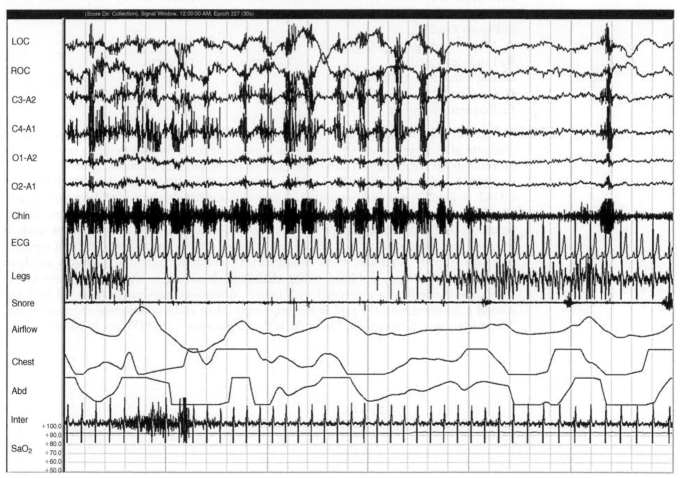

FIGURE E6–1

9. A patient evaluated in a sleep disorders clinic was diagnosed with sleep-related bruxism and primary snoring by overnight PSG. He tried bite guards on and off over the past few years but stopped using them because of repeated episodes of waking with the device out of his mouth. He asks to try a medication to reduce his nocturnal bruxing because of tooth damage and TMJ symptoms. What therapy listed below may help this patient?
   A. Haloperidol
   B. Lithium
   C. Fluoxetine
   D. Flecainide
   E. Clonazepam

ANSWER: **E.**   Clonazepam and methocarbamol are two medications that have been tested in an open study design for pharmacologic management of sleep-related bruxism. From clinical practice, centrally acting benzodiazepines and muscle relaxants have been shown to reduce bruxism-related motor activity. It is worth noting that selective serotonin reuptake inhibitors (SSRIs), antidopaminergic drugs, antipsychotic agents, calcium blockers, amphetamines, and antiarrhythmic drugs can cause secondary bruxism.   (ATLAS2, p 189; Saletu A, Parapaticus S, Saletu B, et al: On the pharmacology of sleep bruxism: placebo-controlled polysomnographic studies with clonazepam, *Neuropsychobiology*. 51:214-225, 2005)

10. A 14-year-old patient is referred to the sleep center by his primary care physician for evaluation of possible RLS. The history includes excessive movements during sleep. Which of the following *best* explains the findings in the leg EMG channel on the 30-second epoch shown in Figure E6–2?
    A. Electrocardiogram (ECG) artifact
    B. Limb-lead artifact
    C. Rhythmic movements
    D. Respiratory flow restriction
    E. Respiratory artifact

ANSWER: **C.**   The findings in the EMG channel are best explained as rhythmic movements. The rate of these events is 34/minute, which makes periodic limb movements unlikely. The movements do not align with either the ECG or the respiratory channels, making ECG and respiratory artifacts unlikely. Because the patient is awake (note the alpha rhythm in the C3-A2 channel), rhythmic movement of one or both legs is the most likely explanation. Rhythmic movement disorder is characterized by repetitive, stereotyped, rhythmic motor behaviors of major muscle groups that occur predominantly during drowsiness or sleep. It is most common in infants (up to 59%) and children (5% at 5 years) but has been reported in adults (usually continued from childhood). In children, common behaviors are head banging, body rocking, and head rolling. Although disturbing to the parents, these movements are generally not associated with injury. Movement rates range from 0.5 to 2 per second (consistent with the rate in the fragment). Most children outgrow the movements. There is no specific treatment for adults with the disorder.   (ICSD3, pp 312-316)

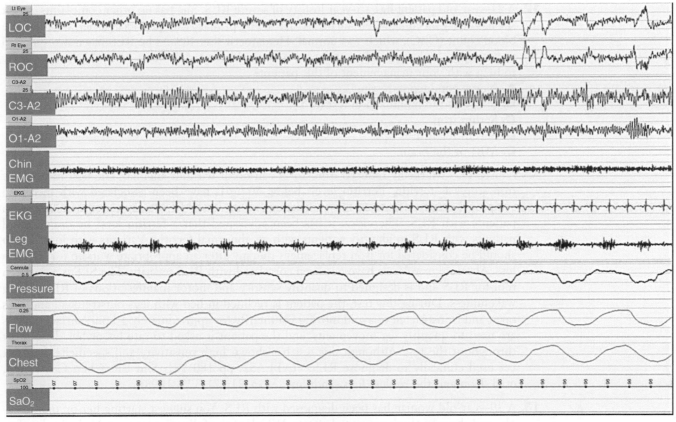

FIGURE E6–2

11. A 21-year-old woman with prior methamphetamine abuse, fibroids with heavy menstrual bleeding, and depression with previous suicide attempt presents with worsening insomnia over the past 5 years. She also has a history of restless legs symptoms since she was a child. She feels that her restless legs symptoms have been worsening over the past few years. Her bed partner reports snoring and violent jerking movements in her sleep. She is currently taking duloxetine 60 mg at bedtime and topiramate. As her sleep physician, what would you do next?

A. Start the patient on zolpidem
B. Start the patient on pramipexole
C. Switch the patient from duloxetine to bupropion
D. Discontinue topiramate
E. Increase the patient's duloxetine from 60 to 90 mg

ANSWER: **C.** Several drugs may induce or exacerbate RLS or PLMS. These include tricyclic or other antidepressants, lithium carbonate, and D2 receptor–blocking agents (neuroleptics). In this case, the patient's antidepressant may have worsened her RLS. Wellbutrin (bupropion) and trazodone are the only two antidepressants that demonstrate dopaminergic activity, so they do not exacerbate RLS and may actually help RLS symptoms. (Lee JJ, Erdos J, Wilkosz MF, et al: Bupropion as a possible treatment option for restless legs syndrome, *Ann Pharmacother.* 43:370-374, 2009)

12. A 21-year-old patient has a 5-year history of severe RLS. She has no other complaints except she has heavy bleeding when she menstruates. Her primary care physician ordered a complete blood count (CBC), which was normal. Hematocrit was 40%. The RLS has not responded to pramipexole therapy. The patient has a family history of diabetes. What test is *most* likely to help with your management of this patient?
    A. Nerve conduction testing
    B. Suggested immobilization test (SIT)
    C. Serum iron
    D. Serum ferritin
    E. MRI of the brain

ANSWER: **D.**   Markedly reduced iron stores can occur without anemia. The best measure of iron stores is ferritin. Ferritin levels below 50 μg/L have been associated with increased symptom severity, decreased sleep efficiency, and increased PLMS associated with arousal in patients with RLS. Therefore, it has been advocated that a ferritin level be drawn in all patients with RLS to identify patients with an abnormal ferritin. Patients with low ferritin should be considered for iron replacement therapy after an appropriate workup for the iron loss. Absolute iron levels have not been correlated with RLS severity. The SIT is a research tool for RLS and is designed to quantify sensory and motor manifestations of RLS during wakefulness. During this test, the patient is reclined in bed with legs outstretched and eyes open and is instructed to avoid moving voluntarily for approximately 1 hour; surface EMGs are used to quantify leg movements, and the patient is asked to rate his or her discomfort throughout the test. Although this test has shown high sensitivity and specificity, it is not yet used clinically to diagnose RLS.   (ATLAS2, pp 180-181; Sun ER, Chen CA, Ho G, et al: Iron and the restless legs syndrome, *Sleep.* 21:371-377, 1998)

13. A 39-year-old woman has been diagnosed with RLS. You suggest starting her on pramipexole, and she asks about unwanted effects. Which of the following is an established side effect of pramipexole when used for the treatment of RLS?
    A. Weight gain
    B. Nausea
    C. Arrhythmias
    D. Tardive dyskinesia
    E. Hypertension

ANSWER: **B.**   In a large, randomized, placebo-controlled trial of pramipexole in patients with RLS, drug-related adverse effects resulting in withdrawal of the study drug occurred in 12.4% of the pramipexole-treated group and in 7.0% of the placebo group. The two most common adverse events in which the frequency was higher in the pramipexole groups compared with placebo were nausea (19.0% vs. 4.7%) and somnolence (10.1% vs. 4.7%). Although somnolence was frequently noted as a side effect, it should be noted that the Epworth Sleepiness Scale (ESS) during the treatment period was not significantly higher in the pramipexole group compared with the placebo group. The risk of sleepiness with pramipexole, especially while driving, appears to be lower in patients with RLS than in patients with Parkinson disease, possibly because of differences in the dose and timing of medication. Abnormal behaviors, such as increased sexual desire and the urge to gamble, have been described as well.   (ATLAS2, Table 11–2.4; Comella CL: Restless legs syndrome: treatment with dopaminergic agents, *Neurology.* 58:87S-92S, 2002; Winkelman JW, Sethi KD, Kushida CA, et al: Efficacy and safety of pramipexole in restless legs syndrome, *Neurology.* 67:1034-1039, 2006)

14. An 11-year-old girl referred for evaluation of insomnia was found to have RLS. Early age of RLS onset is most often associated with which of the following?

A. Uremia

B. Anemia

C. Family history of RLS

D. Small-fiber neuropathy

E. Attention-deficit/hyperactivity disorder (ADHD)

ANSWER: **C.** The prevalence of RLS among first-degree relatives of people with RLS is about three to six times greater than those from the general population. In addition, more than 50% of idiopathic cases report a family history. In most studies, patients with a family history of RLS present at a younger age, before the age of 34 to 45 years, than patients without a family history. In most pedigrees, an autosomal-dominant pattern of inheritance is noted; however, recent genomic studies indicate that multiple genes are likely involved, which supports a pseudo-dominant pattern of inheritance. Uremia, anemia, and small-fiber neuropathy have been associated with secondary RLS. ADHD is highly correlated with RLS in children and suggests a common dopaminergic etiology. (ICSD3, p 284; Konofal E, Cortese S, Marchand M, et al: Impact of restless legs syndrome and iron deficiency on attention-deficit/hyperactivity disorder in children, *Sleep Med.* 8:711-715, 2007)

15. An 8-year-old child is referred with a history of body rocking during sleep diagnosed by the pediatrician, and the parents are concerned about the accuracy of the diagnosis. Which of the following is part of the diagnostic criteria for sleep-related rhythmic movement disorder?

A. Symptoms do not interfere with sleep

B. The movements are not stereotyped

C. The disorder does not impair daytime function

D. Behavior must also occur during the day

E. The movements involve large muscle groups

ANSWER: **E.** The diagnostic criteria for sleep-related movement disorder require the presence of repetitive, stereotyped, and rhythmic motor behaviors that involve large muscle groups and repeat roughly every 1 to 2 seconds during sleep or when the patient is drowsy. These movements may interfere with normal sleep, impair daytime function, or result in injury. (ICSD3, p 312)

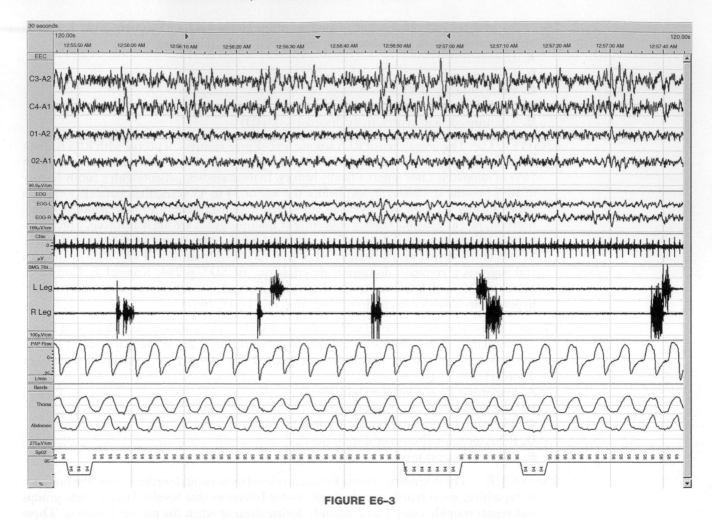

FIGURE E6–3

16. A patient with OSA is having a titration study. Which of the following is noted in the PSG findings in Figure E6–3?
    A. Sawtooth waves
    B. Continuous positive airway pressure (CPAP) overtitration
    C. PLMS
    D. Propriospinal myoclonus
    E. Alternating leg movements in sleep (ALMS)

ANSWER: **C.**   This compressed fragment shows five leg movements 0.5 to 5 seconds in length, which meets the criteria of periodicity (four or more consecutive movements with an inter-movement interval of 4 to 90 seconds). This is consistent with the diagnosis of PLMS, because we can see that the patient is asleep from the EEG data. Sawtooth waves are theta frequency EEG waveforms with a notched morphology that resembles the detailed tooth pattern of saw blades. They are usually seen during REM sleep, which is not noted in the above epoch. CPAP overtitration is unlikely because the positive airway pressure (PAP) flow signal is rounded and relatively constant without evidence of EEG arousal or oxyhemoglobin desaturation. Propriospinal myoclonus is depicted by brief myoclonic jerks seen on relaxed wakefulness and drowsiness, and it disappears on mental activation and sleep onset. This is not the case in the example here because the patient is asleep, and these movements demonstrate periodicity. Alternating leg movements in sleep can be counted when leg movements seen on two different legs occur more than 5 seconds apart with a minimum of four discrete and alternating bursts of leg muscle activity.   (ICSD3, pp 292-299; MANUAL2, Section VII, Movement Rules)

17. A 9-year-old girl is brought in with symptoms of "growing pains" that started 2 months ago and have worsened to the point that she has difficulty falling asleep and staying asleep. Her mother reports that she has always been an "active" sleeper and that when anyone sleeps with her, they remark on being kicked throughout the night. There is no history of snoring, parasomnias, or other sleep complaints. She takes a multivitamin and an antihistamine for seasonal allergies, but otherwise, no past medical conditions are reported. During the day, she is described as "high strung," and she often has difficulty with impulse control. Her pediatrician performed multiple serum tests that were all normal, including a full electrolyte panel; measurement of thyroid-stimulating hormone (TSH), vitamin B_{12}, and folate; and CBC with differential and platelet count. The child is afraid of spending the night in a laboratory, so you recommend a 3-night home test using ankle accelerometry to record leg movements. Figure E6–4 is representative of the findings from night 1. Figure E6–5 is representative of the findings from night 3. From the data, what is the *most* likely cause for the girl's "growing pains"?
  A. Rhythmic movement disorder
  B. Periodic limb movement disorder
  C. RLS
  D. ADHD
  E. Antihistamine use

ANSWER: **C.**   The patient meets the diagnostic criteria for pediatric RLS, given her history of disturbed sleep and actigraphy that demonstrates an elevated periodic limb movement index (PLMI). The symptom of "growing pains" has been found to be prevalent in patients with RLS. The diagnosis of RLS in children requires the same four criteria as in adults, but if the patient is unable to verbally express these symptoms, the condition can be diagnosed if two of the following are apparent: (1) sleep disturbance for age, (2) a biological parent or sibling with RLS, or (3) PSG that demonstrates a PLMI of 5 or more per hour. The number of periodic limb movements varies from night to night but is thought to be pathologic if greater than 5/hr in children and greater than 15/hr in adults. It is found to vary more in those with less severe sleep complaints. The events tend to cluster into episodes that may last several minutes to hours and usually occur during the first half of the night, but they can recur throughout the entire sleep period.   (MANUAL 2, Section VII, Movement Rules)

18. A 56-year-old woman has a 20-year history of RLS that has resulted in severe sleep-onset insomnia. Treatment with nonbenzodiazepine hypnotics (zolpidem, eszopiclone, and zaleplon) has been ineffective. She is started on pramipexole at bedtime and initially had an excellent response. After about 1 week, however, she complains that the insomnia and the RLS have returned, and the latter is more severe than ever. What describes this scenario?
  A. Rebound
  B. Tolerance
  C. Augmentation
  D. Paradoxic response

ANSWER: **C.**   The patient has augmentation, which results in worsening of the RLS symptoms in the evening. With rebound, the symptoms worsen in the morning as the drug effect wears off. *Tolerance* would refer to the medication losing effectiveness and a return of the pretreatment symptoms and severity of symptoms.   (Garcia-Borreguero D, Williams A: Dopaminergic augmentation of restless legs syndrome: the scope of the problem, *Sleep Med.* 12:425-426, 2011)

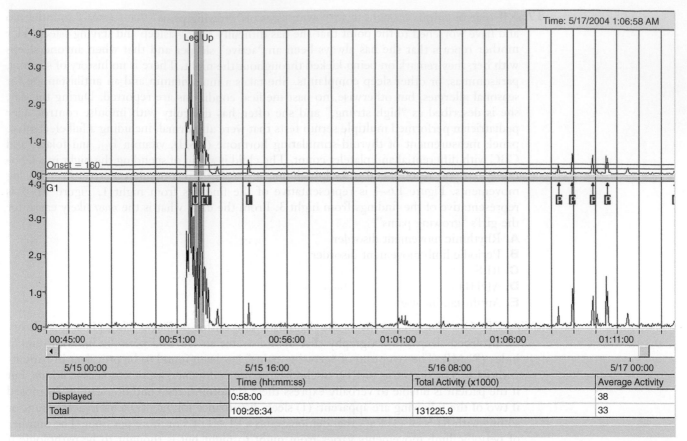

FIGURE E6–4

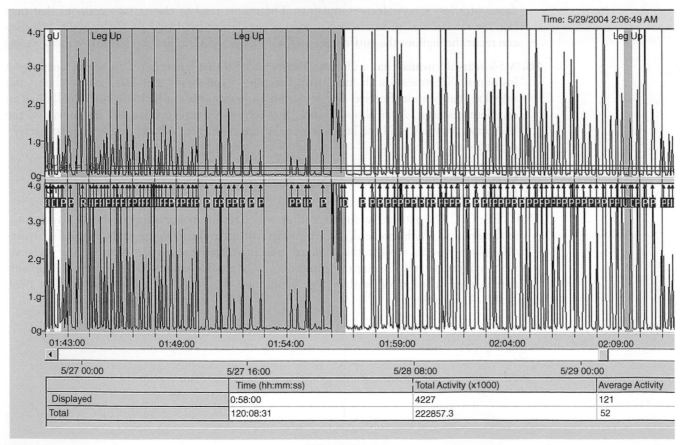

FIGURE E6–5

19. A 42-year-old woman has a 20-year history of RLS that began during her last pregnancy 6 years ago. She is started on levodopa–benserazide at bedtime and initially has an excellent response. After about 1 week, however, she complains that the RLS symptoms have returned, but the restlessness now occurs in the morning and during the daytime. Which of the following is the *best* option at this time?

A. Add an opiate medication at bedtime
B. Increase the nightly dosage of levodopa–benserazide
C. Combine levodopa with a dopamine agonist or benzodiazepine at bedtime
D. Discontinue levodopa–benserazide and replace with a dopamine agonist

ANSWER: **D.** The patient has rebounded. This results in return of the RLS symptoms but at the time medication is wearing off or during the daytime. Because the patient is having an unwanted effect of the medication, it is best to use another medication. (ATLAS2, p 190)

20. A 28-year-old man has a 6-year history of RLS, and both his parents have RLS. At the time of initial diagnosis 4 years previously, he was started on pramipexole. He initially had an excellent response, which continued for 4 years. However, the symptoms have slowly returned. Which of the following is the *best* option at this time?

A. Add an opiate medication at bedtime
B. Increase the nightly dosage of pramipexole
C. Stop pramipexole for 2 weeks, and then restart at a lower dose
D. Add gabapentin

ANSWER: **C.** The patient has developed tolerance to the medication. Often a 2-week drug holiday and restarting at a lower dose are effective in restoring efficacy of treatment. (ATLAS2, p 190)

21. A 48-year-old man, a general in the Air Force, has a 6-year history of severe nightly RLS. At the time of initial diagnosis 4 years previously, he was started on pramipexole. He had an excellent response, and the response has continued for 4 years. However, he states that he frequently has to take long flights as a passenger to air bases around the world, and he develops severe symptoms of motor restlessness when he has to sit. Which of the following is the *best* option at this time?

A. Add an opiate medication before takeoff
B. Add a small dose of pramipexole at takeoff
C. Stop pramipexole for 2 weeks, and then restart at a lower dose
D. Add gabapentin on the morning of the flight

ANSWER: **B.** Some patients with RLS, especially when they are sleep deprived, will have symptoms whenever they are resting or sitting still. Being a passenger in an automobile or airplane or sitting in the audience of an event can result in severe symptoms. Taking a small dose of a dopamine agonist before the onset of expected symptoms can be helpful. (ATLAS2, p 190)

22. A 68-year-old woman has a 40-year history of severe nightly RLS. She was started on pramipexole 5 years previously and had an excellent response, and the response has continued. The patient has been scheduled to have an MRI of her abdomen and refuses to have the test because she had a previous MRI attempt about 10 years before and "freaked out" when she developed distressing motor restlessness while in the machine. She requires the test for evaluation of a possible malignancy. What would you advise?

A. Take a short-acting nonbenzodiazepine hypnotic so she can sleep through the test
B. Add a small dose of pramipexole an hour before the test
C. Stop pramipexole for the 2 weeks before the test
D. Add gabapentin on the morning of the test

ANSWER: **B.** Some patients with RLS have symptoms whenever they are resting or sitting still. Having to lie still for 1 hour can be absolute torture for them. Taking a small dose of the dopaminergic agent before the expected symptoms can be helpful. Nonbenzodiazepine hypnotics have very little effect on RLS symptoms. (ATLAS2, p 190)

23. A 54-year-old man with a history of snoring, observed apnea, severe daytime sleepiness, and a body mass index of 40 is found to have sleep apnea. The apnea-hypopnea index (AHI) is 72 events/hr, and the total arousal index is 65 arousals/hr. The sleep study also showed severe PLMS with a PLMI of 85/hr. On CPAP titration, the apnea is well controlled (the AHI is 4, and the total arousal index is 8), but he continues to have PLMS with a PLMI of 70/hr. He is started on CPAP and pramipexole, and his sleepiness resolves entirely. On follow-up 3 months later, he mentions that his sleep symptoms have resolved but that he had a financial setback and could no longer afford the pramipexole. Since he was last seen, with his increased energy, he had been going to a local casino to gamble, and he was so far in debt that he had to sell his home. What do you advise?

    A. Order an equipment download to ensure that the apnea is well controlled

    B. Stop the pramipexole

    C. Switch him to a less expensive treatment such as generic carbidopa–levodopa

    D. Refer him to a psychiatrist to deal with his gambling addiction

ANSWER: **B.**   Dopamine agonists can result in compulsive or impulsive behaviors that include an addiction to gambling. In this case, the patient could have been started on PAP therapy and then reassessed the residual symptoms from the PLMS before starting a medication. The best course of action at this point is to stop the pramipexole.   (Cornelius JR, Tippmann-Peikert M, Slocumb NL, et al: Impulse control disorders with the use of dopaminergic agents in restless legs syndrome: a case-control study, *Sleep*. 33:81-87, 2010)

24. A 17-year-old girl has been referred for evaluation of severe RLS. She is quite thin but is otherwise healthy. It takes her hours to fall asleep because of severe motor restlessness at bedtime that is relieved temporarily by walking. She is not interested in using medications. Which of the following is *not* helpful in her management?

    A. Referral to a psychologist to treat her with cognitive behavioral therapy

    B. Family history

    C. Menstrual history

    D. Dietary history

    E. GI tract review of symptoms

ANSWER: **A.**   The cause of the probable RLS is not clear. The dietary history in this thin young woman may confirm that she is a vegetarian, and she may therefore be prone to be iron deficient or vitamin B_{12} deficient. The menstrual history may point toward heavy menstrual bleeding, leading to iron deficiency. Family history may point toward a familial cause of the RLS. A GI review of symptoms may point toward celiac disease or Crohn disease, both of which have been associated with RLS.   (ATLAS2, p 179)

25. Electrodes for recording EMG leg movements should be placed two on each leg. The recommended placement for each leg is

    A. Anterior tibialis muscle, 2 to 3 cm apart

    B. Anterior tibialis muscle, 6 to 10 inches apart

    C. Gluteus maximus, 5 to 8 inches apart

    D. One each on opposite sides of the kneecap

ANSWER: **A.**   According to the American Academy of Sleep Medicine, separate channels for each leg are "strongly preferred" because "combining electrodes from the two legs to give one recorded channel may work but could reduce the number of detected limb movements."

26. All of the following rules define a PLMS series *except*
  A. The minimum number of consecutive limb movement events is four
  B. The minimum period length between limb movements to include them as part of the PLMS series is 5 seconds
  C. The maximum period length between limb movements to include them as part of a PLMS series is 60 seconds
  D. Leg movements on two different legs separated by less than 5 seconds between movement onsets are counted as a single leg movement

ANSWER: **C.** According to the American Academy of Sleep Medicine, the maximum period between limb movements to include them in a PLMS series is 90 seconds.

27. The first letters of the four essential criteria for diagnosing RLS spell *URGE*. Which of the following is *not* the correct part of these criteria?
  A. Urge to move limbs
  B. Rest or inactivity precipitates or worsens symptoms
  C. Gastrocnemius pain or tingling
  D. Evening or nighttime appearance or worsening of symptoms

ANSWER: **C.** The *G* in the URGE acronym stands for *getting up* because moving improves the sensation. Although there may be pain or tingling, it is not confined to the gastrocnemius, and it can be any type of discomfort, including the urge to just move the legs. (ATLAS2, p 179)

28. Which of the following statements is *not* true concerning RLS and PLMS?
  A. RLS is diagnosed by history alone; PLMS is diagnosed by PSG alone
  B. PLMS is a subset of RLS; almost all patients with PLMS will also have symptoms suggesting RLS
  C. Patients with PLMS and RLS may respond to the same medications, such as low-dose dopamine agonists and benzodiazepines
  D. Both PLMS and RLS may be associated with restless sleep

ANSWER: **B.** RLS is diagnosed by history alone, and PLMS is diagnosed by PSG alone. About 80% of patients with RLS manifest PLMS, but only about 30% of patients with PLMS have RLS. Both groups may respond to the same medications, and both groups may have restless sleep as a result of leg movements: in RLS, at bedtime; in PLMS, during sleep. (ATLAS2, pp 178-179)

29. All of the following are true about pramipexole *except*
  A. It is a non–ergot dopamine agonist
  B. Dosage adjustment is not necessary in renal insufficiency
  C. It is approved by the US Food and Drug Administration (FDA) for treatment of Parkinson disease
  D. It is FDA approved for treatment of RLS

ANSWER: **B.** Dosage adjustment of pramipexole *is* necessary in patients with renal insufficiency. The other statements are true.

30. A 44-year-old man complains of sleepiness and snoring. He is being treated for severe neuropathic pain related to ankle trauma and takes gabapentin, morphine, eszopiclone, clonazepam, omeprazole, and venlafaxine. A fragment of his overnight sleep study is shown in Figure E6–6. What stage of sleep is shown in this epoch?
  A. W
  B. NI
  C. N3
  D. R

ANSWER: **A.** This 30-second epoch shows high-frequency EEG and slow eye movements, which are characteristic of stage W.

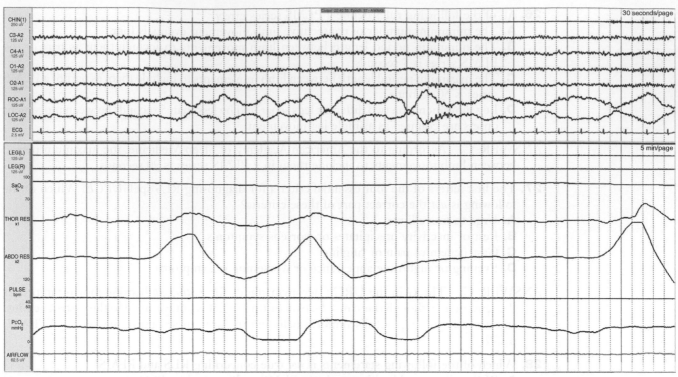

FIGURE E6–6

31. How would you interpret the respiratory abnormality shown in the epoch from Figure E6–6?
  A. It should not be interpreted in this epoch because the patient is awake
  B. It should be scored as central apneas, and it should be indicated that these are an abnormal finding
  C. It should be scored as central apneas, but it is not clinically significant
  D. The epoch shows what is likely voluntary breath holding, and the events should not be scored as central apneas

ANSWER: **B.** The events should be scored as central apneas and should definitely be considered abnormal. Central apneas during wakefulness can be found in patients with Cheyne-Stokes breathing, heart failure, and cerebrovascular disease. They are also seen in patients taking medications that depress breathing, principally opiates. Of all the medications he is taking, the culprit is likely morphine. Opiates are well known to cause central sleep apnea. They blunt the drive to breathe and can actually lead to respiratory acidosis in some cases. (Mogri M, Desai H, Webster L, et al: Hypoxemia in patients on chronic opiate therapy with and without sleep apnea, *Sleep Breath.* 13:49-57, 2009) Note that in 30 seconds, this patient took only three breaths. Patients who manifest central apnea while awake almost always also have central apnea during sleep.

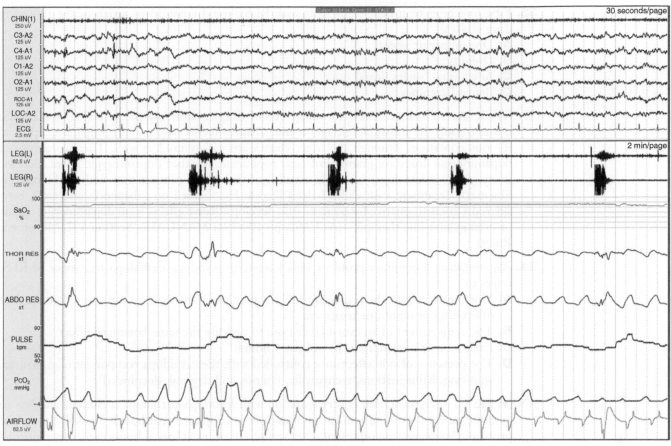

FIGURE E6–7

32. What drug would likely worsen the EMG finding seen in the fragment in Figure E6–7?
A. Pramipexole
B. Metoclopramide
C. Oxycodone
D. Clonazepam

ANSWER: **B.** Figure E6–7 shows PLMS. Metoclopramide is a dopamine antagonist, and it can worsen PLMS. Pramipexole, oxycodone, and clonazepam may be used to treat PLMS. Drugs that can worsen both PLMS and RLS include

○ SSRI antidepressants (mainly worsen PLMS)
○ Tricyclic antidepressants
○ Lithium
○ Dopamine receptor antagonists (e.g., metoclopramide and prochlorperazine, often used as antiemetics)
○ Nicotine
○ Alcohol
○ Caffeine
○ Diphenhydramine

33. First-line drug treatment of patients with RLS should come from which of the following drug classes?
   A. Dopaminergic agents
   B. Opioids
   C. Any alpha-2-delta ligand drug
   D. Benzodiazepines

ANSWER: **A.**   These are the four categories of drugs commonly prescribed to treat RLS; however, only the dopaminergic agents and gabapentin enacarbil are currently FDA approved for this condition, although the other classes are widely used as well. The two approved dopaminergic drugs are pramipexole and ropinirole. Another dopaminergic agent used for many years is levodopa, which is usually prescribed in combination with carbidopa (as Sinemet). Treatment with alpha-2-delta ligands has focused on gabapentin enacarbil, considered a good alternative for patients who develop adverse effects from dopaminergic agents or even as first-line therapy.   (ATLAS2, pp 190-191; MANUAL2, Section VII, Movement Rules)

34. *Augmentation*, a common problem with long-term levodopa–carbidopa treatment of RLS, refers to
   A. Morning rebound, the presence of RLS symptoms that occur de novo as a consequence of evening or nighttime treatment
   B. The requirement of an ever-higher dose to provide the same beneficial effect
   C. Earlier onset of symptoms by at least 4 hours
   D. The presence of side effects not controlled with the carbidopa component (e.g., nausea, vomiting, hallucinations, tachycardia, fatigue, and daytime sleepiness)

ANSWER: **C.**   Augmentation is very common with levodopa–carbidopa treatment and less so with the newer dopamine agonists pramipexole and ropinirole, although it is still a potential problem. Augmentation is present when symptoms occur at least 4 hours earlier than normal plus a shorter latency to symptom onset when at rest, extension of symptoms to other parts of the body, a greater intensity of symptoms, and shorter duration of relief with treatment.

Your New Sleep Technologist

Your trusted sleep tech who has worked with you for 10 years is moving and therefore has resigned. You begin to look for a "seasoned" replacement and decide to include a few scoring exercises and questions as part of the evaluation and qualification process. You provide the job candidate a PSG record that you know includes periodic limb movements.

35. During minutes 200 and 205, there are what appear to be 10 limb movements indicated by an increase in EMG amplitude of 4 μV over baseline, 8 with an increase of 2.5 μV, 12 with an increase of 6 μV, and 16 with an increase of 9 μV. How many limb movements should be scored as "significant"?
   A. 4
   B. 8
   C. 12
   D. 16

ANSWER: **D.**   The minimum amplitude of a limb movement event is an 8-μV increase in EMG voltage above resting EMG.

36. The *minimum* duration of a limb movement event is
   A. 0.05 second
   B. 0.25 second
   C. 0.5 second
   D. 1 second

ANSWER: **C.**   The minimum duration of a limb movement event is 0.5 second.

37. The next 5-minute PSG segment has what appears to be 25 limb movements, although 8 of these have a duration of 12 seconds, 5 have a duration of 15 seconds, and the rest have a duration of 8 seconds. By the 2017 American Academy of Sleep Medicine scoring criteria, how many limb movements should be counted?
   A. 0
   B. 8
   C. 13
   D. 18

ANSWER: **C.** The maximum duration of a limb movement event is 10 seconds.

38. On epochs 100 through 150, a set of 8 periodic limb movements is separated by 4 seconds, a set 2 minutes later of 10 is separated by 10 seconds, and another set 5 minutes later of 8 is separated by 20 seconds. How many PLMS series should be scored?
   A. None
   B. One
   C. Two
   D. Three

ANSWER: **C.** The minimum number of consecutive limb-movement events needed to define a PLMS series is four limb movements. (MANUAL2, Section VII, Movement Rules)

Breathing Disorders

QUESTIONS

Questions 1 through 3 refer to the following scenario:

A patient with Prader-Willi syndrome has a long history of snoring, racing thoughts during periods of sleep disruption, unrefreshing sleep, and occasional bedwetting. His body mass index (BMI) is 43. The following two questions are based on the oximetry channel from an overnight polysomnogram (PSG) (Fig. E7–1).

1. What is the *likeliest* cause of the drops in SaO$_2$?
   A. Position changes
   B. Entry into slow-wave sleep
   C. Loss of tone of muscles that helps maintain upper airway patency
   D. Cheyne-Stokes breathing (CSB) when a patient with heart failure goes into rapid eye movement (REM) sleep

ANSWER: **C.** The timing of the drops in SaO$_2$ is highly regular, first starting at 90 minutes, and is thus likely related to REM sleep. REM-related atonia affecting the upper airways is responsible for the worsening of upper airway obstruction in this obese patient. The pattern is too regular to be explained by change in position. Slow-wave sleep does not occur the entire night and is clustered in the first third of the night. CSB in congestive heart failure (CHF) often disappears during REM sleep. Immediately below are the sleep stage data (Fig. E7–2) added to the above oximetry data.

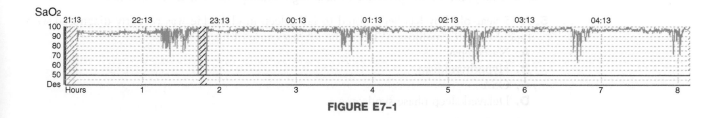

FIGURE E7–1

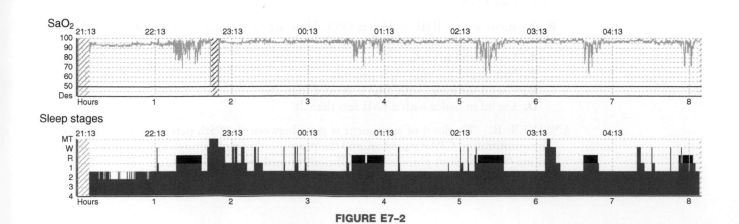

FIGURE E7–2

2. This sleepy patient also has symptoms of depression, and there is consideration of using an antidepressant with alerting properties. Which antidepressant has these features?
A. Amitriptyline
B. Protriptyline
C. Pemoline
D. Imipramine

ANSWER: **B.**   Protriptyline is an antidepressant that has alerting properties, and it has been shown to improve apnea index in patients with OSA by reducing REM sleep. Amitriptyline and imipramine are highly sedating antidepressants. Pemoline is a stimulant that is no longer available because of liver toxicity.

3. If this patient were started on protriptyline for depression, what changes would you expect?
A. Reduction in REM with a change in apnea index
B. Worsening of enuresis
C. Diarrhea
D. Earlier onset on REM but fewer but longer episodes of REM

ANSWER: **A.**   Protriptyline has been evaluated in the treatment of OSA and was used extensively before continuous positive airway pressure (CPAP) was introduced. It is a powerful REM-suppressing agent, and it was felt that its positive effect on sleep-disordered breathing (SDB) was related to REM suppression. It had strong anticholinergic side effects that led to constipation and urinary retention.

4. A patient with abnormal liver enzymes is referred for evaluation of daytime sleepiness. What sleep disorder is *most* likely?
A. Secondary narcolepsy
B. Periodic limb movements in sleep
C. Insomnia
D. OSA

ANSWER: **D.**   About half of patients with nonalcoholic fatty liver disease (NAFLD, also called *nonalcoholic steatohepatitis* [NASH]) have features of sleep apnea.   (Singh et al, 2005) Research in animals indicates that chronic intermittent hypoxia predisposes to liver injury.   (Savransky et al, 2007) The presence of sleep apnea is predictive for the development of NAFLD   (Campos et al, 2008) and for the presence of histologic findings of NAFLD.   (Mishra et al, 2008)

5. A 15-year-old boy has been noted to fall asleep in class. He was recently diagnosed with type 2 diabetes mellitus. What is the *likeliest* cause of his sleepiness?
A. Narcolepsy
B. Hypothyroidism
C. OSA
D. Delayed sleep phase syndrome

ANSWER: **C.**   Although all the choices may cause sleepiness in a teenager, the correct answer is OSA. Obesity is the main cause of type 2 diabetes and is also the most important risk factor for OSA.

6. A patient with a BMI of 34 has OSA. How useful are predictive equations to determine what CPAP pressure will be needed for treatment?
A. Very useful in male patients
B. Not useful for individual patients
C. Useful for males with a BMI greater than 28
D. Useful in males with a BMI less than 28

ANSWER: **B.**   The level of agreement is poor between the 95th percentile pressure obtained by autotitrating CPAP machines and the pressure obtained through various predictive equations (the intraclass correlation coefficient ranged from 0.17 to 0.32).   (Torre-Bouscoulet et al, 2009)

7. Polycystic ovary syndrome (PCOS) is a cause of which sleep disorder?
   A. Insomnia
   B. Sleep apnea
   C. Restless legs syndrome (RLS)
   D. Delayed sleep phase syndrome

ANSWER: **B.**   PCOS is associated with excess production of androgen hormone, which can lead to hirsutism, acne, insulin resistance, hypertension, and anovulation. Sleep apnea is found in 20% to 40% of women with PCOS.   (ATLAS2, p 354)

8. What is the *most* common cause of SDB in children?
   A. Enlarged adenoids and tonsils
   B. Obesity
   C. Retrognathia
   D. Congenital malformations

ANSWER: **A.**   The most common cause of SDB in children is enlarged tonsils and adenoids. In the past few years, however, there has been an increase in the number of cases related to obesity.   (ATLAS2, pp 299–300)

9. In performing sleep studies in children, which procedure is apt to be *least* helpful?
   A. Synchronized digital video
   B. End-tidal PcO_2 measurement
   C. Actigraphy
   D. Oxygen saturation

ANSWER: **C.**   Actigraphy adds little to the evaluation of sleep studies in children. The other choices can provide important information in the diagnosis of breathing and other sleep disorders.

10. Which statement about the association of systemic hypertension and OSA is *true*?
   A. OSA has only been associated with hypertension in obese people
   B. OSA has only been associated with hypertension in people with diabetes
   C. OSA is an independent risk factor for hypertension
   D. OSA is uncommon in treatment-resistant hypertension

ANSWER: **C.**   OSA is a risk factor for development of hypertension independent of BMI. Also, OSA has a high prevalence in patients with treatment-resistant systemic hypertension. Apnea severity, reduced sleep efficiency, and reduced time in REM sleep all correlate with treatment-resistant hypertension.   (Friedman et al, 2010)

11. Which cardiac rhythm abnormality has *not* been described in OSA syndrome (OSAS)?
   A. Atrial fibrillation (AF)
   B. Premature ventricular contractions
   C. Premature atrial contractions
   D. Wolff-Parkinson-White syndrome

ANSWER: **D.**   The first three arrhythmias are associated with OSAS.

12. Which statement about nocturnal angina pectoris is *true*?
   A. It has been linked to OSA
   B. It is a known complication of hypnotic medications
   C. An overnight sleep study is seldom of value in this population
   D. It is most often caused by gastroesophageal reflux

ANSWER: **A.**   In one study, 90% of patients with nocturnal angina pectoris had SDB; therefore, an overnight sleep study is indicated in all patients with nocturnal angina pectoris.   (Franklin et al, 1995)

13. REM-predominant OSA is independently associated with
   A. Daytime sleepiness
   B. Impaired health-related quality of life
   C. Self-reported sleep disruption
   D. None of the above

ANSWER: **D.**   REM-related OSA is mostly seen in women and younger patients. Studies suggest that REM-related OSA does not need treatment with CPAP and that only obstructive events during non-REM (NREM) sleep are associated with excessive daytime sleepiness (EDS) or impaired quality of life. Thus, a patient who complains of EDS but whose sleep study shows only REM-related OSA likely has another cause for the EDS (e.g., insufficient total sleep per 24 hours, medication side effects). However, some caveats apply, especially given that a single-night sleep study may not reflect the patient's regular at-home sleep pattern. In the final analysis, it must be a matter of clinical judgment about whom to treat with CPAP.   (Chami et al, 2010; Ganguly, 2012; Mokhlesi and Punjabi, 2012; Mokhlesi et al, 2014)

Questions 14 through 19 refer to the following case:

A 70-year-old obese woman (BMI = 34) with a history of snoring and sleepiness is referred for a split-night study. On arrival to the sleep lab, she is using nasal oxygen at 3 L/min. She has severe emphysema and has been on supplemental 24-hours-a-day oxygen for several years. The sleep technician notes that the patient's SaO_2 is 90% on oxygen. Without the O_2, her SaO_2 falls to 87%.

14. The technician is unsure what to do and phones to ask if the sleep study should proceed. What should you recommend?
   A. Send the patient home until more information is available
   B. Start the split-night study but without the supplemental O_2
   C. Start the split-night study with the patient using O_2 at 3 L/min
   D. Perform an all-night diagnostic study without the supplemental O_2

ANSWER: **C.**   The important information is that her SaO_2 is only 90% with O_2 at 3 L/min, and it drops to 87% on room air. For safety, the patient should be tested while using oxygen. Thus, answers B and D are incorrect. Answer A is incorrect because additional information is not likely to help in decision making.

15. The study commences while she is using O_2 at 3 L/min. At 4.5 hours into the study, the patient is started on CPAP therapy with 3 L/min O_2 added to the circuit. A four-channel summary is shown below (Fig. E7–3). In regard to CPAP initiation in this patient, what is the *best* answer?
   A. She should have been started on CPAP after 2 hours
   B. She should have been started on ASV at 4.5 hours
   C. She should have been started on bilevel positive-pressure therapy at 4.5 hours into the study
   D. Starting her on CPAP at 4.5 hours was correct

ANSWER: **D.**   Although it is often best to start CPAP after REM has been achieved, some patients do not achieve REM for a variety of reasons. Answer A is incorrect because she was awake the first 2 hours. Answer B is incorrect because there is no indication for ASV here, and the ASV may have induced further hypoventilation. Answer C is incorrect because in a patient with obstructive apnea, the first treatment is CPAP, not bilevel pressure. If CPAP is ineffective, then bilevel or other forms of ventilator assistance can be tried. Answer D is thus the best answer.

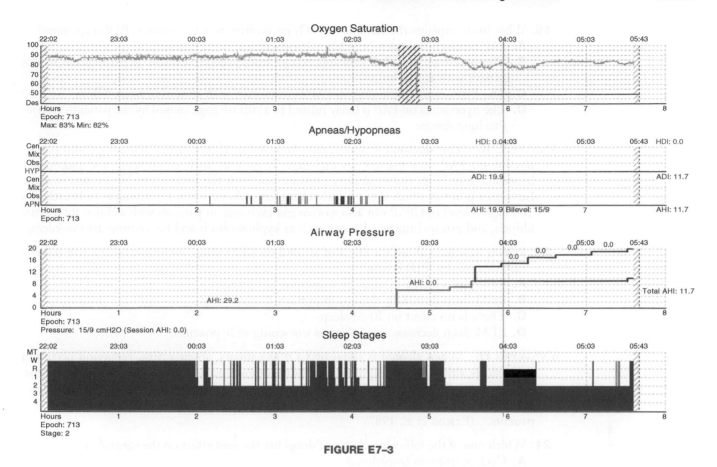

FIGURE E7–3

16. What positive-pressure airway treatment did the patient receive during the titration portion of the study?
  A. CPAP followed by bilevel pressure
  B. Bilevel pressure followed by CPAP
  C. CPAP the entire time
  D. Bilevel pressure the entire time

ANSWER: **A.**   The patient was on CPAP (a single pressure is indicated) followed by bilevel positive pressure (two pressures are indicated).

17. Which statement *best* describes how the patient did on CPAP?
  A. She fell asleep in seconds after starting CPAP
  B. Her apneas continued on CPAP
  C. Her hypoxemia initially worsened on the CPAP (compared with baseline)
  D. She did well on CPAP because the apneas were abolished

ANSWER: **C.**   Clearly, the SaO₂ decreased on CPAP even though the apneas were effectively treated. Thus, apneas were not the cause of her hypoxemia.

18. Which statement *best* describes the situation during the last 2 hours of the study?
  A. The positive-pressure treatment was successful because REM sleep was obtained
  B. The patient's apneas continued
  C. Her hypoxemia remained at an unacceptable level
  D. The patient did well because the apneas were abolished

ANSWER: **C.**   Her SaO₂ decreased on bilevel positive pressure, even though apneas were eliminated. Thus, apneas were not the cause of the hypoxemia. The patient's continued hypoxemia indicates the final settings used in the study were not optimal.

19. What likely explains the changes of SaO_2 on positive airway pressure (PAP) treatment?
  A. PAP resolved the sleep-breathing abnormalities
  B. The hypoxemia on PAP probably results from pressure causing hyperinflation in this patient with emphysema
  C. The hypoxemia continuing on PAP is consistent with comorbid heart failure
  D. The hypoxemia on PAP is likely related to a stiff rib cage caused by the patient's restrictive lung disease

ANSWER: **B.** This question assumes some knowledge of respiratory physiology and pathophysiology. PAP may worsen gas exchange in patients with emphysema and pulmonary hyperinflation. High end-expiratory pressure can push the patient up the pressure-volume curve to a point at which there is little change in volume when she attempts to breathe in. Too high a level of CPAP can also worsen gas exchange in patients with asthma, interstitial fibrosis, and extrapulmonary diseases such as kyphoscoliosis and neuromuscular disorders.

20. Which statement about the effect of alcohol on REM sleep in chronic obstructive pulmonary disease (COPD) is *true*?
  A. REM sleep increases, thereby worsening sleep apnea
  B. REM sleep decreases, thereby improving hypoxemia
  C. There is no effect on REM sleep
  D. REM sleep decreases, and there is worsening of hypoxemia

ANSWER: **D.** When alcohol is taken by COPD patients, about a 50% reduction occurs in REM sleep; although one might expect this to improve gas exchange, gas exchange worsens, and more profound hypoxemia occurs. In addition, the number of premature ventricular contractions increases. Thus, alcohol has very negative effects on sleep in COPD patients. (Easton et al, 1987)

21. Which one of the following classes of drugs has the *least* effect on the control of breathing?
  A. Cyclopyrrolones (zopiclone)
  B. Imidazopyridines (zolpidem)
  C. Pyrazolopyrimidines (zaleplon)
  D. Melatonin MT_1 MT_2 receptor agonist (ramelteon)

ANSWER: **D.** Melatonin receptor agonists have no known effect on the control of breathing. Clinical trials have shown that ramelteon (an MT_1 MT_2 receptor agonist) has no impact on breathing in patients with mild to moderate COPD or mild to moderate OSA. (Kryger et al, 2007, 2008, and 2009)

22. What *best* describes the effect of protriptyline on sleep in patients with OSA?
  A. REM sleep is increased and results in a worsening of sleep apnea
  B. REM sleep decreases, and sleep apnea is improved
  C. There is no effect on sleep architecture
  D. REM sleep decreases, and there is worsening of hypoxemia

ANSWER: **B.** Before the introduction of CPAP, there was interest in compounds that might increase upper airway tone. One such compound was the nonsedating tricyclic antidepressant protriptyline. This drug was found to cause substantial decrease in REM sleep and led to an overall reduction in the apnea-hypopnea index (AHI). (Brownell et al, 1982)

23. What was a major side effect when using protriptyline in sleep-breathing disorders?
  A. Hirsutism
  B. Gynecomastia
  C. Urinary retention
  D. Nasal obstruction

ANSWER: **C.** Principal side effects from protriptyline were urinary retention in patients with large prostate, sexual impotence, and constipation. These anticholinergic side effects led to the medication being seldom used. (Brownell et al, 1982)

24. Mirtazapine (Remeron) has been suggested as a medical treatment for OSAS. What is the suggested mechanism of action?
   A. Increased tone of upper airway muscles
   B. Decreased REM
   C. Increased arousal threshold
   D. Increased hypercapnic drive to breathe

ANSWER: **A.**   Mirtazapine is a tetracyclic piperazinoazepine that enhances both central noradrenergic and serotonergic activity; the drug blocks α_2 receptors and selectively antagonizes serotonin $5HT_2$ and $5HT_3$ receptors. It has been suggested that the loss of upper airway tone in apnea may be related to reduced serotonin activity.   (Marshall et al, 2008)

25. What important factor limits usefulness of mirtazapine in treating OSA?
   A. Cost
   B. Weight gain
   C. Development of polycythemia
   D. Renal failure

ANSWER: **B.**   Weight gain is a common side effect of mirtazapine, and it may actually worsen or cause sleep apnea. The main reason not to use mirtazapine, however, is its lack of efficacy.   (Marshall et al, 2008)

26. A depressed patient is started on mirtazapine to treat her comorbid insomnia. The insomnia worsens substantially within 5 days. What is the *likeliest* cause?
   A. Central apnea
   B. Obstructive apnea
   C. RLS
   D. Rhythmic movement disorder

ANSWER: **C.**   Mirtazapine is one of several antidepressants that can cause RLS. The drug can also cause akathisia. Note that bupropion has not been associated with RLS.   (Hoque et al, 2010)

27. Which statement about progesterone is *not* true?
   A. It is a centrally acting respiratory stimulant
   B. The effect appears to be related to increased chemical (hypoxic and hypercapnic) drive to breathe. CO_2 response
   C. It causes hyperventilation in pregnancy
   D. It may explain a higher prevalence of OSA in premenopausal versus postmenopausal women

ANSWER: **D.**   Progesterone, a female reproductive hormone, is a powerful centrally acting respiratory stimulant. Progesterone levels go up in pregnancy and lead to hyperventilation. Because progesterone levels are higher in premenopausal than in postmenopausal women, sleep apnea is much less common in the former group.

28. Which statement about the use of progesterone in obese patients is *true*?
   A. It decreases awake $PacO_2$ in obesity hypoventilation syndrome (OHS)
   B. It consistently decreases AHI in obstructive sleep apnea (OSA)
   C. Large clinical trials have shown no efficacy in using progesterone to treat sleep apnea in obese patients
   D. Progesterone is the treatment of choice in postmenopausal sleep apnea patients

ANSWER: **A.**   Early clinical trials showed that patients with OHS treated with progesterone had a reduction in PcO_2 during wakefulness. Good clinical trials have not been done to evaluate the effect of progesterone in OHS during sleep.   (Piper, 2010)

29. What statement about alcohol in patients with sleep-breathing disorders is *true*?
    A. It increases upper airway muscle tone
    B. It has no effect in nonapneic snorers
    C. It will improve the overall severity of sleep apnea because of its effect on reducing REM sleep
    D. It may result in acute hypercapnic respiratory failure

ANSWER: **D.**   Alcohol *decreases* the tone of upper airway muscles. Alcohol can definitely worsen sleep apnea even to the point of causing acute respiratory failure.   (Sampol et al, 2010)

30. A STOP-Bang score to identify patients with a high probability of moderate to severe OSA would be
    A. 0 to 2
    B. 3 to 4
    C. 9 to 12
    D. 13 to 16

ANSWER: **B.**   The STOP-Bang questionnaire is a scoring model that consists of eight easily administered yes-or-no questions that spell the acronym *STOP-Bang*. A STOP-Bang score of three or more has shown a high sensitivity for detecting OSA: 93% and 100% for moderate and severe OSA, respectively.   (ATLAS2, p 132; Chung et al, 2008)
The maximum score is 8, and the questions are
    1. S̲noring: Do you snore loudly?
    2. T̲ired: Do you often feel tired, fatigued, or sleepy during the day?
    3. O̲bserved: Has anyone observed you stop breathing during sleep?
    4. Blood p̲ressure: Do you have or are you being treated for high blood pressure?
    5. B̲MI: Is your BMI more than 35?
    6. A̲ge: Is your age over 50 years?
    7. N̲eck circumference (NC): Is it greater than 40 cm?
    8. G̲ender: Is the patient male?

31. Which statement is *true* about sildenafil use in patients who have OSA?
    A. It has no effect on any sleep parameter in patients with OSA
    B. Sildenafil worsens OSA and hypoxemia
    C. It improves AHI but increases hypoxemia
    D. Sildenafil causes pulmonary hypertension

ANSWER: **B.**   Several studies have shown that sildenafil may worsen OSA and nocturnal hypoxemia. The reason for this is not known but may be related to effects on erectile tissue in the nose, resulting in more upper airway obstruction. Sildenafil, a vasodilator, may also increase ventilation-perfusion mismatching and may lower PaO_2. Sildenafil is used not only for erectile dysfunction but also to treat pulmonary hypertension. The author has seen cases of patients being treated for "primary pulmonary hypertension" who actually had OSA, and when apnea was finally diagnosed, the sleep hypoxemia persisted even though the patient was on CPAP.   (Neves et al, 2010)

32. Which of the following medications is *most* likely to be associated with complex sleep apnea?
    A. Morphine
    B. Zopiclone
    C. Clonazepam
    D. Omeprazole

ANSWER: **A.**   Opiates are well known to cause central sleep apnea and complex sleep apnea, which is the manifestation of central apneas when CPAP or bilevel pressure is used to treat OSA. Opiates blunt the chemical drive to breathe and can induce respiratory failure. Patients with complex sleep apnea usually respond to treatment with adaptive servoventilation.   (Mogri et al, 2009)

33. A 14-year-old boy is referred because of heavy snoring at night and disruptive behavior in school. He has a BMI of 35 and grade +1 tonsils. He takes methylphenidate for attention-deficit/hyperactivity disorder. A fragment is shown below from his overnight sleep study (Fig. E7–4). The top window is 30 seconds, and the bottom is 2 minutes. What does this fragment show?

A. The patient is awake, and the fragment shows CSB

B. The patient is in stage R (REM sleep), and the abnormal events are central apneas

C. The patient is in stage R, and the abnormal events are hypopneas

D. The patient is in stage R, and the abnormal breathing events cannot be distinguished between apneas and hypopneas

ANSWER: **D.** Hypopnea is determined from the pressure sensor and apnea from the thermal sensor. It is unclear from this fragment whether the events are apneas because it cannot be accurately determined whether a 90% fall in amplitude occurred in the thermal sensor. Thus, it is best to modify the gain of the signals so we can accurately evaluate the changes in amplitude of the signals. This is shown in Figure E7–5; it is now clear that the thermal sensor excursion (in *blue*) has decreased by about 90% or more from peak thermal sensor excursion (in *red*).

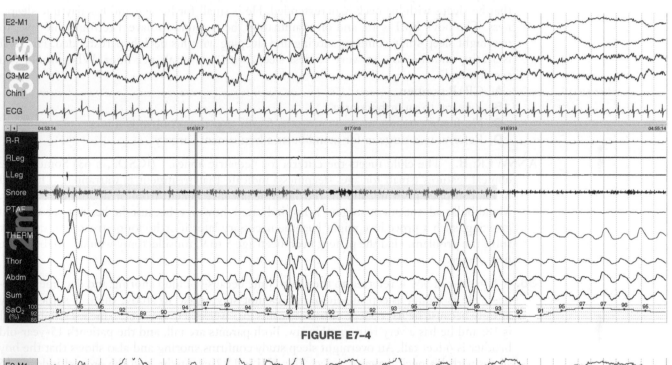

FIGURE E7–4

FIGURE E7–5

34. The above patient's AHI was 4.8 events/hr. What should be the next step in management?

    A. Tonsillectomy

    B. The patient's AHI is too low to confirm a diagnosis of sleep apnea for his age; thus, the focus should be on weight loss

    C. CPAP titration study; encourage the patient to lose weight

    D. Fit the patient for an oral appliance

ANSWER: **C.**   By PSG, pediatric apnea diagnosis requires an AHI of 1 or more with respiratory events associated with hypoxemia, hypercapnia, arousals, or markedly negative esophageal pressure swings. Paradoxic rib cage abdominal motion is also an important feature when present. Because the child has apnea with behavioral and physiologic consequences (hypoxemia), treatment should be instituted. The tonsils are not enlarged, and the cause is likely obesity. It is appropriate to treat this patient with CPAP until weight loss is achieved. Oral appliance therapy is not a viable alternative in this age group. However, if clinically indicated (e.g., a small jaw), orthodontic evaluation should be done.

35. A 12-year-old boy is referred to the sleep clinic because of loud snoring. His parents note that he sleeps with his neck hyperextended. He is small for his age and has daytime sleepiness. The boy's BMI is 18, and on examination, he is found to have a retrognathic jaw. An overnight sleep study confirms snoring and sleeping with his neck hyperextended. His AHI is 1.2/hr, and the boy has very restless sleep, with 6 arousals per hour. What would you recommend?

    A. CPAP titration

    B. Referral to an orthodontist

    C. No further treatment, reassuring the family that the problem is minor

    D. Referral to a surgeon for mandibular advancement surgery

ANSWER: **B.**   The child meets the criteria for pediatric apnea. (ICSD3, p 63) Some of the clinical features (small for age, sleepiness) indicate that treatment is warranted. The child has not stopped growing, and his retrognathic jaw may benefit from orthodontic treatment. Mandibular advancement surgery is not indicated, however, because he has not yet stopped growing; such a procedure might become necessary later if orthodontic treatment does not solve the problem. Had the patient been been age 5 to 9, tonsillectomy would have been the first choice.

36. A 17-year-old boy is referred to the sleep clinic because of loud snoring and daytime sleepiness. He is falling asleep in school and cannot stay awake to study; there is some family anxiety because he has college entrance exams in 3 weeks. He is 5 feet, 2 inches tall; his BMI is 18; and he has a very retrognathic jaw. Both parents are tall, and the patient's 15-year-old brother is 6 feet tall. An overnight sleep study confirms snoring and also shows that the boy sleeps with his neck hyperextended. His AHI is 11.2 events/hr, and the arousal index is 16 arousals/hr. What would you recommend?

    A. CPAP titration and referral to both an orthodontist and an oral-facial surgeon

    B. Referral to an orthodontist to fit the patient for a mandibular advancement device

    C. A stimulant drug approved for this age group

    D. Referral for mandibular advancement surgery

ANSWER: **A.**   The child meets criteria for pediatric OSA. (ICSD3, p 63) The same clinical features as in the previous case (small for age, sleepiness) indicate that treatment is warranted. The extreme sleepiness with the possibility that he will fail his entrance exams mandates early treatment with CPAP but not a stimulant. Because he has probably not stopped growing, his retrognathic jaw may benefit from orthodontic treatment. Maxillary-mandibular surgery may well be indicated but only after he has stopped growing. Thus, it is appropriate to get both the orthodontist and surgeon involved early in the management process.

37. An 18-year-old man with a BMI of 46 has a history of snoring and severe daytime sleepiness. A fragment of his PSG is shown in Figure E7–6. The scoring technologist was not sure whether the electrocardiography (ECG) finding was an artifact. What does the ECG show?

    A. An artifact

    B. Second-degree atrioventricular (AV) heart block, Mobitz I or Wenckebach types

    C. Second-degree AV heart block, Mobitz II type

    D. Third-degree heart block

ANSWER: **C.** The first thing to do is make sure that the ECG finding is real and not artifact. The *circles* in Figure E7–7 show that the ECG artifact in E1-M2 tracks the QRS waves in the ECG; when there is a missed beat on the ECG, no ECG artifact appears in this channel. Thus, the finding is real; an AV block is present. This is a second-degree AV block of the Mobitz II variety. The nomenclature for AV blocks can be confusing. A first-degree block is simply a lengthening of the PR interval. Second-degree block has two types: type 1 is also called *Mobitz I* or *Wenckebach block*, in which the PR interval prolongs in successive beats until a P wave is not conducted; type 2 is also called *Mobitz II*, in which there occur intermittently nonconducted P waves without preceding progressive prolongation of the PR interval. Third-degree heart block occurs when P waves are not followed by conducted beats. (ATLAS2, pp 444–445) This rhythm is not specifically covered in any of the scoring rules (asystole is typically scored only if there is a cardiac pause that exceeds 3 seconds). This event would not have been scored, but it is clearly significant.

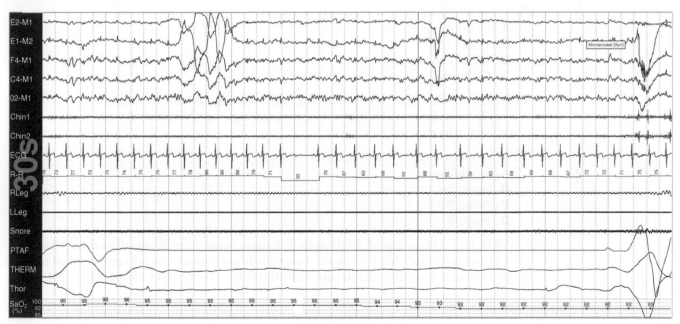

FIGURE E7–6

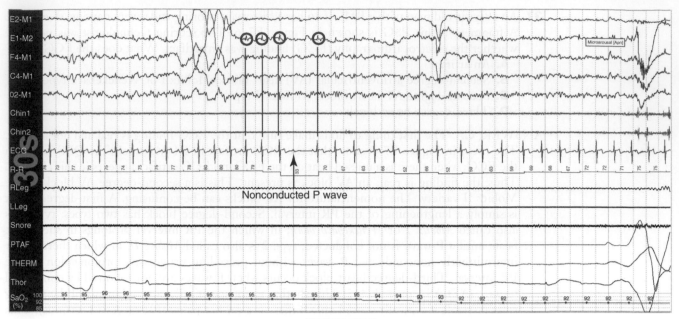

FIGURE E7–7

Questions 38 and 39 refer to the PSG fragment in Figure E7–7.

38. What breathing pattern abnormality is shown?
   A. Central apnea
   B. OSA
   C. Obstructive hypopnea
   D. CSB pattern

ANSWER: **A.**   This is a central apnea. Because of the snoring history, the scoring technologist actually scored it as an obstructive event—a scoring error. Note that there is no effort during the event (the thoracic belt is flat).

39. What sleep stage is shown in this fragment?
   A. Wakefulness
   B. Stage N1
   C. Stage N3
   D. Stage R

ANSWER: **D.**   This is stage R, REM sleep. Eye movements occur along with a mixed-frequency EEG and decreased chin EMG tone. Several bradyarrhythmias have been described in REM sleep in normal subjects and in patients with OSA.   (Holty and Guilleminault, 2011)

40. A 36-year-old hospital cafeteria cook complains that he is very sleepy at work, to the point of falling asleep in the kitchen. He has no symptoms to suggest narcolepsy. His BMI is 46, and an overnight split-night study confirms severe sleep apnea with an AHI of 42; on CPAP at 12 cm H_2O, his AHI is 2. There were no periodic limb movements. He is prescribed CPAP, and at a 3-month follow-up, a data download indicates he used CPAP every night over the 2-week monitoring period, averaging 7.4 hours a night. The machine-calculated AHI was 3. The patient admits that although he feels improved, there is still some daytime sleepiness and a tendency to nod off. He is concerned that he may be fired. What do you recommend next?
- **A.** Repeat overnight PSG
- **B.** PSG followed by a mean sleep latency test (MSLT)
- **C.** Repeat CPAP machine download over the ensuing 2 weeks
- **D.** Clinical trial of modafinil

ANSWER: **D.** Modafinil (and armodafinil) have Food and Drug Administration approval for the improvement of alertness in patients with treated sleep apnea. Additional investigation is unlikely to be helpful.

41. A 46-year-old radio talk show host with a BMI of 39 is diagnosed with OSA; his AHI is 65 events/hr. During his sleep study, severe hypoxemia was evident, with SaO_2 repeatedly dipping to 50%. He also showed many premature ventricular contractions (PVCs) and a 30-second run of ventricular tachycardia. On CPAP at 16 cm H_2O pressure, his AHI is 2 events/hr. The patient is started on CPAP, and he changes his lifestyle, becoming a vegetarian. After losing 30 pounds, he complains of awakening at night and then feeling short of breath. What is your recommendation?
- **A.** Increase CPAP pressure by 2 cm H_2O
- **B.** Switch the patient to an autotitrating machine in the range of 10 to 16 cm H_2O
- **C.** Have the patient undergo an overnight CPAP titration study in the lab
- **D.** Use two-channel monitoring of oronasal airflow and respiratory pressure

ANSWER: **C.** The patient had very severe findings on the original PSG (hypoxemia and cardiac rhythm abnormalities); thus, it is important to know the status of his apnea and whether the CPAP pressure is appropriate. It is likely that he requires less pressure. None of the other options mentioned can determine the level of SaO_2 and whether his cardiac rhythm is problematic.

42. A 51-year-old truck driver with a BMI of 43 is diagnosed with OSA; his AHI is 45, and low SaO_2 on overnight PSG is 60%. There were also many PVCs in the study. On CPAP of 18 cm H_2O pressure, his AHI is 2, and he is started on CPAP at home. Discomfort with the CPAP mask convinces him to have bariatric surgery. After losing 30 lb, he calls to say that he is no longer using CPAP; he believes his apnea has resolved and asks for a letter to his employer stating that he no longer has sleep apnea and does not need CPAP. What is your next step?
- **A.** Write the employer a letter indicating that the patient's apnea has resolved
- **B.** Order a maintenance of wakefulness test (MWT)
- **C.** Repeat an in-lab split-night PSG
- **D.** Start the patient on modafinil

ANSWER: **C.** The patient is a truck driver, and left untreated, he poses a public health risk. He had severe findings on the PSG (hypoxemia and cardiac rhythm abnormalities), and it is thus important to discern whether his apnea has resolved with modest weight loss. You cannot state that his OSA has resolved based on his statement alone. Options B and D cannot determine whether he still has sleep apnea.

43. A 40-year-old woman with a BMI of 60 is referred by a bariatric surgeon before a planned gastric bypass operation. She has history of snoring and hypertension but denies excessive daytime sleepiness. She sometimes awakens with headaches. On examination, you note pitting edema in her legs going up to her knees. She does not think she needs a sleep test. What do you advise?

A. In the absence of daytime sleepiness, it is unlikely that she has sleep-breathing problems; therefore, a sleep study is not needed

B. The patient is at high risk of having OSA and hypoventilation; therefore, an in-lab test is recommended

C. Screening oximetry will suffice to rule out a significant sleep-breathing problem

D. A 2-week trial of autotitrating CPAP with examination of the download is the best next step

ANSWER: **B.** About 50% of patients with a BMI of 40 or more have OSA; this patient's BMI is 60. Also, her risk of OSA is increased by the presence of hypertension. The peripheral edema may be a marker of right-sided cardiac failure, possibly related to hypoventilation. The nocturnal headaches point toward this possibility. The danger for patients with undiagnosed and untreated apnea is risk in the preoperative period, when her breathing control will be likely compromised by anesthetics and analgesics.

44. A 52-year-old woman with a BMI of 20 presents with a history of snoring, excessive sleepiness, and witnessed apneas. She has a history of an Arnold-Chiari malformation. On examination, you note severe retrognathia and the findings shown in Figure E7–8. The PSG showed an AHI of 60 with very severe hypoxemia (low SaO_2 = 55%); about half the apneas were central in origin. She had previously tried fixed-pressure CPAP but noted no improvement in her sleepiness and refuses to try it again. She wants to be treated with an oral appliance. What do you recommend?

A. The patient is an excellent candidate for an oral appliance because of her retrognathia

B. She is not a candidate for an oral appliance but may do well with uvulopalatopharyngoplasty (UPPP) surgery

C. She is not a candidate for an oral appliance, and she should be assessed on a bilevel machine with timed backup or an adaptive servoventilator (ASV) device

D. Oral appliances are not efficacious in patients with retrognathia

ANSWER: **C.** The patient is a very poor candidate for an oral appliance for two reasons: (1) she has many episodes of central apnea (likely related to her Arnold-Chiari malformation), and (2) she has abnormal dentition. She simply does not have a sufficient number of healthy teeth with which to anchor an appliance. UPPP is not likely to be helpful when the problem is retrognathia and the obstruction is in the base of the tongue and not the soft palate. In any case, the patient needs a positive-pressure device that can also treat her central apnea.

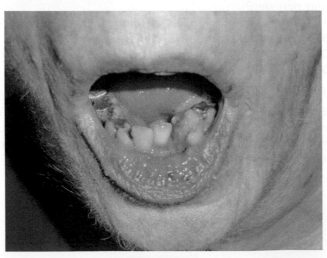

FIGURE E7–8

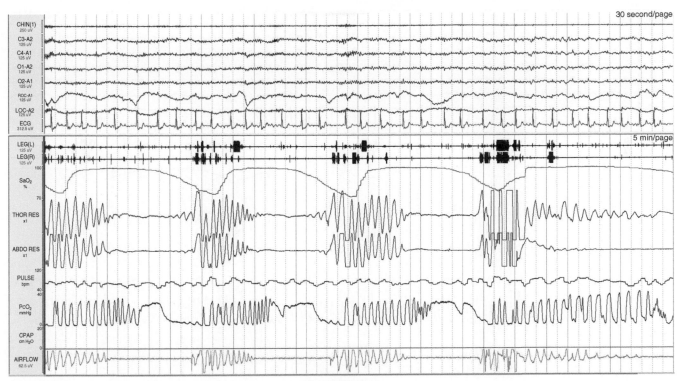

FIGURE E7–9

Questions 45 through 48 are based on Figure E7–9.

45. A 61-year-old man is referred for evaluation of insomnia and nightly episodes of dyspnea. A fragment from his PSG is shown in Figure E7–9. The top window is 30 seconds, and the bottom window 5 minutes. What stage of sleep is shown?
  A. Wakefulness
  B. Stage N2
  C. Stage N3
  D. Stage R

ANSWER: **A.**   This fragment shows that the patient is wide awake. The EEG channels show high frequencies throughout and at times show alpha activity.

46. What does the ECG channel from the fragment show?
  A. Sinus rhythm
  B. AF
  C. First-degree AV heart block
  D. Second-degree AV heart block

ANSWER: **B.**   The rhythm is AF; there are no distinct P waves. The pulse rate in the lower window is "irregularly irregular," the hallmark of AF.

47. What predominant breathing abnormality does the fragment show?
  A. Obstructive apnea
  B. Central apnea
  C. Paradoxic chest wall abdominal movements
  D. Postarousal central apneas that are not scored

ANSWER: **B.**   These are episodes of central apnea. During the apnea episodes, there is little or no movement of the chest wall or abdomen.

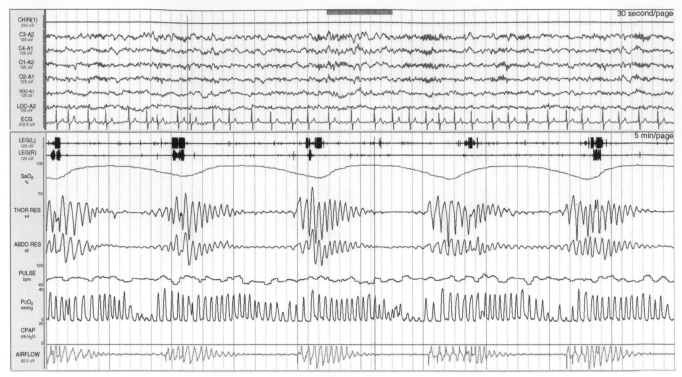

FIGURE E7-10

48. What is the *likeliest* etiology in this patient, who reports awakening short of breath during the night?

   A. Asthma

   B. COPD

   C. Congestive heart failure

   D. Gastroesophageal reflux with aspiration

ANSWER: **C.**   The finding of central apnea during wakefulness is a classic observation in congestive heart failure. This may also be seen in CNS pathologies, for example, after a stroke.   (ATLAS2, p 378)

49. What *best* describes the PSG fragment in Figure E7-10?

   A. CSB

   B. Obstructive apnea with hypercapnia

   C. Central apnea with hypercapnia

   D. Periodic limb movements causing central apnea

ANSWER: **A.**   Some breathing occurs throughout the fragment as shown by the CO_2 trace. The airflow sensor is not as sensitive as the CO_2 sensor in this example; however, the CO_2 stays below 40 mm Hg, so answers B and C are incorrect. Leg movements are not causing the central apneas because they occur during the hyperpneic phase of the CSB pattern and distort the typical waxing and waning of breathing. These findings are commonly seen in heart failure (notice the AF) as well as in patients with renal failure and cerebrovascular disease.

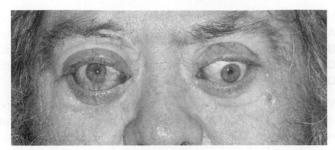

FIGURE E7–11

Questions 50 through 52 refer to Figure E7–11.

50. A 64-year-old retired college professor is referred for evaluation of EDS. In his early 40s, he had an illness for which treatment included radioactive iodine. For the past several years, he has reported "seeing double," and over the past 2 years, he has gained 40 lb. His wife says he snores loudly. What is the *most* likely diagnosis?
  A. Acromegaly
  B. Left orbital tumor
  C. Diabetes mellitus neuropathy
  D. Burned-out Graves disease

ANSWER: **D.** This is an example of burned-out Graves disease with development of hypothyroidism. Radioactive iodine is used to treat hyperthyroidism, and the eye signs (proptosis and asymmetry of eye movements) are consistent with Graves disease. (ATLAS2, p 338) Patients with diabetes who have neuropathy may develop ptosis and weak extraocular muscles but not proptosis.

51. What sleep-breathing disorder will this patient's PSG likely show?
  A. OSA
  B. Central sleep apnea
  C. Continuous hypoventilation
  D. CSB pattern

ANSWER: **A.** Patients with untreated hypothyroidism and a history of snoring are most likely to have OSA. (ATLAS2, p 335)

52. What cardiac findings during sleep would you expect in this patient?
  A. Mean heart rate 80 to 100 beats/min with many PVCs
  B. Mean heart rate 100 to 120 beats/min with episodes of paroxysmal AF
  C. Mean heart rate 50 to 80 beats/min with normal sinus rhythm
  D. Mean heart rate less than 50 beats/min with sinus rhythm

ANSWER: **D.** Sinus bradycardia is a common finding in patients with hypothyroidism. (ATLAS2, p 335)

53. A 35-year-old man is referred with a history of daytime sleepiness, insomnia, mild intermittent snoring, and frequent awakenings from sleep feeling short of breath. Medical history is unremarkable, he has a normal body habitus, and the physical examination results are normal. What would be the *most* likely findings on PSG that includes monitoring with end-tidal PcO_2?
  A. Central apneas, no hypercapnia
  B. Central sleep apnea, hypercapnia
  C. OSA, hypercapnia
  D. OSA, no hypercapnia

ANSWER: **A.** This patient has the clinical features of idiopathic central apnea. Such patients are nonhypercapnic.

54. Which statement about nonhypercapnic central sleep apnea is *incorrect*?
   A. Central sleep apnea is characterized by ventilatory control instability
   B. There is often a decreased responsiveness to hypercapnia
   C. Ventilation during NREM sleep is driven by arterial PcO_2
   D. Central apneas can be precipitated by reduced PcO_2

ANSWER: **B.** In nonhypercapnic central sleep apnea, responsiveness to hypercapnia is increased, not decreased. These patients have ventilatory control instability, and events that lower $PaCO_2$ during sleep may initiate central apneas. Patients with hypercapnic central apneas have decreased responsiveness to hypercapnia.

55. What is the *most* common location of obstruction in patients with OSA?
   A. Nasal airway
   B. Nasopharynx
   C. Oropharynx
   D. Hypopharynx

ANSWER: **C.** The most common site of obstruction is the oropharynx, which includes the retropalatal region and the retroglossal region. However, during sleep, the actual site of obstruction may vary.

56. Which of the following does *not* play a role in cognitive impairment associated with OSA?
   A. Arousals
   B. Intermittent hypoxemia and hypercapnia
   C. Prefrontal cortex dysfunction
   D. Occipital lobe dysfunction

ANSWER: **D.** Sleep disruption related to arousals and also blood gas abnormalities (hypoxemia, hypercapnia) disrupt cellular homeostasis and result in prefrontal cortical dysfunction. This in turn can cause a variety of cognitive impairments that include memory problems, disorganization, poor judgment, and emotional lability.

57. A 45-year-old man has been diagnosed with OSA (AHI = 24 events/hr). His BMI is 26. On a glucose tolerance test, his fasting blood glucose was slightly elevated. Which statement about the relationship between OSA and glucose metabolism is *correct*?
   A. Sleep apnea has no independent effect on glucose metabolism
   B. Sleep apnea may be associated with glucose intolerance and insulin resistance
   C. Sleep apnea does not predispose to the development of type 2 diabetes
   D. Intermittent hypoxemia and arousals have no effect on metabolic function

ANSWER: **B.** OSA is associated with insulin resistance and glucose intolerance and may lead to the development of type 2 diabetes whether the patient is obese or not. Sleep fragmentation and intermittent hypoxemia cause release of cytokines from fat cells, sympathetic activation, and an effect on the hypothalamic-pituitary-adrenal axis that leads to glucose intolerance and insulin resistance.

58. A 40-year-old woman presents with a history of snoring, obesity, and daytime sleepiness. She has a neck circumference (NC) of 43 cm. Which statement about NC and OSA is *correct*?
   A. NC bears no relationship to OSA
   B. NC over 40 cm is predictive of OSA in male patients only
   C. NC over 40 cm is predictive of OSA in female patients only
   D. NC over 40 cm is predictive of OSA in both sexes

ANSWER: **D.** When NC is over 40 cm, there is a sensitivity of 61% and a specificity of 93% for the presence of OSAS in both sexes.

59. Which statement about OSA in females is *incorrect*?
   A. Women are much more overweight than men who have a similar AHI
   B. Women with an AHI over 15 have snoring and daytime symptoms similar to men with a similar AHI
   C. Women with OSA are more likely than men to present with symptoms of insomnia
   D. Women with OSA are less likely than men to be treated for depression

ANSWER: **D.**   There are important differences in the presentation of sleep apnea in men and women. Women are much more likely to present with insomnia, a history of depression, and previous hypothyroidism. At a given AHI, women tend to be more overweight than men.

60. A 42-year-old obese man with a history of snoring and daytime sleepiness is referred to the sleep clinic after a home sleep test that monitored SaO_2, nasal pressure, and chest wall and abdominal motion. The home study was ordered by his family doctor. The patient states he slept very poorly during the study, which showed a respiratory disturbance index (RDI) of 4 events/hr. Which statement about RDI is *incorrect*?
   A. The RDI is the number of apneas and hypopneas plus respiratory event–related arousals (RERAs) per hour of sleep
   B. The RDI is the number of RERAs per hour of sleep
   C. A home sleep test that does not monitor EEG cannot accurately calculate RDI, so a normal RDI cannot be used to exclude OSA
   D. RDI is elevated in patients with upper airway resistance syndrome

ANSWER: **B.**   In this example, the home sleep test resulting in an RDI of 4 cannot be used to exclude the presence of sleep apnea. In home portable studies, the total recording time, rather than actual sleep time, is used as the denominator. If someone were awake for a significant part of the night, the calculated RDI would be an inaccurate reflection of the severity of the patient's sleep-breathing abnormality. The RDI is the number of apneas plus hypopneas plus RERAs per hour of sleep.

61. Which statement about the relationship between hypothyroidism and sleep apnea is *incorrect*?
   A. Hypothyroid patients with sleep apnea may have a reduction in apnea frequency with thyroid hormone replacement
   B. Thyroid hormone replacement in hypothyroid sleep apnea patients does not obviate the use of CPAP
   C. All patients suspected of having sleep apnea should be screened for hypothyroidism
   D. Patients with sleep apnea who continue to be sleepy on adequate PAP should be screened for hypothyroidism

ANSWER: **C.**   Routine screening for hypothyroidism in OSA patients is not indicated unless there are corroborating signs and symptoms. The prevalence of hypothyroidism in OSA is the same as in people without the condition.

62. A 30-year-old man with OSAS (AHI = 30 events/hr) is refusing to use CPAP because he finds it too uncomfortable. He asks why supplemental O_2 cannot be used instead. Which statement about the use of O_2 in OSA is *correct*?
   A. Apnea duration usually increases with oxygen administration
   B. Oxygen treatment may cause hypocapnia
   C. Apnea frequency may increase
   D. There is improvement in daytime sleepiness with oxygen treatment

ANSWER: **A.**   Although supplemental oxygen by nasal cannula is far more comfortable than CPAP, O_2 may prolong apneic episodes and in some patients can lead to hypercapnia. Apnea frequency may decrease with oxygen therapy, but this may simply be caused by longer episodes of each apnea. A potentially positive effect of oxygen is the elimination of bradycardia during apneic events.

63. A 55-year-old man with a BMI of 36, a history of snoring, and witnessed apneas is found to have sleep apnea; his AHI is 40 events/hr, and about 75% of the events are mixed apneas. What should you recommend?
  A. Titration in a lab with a bilevel machine with a backup rate
  B. Titration in a lab with a CPAP machine
  C. Treatment at home with an autotitrating CPAP machine
  D. Titration in a lab with ASV

ANSWER: **B.**   CPAP has been documented to be effective in treating both mixed and obstructive apneas and the central apneas seen in patients with OSA. An unknown proportion of such patients may develop complex sleep apnea and may then require ASV if the left ventricular ejection fraction (LVEF) is greater than 45%.

64. A 51-year-old patient with OSAS and an AHI of 46 is titrated on CPAP with an excellent response at 12 cm H_2O. He is sent home on a CPAP system identical to what he used in the sleep lab. Two weeks later, he contacts the sleep clinic stating that the positive effects have worn off. In the interval, you learn he was switched from captopril to hydrochlorothiazide. What is the *least* likely explanation for the loss of CPAP efficacy?
  A. He has developed a nasal obstruction
  B. He has been using alcohol at home
  C. He is sleeping in a different position at home than he was in the laboratory
  D. His new antihypertensive medication is the problem

ANSWER: **D.**   There is no reason for the medication change to affect CPAP efficacy. You would suspect a medication if it reduced upper airway tone or control of breathing, so one of the three other explanations is more likely. Over a longer interval of time, you should also question possible weight gain.

65. A 56-year-old female patient with sleep apnea is being treated with nasal CPAP and heated humidification. Initially, this setup is very effective. Now she complains of waking up at night with the CPAP mask on the floor, her nose obstructed, and some rhinorrhea. Which treatment approaches for her symptoms would be *least* useful?
  A. Switch from heated to cold pass-over humidification
  B. Examination for the presence of nasal obstruction due to a deviated nasal septum or polyps
  C. Intranasal ipratropium
  D. Antihistamines, topical steroids, or topical nasal saline sprays

ANSWER: **A.**   The cause of nasal symptoms in patients on CPAP is often dryness. She is already on a humidification system that was initially effective, and switching to cold pass-over humidification will likely worsen the situation because such systems actually reduce the relative humidity in the circuit.

66. A 51-year-old man with a BMI of 51 has history of snoring, witnessed apneas, and daytime sleepiness. Medical history includes COPD with a forced expiratory volume in 1 second (FEV_1) of 0.9 L. An overnight PSG shows an AHI of 40 events/hr, AF, and several short runs of ventricular tachycardia. He does not want to use CPAP and asks about upper airway surgery. What do you advise?
  A. A trial of CPAP is not necessary before being considered for surgery
  B. Surgery is not advised because he has several contraindications
  C. Surgery will help the AF
  D. He will be a good candidate for surgery but only if he has failed medical management

ANSWER: **B.**   The patient has several relative contraindications for surgery including morbid obesity, severe pulmonary disease, and unstable cardiovascular status. Most surgeons will not perform upper airway surgery unless there is failure of medical management.

67. A 56-year-old woman with a BMI of 33 has a history of snoring, witnessed apneas, and daytime sleepiness. She is convinced she has sleep apnea (she says the disorder "runs in her family") and wants to proceed directly to surgical therapy. She does not want a sleep test or to even try CPAP but instead asks for a surgical referral. What do you advise?
   A. Given her history, it is reasonable to refer her directly to surgery
   B. Her BMI is a contraindication for surgery
   C. The severity of sleep apnea must be documented before surgical treatment
   D. Her age is a contraindication for surgery

ANSWER: **C.**   The American Academy of Sleep Medicine (AASM) standard of care practice on the surgical management of OSA requires documentation of severity before surgical treatment.

68. Which of the following is *not* a predictor of positive outcome when an oral appliance is used for OSA?
   A. Younger age
   B. Lower BMI
   C. AHI that is lower when sleeping supine
   D. Smaller neck circumference

ANSWER: **C.**   Younger age, lower BMI, and smaller NC are all predictors of positive treatment outcomes when using oral appliances. Patients whose apnea is more severe when supine also tend to do better with an oral appliance.

69. A 50-year-old man with a BMI of 29 had a PSG that showed an AHI of 60 events/hr and low SaO_2 of 55%. He quit using CPAP because it had no effect on his daytime sleepiness. A medical examination by his family doctor showed marked elevation of low-density lipoprotein (LDL) cholesterol and serum triglyceride levels. What can you tell him about the relationship between sleep apnea and these lab results?
   A. Sleep apnea with intermittent hypoxemia increases both LDL cholesterol and triglycerides
   B. CPAP does not change levels of LDL cholesterol or triglycerides
   C. Sleep apnea has no effect on lipid metabolism
   D. The effect of apnea on lipids is only significant in morbidly obese patients

ANSWER: **A.**   OSA increases both LDL cholesterol and triglycerides. This effect is independent of adiposity but seems dependent on the degree of hypoxemia. CPAP reduces LDL cholesterol and triglycerides.

70. A 45-year-old woman with a BMI of 33 had a PSG that showed an AHI of 40 and a low SaO_2 of 60%. She quit using CPAP because it had no effect on her daytime sleepiness. Screening blood tests by her family doctor showed marked elevation of serum alanine aminotransferase (ALT) and aspartate aminotransferase (AST) levels. She has never had more than one alcoholic drink a month. What do you tell her about the relationship between sleep apnea and these lab results?
   A. Sleep apnea with intermittent hypoxemia is associated with NASH
   B. CPAP does not change levels of these enzymes
   C. Sleep apnea has no effect on liver function; the finding is a coincidence
   D. Sleep apnea has not been associated with liver fibrosis

ANSWER: **A.**   Several studies have shown a relationship between NASH and sleep apnea; the effect seems to be related to oxygen desaturation. Hypoxemia results in the release of cytokines, which may initiate the liver injury. Several studies have documented the relationship between sleep apnea and liver fibrosis.

71. A 26-year-old obese woman with a BMI of 48 is referred by her bariatric surgeon for OSA evaluation. She has a history of snoring but no witnessed apneas. In addition to obesity, she has medication-controlled hypertension. She declines to have an overnight sleep study, claiming she feels fine and has no daytime sleepiness. What do you advise her?
    A. Given her lack of symptoms, it is unlikely she has OSA, and a sleep study is unnecessary
    B. Given her BMI, she has at least a 33% chance of having OSA
    C. There are few risks of bariatric surgery, and a sleep study will add little to her management
    D. If she does have sleep apnea, surgery will have no lasting effect on the condition

ANSWER: **B.**   Several studies have examined the relationship between BMI and the presence of OSA. In the Sleep Heart Health Study, the prevalence of OSA was 32% in individuals with a BMI between 32 and 59. Bariatric surgery can be very effective in improving metabolic effects of obesity and can also result in a dramatic reduction of apnea events. Her lack of symptoms does not exclude OSA, and an evaluation is important to reduce risks perioperatively.

72. A 45-year-old woman with a BMI of 33 has a history of snoring and witnessed apneas. She is referred by her cardiologist for evaluation. She recently had a myocardial infarction (MI), and she has a family history of premature death; her father died at 50 years of age of an MI. She does not have high blood pressure. An overnight sleep study shows an AHI of 25, with SaO_2 dropping intermittently into the 70% range. In a follow-up visit, she asks whether there is a relationship between sleep apnea and cardiovascular disease and, given that she is normotensive, whether she is at increased risk. What do you tell her?
    A. In the absence of arterial hypertension, her risk for cardiovascular disease is not increased
    B. Sleep apnea results in the production of several cytokines that have vasoactive and inflammatory properties; these can result in endothelial dysfunction and can lead to cardiovascular disease in the absence of hypertension
    C. Sleep apnea has no effect on mortality
    D. Treatment of sleep apnea has no effect on cardiovascular mortality

ANSWER: **B.**   With sleep apnea, many cytokines are released that can negatively affect cardiovascular morbidity. Sleep apnea has been shown to increase cardiovascular mortality, an increase that can be reversed with CPAP treatment.

73. A 16-year-old student is referred by her family physician because of possible OSA. For approximately 1 year, she has been snoring and taking 2- to 3-hour naps after coming home from school. Her BMI is 34, and she has a family history of sleep apnea. On physical examination, she has central obesity, facial hair on her chin and upper lip, extensive acne, and male pattern hair growth on her lower abdominal area. Her overnight sleep study revealed an AHI of 12. What other diagnosis should you consider?
    A. Cushing disease
    B. Acromegaly
    C. Hypothyroidism
    D. Polycystic ovarian syndrome

ANSWER: **D.**   This is a classic presentation of PCOS, a disorder that affects about 5% to 10% of women of reproductive age (~12–45 years old). Their menstrual cycles are irregular or absent, and they have features of androgen excess that include acne and hirsutism. Such women are likely to have obesity, hypertension, and metabolic abnormalities that include glucose tolerance or diabetes. Women with PCOS are 30 times more likely to have SDB than control participants.   (ATLAS2, pp 354–355)

74. A 12-year-old student has a long history of snoring and witnessed snorting during sleep. His parents state he is a "restless sleeper," but he does not have EDS. He takes methylphenidate and risperidone for attention-deficit/hyperactivity disorder (ADHD). Examination shows that the patient has a small, retrognathic jaw; several of his lower anterior teeth overlap; and he has +2 tonsillar enlargement. An overnight sleep study confirms sleep apnea with an AHI of 8 events/hr. During the night, he hyperextends his neck frequently and is found to struggle while breathing in. He sleeps with his mouth open. What is the next step in management?

   A. Assessment on CPAP

   B. Referral to an ear, nose, and throat (ENT) surgeon for consideration of tonsillectomy and adenoidectomy

   C. Referral to a maxillofacial surgeon

   D. Referral to an orthodontist

ANSWER: **D.**   In this situation, referral to an orthodontist can be life changing. Substantial changes can be made to the jaw anatomy using orthodontics if done before closure of the epiphyseal plates. Orthodontic treatment is much less feasible after a person stops growing (in young men, usually by age 16–18 years). If orthodontia solves the child's sleep-breathing problem, there should be a reassessment of his need for medications to treat ADHD. It is possible that the latter was diagnosed when the symptoms actually were from sleep apnea. If orthodontic treatment is not feasible or effective, referral to a maxillofacial surgeon would be the next step.   (ATLAS2, pp 299–307)

75. A 16-year-old student is seen in your clinic 3 years after being initially diagnosed with OSA. At that time, she had a BMI of 34, +2 tonsillar enlargement, and an AHI of 11; during REM sleep, her AHI was 50. Tonsillectomy was advised; however, the girl's mother, a nurse, started her on a strict diet, and within several months, the snoring and witnessed apneas ceased. In the ensuing 3 years, her weight increased, and all her symptoms returned. On current evaluation, her BMI is now 37, her tonsils are still +2 enlarged, and the new AHI is 25. The patient's pediatrician advises a tonsillectomy. What do you recommend?

   A. Because the patient has enlarged tonsils, they should be removed

   B. Bariatric surgery should be considered

   C. The patient should be evaluated on and treated with CPAP

   D. The patient should be started on a diet, and if that fails, CPAP titration should be considered

ANSWER: **C.**   The patient's clinical course actually gives the correct answer. The fact that the symptoms disappeared when she lost weight suggests her enlarged tonsils were not the cause 3 years ago or at present. She has already failed dieting, and although this should again be strongly recommended, it would not be definitive enough to treat her current sleep apnea. Thus, she should have CPAP titration and be treated with CPAP. Bariatric surgery would be overly aggressive at this time.

76. A 29-year-old woman who is 36 weeks pregnant is referred for evaluation of EDS. She has developed preeclampsia with arterial hypertension, proteinuria, and gestational diabetes. Her BMI was 36 before pregnancy. Her obstetrician is concerned that if she does have sleep apnea, CPAP treatment would be "too dangerous" during pregnancy and might harm the developing baby. Overnight PSG shows an AHI of 40 events/hr with frequent drops of SaO_2 into the mid-80s. What do you recommend?

   A. Immediate delivery of the baby by cesarean section if necessary to treat the preeclampsia

   B. Immediate bed rest without treatment of the sleep apnea until the baby is delivered

   C. Antihypertensive medication to treat the high blood pressure and proteinuria

   D. Immediate CPAP titration and CPAP treatment

ANSWER: **D.**   It is far more dangerous to the developing baby to leave the mother's OSA untreated. The repetitive episodes of hypoxemia are likely harmful. After starting CPAP, the mother should be followed closely to see if preeclampsia improves; if not, early delivery of the baby may be necessary.

77. Which statement about SDB in pregnancy is *incorrect*?
   A. Pregnant women with sleep apnea will usually show improvement in the AHI after the baby is delivered
   B. The incidence of SDB in pregnant women is very low
   C. The severity and frequency of snoring increase as pregnancy progresses
   D. CPAP compliance is poor in pregnant women with sleep apnea

ANSWER: **D.** Surprisingly, CPAP is well tolerated in pregnant women, and compliance is generally good. Women who have sleep apnea diagnosed before pregnancy or early on in pregnancy may require CPAP treatment at about 24 weeks of gestation.

78. Which statement about management of the morbidly obese sleep apnea patient immediately after bariatric surgery is *incorrect*?
   A. Extubation should only be performed when the patient is fully awake and alert and has return of neuromuscular function
   B. Removal of the endotracheal tube should only be performed in the operating room, postanesthesia recovery area, or special care area where monitoring is available
   C. The patient should be maintained in the supine position
   D. The patient should be started on CPAP immediately after extubation

ANSWER: **C.** The patient should be maintained in a lateral or semiupright position postoperatively. Supine position presents the greatest risk. The patient should be followed closely in the first 24 postoperative hours, when a combination of REM rebound sleep and analgesic medications can have detrimental effects on sleep breathing.

79. Which statement about the relationship between sleep apnea and cardiovascular disease is incorrect?
   A. Untreated sleep apnea increases the risk of recurrent atrial fibrillation after cardioversion
   B. OSA is uncommon in patients with nocturnal angina pectoris
   C. Sleep apnea can induce severe bradyarrhythmias even in a normal heart
   D. In congestive heart failure, both obstructive and central apneas can occur

ANSWER: **B.** The vast majority of patients with nocturnal angina pectoris are found to have OSA.

80. A 64-year-old patient is referred by his cardiologist to evaluate severe sleep-onset insomnia and paroxysmal nocturnal dyspnea. His left ventricular ejection fraction is very low, at 18%. An overnight sleep study shows classic CSB virtually the entire night, with long episodes of central apnea in each cycle. Which statement about the treatment of this patient is *incorrect*?
   A. Treating the underlying heart failure is paramount
   B. ASV seems to be the most effective therapy for these patients
   C. Oxygen inhalation reduces the apnea index by about half in these patients
   D. Theophylline reduces the AHI by about 50% in this population but is seldom used because of potential arrhythmogenic effects

ANSWER: **B.** The use of PAP in heart failure OSA patients is controversial. The original CanPAP publication indicated that there was no benefit from CPAP in this population and that overall, there may have been harm. (Bradley et al, 2005) However, further analysis showed CPAP responders did well, but nonresponders had a higher mortality rate than the control participants. It turns out that about 50% of patients with heart failure and central sleep apnea respond to CPAP. Thus, it is very important to document a positive effect of CPAP before committing to long-term therapy. The Adaptive Servo-Ventilation for Central Sleep Apnea in Systolic Heart Failure (SERVE-HF) study reported that ASV can increase the mortality rate in such patients if LVEF is less than 45%. (Cowie et al, 2015)

81. What channels are used in a portable sleep study, level 3?
   A. The same channels as with a PSG performed in the sleep lab
   B. Oximetry, abdomen or chest movement, airflow, pulse
   C. Oximetry and pulse or ECG
   D. The same channels as an in-lab PSG with the exception of EEG

ANSWER: **B.**   There are four recognized levels of sleep monitoring.   (Collop et al, 2007)

   Level 4—Unattended by a sleep technician; it records one or two channels, usually oximetry and pulse.

   Level 3—Unattended with four to seven channels; minimum would be airflow, abdomen or chest movement, oximetry, and ECG or pulse. Ventilation is measured with respiratory movement and airflow. This is the most common level for a home or portable sleep study.

   Level 2—Full unattended PSG (seven or more channels), with the same or similar channels as in a regular PSG (i.e., it includes EEG, EOG, and EMG).

   Level 1—Full attended PSG (seven or more channels). This is the standard in-lab PSG.
   Whereas levels 2, 3, and 4 are "portable," only level 3 is feasible for diagnosing OSA (4 is insufficient, and 2 is impractical). Note that level 3 does not include channels for staging sleep (i.e., there is no EEG, EOG, or EMG). Portable studies are gaining traction now that Medicare has approved them for reimbursement. In most cases, level 3 is sufficient for diagnosing clinically significant OSA.

82. Which sleep-related diagnoses are *not* recommended for study with unattended portable monitoring?
   1. OSA in a commercial trucker who is otherwise healthy
   2. Narcolepsy in a 15-year-old girl
   3. Central sleep apnea in 65-year-old patient with congestive heart failure
   4. Central sleep apnea in 40-year-old patient taking opiates

   A. 1 and 2
   B. 3 and 4
   C. 2, 3, and 4
   D. All of the above

ANSWER: **C.**   "Portable Monitoring (PM) may be used as an alternative to PSG for the diagnosis of OSA in patients with a high pretest probability of moderate to severe OSA. PM is not appropriate for the diagnosis of OSA in patients with significant comorbid medical conditions that may degrade the accuracy of PM."   (Collop et al, 2007) PM is not appropriate to diagnose central apnea or narcolepsy.

83. What is the mean BMI of patients with OSAS?
   A. 25 to 30
   B. 30 to 35
   C. 35 to 40
   D. >40

ANSWER: **B.**   In one large study of 5163 new patients (3679 men and 1484 women) referred to a center for SDB, the mean BMI was 32.2. A statistical increase in BMI was also seen over the 9-year period of the study (1995–2004; an increase of 3.4 BMI units for women and 1.7 BMI units for men). The authors concluded that "the BMI in patients referred to a sleep disorders center … has increased significantly over 9 years. Recent obesity trends may contribute to the increase in the number of patients with SDB."   (Banno et al, 2005)

84. Which of the following is *least* likely to be associated with OSA?
   A. Nasal obstruction
   B. Enlarged tonsils
   C. Receding lower jaw
   D. Protruding lower jaw

ANSWER: **D.**   Each of these conditions can be associated with OSA, but a protruding jaw is the least likely. With nasal obstruction, the patient may have to switch to mouth breathing, which makes upper airway obstruction more likely. Enlarged tonsils are a common cause of sleep apnea, especially in children. A receding jaw is most often a sign of retrognathia; this condition may be associated with scalloping of the tongue because the tongue is too large for the oral cavity.

85. Among patients with SDB, all of the following tend to be increased in REM sleep over non-REM sleep *except*
   A. Oxygen desaturation
   B. Heart rate
   C. Central apneas
   D. End-tidal PcO_2

ANSWER: **C.**   Figure E7–12 shows an all-night hypnogram with REM-related desaturation. Profound oxygen desaturation and increased heart rate occur during REM sleep (*black bars*). End-tidal PcO_2 (not shown) also often increases during REM caused by atonia of some respiratory muscles (excluding the diaphragm). These data are from a 35-month-old child with loud snoring, witnessed apneas, and restless sleep. The patient had enlarged tonsils and a strong family history of apnea. Among adults, REM-related hypoxemia appears to be more common in women than in men. Central apneas in patients with primary central sleep apnea most often occur during stages N1 and N2 sleep and are rare during stages N3 and R. (ICSD3, pp 89–93)

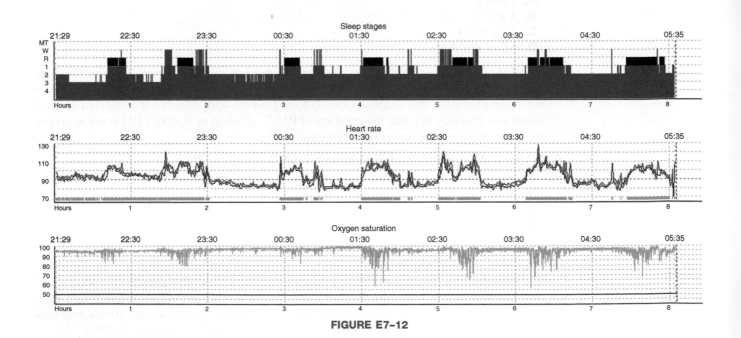

FIGURE E7–12

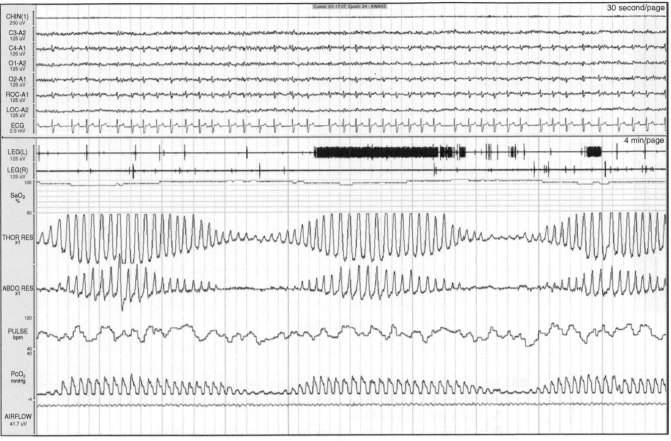

FIGURE E7–13

86. Figure E7–13 shows classic CSB in a patient with congestive heart failure. Other features suggested in this epoch include all but which one of the following?
A. Hypoventilation
B. Mouth breathing
C. AF
D. REM sleep

ANSWER: **A.**   The PcO₂ channel actually shows hyperventilation because the end-tidal PcO₂ is significantly less than 40 mm Hg. Mouth breathing is suggested by the flat nasal pressure curve (airflow). REM sleep is suggested by the low-voltage, mixed-frequency EEG and flat chin EMG. Finally, the patient displays typical AF in the ECG channel.

87. Which of the following low-high filter settings is recommended for respiratory channels?
A. 0 to 15 Hz
B. 0.3 to 35 Hz
C. 0.3 to 70 Hz
D. 10 to 100 Hz

ANSWER: **A.**   The settings in answer B are recommended for EEG and EOG, those in answer C are for ECG, and those in answer D are for EMG and snoring.   (MANUAL2)

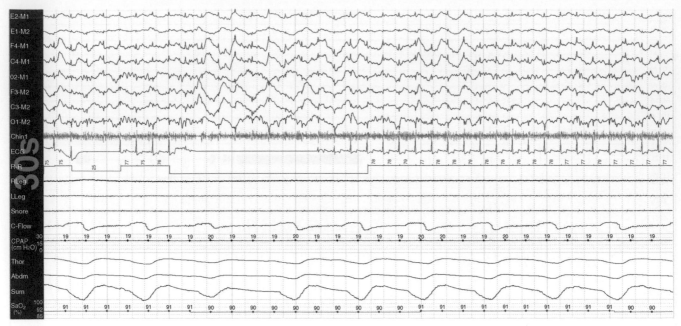

FIGURE E7–14

88. Your sleep technician is confronted with an abnormal ECG rhythm strip that suggests asystole (Fig. E7–14). What might the tech do to determine if it is an artifact?
   A. Use a stat 12-lead ECG
   B. Go into the patient's room and determine true pulse, blood pressure, and any symptoms
   C. Review the epoch with increased sensitivity
   D. Add another ECG lead, and monitor two leads for the duration of the study

ANSWER: **C.** Flatline ECG is always a concern, although it is usually a technical (as opposed to a patient) problem. In this case, it may be from amplifier damping. To be certain the problem is not asystole, the technician reviewed the same epoch with increased sensitivity to the EEG and eye channels. The increased sensitivity nicely shows the ECG artifact in both EEG and eye leads. (Although it may not have been obvious at the time, we can also see a tiny ECG artifact in E2-M1 before the sensitivity was increased.) The default montage shows PTAF and THERM channels but not C-flow. Because the patient was on CPAP at the time, both PTAF and THERM should have been turned off and flatlined. It is assumed that the technician did turn off the PTAF channel but left the THERM channel on and that the THERM lead was somewhere on the bed; hence, THERM also picked up the ECG artifact (Fig. E7–15).*

89. A patient on multiple pain medications has the PSG tracing shown in Figure E7–16. What is the main finding in this fragment?
   A. Post–periodic limb movement (PLM) arousal central apneas
   B. Obstructive apnea
   C. Central apnea
   D. The CPAP pressure is too high

ANSWER: **C.** The patient has central events with either no movement or minimal movement seen in the two effort belts (Thor and Abdm). This is a common finding in patients taking opiates. There is no snoring. This is not post-PLM arousal central apnea because of the timing of events. It is more likely that the leg movements are related to apnea termination.

---

*Thanks to Allen Boone, RPSGT, Associate Clinical Director, Sleep Services, SleepMed, Inc., for assistance with this interpretation.

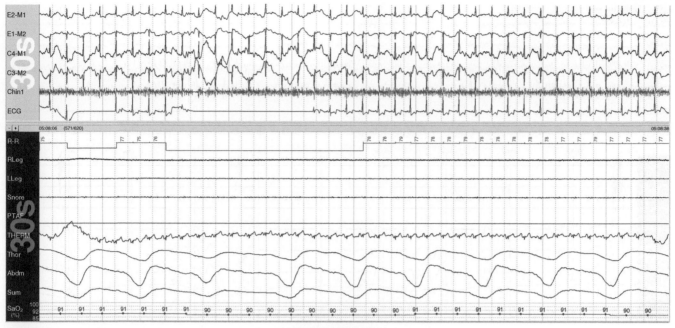

FIGURE E7–15

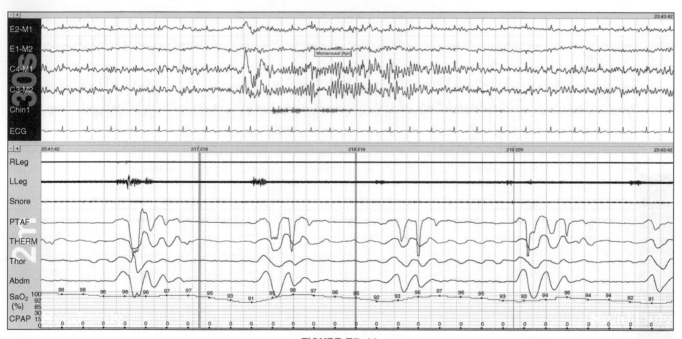

FIGURE E7–16

90. A patient on multiple medications for severe hip pain has an overnight sleep study. Below is a fragment of the sleep study (Fig. E7–17). What does the PSG fragment show?

A. Because the patient is awake, these episodes in the C-flow channel can be ignored

B. The patient should be started on CPAP

C. The episodes in the C-flow channel are obstructive apneas

D. Abnormalities in the C-flow channel may be related to medications and should not be ignored

ANSWER: **D.**   This is the correct answer by a process of elimination and careful inspection of all the channels. Even though the patient is awake, there is hypoxemia with the abnormal breathing events. The epoch shows 5 minutes of data, and there are about 25 breaths. Thus, the overall breathing frequency is 5 breaths/min, a low frequency most often found in patients on opiates. Answer B is incorrect because the patient is on CPAP; this is indicated by the bottom channel that actually displays the values and the C-flow channel. Answer C is incorrect because the episodes of apnea are not obstructive.

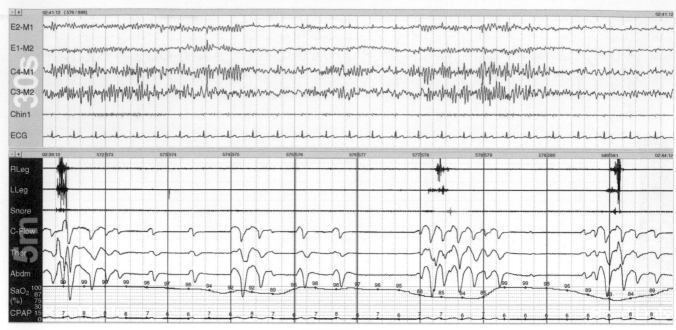

FIGURE E7–17

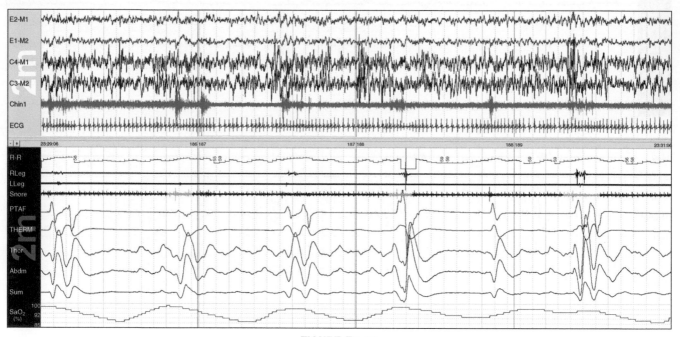

FIGURE E7–18

91. A 10-year-old boy with enlarged tonsils is being evaluated for snoring and insomnia. What does his PSG fragment show (Fig. E7–18)?

    A. All the episodes are obstructive apneas

    B. All the episodes are central apneas

    C. There are central and obstructive apnea episodes

    D. There are central, obstructive, and mixed apnea episodes

ANSWER: **D.**   There are six apnea episodes in the fragment. The first apnea is mixed; the second, third, fifth, and sixth are obstructive; the fourth is central. It is important to remember that upper airway obstruction can result in different apnea types.   (MANUAL2)

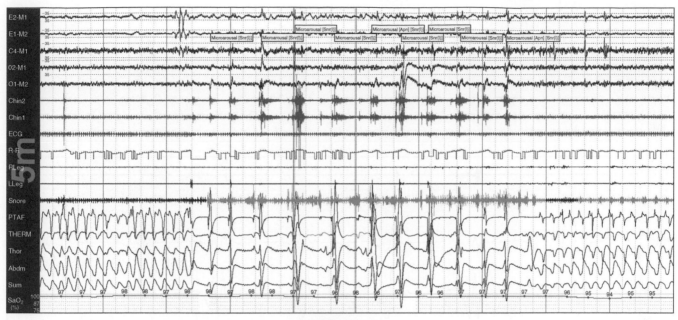

FIGURE E7-19

92. A 32-year-old man is referred for PSG to evaluate a suspected sleep disorder. He has symptoms of snoring, unrefreshing sleep, daytime sleepiness, and witnessed apneas. He has also been told he makes loud moaning noises during sleep. Figure E7–19 shows a 5-minute fragment of his PSG. What is the patient's diagnosis?
   A. OSA
   B. Central sleep apnea
   C. Biot respiration
   D. None of the above

ANSWER: **D.**   Although superficially these episodes resembled central apneas (apparent lack of airflow and lack of effort), there are three clues that this is not a central apnea: there is no change in SaO_2; there is significant noise in the snore channel (during central apnea, there should be little noise except at apnea termination); and there is a history of moaning during sleep. The diagnosis is catathrenia or sleep-related moaning, and the findings in this case are typical. Notice the eye movements about a quarter of the way into the epoch. The moaning typically (but not always) occurs during REM sleep.   (ICSD3, p 141)

93. What is the *most* common sleep-breathing abnormality after acute ascent to high altitude?
   A. Continuous hypoventilation
   B. Obstructive apnea
   C. Periodic breathing
   D. Biot respiration

ANSWER: **C.**   After acute ascent to high altitude, the most common breathing abnormality is CSB, a periodic breathing pattern. The cycle duration is usually short, often 20 to 30 seconds, and each cycle may contain only 3 or 4 breaths. Frequently, the breathing pattern normalizes during REM sleep.

94. What is the *most* common awake breathing abnormality in a thin patient taking opiates?
   A. Continuous hypoventilation
   B. Obstructive apnea
   C. Periodic breathing
   D. Biot respiration

ANSWER: **D.**   Biot respiration is an abnormal breathing pattern characterized by clusters of several irregular breaths followed by regular or irregular periods of apnea. Biot respiration is often found, in wakefulness and in sleep, in patients taking opiates (Fig. E7–20).

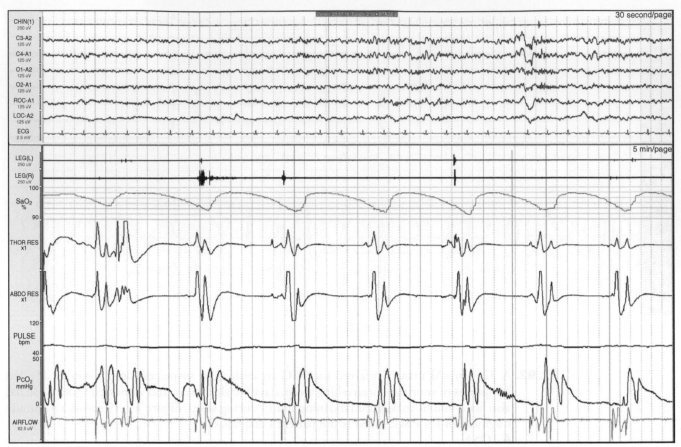

FIGURE E7–20

95. The hypoxic ventilatory response in sleep is
   A. Increased in NREM sleep compared with wakefulness
   B. Triggered at 96% oxygen saturation
   C. Reduced more in REM sleep (stage R) than in NREM sleep (stages N1, N2, and N3)
   D. A slowing of breathing rate to conserve air

ANSWER: **C.**   The hypoxic ventilatory response is the change in ventilation that occurs when hypoxemia is sensed by the carotid bodies. The response decreases with sleep and is virtually absent in REM sleep. This must be differentiated from the arousal response to hypoxemia, which is less predictable; hypoxemia may not cause arousal even when SaO_2 is about 70% during REM sleep.

96. During wakefulness, the upper airway dilator muscles (e.g., genioglossus and tensor palatini) in OSA patients are
   A. More relaxed than in normal subjects
   B. More active than in normal subjects
   C. As active as in normal subjects
   D. Infiltrated by fat and therefore flaccid

ANSWER: **B.**   Because apnea patients often have upper airway obstruction, to maintain airflow, the upper airway dilator muscles are more active than in normal subjects.   (Horner, 2007)

97. Compared with wakefulness, which of the following is *true* about NREM sleep (stages N1, N2, and N3)?
  A. Functional residual capacity (FRC) is increased
  B. Residual volume (RV) is increased
  C. The upper airway is narrowed
  D. $PacO_2$ is decreased

ANSWER: **C.**   With sleep, the main mechanical changes are related to upper airway narrowing. FRC and RV may be reduced. With sleep, usually a small but measurable *increase* in $PacO_2$ occurs from withdrawal of the stimulus to breathe.

98. Which of the following might explain the changes in FRC during sleep?
  A. Relaxation of the intercostal muscles
  B. Increased tone of the accessory expiratory muscles
  C. Increased sensitivity to CO_2
  D. Diaphragmatic muscle hypotonia

ANSWER: **D.**   FRC usually decreases during sleep. Possible explanations include reductions in the tone of the diaphragm leading to a rostral movement of the diaphragm and abdominal contents, which thus reduces FRC. Other possible mechanisms are decreased lung or thoracic compliance. Intercostal muscle tone is actually increased in sleep.

99. Which of the following *best* predicts arousals from sleep caused by upper airway narrowing or complete airway occlusion?
  A. The $PacO_2$ nadir
  B. The SaO_2 rate of decline
  C. The end-tidal CO_2 level
  D. The esophageal pressure nadir

ANSWER: **D.**   The final common pathway that occurs when arousal is initiated (by hypoxia, hypercapnia, and increased resistance) is the level of ventilatory effort, which is best measured by esophageal pressure.

100. Which statement about arousal and coughing during sleep is *incorrect*?
  A. In normal subjects, sleep suppresses coughing
  B. In chronic lung disease, coughing is not suppressed by sleep
  C. In humans, there is no difference between REM and NREM sleep in arousal from irritating pulmonary stimuli
  D. Coughing has been shown to only occur after arousal or during wakefulness in both healthy individuals and in those with lung disease

ANSWER: **B.**   Sleep inhibits coughing in both normal subjects and in patients with lung disease.

101. A patient with severe COPD has overnight oximetry. What is a likely contributor to the episodes of oxygen desaturation?
  A. Aspiration of gastric fluid into the lung
  B. Ventilation-perfusion mismatching
  C. Loss of muscle tone in the diaphragm
  D. OSA

ANSWER: **B.**   Patients with severe COPD use their accessory muscles of respiration to help maintain ventilation. During REM sleep, these muscles lose tone and ventilation decreases, worsening ventilation-perfusion mismatching.

102. Which statement about upper airway physiology is *incorrect*?
  A. Increased lung volumes decrease upper airway resistance
  B. During sleep, the tone of upper airway muscles decreases less than the tone of the diaphragm
  C. The loss of the wakefulness stimulus contributes to the loss of upper airway muscle tone with sleep onset
  D. Upper airway resistance increases with sleep onset

ANSWER: **B.** With sleep comes a drop in upper airway muscle tone, resulting in increased upper airway resistance. The reduction in tone of the upper airway muscles is relatively greater than that of the diaphragm.

103. Activity of which muscle *best* correlates with increased airway resistance at sleep onset?
  A. Tensor palatini
  B. Genioglossus
  C. Palatoglossus
  D. Levator palatini

ANSWER: **A.** Because the pharynx is used for speech, breathing, eating, and drinking, the muscles of the upper airway serve several functions. The tensor palatini has tonic activity, and it tenses the soft palate. The levator palatini contracts during swallowing. During swallowing, these two muscles together elevate the palate and thus occlude the passage and prevent entry of food and liquid into the nasopharynx. Of the muscles listed, only the tensor palatini demonstrates tonic activity; with sleep comes a decrease in this activity, leading to an increase in upper airway resistance and a compensatory rise in genioglossus activity.

104. All of the following are true about congenital central hypoventilation syndrome (CCHS) *except*
  A. It manifests decreased sensitivity to hypercapnia and hypoxemia during sleep
  B. Is associated with Hirschsprung disease, tumors of neural crest origin, and autonomic dysregulation
  C. It is related to mutations in the human *PHOX2B* gene
  D. In the majority of cases, the disease becomes manifest after the first 6 months of life

ANSWER: **D.** CCHS is usually present from birth. Per the ICSD3: "Although the condition is termed *congenital*, some patients [but not the majority] with a *PHOX2B* genotype may present phenotypically later in life (and even in adulthood), especially in the presence of a stressor such as general anesthesia or a severe respiratory illness." (ICSD3, pp 113–117)

105. A 4-month-old child is brought to the emergency department by EMS. A half hour earlier, his mother observed him "stop breathing to the point that he became blue and unresponsive." By the time the paramedics arrived, he was responsive, and now in the ED, his examination results are normal. His medical history to this point has been unremarkable. The *most* accurate diagnosis is
  A. Either obstructive or central sleep apnea (a PSG is needed to differentiate these)
  B. Acute upper airway obstruction caused either by material (e.g., mucus) or by vocal cord adduction
  C. Apparent life-threatening event (ALTE)
  D. Voluntary hypoventilation of childhood

ANSWER: **C.** ALTE is a specific diagnosis that requires thorough evaluation. It is defined as an event of apnea that is frightening to the caregiver, usually because the child turns blue, becomes unresponsive, or both. ALTE does not presage sudden infant death syndrome (SIDS; years ago, ALTE was called *near-miss SIDS*, a term that has since been abandoned.) ALTE may be due to a variety of causes, including upper airway obstruction (from material such as mucus or vomit), seizures, or a cardiorespiratory abnormality. Obstructive and central sleep apneas occur during sleep and are not in the differential, although workup may include an overnight PSG. Patients with severe cases of ALTE, such as this one, should be admitted to the hospital for overnight observation and further evaluation. (Hall and Zalman, 2005)

106. All of the following are *true* about SIDS *except*

    A. The stage of increased risk of SIDS begins at 2 months of age

    B. The sleeping surface should be firm, without toys or pillows or blankets

    C. The infant's head should remain uncovered

    D. The child should be placed in bed in the prone position

ANSWER: **D.** The child should be placed in the supine (face-up) position. Changing from prone to supine sleep has led to a decreased incidence of SIDS.

REFERENCES

American Academy of Sleep Medicine. *International classification of sleep disorders*, ed 3. Darien, Ill.: American Academy of Sleep Medicine; 2014.

American Academy of Sleep Medicine. *The AASM manual for the scoring of sleep and associated events: rules, terminology and technical specifications, Version 2.1.* Darien, Ill.: American Academy of Sleep Medicine; 2014.

Banno K, Walld R, Kryger MN. Increasing obesity trends in patients with sleep-disordered breathing referred to a sleep disorders center. *J Clin Sleep Med.* 2005;1:364–366.

Bradley TD, et al. Continuous positive airway pressure for central sleep apnea and heart failure. *N Engl J Med.* 2005;353:2025–2033.

Brownell LG, West P, Sweatman P, et al. Protriptyline in obstructive sleep apnea: a double-blind trial. *N Engl J Med.* 1982;307(17):1037–1042.

Campos GM, Bambha K, Vittinghoff E, et al. A clinical scoring system for predicting nonalcoholic steatohepatitis in morbidly obese patients. *Hepatology.* 2008;47(6):1916–1923.

Chami HA, Baldwin CM, Silverman A, et al. Sleepiness, quality of life, and sleep maintenance in REM versus non-REM sleep-disordered breathing. *Am J Resp Crit Care Med.* 2010;181:997–1002.

Chung F, Yegneswaran B, Liao P, et al. STOP questionnaire: a tool to screen patients for obstructive sleep apnea. *Anesthesiology.* 2008;108:812–821.

Easton PA, West P, Meatherall RC, et al. The effect of excessive ethanol ingestion on sleep in severe chronic obstructive pulmonary disease. *Sleep.* 1987;10(3):224–233.

Franklin KA, Nilsson JB, Sahlin C, Näslund U. Sleep apnoea and nocturnal angina. *Lancet.* 1995;345(8957):1085–1087.

Friedman O, Bradley TD, Ruttanaumpawan P, Logan AG. Independent association of drug-resistant hypertension to reduced sleep duration and efficiency. *Am J Hypertens.* 2010;23(2):174–179.

Ganguly G. The clinical dilemma: to treat or not to treat REM-related obstructive sleep apnea? *Sleep.* 2012;35:755.

Hall KL, Zalman B. Evaluation and management of apparent life-threatening events in children. *Am Fam Physician.* 2005;71(12):2301–2308.

Holty JE, Guilleminault C. REM-related bradyarrhythmia syndrome. *Sleep Med Rev.* 2011;15(3):143–151.

Hoque R, Chesson AL Jr. Pharmacologically induced/exacerbated restless legs syndrome, periodic limb movements of sleep, and REM behavior disorder/REM sleep without atonia: literature review, qualitative scoring, and comparative analysis. *J Clin Sleep Med.* 2010;6(1):79–83.

Horner RL. Respiratory motor activity: influence of neuromodulators and implications for sleep disordered breathing. *Can J Physiol Pharmacol.* 2007;85:155–165.

Kryger MH, Avidan A, Berry R. *Atlas of clinical sleep medicine*, ed 2. Philadelphia: Saunders; 2014.

Kryger M, Roth T, Wang-Weigand S, Zhang J. The effects of ramelteon on respiration during sleep in subjects with moderate to severe chronic obstructive pulmonary disease. *Sleep Breath.* 2009;13(1):79–84.

Kryger M, Wang-Weigand S, Roth T. Safety of ramelteon in individuals with mild to moderate obstructive sleep apnea. *Sleep Breath.* 2007;11(3):159–164.

Kryger M, Wang-Weigand S, Zhang J, Roth T. Effect of ramelteon, a selective MT(1)/MT (2)-receptor agonist, on respiration during sleep in mild to moderate COPD. *Sleep Breath.* 2008;12(3):243–250.

Marshall NS, Yee BJ, Desai AV, et al. Two randomized placebo-controlled trials to evaluate the efficacy and tolerability of mirtazapine for the treatment of obstructive sleep apnea. *Sleep.* 2008;31(6):824–831.

Mishra P, Nugent C, Afendy A, et al. Apnoeic-hypopnoeic episodes during obstructive sleep apnoea are associated with histological nonalcoholic steatohepatitis. *Liver Int.* 2008;28(8):1080–1086.

Mogri M, Desai H, Webster L, et al. Hypoxemia in patients on chronic opiate therapy with and without sleep apnea. *Sleep Breath.* 2009;13(1):49–57.

Mokhlesi B, Finn LA, Hagen EW, et al. Obstructive sleep apnea during REM sleep and hypertension. results of the Wisconsin sleep cohort. *Am J Respir Crit Care Med.* 2014;190(10):1158–1167.

Mokhlesi B, Punjabi N. "REM-related" obstructive sleep apnea: an epiphenomenon or a clinically important entity? *Sleep.* 2012;35:5–7.

Neves C, Tufik S, Monteiro MA, et al. The effect of sildenafil on sleep respiratory parameters and heart rate variability in obstructive sleep apnea. *Sleep Med.* 2010;11(6):545–551.

Piper A. Obesity hypoventilation syndrome: therapeutic implications for treatment. *Expert Rev Respir Med.* 2010;4(1):57–70.

Sampol G, Rodés G, Ríos J, et al. Acute hypercapnic respiratory failure in patients with sleep apneas. *Arch Bronconeumol.* 2010;46(9):466–472.

Savransky V, Nanayakkara A, Vivero A, et al. Chronic intermittent hypoxia predisposes to liver injury. *Hepatology.* 2007;45(4):1007–1013.

Singh H, Pollock R, Uhanova J, et al. Symptoms of obstructive sleep apnea in patients with nonalcoholic fatty liver disease. *Dig Dis Sci.* 2005;50(12):2338–2343.

Torre-Bouscoulet L, Castorena-Maldonado A, López-Escárcega E, et al. Agreement between 95th percentile pressure based on a 7-night auto-adjusting positive airway pressure trial vs. equation-based predictions in sleep apnea. *J Clin Sleep Med.* 2009;5(4):311–316.

Sleep in Other Disorders

QUESTIONS

Neurologic

1. A 34-year-old healthy patient without any symptoms in the daytime displays dystonic posturing, open eyes, and rapid pulse every night during sleep, with an episode length of 40 and 50 seconds. The patient has no recollection of these events the next morning. What is the *most* likely diagnosis?
A. Paroxysmal nocturnal dystonia
B. Rapid eye movement (REM) sleep behavior disorder
C. Confusional arousals
D. Sleep terrors

ANSWER: **A.** This history is consistent with paroxysmal nocturnal dystonia, in which a patient will have periods of odd posturing during the night. This disorder is believed to be a disorder of nocturnal frontal lobe epilepsy (NFLE), at times confirmable via nocturnal video polysomnography (PSG) monitoring with specialized electroencephalograph (EEG) recordings. (ICSD3, p 345, Sleep-Related Epilepsy)

2. The above-mentioned patient's problem is currently classified as which of the following?
A. REM parasomnia
B. Non-REM (NREM) parasomnia
C. Anxiety disorder
D. Epilepsy disorder

ANSWER: **D.** As noted in the answer to question 1, paroxysmal nocturnal dystonia is considered a subset of epilepsy with abnormal video PSG and EEG findings to support this conclusion.

3. An otherwise healthy patient complains of a lifelong history of a single, violent "electric-like" body jerk that sometimes occurs at sleep onset. What is the diagnosis?
A. Fragmentary myoclonus
B. Persistent benign sleep myoclonus of infancy
C. Hypnic jerk
D. Hypnagogic foot tremor

ANSWER: **C.** What the patient is describing is a hypnic jerk, also known as a *sleep start*. In the ICSD3, this is classified in the category of "Sleep-Related Movement Disorders, Isolated Symptoms, and Normal Variants." These are sudden, brief contractions of the body that occur at sleep onset, often associated with a sensation of falling. This is not persistent benign sleep myoclonus of infancy; this disorder, manifested by myoclonic jerks that occur during sleep in infants, typically begins at birth and resolves spontaneously by 6 months. Hypnagogic foot tremor and alternating leg muscle activation both can occur at sleep-wake transitions or during light NREM sleep. PSG shows recurrent EMG potentials in one or both feet that are in the myoclonic range of longer than 250 ms. Propriospinal myoclonus at sleep onset is a disorder of recurrent, sudden muscular jerks in the transition from wake to sleep and is often associated with insomnia.

4. How would you treat this patient?
   A. Confirm the diagnosis by PSG and then treat with anticonvulsants
   B. Offer reassurance about the benign nature of the condition
   C. Start the patient on pramipexole at night
   D. Order a PSG to better evaluate the diagnosis

ANSWER: **B.**   Because hypnic jerks are common and benign and have no known negative consequences, reassurance is the goal of management. Such patients often worry they have epilepsy. These patients do not require a diagnostic PSG.

5. In humans, epileptic seizures are more common in REM sleep
   A. True
   B. False

ANSWER: **B.**   False. Epileptic seizures least commonly occur in REM sleep. Whereas stage N3 sleep activates interictal discharges, lighter stages of NREM sleep promote seizures.   (ATLAS2, p 195; Minecan D, Natarajan A, Marzec M, Malow B: Relationship of epileptic seizures to sleep stage and sleep depth, *Sleep.* 25[8]:899–904, 2002)

6. Which structures are active in maintaining wakefulness?
   A. Galanin (Gal) neurons
   B. Histamine neurons
   C. Gamma aminobutyric acid (GABA) neurons
   D. Ventrolateral preoptic nucleus (VLPO)

ANSWER: **B.**   Histamine produced by the tuberomammilary nucleus is an alerting agent. Remember that antihistamines that cross the blood brain barrier are sedating.   (ATLAS2, pp 22)

7. Although scalp electrodes may not demonstrate NFLE, a clinical history of all of the following is consistent with this diagnosis *except*
   A. Attacks persist into adulthood
   B. Attacks are stereotyped
   C. Attacks occur several times in one night
   D. Attacks occur mostly during REM sleep
   E. Dystonic posturing may be associated with the attacks

ANSWER: **D.**   This parasomnia occurs primarily in NREM sleep, with 60% of episodes out of N2 sleep.   (ATLAS2, Ch 11.3–1, p 207)

8. REM sleep behavior disorder has not been reported in patients with multiple sclerosis (MS)
   A. True
   B. False

ANSWER: **B.**   False. Patients with MS can have several sleep disorders, including REM sleep behavior disorder, hypersomnia, sleep paralysis, RLS, and REM-related sleep apnea.   (ATLAS2, pp 226 and 228)

9. Parkinson disease involves degeneration of dopamine neurons in the substantia nigra and may be preceded by years with which of the following?
   A. Sleepwalking
   B. Central sleep apnea
   C. REM sleep behavior disorder (RBD)
   D. Sleep-related rhythmic movement disorder

ANSWER: **C.**   Symptoms of RBD may precede the other symptoms of Parkinson disease; patients with Parkinson disease are also prone to insomnia, nightmares, RLS, and sleep-disordered breathing.   (ATLAS2, pp 213–216)

10. Hypersomnolence in Alzheimer disease is associated with loss of which neurons in the basal forebrain?
   A. Melatonin
   B. Dopamine
   C. Acetylcholine
   D. Gamma aminobutyric acid (GABA)
   E. Serotonin

ANSWER: **C.** Degeneration of the cholinergic neurons in the nucleus basalis of Meynert are thought to play in important role in the many sleep problems of patients with Alzheimer dementia. (ATLAS2, pp 223–226)

11. Secondary forms of RBD generally involve neurologic disease that affects which neuroanatomic region?
   A. The cortex
   B. The thalamus
   C. The brainstem
   D. The spinal cord
   E. Peripheral nerves

ANSWER: **C.** The location of the system that leads to muscle atonia in REM is in the pontine tegmentum. (ATLAS2, p 217)

12. Secondary forms of RLS and periodic limb movement disorder (PLMD) occur with a number of neurologic disorders that affect all of the following *except*
   A. Dopamine neurons
   B. The frontal cortex
   C. The motor pathways
   D. The brainstem
   E. Peripheral nerves

ANSWER: **B.** (ATLAS2, pp 180–183)

13. Obstructive sleep apnea (OSA) is thought to precipitate stroke for all of the following reasons *except*
   A. Increased atrial fibrillation
   B. Increased diabetes
   C. Increased hypertension
   D. Increased vascular malformations
   E. Increased atherosclerosis

ANSWER: **D.** OSA is associated with several comorbidities that may lead to stroke. (ATLAS2, pp 328–334)

14. Studies demonstrate what percentage of patients with stroke or transient ischemic attack (TIA) are noted to have OSA?
   A. 20% to 30%
   B. 30% to 40%
   C. 40% to 50%
   D. 50% to 60%
   E. 60% to 70%

ANSWER: **E.** (Johnson KG, Johnson DC: Frequency of sleep apnea in stroke and TIA patients: a meta-analysis, *J Clin Sleep Med.* 6:131–137, 2010)

15. In what stages of sleep or wakefulness are seizures more likely to occur?
   A. Wake > NREM > REM
   B. NREM > Wake > REM
   C. Wake > REM > NREM
   D. REM > Wake > NREM

ANSWER: **B.** (ATLAS2, p 195; Benbadis SR: Epileptic seizures and syndromes, *Neurol Clin.* 19:251–270, 2001)

Psychiatric

16. In what proportion of schizophrenic patients does insomnia occur?
  A. 10%
  B. 20%
  C. 30%
  D. 40%

ANSWER: **D.** Insomnia is quite common in schizophrenia. (Palmese LB, DeGeorge PC, Ratliff JC, et al: Insomnia is frequent in schizophrenia and associated with night eating and obesity, *Schizophr Res.* 133[1–3];238–243, 2011)

17. What EEG sleep changes are found in major depressive disorder?
  A. Short REM latency
  B. Increased slow-wave (N3) sleep
  C. Decreased REM sleep time
  D. Short first REM period
  E. Decreased N2 sleep

ANSWER: **A.** Reduced REM latency and increased REM during the first half of the night are common in depression. (ATLAS2, Table 17–2, p 366; Benca RM, Obermeyer WH, Thisted RA, Gillin JC: Sleep and psychiatric disorders. A meta-analysis, *Arch Gen Psychiatry.* 49:651–668, 1992)

18. Most antidepressant medications have what characteristic effect on sleep?
  A. Increased slow-wave (N3) sleep
  B. Prolonged REM sleep latency
  C. Increased proportion of REM sleep
  D. Suppressed dreaming
  E. Improved RLS symptoms

ANSWER: **B.** The most consistent finding is a reduction of REM sleep. (ATLAS2, Table 17–2, p 367; Wilson S, Argyropoulos S: Antidepressants and sleep: a qualitative review of the literature, *Drugs.* 65[7]:927–947, 2005)

19. The following statements accurately describe the relationship between depression and sleep complaints *except*
  A. Insomnia is a risk factor for the subsequent development of depression.
  B. 80% of patients with depression have sleep-related complaints.
  C. The appearance of insomnia precedes the onset of depression more often than it occurs following the onset of depression.
  D. Early morning awakening is more commonly reported than difficulty in falling asleep.

ANSWER: **A.** Insomnia and abnormalities in sleep architecture are common in depression. (ATLAS2, p 365; Perlis ML, Giles DE, Buysse DJ, et al: Which depressive symptoms are related to which sleep electroencephalographic variables? *Biol Psychiatry.* 42:904–913, 1997)

20. PSG changes in schizophrenia include the following *except*
  A. Increased REM sleep latency
  B. Decreased slow-wave sleep (SWS)
  C. Increased REM density
  D. Poor sleep efficiency

ANSWER: **A.** Decreased REM sleep latency and increased REM density are found in schizophrenia and depression. (ATLAS2, p 368; Monti JM, Monti D: Sleep in schizophrenia patients and the effects of antipsychotic drugs, *Sleep Med Rev.* 8[2]:133–148, 2004)

21. Which of the following sleep "therapies" has demonstrated the longest duration of benefit in depression?
  A. REM sleep deprivation
  B. Total sleep deprivation
  C. Sleep deprivation for the first half of the night
  D. Sleep deprivation for the second half of the night

ANSWER: **A.** (ATLAS2, p 366; Reynolds CF 3rd, Kupfer DJ: Sleep research in affective illness: state of the art circa 1987, *Sleep*. 10:199–215, 1987)

22. Which of the following acute changes after trauma are associated with the subsequent development of PTSD?
  A. Dream enactment
  B. Fragmented REM sleep
  C. Increased N1 sleep
  D. Decreased N2 sleep

ANSWER: **B.** (ATLAS2, p 368; Mellman TA, Bustamante V, Fins AI, et al: REM sleep and the early development of posttraumatic stress disorder, *Am J Psychiatry*. 159:1696–1701, 2002)

23. Sleep-related panic attacks
  A. Arise out of REM sleep
  B. Arise out of stage 2 and 3 sleep
  C. Are more frequent than daytime panic attacks
  D. Are usually associated with vivid dreams
  E. Usually follow traumatic events during the preceding day

ANSWER: **B.** (Mellman TA: Sleep and anxiety disorders, *Psychiatr Clin North Am*. 29[4]:1047–1058, 2006)

24. Insomnia is temporally associated with the appearance of an anxiety disorder predominantly in which way?
  A. Before the anxiety disorder
  B. Concurrently or after the anxiety disorder
  C. There is no dominant temporal relationship

ANSWER: **B.** (Ohayon MM, Roth T: Place of chronic insomnia in the course of depressive and anxiety disorders, *J Psychiatr Res*. 37[1]:9–15, 2003)

25. Which of the following psychiatric disorders has been *most* strongly observed in patients with OSA?
  A. Depressive disorders
  B. Anxiety disorders
  C. Psychotic disorders
  D. Dementia
  E. Drug abuse

ANSWER: **A.** Depression symptoms are very common in OSA, especially in female patients. (Sharafkhaneh A, Giray N, Richardson P, et al: Association of psychiatric disorders and sleep apnea in a large cohort, *Sleep*. 28[11]:1405–1411, 2005)

26. Which of the following antidepressant medications is *least* likely to suppress REM sleep?
  A. Bupropion
  B. Fluoxetine
  C. Imipramine
  D. Citalopram
  E. Venlafaxine

ANSWER: **A.** (ATLAS2, Table 17–3, p 367; Nofzinger EA, Reynolds CF 3rd, Thase ME, et al: REM sleep enhancement by bupropion in depressed men, *Am J Psychiatry*. 152[2]:274–276, 1995)

27. Which of the following antidepressant medications is considered *most* sedating?
A. Bupropion
B. Fluoxetine
C. Protriptyline
D. Mirtazapine
E. Venlafaxine

ANSWER: **D.** (Versiani M, Moreno R, Ramakers-van Moorsel CJ, Schutte AJ: Comparative Efficacy Antidepressants Study Group. Comparison of the effects of mirtazapine and fluoxetine in severely depressed patients, *CNS Drugs.* 19[2]:137–146, 2005)

28. Which of the following treatments has little or no effect on sleep quality in patients with chronic obstructive pulmonary disease (COPD)?
A. Oxygen
B. Theophylline
C. Nicotine
D. Alcohol

ANSWER: **A.** The answer is oxygen. Although oxygen improves gas exchange, it has little effect on sleep structure or arousal frequency. The other factors mentioned can worsen sleep. (Fleetham J, West P, Mezon B, et al: Sleep, arousals, and oxygen desaturation in chronic obstructive pulmonary disease. The effect of oxygen therapy, *Am Rev Respir Dis.* 126[3]:429–433, 1982; Roth T: Hypnotic use for insomnia management in chronic obstructive pulmonary disease, *Sleep Med.* 10[1]:19–25, 2009)

29. In which disorder does pain classically occur 1 to 2 hours after sleep onset?
A. Bone cancer
B. Duodenal ulcer disease
C. Rheumatoid arthritis
D. Fibromyalgia

ANSWER: **B.** Patients with duodenal ulcers do not inhibit gastric acid secretion in the first 2 hours after sleep.

30. Which statement is *most* correct about the relationship between hypothyroidism and OSA?
A. Thyroid treatment may worsen heart disease in untreated patients with OSA
B. Few patients with hypothyroidism have OSA
C. Thyroid therapy increases the apnea index in untreated patients with OSA
D. OSA is present only when microglossia is a side effect of hypothyroidism

ANSWER: **A.** In hypothyroid patients with OSA, the apnea index does not decrease significantly in all when euthyroidism is achieved. Treatment of hypothyroidism with thyroxine in the presence of sleep apnea is potentially hazardous and may lead to cardiovascular complications such as nocturnal angina and cardiac arrhythmias. Management should include continuous positive airway pressure (CPAP) and low-dose thyroxine. (Grunstein RR, Sullivan CE: Sleep apnea and hypothyroidism: mechanisms and management, *Am J Med.* 85:775–779, 1988)

31. In patients with heart failure and resultant Cheyne-Stokes respiration, when do the arousals typically occur?
A. During a peak of hyperpnea
B. At the end of a central apnea
C. At the onset of apnea
D. During hypopnea

ANSWER: **A.** Arousal occurs during the peak of hyperpnea (as does maximal oxygen desaturation) in heart failure. (ATLAS2, pp 322–324)

32. What treatment has been shown to improve Cheyne-Stokes breathing in heart failure?
   A. Oxygen
   B. Temazepam
   C. Medroxyprogesterone acetate
   D. Protriptyline

ANSWER: **A.**   Oxygen has been shown to both improve CSB and sleep quality.   (Hanly PJ, Kinnear WJ, Starling R, et al: The effect of oxygen on respiration and sleep in patients with congestive heart failure, *Ann Intern Med.* 111[10]:777–782, 1989) Temazepam improved sleep but had no effect on CSB.   (Biberdorf DJ, Steens R, Millar TW, Kryger MH: Benzodiazepines in congestive heart failure: effects of temazepam on arousability and Cheyne-Stokes respiration, *Sleep.* 16[6]:529–538, 1993)

33. Which statement is *true* about the time of death secondary to cardiovascular causes?
   A. Death rate peaks in the morning
   B. Death rate peaks just after noon
   C. Death rate peaks in the beginning of the night
   D. Death rate peaks in the middle of the night

ANSWER: **A.**   Many studies have examined the time of death, and it seems to be in the early morning hours. And indeed, many cardiovascular comorbidities have serious events at this time. The exact pathogenesis is unknown but could be related to a surge in sympathetic tone, which in turn may be initiated by arousal from sleep.

34. Acute nocturnal asthma attacks often occur during which stage of sleep?
   A. N1
   B. N2
   C. N3
   D. REM

ANSWER: **C.**   (Bellia V, Cuttitta G, Insalaco G, et al: Relationship of nocturnal bronchoconstriction to sleep stages, *Am Rev Respir Dis.* 140[2]:363–367, 1989)

35. Possible mechanisms for nocturnal asthma in OSA include all of the following *except*
   A. Increased parasympathetic tone
   B. Increased sympathetic tone
   C. Inflammatory effects
   D. Impact of obesity
   E. Gastroesophageal reflux disease (GERD)

ANSWER: **B.**   (Emilsson ÖI, Bengtsson A, Franklin KA, et al: Nocturnal gastro-oesophageal reflux, asthma and symptoms of OSA: a longitudinal, general population study, *Eur Respir J.* 41[6]:1347–1354, 2013)

36. In the overlap syndrome (patients with COPD and OSA), which of the following statements is *most* correct?
   A. Almost all patients with overlap syndrome have severe COPD
   B. Pulmonary hypertension occurs mainly in those patients with severe airflow obstruction
   C. Prevalence of OSA is higher in the COPD population than in normal controls
   D. Overlap syndrome patients have higher intensive care unit (ICU) admission rates than OSA patients without COPD

ANSWER: **D.**   (Weitzenblum et al: Proceedings of American Thoracic Society, Feb 15, 2005, pp 237–241)

37. In obesity hypoventilation syndrome (OHS), carbon dioxide retention mechanisms include which of the following?

   A. Blunted hypoxic and hypercapnic drives to breathe

   B. Associated OSA

   C. Mechanical load of obesity

   D. Reduced inspiratory muscle strength

   E. All of the above

ANSWER: **E.**   Hypoventilation in this syndrome is multifactorial.   (Mokhlesi B, Tulaimat A: Recent advances in obesity hypoventilation syndrome, *Chest.* 132:1322–1336, 2007)

Call From the Scoring Technologist

At 8 AM, you receive a call from the scoring tech, who is concerned about an electrocardiogram (ECG) from the night before. The patient is a 68-year-old woman with a history of heart disease, arthritis, and GERD. You are able to bring up her study on the computer, an epoch of which is shown in Figure E8–1.

38. What is the underlying cardiac rhythm?

   A. Sinus rhythm

   B. Sinus arrhythmia

   C. Third-degree heart block

   D. Atrial fibrillation (AF)

ANSWER: **D.**   Absence of P-waves and slight variability in the R-R interval indicate the rhythm is AF. ECG abnormalities should be examined systematically. First, pay attention to the epoch length, which in this example is 30 seconds. Determine the overall rate, here in the mid-60s, and then determine the underlying rhythm. Nowhere do you see a P-wave. The width of the underlying QRS is narrow, indicating origin in the atria or high up in the atrioventricular (AV) node. The rate is somewhat slow for AF, but the patient was taking digoxin, which slows the rate.

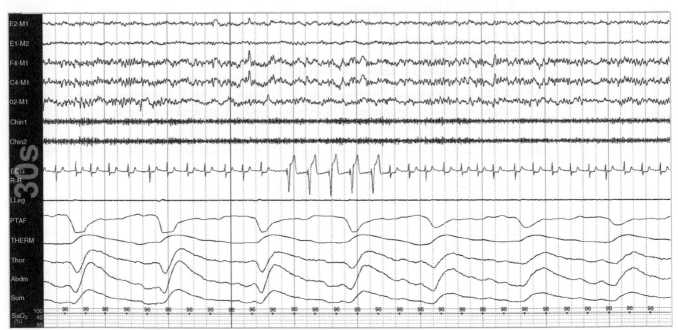

FIGURE E8–1

39. What is the five-beat abnormal cardiac rhythm in the middle of this 30-second epoch?
   A. Ventricular fibrillation
   B. Ventricular tachycardia
   C. Supraventricular tachycardia with aberrant conduction
   D. Indeterminate arrhythmia

ANSWER: **D.**   It is difficult to ascertain the rhythm in this five-beat run. Answers A, B, and C are incorrect because those diagnoses should result in a wider QRS *and* because there really is no tachycardia.

40. What can be done to improve the diagnostic accuracy of the ECG in Figure E8–1?
   A. Examine a 2-minute epoch
   B. Decrease the high-frequency filter
   C. Increase the high-frequency filter
   D. Increase amplitude of the ECG

ANSWER: **C.**   There are two options to improve ECG accuracy on a PSG: (1) examine a shorter epoch (thus answer A is incorrect) or (2) examine the same data but with an increased high-frequency filter setting. This latter option allows a higher resolution and assumes that the sampling rate of the ECG was the desirable 500 Hz. Increasing the amplitude of the ECG will not really help here. Figure E8–2 shows a shorter epoch (15 seconds) followed by an enlargement of the aberrant rhythm sequence (Fig. E8–3). It is now apparent that this is a paced rhythm, originating from an implanted ventricular pacemaker. The pacemaker starts firing when there is a longer-than-desired interval after the last nonpaced QRS, and it ceases firing when the intrinsic fibrillation rate increases. (Note that in the 15-second epoch, the distance between the last fibrillation QRS and first paced beat is longer than the interval between the last paced beat and next fibrillation QRS; see Fig. E8–2.)

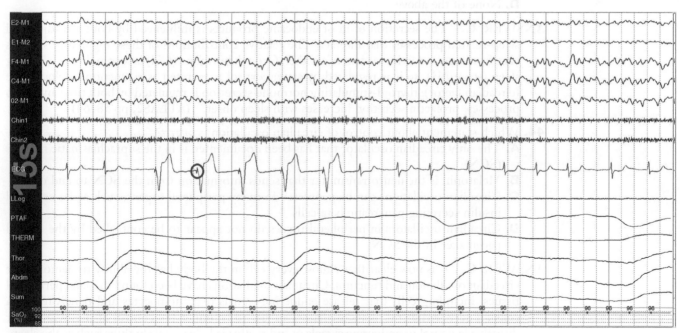

FIGURE E8–2

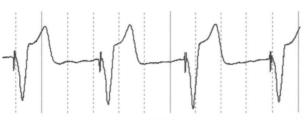

FIGURE E8–3

41. Which statement about sleep and infections is *most* correct?
  A. After infectious challenge, animals that exhibit robust NREM sleep have better survival
  B. Sleep deprivation has no effect on response to influenza vaccination
  C. The acute phase response to inflammation does not include changes in sleep
  D. There is no sleep abnormality in early human immunodeficiency virus (HIV) infection

ANSWER: **A.** Animals that exhibit robust NREM sleep have better survival in response to infection. Sleep has been shown to be an important component of the acute phase response to inflammation. Sleep deprivation has been shown to affect the rapidity of antibody response after influenza vaccination. In early HIV infection, before the onset of acquired immune deficiency syndrome (AIDS), an increase in stage 4 sleep occurs in the latter part of the night, a time usually devoid of SWS. (ATLAS2, pp 42–43)

42. Which cytokine is not involved in the acute phase response and sleep regulation?
  A. Interleukin-1β
  B. Interleukin-6
  C. Tumor necrosis factor alpha
  D. Ghrelin

ANSWER: **D.** Ghrelin is not involved in the acute phase response, nor is it involved in sleep regulation. The other entities are involved in both sleep regulation and the acute phase response. (ATLAS2, Table 3.5–1, p 42)

43. The regulation of hormonal release in *most* components of the endocrine system is modulated by
  A. Mainly circadian processes
  B. Mainly sleep processes
  C. Interacting circadian and sleep processes
  D. None of the above

ANSWER: **C.** The secretion of most endocrine products is influenced by both circadian and sleep-related processes that interact. The relative contributions of these regulatory systems vary from one endocrine system to another. Growth hormone (GH) is secreted mostly during sleep (stage N3), so it is regulated by state; cortisol is secreted as a function of clock time (circadian factor); thyroid-stimulating hormone secretion is regulated by both time and sleep processes; prolactin secretion increases with sleep onset. (ATLAS2, pp 58–64)

44. Which statement about control of circadian oscillation is *correct*?
  A. The only circadian oscillator that has been documented is in the suprachiasmatic nucleus (SCN)
  B. Melatonin is the neurotransmitter that sends information from the SCN to end organs
  C. Circadian oscillations can be generated in many peripheral organs, such as fat cells and insulin secreting pancreatic beta cells
  D. Circadian oscillators in peripheral tissues do not appear to be controlled by the central pacemaker in the SCN

ANSWER: **C.** It is now clear that almost every cell in the body has the ability to demonstrate circadian oscillation and function. Circadian oscillations have been found in many peripheral tissues, including cells that release endocrine signals (e.g., adipocytes and pancreatic beta cells). These peripheral tissue oscillators appear to be under the control of the SCN either directly via neural or endocrine signals or indirectly via behavioral rhythms such as the sleep-wake cycle or the timing of feeding. (ATLAS2, pp 34–37)

45. Which statement about the timing of GH release is *correct*?
  A. GH is secreted primarily during physical activity
  B. The most reproducible pulse of GH secretion occurs shortly before awakening in the morning
  C. In men, the sleep-onset GH pulse is generally the largest secretory pulse observed
  D. The GH spike in secretion at night is linked to REM sleep

ANSWER: **C.** The 24-hour plasma GH levels are stable and low levels but are abruptly interrupted by bursts of secretion. The most reproducible pulse is shortly after falling asleep. In men, the sleep-onset pulse is the largest—and often the only—burst in secretion. In women, daytime GH pulses are more frequent, and the sleep-associated pulse, although still present, does not account for most of the GH secretion. A burst in GH secretion occurs with a sleep onset whether sleep is advanced, delayed, or interrupted and then resumed. (ATLAS2, p 59)

46. Which statement about the relationship between SWS and GH secretion is *incorrect*?
  A. Peak GH release occurs within minutes of the onset of SWS
  B. Gamma-hydroxybutyrate (GHB), which increases SWS, results in increases in GH secretion
  C. Sedative hypnotics (benzodiazepines and imidazopyridines) that do not increase SWS do not increase nocturnal GH release
  D. The relationship between GH secretion and SWS is stronger in men than in women

ANSWER: **C.** There does appear to be a tight linkage between the production of GH and SWS, and compounds that increase the amount of SWS, for example, GHB, increase the production of GH. Athletes have been known to use GHB as a means of increasing GH production to improve their athletic performance. (ATLAS2, p 59)

47. Which statement about cortisol levels and sleep is *incorrect*?
  A. The plasma levels of cortisol are highest in the early morning
  B. The plasma levels of cortisol are lowest in the late evening and early part of the sleep period
  C. Sleep is normally initiated when corticotropic activity is quiescent
  D. Sleep onset is associated with a burst of cortisol secretion

ANSWER: **D.** Cortisol secretion is primarily related to the circadian system (clock time) and is not affected much by whether sleep occurs. It is believed that sleep actually inhibits cortisol secretion, but this inhibition may be difficult to demonstrate because cortisol levels are already low at normal sleep time. One clinically useful test of adrenal function is to measure cortisol levels at midnight and in the morning. A very high midnight cortisol level and loss of circadian variability (the morning cortisol level remains high) are supportive of a diagnosis of Cushing syndrome, a disorder in which the adrenals produce too much cortisol. This can be due to a tumor: an adenoma in the pituitary that produces too much adrenocorticotropic hormone (ACTH), a tumor that produces ectopic ACTH (e.g., small cell lung cancer), or a tumor of adrenal tissue. (ATLAS2, p 59)

48. Which statement about sleep and thyroid hormone secretion is *incorrect*?
  A. Daytime levels of plasma TSH are low and relatively stable
  B. There is a rapid elevation in TSH level starting in the early evening
  C. The highest level of TSH occurs at the beginning of the sleep period
  D. Sleep deprivation results in a suppression of TSH secretion

ANSWER: **D.** During sleep deprivation (Fig. E8–4), nocturnal TSH secretion is increased by as much as 200% over the levels observed during nocturnal sleep. Thus, sleep inhibits TSH secretion, and sleep deprivation relieves this inhibition. (ATLAS2, p 59)

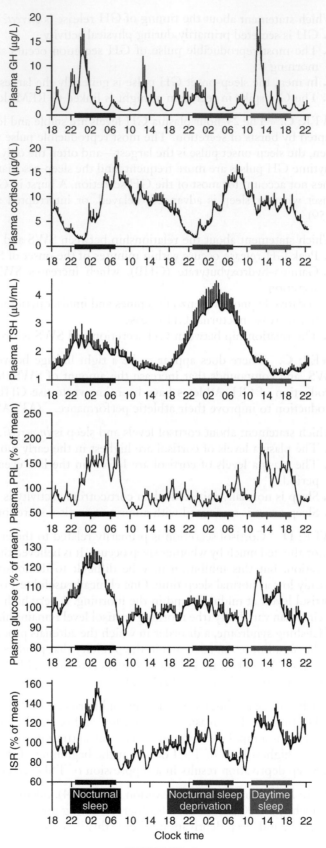

FIGURE E8–4

49. Which statement about sleep and glucose regulation is *incorrect*?
   A. During sleep, glucose levels typically increase
   B. During sleep, there is a drop in glucose use by the brain
   C. During NREM sleep, a substantial reduction occurs in cerebral glucose metabolism
   D. Glucose use during REM sleep exceeds glucose use during NREM sleep

ANSWER: **A.**   Despite a relative fast during sleep, blood glucose levels remain constant or only decrease minimally. In contrast, during a daytime fast, blood glucose falls. These findings can be explained by a relative decrease in glucose tolerance together with a decrease of glucose utilization.   (ATLAS2, p 59)

50. Which statement about appetite-regulating hormones is *incorrect*?
   A. Leptin levels increase in response to acute caloric shortage
   B. Leptin is produced by adipocytes
   C. Orexins have wakefulness-promoting effects and stimulate intake of food
   D. Ghrelin levels increase before mealtime

ANSWER: **A.**   Knowledge about these compounds is critical. Leptin, produced by fat cells, is an appetite-suppressing hormone. Ghrelin, produced by gastric cells, promotes hunger. Orexin stimulates food intake and leads to wakefulness (remember that narcoleptics are deficient in orexin, also called *hypocretin*). Orexin is inhibited by leptin and stimulated by ghrelin.   (ATLAS2, pp 56–58)

51. What statement about chronic sleep deprivation on metabolism is *incorrect*?
   A. Sleep deprivation results in improved glucose tolerance
   B. Sleep deprivation results in increased ghrelin levels
   C. Sleep deprivation results in reduced leptin levels
   D. Sleep deprivation results in weight loss

ANSWER: **A.**   Sleep deprivation results in reduced leptin and increased ghrelin, which increase appetite. These result in changes that would lead to obesity and insulin resistance. This is a very important topic and impacts several aspects of sleep medicine.   (ATLAS2, pp 56–58)

Printed and bound by CPI Group (UK) Ltd, Croydon, CR0 4YY

03/10/2024

01040305-0007